A Case Approach to Perioperative Drug-Drug Interactions

Catherine Marcucci • Michael P. Hutchens
Erica D. Wittwer • Toby N. Weingarten
Juraj Sprung • Wayne T. Nicholson
Kirk Lalwani • David G. Metro • Randal O. Dull
Christopher E. Swide • F. Jacob Seagull
Jeffrey R. Kirsch • Neil B. Sandson
Editors

A Case Approach to Perioperative Drug-Drug Interactions

Springer

Editors
Catherine Marcucci, MD
Philadelphia Veterans Affairs Med Center
Anesthesia Services Department
Philadelphia, PA
USA

Michael P. Hutchens, MD
Oregon Health and Science University
Department of Anesthesiology
Portland, OR
USA

Erica D. Wittwer, MD, PhD
Mayo Clinic
Department of Anesthesiology
Rochester, MN
USA

Toby N. Weingarten, MD
Mayo Clinic
Department of Anesthesiology
Rochester, MN
USA

Juraj Sprung, MD, PhD
Mayo Clinic
Department of Anesthesiology
Rochester, MN
USA

Wayne T. Nicholson, MD, PharmD, MSc
Mayo Clinic
Department of Anesthesiology
Rochester, MN
USA

Kirk Lalwani, MD
Oregon Health and Science University
Department of Anesthesiology and
Perioperative Medicine
Portland, OR
USA

David G. Metro, MD
University of Pittsburgh School of Med
Liliane S. Kaufmann Building
Department of Anesthesiology
Pittsburgh, PA
USA

Randal O. Dull, MD, PhD
University of Illinois at Chicago
Department of Anesthesiology
Chicago, IL
USA

Christopher E. Swide, MD
Perioperative Medicine,
Oregon Health and Science University
Department of Anesthesiology
Portland, OR
USA

F. Jacob Seagull, PhD
University of Michigan Medical School
Department of Learning Health Sciences
Ann Arbor, MI
USA

Jeffrey R. Kirsch, MD
Department of Anesthesiology
and Perioperative Medicine
Professor and Chair
Portland, OR
USA

Neil B. Sandson, MD
University of Maryland Medical System
VA Maryland Health Care System
Department of Psychiatry
Baltimore, MD
USA

ISBN 978-1-4614-7494-4 ISBN 978-1-4614-7495-1 (eBook)
DOI 10.1007/978-1-4614-7495-1

Library of Congress Control Number: 2015949508

Springer New York Heidelberg Dordrecht London

Printed on acid-free paper

Springer Science+Business Media LLC New York is part of Springer Science+Business Media
(www.springer.com)

The editors wish to thank the following people for their support, patience, and love throughout this project and for being an enduring source of inspiration:

Charlie and Lisa Sandson

Alison Woodcock; Louise Postman, MD;
Noah, Oliver, and Sylvan Hutchens

James Wittwer; Travis and Kylee Wittwer

Melisa Weingarten; Chloe, Elise, and Ben Weingarten

Jasminka Sprung

Jo Ann Nicholson

Seema Lalwani; Nikita and Rohan Lalwani

Maria Metro; Luke, Nicholas, and Emily Metro

Ann Marie Canelas, MD; Gabriella, Isabella,
and Katherine-Grace Dull

Sharon Kenny; Joseph, Erin, and Thomas Swide

Judy Smith; Daniel Seagull

Robin Kirsch; Jodi, Alan, and Erica Kirsch

Foreword

Drug–drug interactions (DDIs) comprise a category of medical mysteries that are, to say the least, perplexing to anesthesia providers. Despite their very real potential to cause major morbidity and even death to patients, they have generally failed to generate the sizzle of recognition associated with major discoveries in medicine. Why is this? Is it because the potential numbers of DDIs are too large or perhaps too ill-defined to stimulate anesthesia providers to care? Is it because we don't have sufficient epidemiologic studies to document the extent and severity of DDIs? Do they cause harm that is observed by individual providers so infrequently that they don't generate interest in learning about them?

All of these issues may be at play, but I suspect that many trainees and colleagues in anesthesia find there are so many hypothetical DDIs – and they personally observe any bad outcomes so infrequently – that they don't put effort into learning about them except to superficially be aware of the general concept. Is my observation real or perceived? It's hard to say for certain, but let's take the example of herbal medications and potential DDIs. Most anesthesia providers are aware that there are herbal medications that can alter drug metabolism. Ironically, because most anesthesia providers don't observe significant DDIs associated with these medications, few pay much attention to them. When major DDIs associated with herbal medications occur, they often are surprising to anesthesia providers, and more often than not, these events are written off as rarities that the providers will likely never again encounter.

I believe that past perceptions will change. DDIs matter, and they will matter more as the medical world advances. More drugs and herbal products lead to more potential DDIs. Emerging technologies and the growing spread of integrated health care-related electronic medical records offer opportunities to incorporate algorithms and other software identification pathways to warn unsuspecting anesthesia providers of potential DDIs. It would be so simple to have an electronic screen warning displayed whenever a potential DDI-associated medication was part of a patient's care.

Even in this advanced health care world, anesthesia providers will have to be able to understand basic DDI issues. That's where this wonderful new text becomes valuable. The unique use of case studies and subsequent detailed chapters provide anesthesia providers with several ways, both entertaining and scientific, to learn more about these increasingly important DDI issues. Ultimately, the outcomes of our patients are at stake, and the safe care of our patients is why we are anesthesia providers. Congratulations to the team for putting together such an outstanding and valuable resource for our patients and their providers.

Mark A. Warner, MD

Preface

What do you want me to do?

To watch for you while you're sleeping?
Well please don't be surprised
When you find me dreaming too.

—Robert Hunter

Anesthesia providers rest their notion of safe, quality care on constant and inquisitive vigilance. In the operating room, we react and change anesthetic parameters to subtle changes in the pitch of the pulse oximeter signal, the sound of the ventilator or respiratory circuit, the look of the blood in the surgical field, the tone of voice around the operating table, or any other of a thousand cues in a complex environment. We believe that this attention to detail serves our patients and improves outcomes, and we fear missing something big – metaphorically, being caught sleeping.

Yet those of us who have focused on the perioperative implications of drug–drug interactions (DDIs) frequently describe our introduction to the field as having our eyes opened, of being "turned on" to something new and important. Although DDIs occur frequently in both inpatients and outpatients and are often morbid or even mortal, most of us rely daily on knowledge of pharmacodynamic interactions (eg. two drugs affecting the same receptor) and rarely consider DDIs as potential sources of harm to the patient.

It is time for all of us to wake up to DDIs. Indeed, in this era of 80-hour workweeks for medical trainees, many of us owe our arousability to a single DDI. The phenelzine-meperidine DDI that killed young Libby Zion directly led to the adoption of work hour restrictions – and better sleeping and waking for a generation of resident physicians.

We hope this book will be a gentle, comprehensive introduction to an important concept. We have chosen a case-based format to introduce potentially dry concepts, with each case backed by referenced discussion and take-home points. None of the cases presented here are based on hypotheticals from *in vitro* data alone. Particularly severe interactions are highlighted as the "**Fatal Forty**." In addition, however, detailed mechanistic chapters cover important concepts in depth, offering a second level of knowledge for the interested reader. Finally, comprehensive tables are clearly separated from the text and easily found in the back of the book, allowing use of this book as a reference as well. If you just want to get started now, flip to the cases and read at random. I am confident they will pique your curiosity and start you on a path. If not, there is a more comprehensive "how to use this book" chapter immediately following this preface. Regardless of how you use the book, we welcome you to a fascinating and complex new world and wish you and your patients pleasant awakenings.

Michael P. Hutchens, MD

Acknowledgments

This book is being given as a gift to the Foundation for Anesthesia Education and Research (FAER) and to the national and international anesthesia communities. It is our belief that increased awareness, knowledge, and insight regarding the drug–drug interactions we face in the practice of anesthesiology and perioperative medicine will result in safer and better care for patients.

The project has required an enormous and sustained effort. Many individuals, including anesthesiologists, anesthetists, pharmacologists, pharmacists, and other clinicians, have generously given their time and energy to research and write the case scenarios. We are grateful for these contributions.

Among our colleagues, we must, first and foremost, acknowledge and thank our students, residents, and other junior colleagues for their interest, enthusiasm, and discipline. They were the inspiration that drove this project. We also acknowledge the Cardiac and Surgical Intensive Care Unit (8CSI) at Oregon Health & Science University for their never-ending and driving curiosity.

We further thank a number of individuals for their unique contributions, especially Theresa Hanson at the Mayo Clinic for her superb energy and diligent assistance with this manuscript. She is something of a miracle worker, who can apparently get any permission or authorization from any source in zero time. We thank Kathryn Riccio at the University of Pittsburgh for helping us track authors and affiliations, and Vincent L. Hoellerich, MD, and Anthony Silipo, DO, for soliciting early and helpful reviews of the material and cases.

Our sincerest thanks goes to Matthew DeCaro, MD, at Thomas Jefferson University and Kevin Cleveland, PharmD, at Idaho State for generously taking time away from their own specialties to contribute to ours. We are always grateful to have Dr. DeCaro act as our cardiology editor!

A special thanks and acknowledgment goes to David K. Miller, Esq., principal at Miller & Wagner, for generously contributing his time and expertise to do our legal section and to Mark Warner, MD, for writing our foreword.

We would also like to thank several busy academic anesthesiologists and friends for taking a special interest in this project, sending us ideas and suggestions, and shepherding a number of topics through to completion at their respective institutions:

Nabil M. Elkassabany, MD, and Jonathan Gavrin, MD, at the University of Pennsylvania; Jonathan Anson, MD, at Penn State Hershey Medical Center; Michael Bishop, MD, at the University of Washington; Roman Sniecinski, MD, at Emory; Christine Formea, PharmD, at the Mayo Clinic; Daniel W. Johnson, MD, at the Massachusetts General Hospital; and Angela Kendrick, MD, Kimberly Mauer, MD, and Ansgar Brambrink,MD PhD, at Oregon Health and Science University.

We are grateful to a number of chairpersons for fostering a spirit of academic interest and inquiry at their institutions and for supporting their people's efforts on this book: Lee A. Fleisher, MD, at the University of Pennsylvania; Jeanine Wiener-Kronish, MD, at the Massachusetts General Hospital; James Zaidan, MD, at Emory; Bradley J. Narr, MD, at the Mayo Clinic; David Schwartz, MD, at the University of Chicago-Illinois; and John Williams, MD at the University of Pittsburgh Medical Center. Although he did not contribute directly to the manuscript, we have long admired and referenced the truly groundbreaking and pioneering drug-drug interaction work of Evan Kharasch, MD PhD. There is the tiniest of jokes buried deep in the pages in this book and we think that probably only Dr. Kharasch will recognize it (hint: it has to do with the Fatal Forty).

Also, we would like to thank our entire team of Springer editors and production people, including but not limited to Shelley Reinhardt, Michael D. Sova, Asja Parrish, Rebekah Amos, Richard Lansing, as well as Jeffrey Taub and Rajan Bharatwaj, for their patience, diligence, stamina and ongoing faith in our project. It was a complicated process, but we got it done, and we are very grateful to all the Springer folks for hanging in there with us.

Of course, it also goes without saying that I personally have been continually grateful and humbled by the astounding knowledge, tolerance, and patience of all of my coeditors. I am honored to be in this group! I would like to give special acknowledgment to three of my editorial colleagues: Jeffrey R. Kirsch, MD, for his attention, dedication, support, and patience, as well as for his energy and expertise in developing this manuscript; Erica D. Wittwer, MD PhD, who was the only member of group to undertake full editorial duties while a busy resident and fellow and whose work was nothing short of great at all times; and finally Neil B. Sandson, MD. The anesthesiology community will benefit greatly from Dr. Sandson's knowledge, commitment, and generosity. Without him, this project simply and literally would not have been possible.

Catherine Marcucci, MD

Contents

Part XII. Drug–Drug Interactions Involving Cardiovascular Medications

Contributors

Phillip Adams, DO Department of Anesthesiology, University of Pittsburgh Medical Center, Pittsburgh, PA, USA

Alfredo Aguiar, MD Department of Anesthesiology, University of Utah SOM, Salt Lake City, UT, USA

Jonathan Anson, MD Department of Anesthesiology, Penn State Milton S. Hershey Medical Center, Hershey, PA, USA

Miya Asato, MD Division of Child Neurology, Department of Pediatrics and Psychiatry, Children's Hospital of Pittsburgh, Pittsburgh, PA, USA

Dawn L. Baker, MD, MS Department of Anesthesiology, University of Utah, Salt Lake City, UT, USA

Ryan D. Ball, MD Department of Anesthesiology, University of Pittsburgh Medical Center, Pittsburgh, PA, USA

Brian C. Bane, MD Anesthesia Element, RAF Lakenheath, Suffolk, UK

David W. Barbara, MD Department of Anesthesiology, Mayo Clinic, Rochester, MN, USA

Shawn T. Beaman, MD Department of Anesthesiology, University of Pittsburgh School of Medicine, Pittsburgh, PA, USA

Michael W. Best, MD Department of Anesthesiology, University of Pittsburgh Medical Center, Pittsburgh, PA, USA

Nikhil K. Bhatnagar, MD Department of Anesthesiology, University of Pittsburgh Medical Center, Pittsburgh, PA, USA

Nathaniel Birgenheier, MD Department of Anesthesiology, University of Utah School of Medicine, Salt Lake City, UT, USA

Michael J. Bishop, MD Department of Anesthesiology, University of Washington School of Medicine, Seattle, WA, USA

Brian Blasiole, MD, PhD Department of Anesthesiology, Children's Hospital of Pittsburgh of UPMC, Pittsburgh, PA, USA

Katarina Bojanić, MD Division of Neonatology, Clinical Hospital Merkur, Zagreb, Croatia

Richard Levi Boortz-Marx, MD, MS Department of Anesthesiology, University of North Carolina, Chapel Hill, NC, USA

Karen Boretsky, MD Department of Anesthesiology, University of Pittsburgh Medical Center, Pittsburgh, PA, USA

Charles Boucek, MD Department of Anesthesiology, University of Pittsburgh Medical Center, Pittsburgh, PA, USA

Ansgar M. Brambrink, MD, PhD Department of Anesthesiology and Perioperative Medicine, Oregon Health and Science University, Portland, OR, USA

James Gordon Cain, MD, MBA, FAAP Department of Anesthesiology, Children's Hospital of Pittsburgh of UPMC, Pittsburgh, PA, USA

Ann Marie Canelas, MD Department of Anesthesiology, University of Illinois at Chicago, Chicago, IL, USA

Scott W. Cantwell, MD Kansas Professional Anesthesia & Pain Management Specialists, Wichita, KS, USA

Tara C. Carey, BA, MD Department of Anesthesiology and Perioperative Medicine, Brigham and Women's Hospital, Boston, MA, USA

Thomas M. Chalifoux, MD Department of Anesthesiology, Magee-Womens Hospital Anesthesiology, University of Pittsburgh School of Medicine, Pittsburgh, PA, USA

Lisa Chan, MD Department of Pediatric Cardiac Anesthesiology, Memorial Regional Hospital, Hollywood, FL, USA

Jeff Chen, MD Sierra Anesthesia, Inc., Reno, NV, USA

Rani Chovatiya, MD Department of Anesthesiology, University of Illinois Medical Center, Chicago, IL, USA

Clint Christensen, MD Department of Anesthesiology, University of Utah School of Medicine, Salt Lake City, UT, USA

Franklyn P. Cladis, MD, FAAP Department of Anesthesiology, The University of Pittsburgh School of Medicine, Children's Hospital of Pittsburgh of UPMC, Pittsburgh, PA, USA

Kevin W. Cleveland, PharmD Idaho Drug Information Service, Idaho State University College of Pharmacy, Pocatello, ID, USA

Norman A. Cohen, MD Department of Anesthesiology and Perioperative Medicine, Oregon Health & Science University, Portland, OR, USA

Dustin Coyle, MD Department of Anesthesiology, University of Utah, Salt Lake City, UT, USA

Patricia L. Dalby, MD Department of Anesthesiology, Magee-Womens Hospital, University of Pittsburgh School of Medicine, Pittsburgh, PA, USA

Matthew DeCaro, MD, FACC, FACP Coronary Care Unit, Thomas Jefferson University Hospital, Jefferson Medical College, Philadelphia, PA, USA

Jennifer DeCou, MD Department of Anesthesiology, University of Utah School of Medicine, Salt Lake City, UT, USA

Anna Dubovoy, MD Department of Anesthesiology, University of Michigan Hospital Center, Ann Arbor, MI, USA

Elizabeth Duggan, MD Department of Anesthesiology, Emory University School of Medicine, Atlanta, GA, USA

Randal O. Dull, MD, PhD Department of Anesthesiology, University of Illinois at Chicago, Chicago, IL, USA

Bruce T. Dumser, MD Anesthesiology Consultants of Walla Walla, Walla Walla, WA, USA

J. Andrew Dziewit, MD Department of Anesthesia and Perioperative Medicine, Crozer Chester Medical Center, Upland, PA, USA

Jennifer Egan, MD Department of Anesthesia, Indiana University School of Medicine, Indianapolis, IN, USA

Mariam M. El-Baghdadi, MD Private Practice, Houston, TX, USA

Nabil M. Elkassabany, MD Section of Orthopedic Anesthesiology, Department of Anesthesiology and Critical Care, University of Pennsylvania, Wayne, PA, USA

Stephen Esper, MD, MBA Department of Anesthesiology, University of Pittsburgh Medical Center, Pittsburgh, PA, USA

Stacy L. Fairbanks, MD Department of Anesthesiology, University of Colorado, Denver, Denver, CO, USA

Byron Douglas Fergerson, MD Department of Anesthesiology, University of California, San Diego, San Diego, CA, USA

Matthew Patrick Feuer, MD Department of Anesthesiology, Frederick Memorial Hospital, Frederick, MD, USA

Randall Flick, MD Department of Anesthesiology, Mayo Clinic, Rochester, MN, USA

Christine M. Formea, PharmD, BCPS Pharmacy Research, Mayo Clinic, College of Medicine, Rochester, MN, USA

Patrick J. Forte, MD Department of Anesthesiology, University of Pittsburgh Medical Center, Pittsburgh, PA, USA

Eric Fox, BA College of Medicine, Oregon Health and Science University, Portland, OR, USA

Charles Galaviz, MD Department of Anesthesiology, University of Utah, Salt Lake City, UT, USA

Theresa A. Gelzinis, MD Department of Anesthesiology, University of Pittsburgh Medical Center, Pittsburgh, PA, USA

Brian Gierl, MD Department of Anesthesiology, University of California San Diego, San Diego, CA, USA

Stephen J. Gleich, MD Department of Anesthesiology, Mayo Clinic, Rochester, MN, USA

Benjamin S. Gmelch, MD Department of Anesthesiology, University of Utah School of Medicine, Salt Lake City, UT, USA

Tammara S. Goldschmidt, MD Department of Anesthesiology, University of Illinois, Chicago, IL, USA

Julio A. Gonzalez-Sotomayor, MD Pain Division, Department of Anesthesiology and Perioperative Medicine, Oregon Health and Science University, Portland, OR, USA

Cornelius B. Groenewald, MD, ChB Department of Anesthesiology & Pain Medicine, Seattle Children's Hospital and the University of Washington, Seattle, WA, USA

Allen N. Gustin, MD, FCCP Department of Anesthesia and Critical Care, University of Chicago Pritzker School of Medicine, Chicago, IL, USA

Ferenc E. Gyulai, MD Department of Anesthesiology, University of Pittsburgh Medical Center, Pittsburgh, PA, USA

John Hache, MD Department of Anesthesiology, University of Pittsburgh Medical Center, Pittsburgh, PA, USA

Emily Hagn, MD Department of Pain Management, University of Utah School of Medicine, Salt Lake City, UT, USA

Denise M. Hall Burton, MD Department of Anesthesiology, Children's Hospital of Pittsburgh, University of Pittsburgh Medical Center, Pittsburgh, PA, USA

Matthew Hart, MSN, CRNA Department of Anesthesiology & Perioperative Medicine, Oregon Health and Science University, Portland, OR, USA

William Hartman, MD, PhD Department of Anesthesiology, Mayo Clinic, Rochester, MN, USA

Nicole Henwood, MD West Chester Anesthesia Associates, West Chester, PA, USA

James Hilliard, MSN, CRNA Department of Anesthesiology and Perioperative Medicine, Oregon Health and Science University, Portland, OR, USA

Ibtesam A. Hilmi, MB, CHB, FRCA Department of Anesthesiology, UPMC-Presbyterian Hospital, University of Pittsburgh Medical Center, Pittsburgh, PA, USA

Bryan C. Hoelzer, MD Department of Anesthesiology, Mayo Clinic, Rochester, MN, USA

Mayumi Horibe, MD Department of Anesthesiology & Pain Medicine, University of Washington, Seattle, WA, USA

Michael P. Hutchens, MD Department of Anesthesiology & Perioperative Medicine, Oregon Health & Science University, Portland, OR, USA

James W. Ibinson, MD, PhD Department of Anesthesiology, University of Pittsburgh School of Medicine, Pittsburgh, PA, USA

Norah Janosy, MD Department of Anesthesiology, The Children's Hospital, Aurora, CO, USA

Nikki Jaworski, MD Department of Anesthesiology & Perioperative Medicine, Oregon Health & Science University, Portland, OR, USA

Arun L. Jayaraman, MD, PhD Department of Anesthesiology, Columbia University Medical Center, New York, NY, USA

Barbara Jericho, MD Department of Anesthesiology, University of Illinois Hospital and Health Sciences System, University of Illinois-Chicago, Chicago, IL, USA

James A. Jernigan, MD Department of Anesthesia - PGY3, University of Pittsburgh Medical Center, Pittsburgh, PA, USA

Daniel W. Johnson, MD Department of Anesthesia, Critical Care & Pain Medicine, Massachusetts General Hospital, Boston, MA, USA

Edward A. Kahl, MD Department of Anesthesiology and Perioperative Medicine, Oregon Health and Science University, Portland, OR, USA

A. Murat Kaynar, MD, MPH Departments of Critical Care Medicine and Anesthesiology, University of Pittsburgh School of Medicine, Pittsburgh, PA, USA

Angela Kendrick, MD Department of Anesthesiology and Perioperative Medicine (APOM), Doernbecher Children's Hospital, Oregon Health and Science University, Portland, OR, USA

Scott Kennedy, MD Columbia Anesthesia Group, Vancouver, WA, USA

Janice Kim, MD Department of Anesthesiology, Children's Hospital Colorado, University of Colorado School of Medicine, Aurora, CO, USA

Jeffrey R. Kirsch, MD Department of Anesthesiology & Perioperative Medicine, Oregon Health & Science University, Portland, OR, USA

Jonathon E. Kivela, MD Department of Anesthesiology, Mayo Clinic, Rochester, MN, USA

Ines P. Koerner, MD, PhD Department of Anesthesiology & Perioperative Medicine, Oregon Health & Science University, Portland, OR, USA

Lavinia Kolarcyzk, MD Department of Anesthesiology, University of North Carolina, Chapel Hill, NC, USA

Rachel Koll, MD Department of Anesthesiology, Cincinnati Children's Hospital Medical Center, Cincinnati, OH, USA

Helga Komen, MD Department of Anesthesiology and Critical Care Medicine, University Hospital Rijeka, Rijeka, Croatia

Robert G. Krohner, MD Department of Anesthesiology, Magee-Womens Hospital of UPMC, University of Pittsburgh School of Medicine, Pittsburgh, PA, USA

Matthew M. Kumar, MD Department of Anesthesiology & Critical Care Medicine, Mayo Clinic, Rochester, MN, USA

Richard J. Kuwik, MD Department of Anesthesiology, University of Pittsburgh Medical Center, Pittsburgh, PA, USA

Kirk Lalwani, MD, FRCA, MCR Department of Anesthesiology & Perioperative Medicine, Oregon Health and Science University, Portland, OR, USA

Robert Scott Lang, MD Department of Anesthesiology, University of Pittsburgh Medical Center, Pittsburgh, PA, USA

Dean Laochamroonvorapongse, MD Department of Anesthesiology and Perioperative Medicine, Oregon Health and Science University, Portland, OR, USA

Christine A. Kenyon Laundre, MD Anesthesiology Associates of Wisconsin, Milwaukee, WI, USA

Vincent Lew, MD Department of Anesthesia & Perioperative Care, University of California, San Francisco, San Francisco, CA, USA

Pulsar Li, DO Department of Anesthesiology, University of Pittsburgh Medical Center, Pittsburgh, PA, USA

Charles Lin, MD Department of Anesthesiology, University of Pittsburgh Medical Center, Pittsburgh, PA, USA

Steven S. Liu, MD Department of Anesthesiology and Critical Care, University of Pennsylvania, Philadelphia, PA, USA

Jessica D. Lorenz, MD Department of Anesthesiology, Mayo Clinic, Rochester, MN, USA

Joseph A. Lovely, PharmD, BCPS Department of Pharmacy Services, St. Marys Hospital, Mayo Clinic, Rochester, MN, USA

Kitling M. Lum, RN, BSN, CCRN-CSC Cardiac and Surgical Intensive Care Unit, Oregon Health and Science University, Portland, OR, USA

Elizabeth Macri, MD Department of Neurology, Presbyterian Medical Group, Albuquerque, NM, USA

Michael Mangione, MD Department of Anesthesiology, University of Pittsburgh School of Medicine, VA Pittsburgh Healthcare System, Pittsburgh, PA, USA

Ana Maria Manrique, MD Department of Anesthesiology, Children's Hospital of Pittsburgh, Pittsburgh, PA, USA

Catherine Marcucci, MD Anesthesia Services Department, Philadelphia Veterans Affairs Medical Center, Philadelphia, PA, USA

Joško Markić, MD, MSc Pediatric Intensive Care Unit, Department of Pediatrics, University Hospital of Split, Split, Croatia

Koshy M. Mathai, MD Division of Pain Management, Department of Neurosurgery, West Virginia University, Morgantown, WV, USA

Kimberly Mauer, MD Department of Anesthesiology & Perioperative Medicine, Oregon Health and Science University, Portland, OR, USA

Justin McCray, MD Department of Anesthesiology, University of Pittsburgh Medical Center, Pittsburgh, PA, USA

Kristen B. McCullough, PharmD, BCPS, BCOP Department of Pharmacy Services, Mayo Clinic, Rochester, MN, USA

Li Meng, MD, MPH Department of Anesthesiology, University of Pittsburgh School of Medicine, Pittsburgh, PA, USA

Matthias J. Merkel, MD, PhD Department of Anesthesiology & Perioperative Medicine, Oregon Health and Science University, Portland, OR, USA

Julije Meštrović, MD, PhD Pediatric Intensive Care Unit, Department of Pediatrics, University Hospital of Split, Split, Croatia

David G. Metro, MD Department of Anesthesiology, University of Pittsburgh School of Medicine, Pittsburgh, PA, USA

David K. Miller, JD Miller & Wagner, LLP, Portland, OR, USA

Jessica Miller, MD Oregon Anesthesiology Group, Providence St. Vincent's Hospital, Portland, OR, USA

Brian Mitchell, MD Department of Anesthesiology and Perioperative Medicine, Oregon Health and Science University, Portland, OR, USA

Richard C. Month, MD Department of Anesthesiology and Critical Care, University of Pennsylvania Health System, Philadelphia, PA, USA

Chad D. Moore, PhD Department of Pharmacology and Toxicology, University of Utah, Salt Lake City, UT, USA

Stephanie Neuman, MD Department of Anesthesiology, Gundersen Lutheran, La Crosse, WI, USA

Wayne T. Nicholson, MD, PharmD, MSc Department of Anesthesiology, Mayo Clinic, Rochester, MN, USA

L. Michele Noles, MD Department of Anesthesiology & Perioperative Medicine, Oregon Health and Science University, Portland, OR, USA

Heather Norvelle, PharmD, BCPS Department of Infectious Diseases and Critical Care, Oregon Health and Science University, Portland, OR, USA

Nenna Nwazota, MD Department of Anethesiology, Baylor College of Medicine, Houston, TX, USA

L. Lazarre Ogden, MD Department of Anesthesiology, University of Utah, Salt Lake City, UT, USA

Andrew Oken, MD Operative Care Division, Portland VAMC, Portland, OR, USA

Michael D. Olson, PA-C Department of Otolaryngology, Mayo Clinic, Rochester, MN, USA

Kristin Ondecko Ligda, MD Department of Anesthesiology, UPMC Mercy Hospital, University of Pittsburgh Medical Center, Pittsburgh, PA, USA

Todd M. Oravitz, MD Department of Anesthesiology, University of Pittsburgh School of Medicine, Pittsburgh, PA, USA

Steven L. Orebaugh, MD Department of Anesthesiology & Critical Care, University of Pittsburgh School of Medicine, Pittsburgh, PA, USA

Nathan G. Orgain, MD Department of Anesthesiology, University of Utah, Salt Lake City, UT, USA

Mehmet S. Ozcan, MD, FCCP Department of Anesthesiology, The University of Oklahoma Health Sciences Center, Oklahoma City, OK, USA

Lauren Partyka, MD Department of Anesthesiology, University of Pittsburgh Medical Center, Pittsburgh, PA, USA

Nikhli Patel, MD Department of Anesthesiology, University of Illinois at Chicago, Chicago, IL, USA

Shreya Patel, MD Department of Anesthesiology, University of Arizona College of Medicine, Phoenix, AZ, USA

Erin B. Payne, MD Preoperative Assessment Clinic, University of Michigan Health System, Plymouth, MI, USA

Elizabeth Pedigo, MD Department of Anesthesiology and Perioperative Medicine, Oregon Health and Science University, Portland, OR, USA

Kelly T. Peretich, MD Department of Anesthesiology, University of Pittsburgh Medical Center, Pittsburgh, PA, USA

Adrian Pichurko, MD Department of Anesthesiology, University of Illinois, Chicago, IL, USA

Raymond M. Planinsic, MD Department of Anesthesiology, University of Pittsburgh School of Medicine, Pittsburgh, PA, USA

Branka Polić, MD, MSc Pediatric Intensive Care Unit, Department of Pediatrics, University Hospital of Split, Split, Croatia

Thomas P. Pontinen, MD Department of Anesthesiology, University of Illinois Hospital and Health Sciences System, Chicago, IL, USA

Syed M. Quadri, DO Department of Anesthesiology, University of Illinois at Chicago College of Medicine, Chicago, IL, USA

Jennifer A. Rabbitts, MB, ChB Department of Anesthesiology, Seattle Children's Hospital and University of Washington, Seattle, WA, USA

Avinash Ramchandani, MD Pain Care Physicians, Board Certified in Physical Medicine & Rehabilitation, Austin, TX, USA

Bryan J. Read, MSN, CRNA Department of Anesthesiology and Perioperative Medicine, Oregon Health and Science University, Portland, OR, USA

Scott Richins, MD Pikes Peak Anesthesia Associates, Colorado Springs, CO, USA

Nashaant N. Rizk, MD Department of Anesthesiology, University of Pittsburgh Medical Center, Pittsburgh, PA, USA

Ryan Romeo, MD Department of Anesthesiology, University of Pittsburgh School of Medicine, Pittsburgh, PA, USA

Danielle Roussel, MD Department of Anesthesiology, University of Utah, Salt Lake City, UT, USA

John C. Sanders, MBBS, FRCA Department of Anesthesiology, Shriners Hospitals for Children, Salt Lake City, UT, USA

Neil B. Sandson, MD Department of Psychiatry, University of Maryland Medical System, Baltimore, MD, USA

Department of PsychiatryVA Maryland Health Care System, Baltimore, MD, USA

Federica Scavonetto, MD Department of Anesthesiology, Mayo Clinic, Rochester, MN, USA

Paul Schipper, MD, FACS, FACCP Section of General Thoracic Surgery, Division of Cardiothoracic Surgery, Department of Surgery, Oregon Health and Sciences University, Portland, OR, USA

Nicole Scouras, MD Department of Anesthesiology, University of Pittsburgh Medical Center, Pittsburgh, PA, USA

F. Jacob Seagull, PhD Department of Learning Health Sciences, University of Michigan Medical School, Ann Arbor, MI, USA

William A. Shakespeare, MD Department of Anesthesiology, Mayo Clinic, Rochester, MN, USA

Joseph C. Shy, MD Department of Anesthesiology, University of Pittsburgh Medical Center, Pittsburgh, PA, USA

Michael J. Sikora, MD Department of Anesthesiology, Cincinnati Children's Hospital Medical Center, Cincinnati, OH, USA

Anthony T. Silipo, DO Department of Anesthesiology, University of Pittsburgh Medical Center, Magee Women's Hospital and Presbyterian Medical Center, Pittsburgh, PA, USA

Sara M. Skrlin, MD Department of Anesthesiology and Perioperative Medicine, Oregon Health and Science University, Portland, OR, USA

Roman M. Sniecinski, MD Division of Cardiothoracic Anesthesia, Department of Anesthesiology, Emory University School of Medicine, Atlanta, GA, USA

Juraj Sprung, MD, PhD Department of Anesthesiology, Mayo Clinic, Rochester, MN, USA

Kelly N. Stafford, BSN, CCRN, CSC Cardiac & Surgical ICU, Oregon Health and Science University, Portland, OR, USA

Kathirvel Subramaniam, MD Department of Anesthesiology, University of Pittsburgh Medical Center, Presbyterian Hospital, Pittsburgh, PA, USA

Arun Subramanian, MBBS Department of Anesthesiology, Mayo Clinic, Rochester, MN, USA

Erin A. Sullivan, MD Department of Anesthesiology, University of Pittsburgh Medical Center, Pittsburgh, PA, USA

Hans P. Sviggum, MD Department of Anesthesiology, Mayo Clinic College of Medicine, Rochester, MN, USA

Christopher E. Swide, MD Department of Anesthesiology & Perioperative Medicine, Oregon Health & Science University, Portland, OR, USA

Thomas N. Talamo, MD Department of Anesthesiology, University of Pittsburgh Medical Center, Pittsburgh, PA, USA

Joseph F. Talarico, DO Department of Anesthesiology, UPMC Presbyterian, University of Pittsburgh Medical Center, Pittsburgh, PA, USA

Kenichi Tanaka, MD, MSc Department of Anesthesiology, University of Pittsburgh Medical Center, Pittsburgh, PA, USA

Devin C. Tang, MD MedStar Harbor Hospital, Baltimore, MD, USA

Jerusha Taylor, PharmD, BCPS Department of Pharmacy, Oregon Health and Science University, Portland, OR, USA

Leelee Thames, MD Oregon Anesthesiology Group, Portland, OR, USA

Solina Tith, MD Department of Anesthesiology and Pain Medicine, University of Washington, Seattle, WA, USA

Brian D. Tompkins, MD Department of Anesthesiology and Critical Care, University of Pennsylvania Health System, Philadelphia, PA, USA

Nicole L. Varela, MD Department of Anesthesiology, Winona Health, Winona, MN, USA

Giorgio Veneziano, MD Department of Anesthesiology & Pain Medicine, University of Pittsburgh Medical Center, Columbus, OH, USA

Jessica Voge, MD Department of Obstetrics & Gynecology, Oregon Health and Science University, Portland, OR, USA

Crystal B. Wallentine, MD Department of Anesthesiology, University of Utah School of Medicine, Salt Lake City, UT, USA

Audra M. Webber, MD Department of Anesthesiology, Kosair Children's Hospital, Louisville, KY, USA

Guy Weinberg, MD Department of Anesthesiology, University of Illinois, Chicago, IL, USA

Melisa N. Weingarten, RN, MS Patient Education, Mayo Clinic, Rochester, MN, USA

Toby N. Weingarten, MD Department of Anesthesiology, Mayo Clinic, Rochester, MN, USA

Department of Anesthesiology, Mayo Clinic College of Medicine, Rochester, MN, USA

Tasha L. Welch, MD Department of Anesthesiology, Mayo Clinic College of Medicine, Rochester, MN, USA

Corinne Wisdo, DPM Dunes Podiatry, Murrells Inlet, SC, USA

Erica D. Wittwer, MD, PhD Department of Anesthesiology, Mayo Clinic, Rochester, MN, USA

Michael Wollenberg, MD Department of Anesthesiology & Perioperative Medicine, Oregon Health and Science University, Portland, OR, USA

Lei Wu, MD Department of Radiology, USC Medical Center in Los Angeles, Los Angeles, CA, USA

Joseph J. Yurigan, DO Department of Anesthesiology, University of Pittsburgh Medical Center, Pittsburgh, PA, USA

James Zaidan, MD Department of Anesthesiology, Emory University School of Medicine, Stone Mountain, GA, USA

Ahmed F. Zaky, MD, MPH Department of Anesthesiology and Pain Medicine, VA Puget Sound Health Care Center/University of Washington, Seattle, WA, USA

Introduction to Drug–Drug Interactions

Let's Start at the Very Beginning: Overcoming Fear and Gaining Mastery of Drug–Drug Interactions

1

F. Jacob Seagull PhD, Christopher E. Swide MD and Catherine Marcucci MD

Abstract
This discusses the layout and best use of the book.

Our primary design concept in the development of cases and didactic material for this book on drug–drug interactions (DDIs) has been that of a level and lighted pathway. We believe that pharmacology in general is a subject that is dense and a little scary at times for many medical professionals, including physicians. We have ruefully learned from our trainees and students that the subject of DDIs proves that it is possible to be both **scared** and **bored** at the same time! Therefore, from the beginning, we felt that what was needed was a lighter, brighter way to travel into and through the material as well as easy places and ways to stop and browse the material. After all, if you're going to go down a path through a dark forest, you need a flashlight, or better yet, a whole suitcase of flashlights. This book is a serious book on a serious subject, but we decided from the get-go to write the most accessible and friendly pharmacology book we could come up with.

F.J. Seagull PhD (✉)
Department of Learning Health Sciences, University of Michigan Medical School, Ann Arbor, MI, USA
e-mail: jseagull@umich.edu

C.E. Swide MD
Perioperative Medicine, Oregon Health and Science University, Department of Anesthesiology, Portland, OR, USA

C. Marcucci MD
Anesthesia Services Department, Philadelphia Veterans Affairs Medical Center, Philadelphia, PA, USA

C. Marcucci et al. (eds.), *A Case Approach to Perioperative Drug-Drug Interactions*, DOI 10.1007/978-1-4614-7495-1_1

There are over 11,000 FDA-approved prescription drugs containing over 1300 unique active ingredients, yielding somewhere between 1.75 million and 121 million combinations of two prescription drugs. These are ridiculous numbers and, clearly, a brute force attack on the problem of DDIs will not be a useful strategy. Instead, the best approach is one comprised of simple, small steps.

This book starts by reviewing some of the core concepts of the fraternal twins of pharmacology--pharmacodynamics and pharmacokinetics. However, the reader should not be afraid. These are short, easy-to-read explanations and reviews and these chapters are heavy on accessibility and relevant examples as well as simple drawings and figures. This material is light on the stuff that makes everybody want to put a pharmacology book down.

Core Concepts in Pharmacodynamic Interactions presents the classic paradigm that while pharmacokinetics describes what the body does to drugs, pharmacodynamics describes what drugs to do the body. This is a very comfortable, easy place for anesthesia providers to launch their DDI studies. It is familiar territory—this is what we do every day, we give a drug and we see what happens. The authors review basics such as ligand-binding, the types of pharmacodynamic interactions, and the main receptors involved in pharmacodynamic DDIs.

Core Concepts in Pharmacokinetic Interactions follows next. This essay serves as the starting point for the discussion of how the body processes and interacts with drugs, including absorption, distribution, metabolism, and elimination. These key pharmacokinetic concepts include the cytochrome P450 (CYP) system, and the roles played by substrates, inhibitors, and inducer in drug interactions.

We next present a **Brief Review of CYP450 Enzymes and UGTs.** This is a compilation and summary of the each of the major enzymes involved in oxidative (Phase I) metabolism. We have nicknamed each of the enzymes to indicate what their primary business is and to help the reader remember and discriminate between them. A mastery of the P450 enzymes is important as they are prime actors in the occurrence of metabolic DDIs—at least the pharmacokinetic DDIs that involve metabolism. This is how and where drugs are metabolized. These enzymes can also be inhibited and induced by medications, foods, and other substances, such as smoked tobacco. We have also included a short discussion of uridine 5′-diphospho-glucuronosyl transferases (UGTs), which is a family of enzymes much like the P450 enzymes that does the work of conjugative (Phase II) metabolism.

P-glycoprotein and OATP Transporters is a short and easy-to-understand section that introduces two main drug transport systems that factor heavily in DDIs involving absorption. Like the P450 and UGT enzymes, the organic anion transporting polypeptides (OATPs) are transporters that have substrates, inducers, and inhibitors.

The next section is **The "Fatal" Forty.**[1] This section is our personal favorite. It is a compilation of forty commonly prescribed drugs whose interactions, if mastered to any reasonable degree, would form a robust and permanent knowledge of DDI principles that can serve as a foundation for further and future study. If you can master the **Fatal Forty**, you will eventually gain ongoing mastery and currency in the larger DDI universe. In business and manufacturing, the Pareto principle states that 80% of events are caused by 20% of the causes. In pharmacokinetics, the **Fatal Forty** is the very small percent of drugs that are involved in a disproportionate number of adverse DDIs. We present approaches to the mastery of these drugs and their DDIs by further organizing them into smaller groups based on clinical use or DDI mechanism.

The **Six Patterns of Pharmacokinetic DDIs** is designed to further demystify the cytochrome P450 enzymes and the interactions they are involved in. There are really only six basic types of interactions between enzymes, substrates, inducers, and inhibitors. They are presented here in short and simple form.

In **The Problem with the DDI Software: A Procrustean Dilemma,** we present our arguments against an over reliance on both commercial and institutional DDI software. These can be valuable adjuncts in careful management of perioperative DDIs, but we believe the best defense against avoidable and untoward DDIs is an educated clinician who has taken the time and made the effort to acquire a fund of knowledge and true understanding of the DDI universe.

Pharmacogenomics provides background for the several drug–gene interactions included in the book. This piece is also a general primer on what may be a new paradigm in anesthetic and medical practice and how medicine will be practiced in the future.

In **Pharmacoepidemiology of Drug Interactions,** we discuss how and why anesthesiologists encounter DDIs. An appreciation of the unique challenges and situations faced by perioperative providers as well as how the high-risk perioperative period and pain setting puts our patients at risk for DDIs will help motivate the DDI student and validate the need to dedicate ongoing time and attention to the subject.

The final didactic piece is a brief legal section entitled **The Lawyers Can Read, Too**. This is an admittedly light title for a very serious subject. Again, we are very

---

[1] The editors wish to acknowledge that use of the term "**The Fatal Forty**" in no way implies that any of the cited drugs is a lethal agent. Every drug on this list can be and has been safely, appropriately, and effectively utilized by providers and provided therapeutic benefit to patients. We also acknowledge that even when any of these drugs is involved in a DDI, the likelihood of an outcome as dire as fatality is small. Rather, the "**Fatal Forty**" name is employed solely as a motivational stratagem to highlight for our readers and students certain drugs that are especially worthy of consideration due to known involvement in clinically significant drug interactions, either by virtue of their prevalence or severity of the interactions in question. The term "**Fatal Forty**" is employed in the educational context that failure to learn and consider the potential well-recognized DDIs associated with these drugs would prove fatal to the student's ultimate innate mastery of this most important arena of patient safety.

grateful to David K. Miller, Esq. for providing actual legal case material from his files and generously providing his time to write them up for us. The inclusion of a legal section may seem unusual for a pharmacology textbook, but this is first and foremost a *clinical* pharmacology book. Reading the cases of actual patients that have come to serious or mortal harm, due to their clinician's failure to recognize and appreciate DDIs, is sobering. Hopefully, it will provide the reader with a compelling motivation to read further and dig deeper into the material.

After the didactic material, we begin to introduce DDI exemplars in the **Case Vignettes** sections. With the single exception of the QT-prolongers, the DDIs are grouped by drug classification, starting with the drugs we most commonly use. Each section is prefaced by an Introduction highlighting the editors' own DDI experiences, general practice considerations, or (in the case of the QT-prolongers) the always-valuable refresher on the effects of drugs on cardiac conduction.

The vignettes are brief and can each be read or reviewed in ten minutes or less. Each vignette presents a single DDI or a tightly-linked DDI pair. The vignettes are arranged generally from the simplest and most straightforward DDIs to more complex and/or less well-understood interactions. We have included an abstract giving the drug pair and main clinical effect of the DDI. The clinical case is followed by a discussion of the pertinent pharmacological issues and summarized in both bullet and tabulated form.

All of the vignettes, unless otherwise noted, are based on clinical reports of interactions known to occur in humans or on personal communications.[2] They were written by working clinicians---physicians, anesthetists, nurses, and clinical pharmacists and pharmacologists. The authors were asked, if possible, to write up cases that were of particular interest to them or of which they had personal knowledge. We believe this will make the material more interesting and less dry and also provide a key to developing expertise in DDIs. People believe facts, but they remember stories and it is known that recognition-based priming is a hallmark of expertise in complex, uncertain environments. Put another and much simpler way, we would be delighted to hear someday that a clinician or student said to a colleague, "Don't you remember—that was **The Bawling Baby**?"

Each didactic essay and clinical case in the book is designed to be a self-contained learning module, so there is really no bad place to begin your DDI studies. Mastering DDIs is really all about mastering your *fear* of DDIs. So, if you are a newcomer to DDIs or have limited time, we recommend you start by reading the Core Concepts chapters (remember, they are short!) to create a good foundation, and then the introductions to the P450 enzymes, and the **Fatal Forty**. Study the **Fatal Forty** several times and then think about and start to develop your own "**Top Ten**" list.

If you do not have time or otherwise cannot do that or, despite of our best efforts, you are still intimidated, look at our compilation of DDIs for both junior and senior anesthesia trainees below and start working on those. They have been selected by an anes-

[2] Animal and in vitro DDI data and studies are both valuable from a scientific viewpoint as well as fascinating, however they are beyond the scope of this clinical handbook. Also, although these studies are often the precursors to understanding and recognizing corresponding or similar DDIs in humans, this is not necessarily always the case.

thesiology program director for their relevance and accessibility. If you cannot spend ten minutes on a case, spend just five minutes and then invest the second five minutes reviewing it later. You will eventually gain a familiarity and knowledge not just of the drug pairs that are presented in the cases, but with the broader associations, classifications, and mechanisms of DDIs. Take your top ten list and try to place into the routine of your clinical practice—for example, if smoked tobacco is on your list (a CYP1A2 inducer), make a list of CYP1A2 substrates (eg, caffeine and cyclobenzaprine) and for one week, make a special effort to scan the medication list of every patient who has "quit" smoking before coming to the operating room. Try to discuss one DDI case a day with your attendings or colleagues. Before each induction of anesthesia, stop a minute and think about whether any of the patient's preexisting medications may have caused a catecholamine-depleted state. Start considering DDIs in the differential diagnosis of common anesthesia issues, such as apparent local anesthetic toxicity. Make friends with your clinical pharmacists and pharmacologists! They are a wealth of information and knowledge and will be delighted to sit down and talk about drugs and drug interactions with you. Feel free to harbor suspicions and hold grudges.

Once you have developed a familiarity with DDIs and built a personal list of the most relevant drugs and DDIs, start working on maintaining currency with the DDI literature. We consider PubMed to be the most powerful DDI software program out there.[2] We recommend sitting down at the computer once a month to look at the emerging literature, so just type in your drug of interest and a simple search term, such as "P450" or "drug interactions" and see what comes up. The field of DDIs and drug–gene interactions is rapidly expanding and there will be new information and studies every month. As noted above, if you are not an expert, we recommend that you concentrate on human studies and case reports as these will contribute the most to your clinical practice.

If you are expert in pharmacology or are already knowledgeable about DDIs, this book will make an easy and fun refresher for airports or your daily commute. We are also hopeful the didactics and cases will be of use to you for your own lectures and presentations to pharmacology and pharmacy students and perioperative clinicians at all levels. Read the book with an eye to borrowing cases and the **Fatal Forty** approaches to motivate your students and trainees and raise their awareness of DDIs. We feel the book, with its concise tables, also makes a good pocket reference. We welcome input and feedback, so please feel free to contact us with comments and suggestions![3]

A DDI reading list for the CA-1:

- **That Sums It Up**—additive nature of minimum alveolar concentration of volatile anesthetics
- **Hot Stuff!**—triggering drugs, ryanodine receptor, malignant hyperthermia
- **1+1+1+1=?**—variable effects of alcohol and sedatives
- **Riding the Rollercoaster**—additive effects of vasoactive substances
- **How to Successfully Occlude an Intravenous Line**—chemical precipitation of an induction agent and succinylcholine in an intravenous line
- **Lipid Lifesaver**—the interaction of local anesthetics and lipid emulsion

[3] Sandson.marcucci@comcast.net

- **Comfortably Numb**—the additive effects of local anesthetics
- **The Topic of the Day**—inhibited metabolism of lidocaine causing seizures
- **Blocked Again**—repeated doses of succinylcholine
- **Irreversibility Sux**—neostigmine-succinylcholine interaction
- **Keep an "Ion" the Twitches**—magnesium, neuromuscular blockade
- **Relax, It's Only Gentamicin**—interaction of aminoglycoside antibiotics and volatile anesthetics at the neuromuscular junction
- **A Delayed Surgeon Is a Dismayed Surgeon**—combined effects of volatile anesthetics on somatosensory-evoked potentials
- **Doggone It–The Case Is Cancelled**—interaction of midazolam and HIV drugs
- **The Worry That's Always With Us: Now I'm Depressed**—interaction of benzodiazepines, opioids, and propofol
- **The Wakeup Call: 2 AM Trauma**—interaction of cocaine and ß-blockers
- **Shiver Yes, Die No**—interaction of meperidine and monoamine oxidase inhibitors
- **The Lawyers Can Read, Too: Cases from the Courtroom**

A DDI reading list for the CA-2 or CA-3:

- **The Hemodynamic Hole**—general anesthetics, ACE inhibitors, and angiotensin receptor blockers
- **Alpha-2 to the Rescue but Beware Bradycardia**—α_2-agents and anesthetic requirements
- **Bounce Back**—ultrametabolism of ondansetron
- **LOL-LOL: Little Old Lady—Lots of Lido**
- **Stop Moving**—phenytoin induction of vecuronium
- **Misusing Mom's Meds**—catecholamine depletion and indirect-acting sympathomimetics
- **Dexy's Midnight Spinal**—dexmedetomidine and bupivacaine spinal
- **TPN (I): A Review and Two Interactions**
- **Garlic II: A Girl Named Allicin**
- **The Lawyers Can Read, Too: Cases from the Courtroom**

References

1. Benet LZ. Pharmacokinetics: basic principles and its use as a tool in drug metabolism. In: Mitchell JR, Horning MG, editors. Drug metabolism and drug toxicity. New York: Raven Press; 1984. p. 199.
2. US National Library of Medicine, National Institutes of Health. http://www.ncbi.nlm.nih.gov/sites/entrez. Last accessed 21 Sept 2012.

Pharmacodynamic Interactions: Core Concepts

2

Erica D. Wittwer MD, PhD
and Wayne T. Nicholson MD, PharmD, MSc

Abstract
This chapter discusses the essential terms and concepts pertaining to the relationship between the concentration of a drug at the end-organ site and the degree of drug effect. This subset of pharmacology is known as **pharmacodynamics**.

Introduction to Pharmacodynamics

Pharmacodynamics is commonly described as "what a drug does to the body" and this concept includes biochemical and physiological actions resulting from the administration of a drug. In contrast, *pharmacokinetics* describes "what the body does to a drug" (ie, absorption, distribution, metabolism, or excretion). Pharmacodynamics describes the relation between the concentration of drug at the effect site and the degree of the resulting drug effect. Dose-response relations may demonstrate the pharmacodynamic effects of a single drug or allow comparison of different drugs. Graphic illustrations often show the relations between dosage along the x-axis and the degree of the response to the drug (efficacy) along the y-axis. The effects may be intended (therapeutic), unintended (adverse effects), or supratherapeutic (toxicity). Clinically, the drug concentration is targeted for the therapeutic window through proper dosage, thereby maximizing therapeutic effects while minimizing adverse effects (Fig. 2.1).

E.D. Wittwer MD, PhD (✉) • W.T. Nicholson MD, PharmD, MSc
Department of Anesthesiology, Mayo Clinic, Rochester, MN, USA
e-mail: Wittwer.erica@mayo.edu

C. Marcucci et al. (eds.), *A Case Approach to Perioperative Drug-Drug Interactions*, DOI 10.1007/978-1-4614-7495-1_2

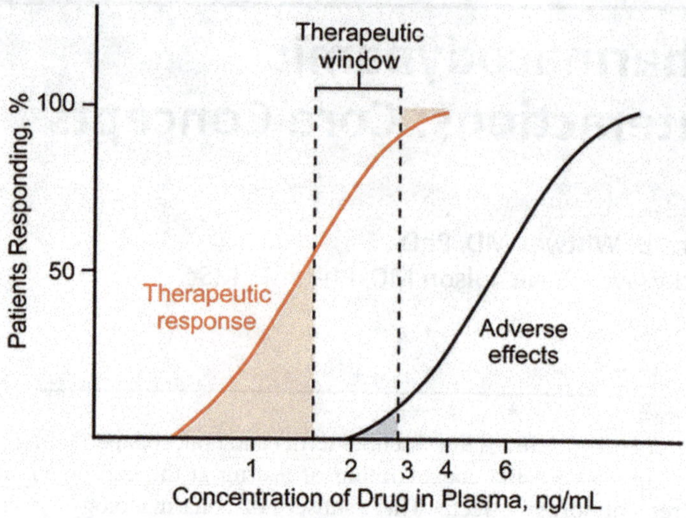

Fig. 2.1 The relation of the therapeutic window of drug concentration to the therapeutic and adverse effects in the patient population. The ordinate is linear; the abscissa is logarithmic [Adapted from Blumenthal DK, Garrison JC. Pharmacodynamics: molecular mechanisms of drug action. In: Brunton LL, Chabner BA, Knollmann BC, editors: Goodman & Gilman's The Pharmacological Basis of Therapeutics. 12th ed. New York, McGraw-Hill Medical, 2011, pp. 41–72. With permission from McGraw-Hill]

Pharmacodynamics also includes the ligand–receptor interactions that result in drug action. The *affinity* of a ligand or a drug for a receptor is the strength of the attraction for a receptor and ligand to bind; the affinity has a degree of *specificity.* Specificity may not be absolute for a given receptor, and a single drug may have affinity for several completely different types of receptor classes. In the case of diphenhydramine, affinity for the completely unrelated histamine and muscarine receptors is seen. By comparison, ondansetron has a greater specificity, showing affinity and selectivity for the 5-hydroxytryptamine$_3$ (5-HT$_3$) receptor subtype over other serotonin subtypes.

However, ligand affinity alone does not fully explain single drug action. After a ligand is bound to a receptor, the drug may act as an *agonist* (able to cause a full effect), a partial agonist (able to cause a submaximal effect), or an *antagonist* (occupying the receptor but not causing an effect). Although antagonists have affinity for a receptor and lack efficacy, their ability to act pharmacologically is to competitively or noncompetitively interfere with the action of an agonist.

An example of direct competitive antagonism is the interaction between nondepolarizing neuromuscular blocking drugs (NMBDs) and the acetylcholine receptors (nicotinic cholinergic receptors). NMBDs compete for receptor occupancy with acetylcholine and interfere with the binding of acetylcholine to the receptor, preventing a muscle contraction. An NMBD must occupy 75% to 80% of the receptors to cause clinically significant paralysis. The drug action is terminated through metabolism over time, however; reversal of blockade can be facilitated indirectly with administration of an acetylcholinesterase inhibitor. These drugs bind with acetylcholinesterase and prevent the degradation of endogenous acetylcholine. This prevention increases the amount of acetylcholine available at the nicotinic receptors to compete with the neuromuscular blockers for binding. Because acetylcholine does not have absolute specificity for neuromuscular nicotinic receptors, a muscarinic antagonist needs to be coadministered to prevent parasympathetic adverse effects.

Receptor occupancy in an organ or enzyme system also assists in dictating drug action, and the effects are limited when either system reaches a saturation point. In this example, when a patient is paralyzed with an NMBD and demonstrates no muscle twitches when stimulated with a nerve stimulator, nearly all of the receptors are occupied. At this point, further administration of the NMBD does not confer additional efficacy. This clinical result is often referred to as a pharmacologic *ceiling effect.*

At full blockade, administration of a cholinesterase inhibitor is not effective because the degree of receptor occupation cannot be overcome by the endogenous increase in acetylcholine. Therefore, effective reversal of neuromuscular blockade is often achieved after the NMBD effect has begun to wane and the patient has at least one twitch return when stimulated with a train-of-four stimulus. Endogenous levels of acetylcholine as a result of acetylcholinesterase inhibition are then adequate to compete with the NMBD, thus allowing for muscle function recovery. Of note, the clinician needs to consider the duration of action of the administered NMBD when giving a reversal agent because re-paralysis is possible. If the duration of action of the reversal agent is shorter than that of the NMBD, the action of the NMBD continues after the cholinesterase inhibitor is no longer effective.

The effect of competitive antagonists can be overcome by increasing the concentration of the agonist, whereas the effect of noncompetitive antagonists cannot be overcome. Noncompetitive interactions are bound irreversibly or these ligands disassociate very slowly from the receptor (Fig. 2.2). Where irreversible interactions occur, a new receptor must be produced. Phenoxybenzamine is an example of a noncompetitive α-antagonist.

Receptors act as the mediators for many pharmacodynamic effects. The four main receptor families are ligand-gated ion channels, G protein-coupled receptors, enzyme-linked receptors, and intracellular receptors (Fig. 2.3). The majority of the receptors relevant in drug action are G protein–coupled receptors, including opioid (μ, κ, and δ subtypes), substance P, dopamine, serotonin, histamine$_1$ (H_1), cannabinoid, and muscarinic cholinergic and γ-aminobutyric acid$_B$ ($GABA_B$) receptors. The acetylcholine receptor (nicotinic cholinergic receptor) is an example of a ligand-gated ion channel, as are the N-methyl-D-aspartate (NMDA) and $GABA_A$ receptors. Enzyme-linked and intracellular receptors are less commonly drug targets. Enzyme-linked receptors include the natriuretic peptide receptor and epidermal growth factor receptors. Estrogen, mineralocorticoid, and thyroid hormone receptors are examples of intracellular receptors.

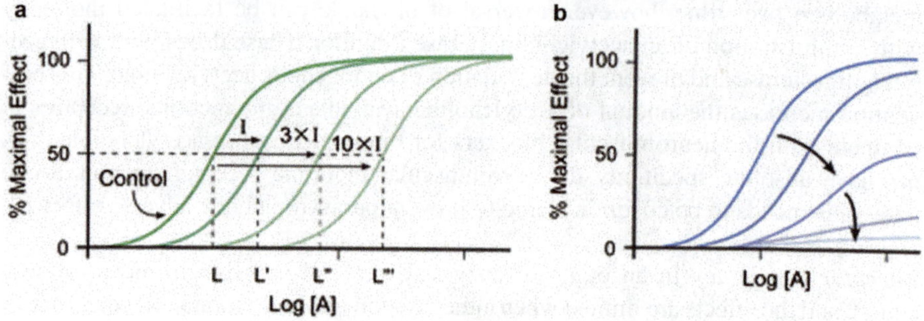

Fig. 2.2 Mechanisms of receptor antagonism. A, Competitive antagonism occurs when agonist A and antagonist I compete for the same binding site on the receptor. Response curves for the agonist are shifted to the right in a concentration-related manner by the antagonist, such that the EC50 (the concentration of drug that gives half maximal effect) for the agonist increases (ie, L vs L′, L", and L′′′) with the concentration of the antagonist. B, If the antagonist binds to the same site as the agonist but does so irreversibly or pseudoirreversibly (slow dissociation but no covalent bond), it causes a shift of the dose-response curve to the right, with further depression of the maximal response [Adapted from Blumenthal DK, Garrison JC. Pharmacodynamics: molecular mechanisms of drug action. In: Brunton LL, Chabner BA, Knollmann BC, (Eds.). Goodman & Gilman's The Pharmacological Basis of Therapeutics. 12th ed. New York, McGraw-Hill Medical, 2011, pp. 41-72. With permission from McGraw-Hill]

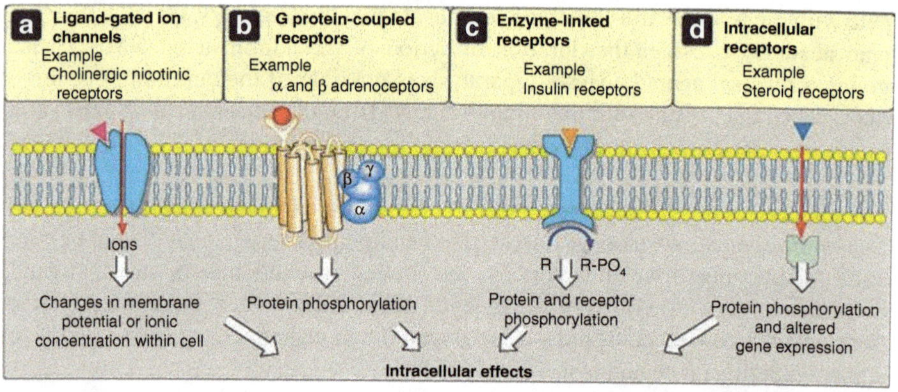

Fig. 2.3 Transmembrane signaling mechanisms. A, Ligand binds to extracellular domain of a ligand-gated channel. B, Ligand binds to a domain of a serpentine receptor, which is coupled to a G protein. C, Ligand binds to the extracellular domain of a receptor that activates a kinase system. D, Lipid-soluble ligand diffuses across the membrane to interact with its intracellular receptor [Adapted from Finkel R, Clark MA, Cubeddu LX, (Eds.). Pharmacology, 4th ed. Philadelphia, PA: Lippincott Williams & Wilkins, 2009. With permission from Wolters Kluwer Health]

Tolerance is the development, over time, of a resistance to the effects of a drug. An increased amount of the drug must be administered to achieve the same level of effect that was achieved earlier with less drug. Pharmacodynamically, this resistance may be due in part to receptor re-regulation. Continuous exposure to drugs may cause receptor upregulation or downregulation and result in a change of overall receptor density. Tolerance may be to a single agent or to other drugs of a similar class or with a similar mechanism—a phenomenon often referred to as *cross-tolerance*. Cross-tolerance between two different drugs may be complete (ie, similar in degree of tolerance) or incomplete (ie, tolerance is reduced in degree).

An important point of consideration is that tolerance may also build up toward one effect of a drug and not another effect. As the dose is increased to achieve the same desired effect, other effects may increase in intensity. A classic example is opioid use. Persons taking opioids on a long-term basis eventually have tolerance to the medication's analgesic, or pain-relieving, effect, thereby requiring increased doses over time. However, tolerance does not develop to all the opioid effects, for example, adverse effects of opioids include constipation, and tolerance to opioid-induced constipation does not develop as it does toward the analgesic effect.

Tolerance is not the same as *addiction* or *dependence*. Dependence is physiological and often seen on cessation of a drug, eliciting a withdrawal syndrome. Opioids can cause both tolerance and dependence and, given enough time, these effects are expected pharmacologically. Addiction, however, is a psychological phenomenon and the drug becomes the focus of behavior. Although a patient may present with tolerance, dependence, and addiction to an opioid, addiction is not a regularly expected pharmacologic outcome in pain management.

Tolerance also should be differentiated from *tachyphylaxis*. Although tolerance develops gradually during long-term administration, tachyphylaxis is a rapid decrease in drug effect that may begin with the initial drug administration. Transdermal nitroglycerin is an example of a drug that undergoes tachyphylaxis and requires drug-free intervals because of the decrease in effect.

Pharmacodynamic interactions occur when two or more drugs are given concomitantly. An *additive* interaction occurs when the combined effect of two drugs equals the sum of their individual effects. By comparison, *synergy* is an important concept in pharmacodynamics and in understanding drug interactions. These interactions may occur unwittingly or drug properties may be taken advantage of to increase a desired effect. Synergy occurs when two drugs are combined in therapy and produce a pharmacologic effect greater than the sum of their individual effects. The degree of respiratory depression observed as a result of concomitant administration of midazolam and fentanyl is an adverse effect that demonstrates synergism. In contrast, the synergistic effect on sedation is desirable in many situations. When considering hypnosis and immobility in anesthesia, the clinician needs to be aware that drug combinations that act at the same receptor are likely to act in an additive manner; drugs that act at different receptors are more likely to act synergistically.[1]

Drug combinations that result in antagonistic interactions also deserve consideration. *Antagonism* occurs when the combined effect of two drugs is less than the sum of their individual effects. Commonly, when antagonism is considered, one drug is administered to decrease the effect of another, as in the case of naloxone reversal of an opiate. However, antagonism also occurs when the effect of two drugs administered together is greater than the effect of either drug alone but is less than the projected additive effect of each drug. This response is often described as an *infra-additive interaction*. The combination of isoflurane and nitrous oxide results in an infra-additive interaction since the combination produces less than an additive effect on hypnosis but more than the effect of either agent alone.[1]

Knowledge of the individual types of interactions (synergy, additive, or antagonistic) enables complex interactions to be broken down and understood in a more thorough level. Such improved understanding may be used to recognize and, hopefully, to predict and prevent adverse drug interactions.

Reference

1. Hendrickx JF, Eger 2nd EI, Sonner JM, et al. Is synergy the rule? A review of anesthetic interactions producing hypnosis and immobility. Anesth Analg. 2008;107:494–506.

Pharmacokinetic Interactions: Core Concepts

3

Erica D. Wittwer MD, PhD
and Wayne T. Nicholson MD, PharmD, MSc

Abstract
This chapter discusses the essential terms and concepts pertaining to how the body processes drugs. This subset of pharmacology is known as **pharmacokinetics**.

Introduction to Pharmacokinetics

Pharmacokinetics describes what the body does to a drug. This subject is in contrast to *pharmacodynamics*, which is the relation between the concentration of drug at the effect site and the degree of the resulting drug effect. Pharmacokinetics starts with the introduction of a drug into the body, beginning with absorption and followed by drug distribution, metabolism, and, finally, excretion. Many drug–drug interactions (DDIs) involve pharmacokinetics that may lead to adverse drug effects.

Drug administration occurs through several possible routes, including oral, intravenous, rectal, sublingual, subcutaneous, inhalation, and transdermal. Aside from intravenous (IV) administration, all other routes require that the drug be absorbed. *Bioavailability* refers to the fraction of the drug dose that reaches the systemic circulation after administration, and it is often dependent on the route of administration. By definition, drugs administered intravenously have 100% bioavailability; drugs delivered through other routes may have a lower percentage of bioavailability. This comparison is especially true for drugs administered orally and rectally. A reduction in systemically available drug may be caused by reduced absorption in the gastrointestinal tract or by first-pass metabolism (high hepatic extraction before the drug enters the systemic circulation), or both. Bioavailability is the basis for the

E.D. Wittwer MD, PhD (✉) • W.T. Nicholson MD, PharmD, MSc
Department of Anesthesiology, Mayo Clinic, Rochester, MN, USA
e-mail: Wittwer.erica@mayo.edu

C. Marcucci et al. (eds.), *A Case Approach to Perioperative Drug-Drug Interactions*, DOI 10.1007/978-1-4614-7495-1_3

discrepancy between plasma levels after an oral dose and after an IV dose. Morphine is a good example of a drug that has a reduced oral bioavailability: 30 mg of orally administered morphine is required to equal the effect of 10 mg of morphine given intravenously.

Absorption from the gastrointestinal tract can be altered by food intake through changes in gastric emptying time, gastric pH, alteration of enzyme function, or interactions with drug transport mechanisms. Two drug transporters involved in drug interactions are P-glycoprotein (P-gp) and organic anion-transporting peptide (OATP). P-gp is an efflux transporter that actively pumps substrates into the intestinal lumen. Inhibition of P-gp allows an increased plasma concentration secondary to increased absorption. For example, the bioavailability of cyclosporine is increased after P-gp inhibition. OATP, however, is an influx pump that transports substrates into intestinal enterocytes. Here, grapefruit juice decreases absorption of fexofenadine by inhibition of intestinal OATP.[1] In addition, drug absorption may be modified through alteration of intestinal cytochrome P450 3A (CYP3A). In this case, grapefruit juice can inhibit CYP3A, allowing increased bioavailability of oral midazolam that otherwise would be metabolized before absorption with this enzyme.[2]

After a single dose of a drug, the plasma concentration begins to increase as the drug is absorbed (Fig. 3.1). The highest plasma concentration achieved is the ***peak concentration***. After reaching this peak, the plasma concentration begins to decrease because of drug distribution, metabolism, and clearance. When a second dose is administered, the plasma concentration again increases and peaks. This second peak may be higher than the first, depending on the time interval between the first and second doses (Fig. 3.2). When drugs are dosed at a given interval, the minimum concentration before the next dose is called the *trough*. Drug trough values are

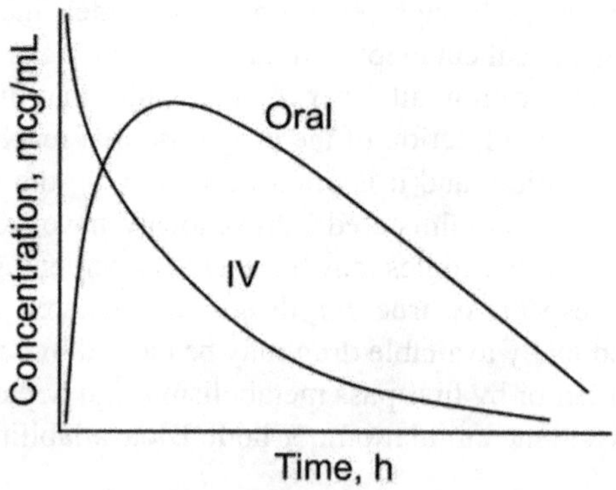

Fig. 3.1 Schematic representation of pharmacokinetic profiles for intravenous (IV) and oral doses [Adapted from Gunaratna C. Drug metabolism and pharmacokinetics in drug discovery: a primer for bioanalytical chemists, part II. Current Separations [Internet]. 2001;19(3):87–92. Available from: http://www.currentseparations.com/issues/19-3/19-3e.pdf. with permission from Bioanalytical Systems, Inc]

Fig. 3.2 Predicted plasma concentrations of a drug given as (A) a continuous infusion of two units of drug daily, (B) an injection of one unit of drug twice daily, or (C) an injection of two units of drug once daily. 1/2 indicates rapid injection of drug [Adapted from Finkel R, Clark MA, Cubeddu LX (Eds.). Pharmacology, 4th ed. Philadelphia, PA: Lippincott Williams & Wilkins, 2009. With permission from Wolter Kluwers Health]

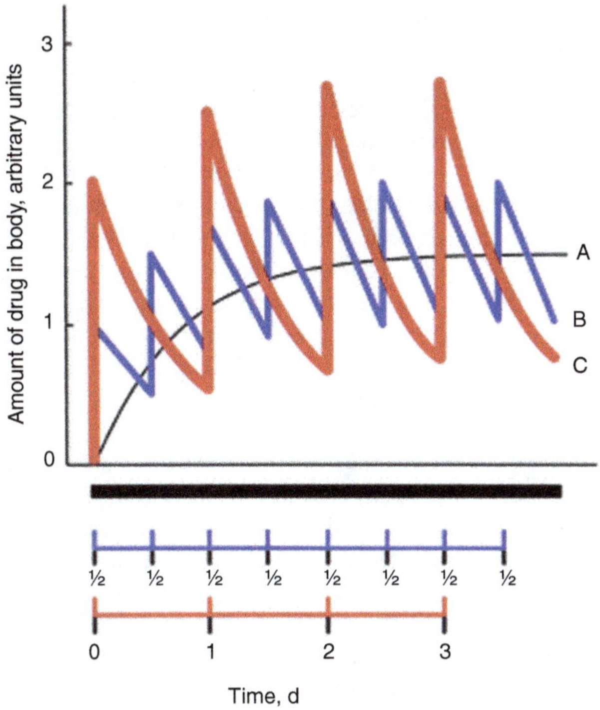

especially important when a certain level of drug must be maintained for therapeutic effect, such as with antibiotics or antiepileptics.

Drug distribution involves the spread of drug throughout the body. Distribution between the intravascular space and the tissues in the body depends on tissue perfusion, as well as the chemical properties of the drug that dictate protein binding, ionization, and lipid solubility. The apparent volume of distribution is the hypothetical volume that a given dose of drug has to be diluted to achieve the resulting plasma concentration:

Volume of distribution=drug dose/plasma concentration

A drug that leaves the intravascular space and enters tissue compartments has a larger volume of distribution more readily than a drug that remains primarily intravascular. Warfarin, for example, is highly protein-bound and thus stays primarily in the intravascular space and has a small volume of distribution (0.14 L/kg).[3] In contrast, digoxin undergoes less protein binding and has a large volume of distribution (4-7 L/kg).[4]

Acidic drugs, such as warfarin, tend to bind more extensively with albumin; basic drugs tend to bind with α_1–acid glycoprotein and lipoproteins. Drug interactions may occur when two drugs that are both protein-bound are administered together, thereby increasing the free (unbound) fraction of one or both of the drugs. An increase in unbound drug may increase both the desired effect and adverse effects and may result in toxicity. A decrease in protein available to bind a drug may also affect the drug pharmacokinetics. It may cause an increase in unbound fraction of drug and increase the volume of distribution while also increasing the free drug available for metabolism and excretion, which may increase drug clearance. Such conditions as chronic disease, liver failure, malnutrition, nephrotic syndrome, and heart failure may lead to decreased protein levels. Although these drug-protein-interactions are frequently considered, they clinically are of reduced importance since a new steady state concentration is often achieved after the interaction.[5] The overall clinical significance of this interaction likely depends on the inherent toxicity and clearance of the drug.

The acid–base properties of a drug also affect the degree of ionization that occurs at a given pH. Only the un-ionized form of a drug can pass through cell membranes. An increase in the un-ionized form will increase drug distribution; an increase in the ionized form will decrease distribution. This relation explains why infiltration of local anesthetics at the site of infection is less efficacious. Local anesthetics are weak bases and infection creates an acidosis, thereby increasing the ionized form of the drug and decreasing the amount of drug available to cross the cell membrane to the site of action. High lipid solubility also increases the volume of distribution because the drug tends to leave the intravascular space. Fentanyl is more lipid soluble than morphine and has a faster onset of action and greater volume of distribution than morphine.

Initially, a drug is distributed to areas with high blood flow, but over time, the drug redistributes to other areas as the concentration gradients change. One area of high blood flow is the brain, the site of action for IV anesthetics. Thus, IV anesthetics initially distribute quickly to their site of action, but the action is terminated by redistribution of drug from the brain, away from the effect site. With repeated drug administration or continuous infusion, the areas into which a drug redistributes may become saturated and the drug effect will continue for an increased length of time. Metabolism, rather than redistribution, becomes the primary mechanism for termination of drug action.

The action of drug metabolism has a large potential for drug–drug interactions. Drugs may compete for the same route of metabolism or a drug may alter the metabolism of another drug. Drug metabolism is divided primarily into two categories: Phase I reactions and Phase II reactions. Phase I reactions involve oxidation, reduction, or hydrolysis of substrates both endogenous (steroid hormones) and exogenous (drugs) through such enzymes as the cytochrome P450 (CYP) enzymes. The CYP family of enzymes is responsible for a large majority of drug metabolism.

Phase II reactions involve drug conjugation through glucuronidation, acetylation, sulfation, methylation, and glutathione conjugation. Drug interactions may occur simply because of interference. When two drugs are metabolized through the same enzyme system coadministered, one or both of the drugs may be metabolized at a slower rate (competitive inhibition). This slower metabolism rate results in increased drug plasma concentrations and, possibly, increased drug effect or toxicity due to the reduced metabolism. Drug interactions may also be more complex. Some enzyme substrates act as enzyme inducers; they cause an increase in enzyme activity resulting in increased metabolism of substrates for that enzyme. Conversely, a drug may act to inhibit an enzyme, decreasing the enzyme activity and resulting in decreased substrate metabolism (noncompetitive inhibition). Enzyme inhibition is a relatively rapid process, beginning with the first dose of the inhibitor, and cessation of inhibition is related to the half-life of the inhibiting drug.[6] The time course of induction is more complex because the primary method of induction is increased enzyme production. Thus, induction requires enzyme synthesis for onset, which may take days to weeks, and enzyme degradation for offset.[7]

The CYP3A subfamily includes the CYP3A4, CYP3A5, and CYP3A7 isoenzymes. Collectively, they are responsible for 50% of the biotransformation of drugs that undergo oxidative metabolism.[8] However, depending on the drug, there can be differential ability for each isoenzyme on metabolism.[9] The frequently discussed 3A4 enzyme is usually considered the major determinant in this metabolism, however, 3A5 may have an equally large contribution in some cases.[8] CYP3A7 has little or no role in adult metabolism because it is present primarily in fetal hepatic tissue. Intestinal and hepatic CYP3A is subject to both inhibition and induction through relatively common medications. Many drugs cause varying degrees of inhibition ranging from a clinically insignificant to a marked reduction of CYP3A activity. Potent inhibitors include clarithromycin, itraconazole, and ketoconazole. CYP3A inducers include rifampin, carbamazepine, and St. John's wort, among others. Coadministration of carbamazepine with valproic acid can reduce the concentration of valproic acid by approximately 50% through induction of CYP2C9 and multiple phase II enzymes.[10] In addition, coadministration of carbamazepine can substantially reduce oral contraceptive levels through induction of CYP3A.[11]

When considering enzyme induction, clinicians need to note whether the drug of interest is inactivated with metabolism, has an active metabolite, or is a prodrug (ie, becomes active with metabolism). A drug that is inactivated with metabolism has a reduced effect when coadministered with an enzyme inducer because the drug is metabolized more extensively. However, if the drug has an active metabolite or is a prodrug, coadministration with an inducer may actually increase drug effect. The opposite is true for coadministration with an enzyme inhibitor. In this clinical situation, a drug inactivated by metabolism may have an increased effect when administered with an inhibitor; a drug with an active metabolite or a prodrug may have a decreased effect.

The CYP2D6 enzyme also undergoes inhibition with such medications as some of the selective serotonin reuptake inhibitors and serotonin-norepinephrine reuptake inhibitors, several antipsychotics, and some cardiac medications. Tamoxifen, a medication used in treatment of breast cancer, is metabolized through CYP2D6 to endoxifen, an active metabolite that is a potent antiestrogen. Inhibition of CYP2D6 can decrease the endoxifen levels and is potentially related to an increased recurrence of breast cancer. One study showed that venlafaxine did not reduce endoxifen concentration, and sertraline and citalopram reduced endoxifen concentrations slightly. The study also showed that fluoxetine and paroxetine are strong inhibitors and reduce endoxifen concentrations significantly.[12]

When considering inhibition and induction of enzymes, since outcomes may be toxicological, clinicians need to realize that much of the data are derived from in vitro studies, retrospective data analysis, or case reports. *In vitro* data do not necessarily correlate with *in vivo* action, and an effect that may be present with *in vitro* studies may not result in a clinically significant effect.

Drug metabolism is affected by differences in enzyme genotype, which may result in different levels of enzyme function. ***Pharmacogenomics*** is the study of genetic differences in drug metabolism and drug response. Persons may be poor, intermediate, extensive, or ultra-rapid metabolizers depending on the respective enzyme. Similar to the dependence of the impact of an inducer or inhibitor on drug effect, the impact of genotype on drug effect is dependent on whether the active form of the drug is the parent drug or the drug metabolite. If the parent drug is active with an inactive metabolite, poor metabolizers will have increased drug effect, extensive metabolizers will have the expected effect, and ultra-rapid metabolizers will have decreased effect. The CYP2D6 enzyme has various genotypes that result in poor, intermediate, extensive, and ultra-rapid metabolism. β-Blockers, including metoprolol and carvedilol, are metabolized through CYP2D6. Because the parent drug is the active compound, poor metabolizers have increased effect and may have excessive blockade and ultra-rapid metabolizers have decreased active agent at the effect site.

With a prodrug, the converse occurs and poor metabolizers have decreased drug effect; extensive metabolizers, normal effect; and ultra-rapid metabolizers, increased effect. Codeine is an example of a prodrug, and it is metabolized through CYP2D6 to the active compound, morphine. Poor metabolizers have less active agent at the effect site and less effective analgesia, whereas ultra-rapid metabolizers have increased active agent at the effect site with a possibility of toxicity.

Total drug clearance is a combination of drug elimination and metabolism. Drugs are eliminated from the body via both renal and nonrenal routes. Nonrenal routes include hepatic (biliary excretion), gastrointestinal (fecal), and skin (secretion). Renal clearance occurs as the kidneys remove drugs from the plasma by filtration or active secretion and is described in units of plasma volume that are cleared of the drug over time (L/h). Changes in renal function can impact the ability of the kidneys to clear drugs. Famotidine, a commonly used histamine$_2$ receptor antagonist, requires dose reduction or increased time between doses when renal function is impaired.

Glomerular filtration rate is a useful measure of kidney function, and creatinine clearance rate is a surrogate measure for the glomerular filtration rate. Exact measurement of creatinine clearance requires 24-hour urine collection and is not often performed. Various methods can be used to estimate creatinine clearance, including the Cockcroft-Gault formula, which uses age, body mass, sex, and serum creatinine concentration, as well as the Modification of Diet in Renal Disease formula, which uses age, sex, race, and serum creatinine concentration. Drug interactions may occur at the level of the kidneys through drug impairment of renal function and alterations in drug secretion. Probenecid, an antigout agent, is an example of a drug that interferes with secretion of another drug. It impairs the tubular secretion of penicillin and is used therapeutically to reduce the required dosing interval of penicillin.

As noted, drug clearance is measured as volume of plasma cleared per unit of time. ***Half-life*** also describes the decrease in drug concentration and is defined as the length of time required to reduce the plasma concentration by 50%. After two half-lives, 25% of the original drug concentration remains; after three half-lives, 12.5% remains. The concept of half-life implies that a drug follows first-order kinetics, where the rate of drug concentration decline is proportional to the concentration of the drug. Most drugs undergo first-order kinetics. Drugs also may follow zero-order kinetics, in which the rate of decline of drug concentration proceeds at a constant rate, independent of drug concentration in plasma. Fortunately, few drugs undergo zero-order kinetics because once the respective enzyme system is saturated, small dosage changes can cause much greater changes in plasma concentrations.

Context-sensitive half-time describes the time for the plasma concentration of a drug to decrease by half after a continuous infusion of the drug is discontinued. The half-time varies on the basis of the infusion duration. In general, the context-sensitive half-time increases as the duration of the infusion increases and is due to a decreasing ability for the agent to undergo redistribution. With some drugs, the increase is clinically significant and with others, it is not. The half-time of fentanyl changes markedly with increased infusion duration; the half-time of remifentanil is unaffected by infusion duration (Fig. 3.3).

Of importance, much of what is known about the pharmacokinetics of a given drug may have been determined in a small, healthy population and may not be generalizable to a specific patient or patient population. Changes in physiology, pathology, and concomitant drug administration often alter the absorption, distribution, metabolism, and excretion of a given drug, causing adverse effects or toxicity. Consideration also should be given to the normal variations seen in different age groups, such as pediatric and geriatric patients, that cause pharmacokinetic changes.

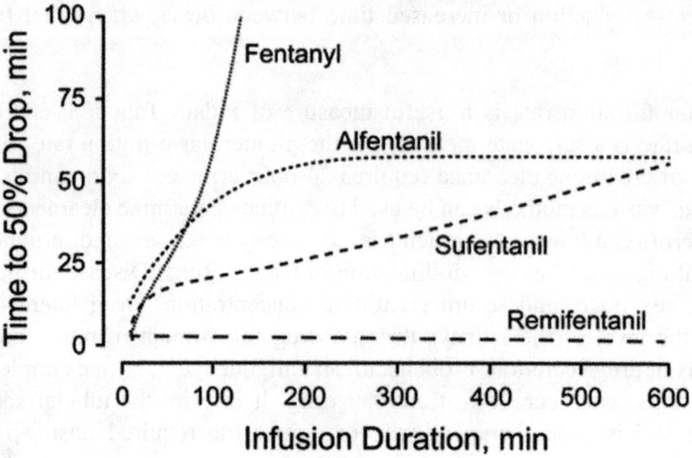

Fig. 3.3 A simulation of the time necessary to achieve a 50% decrease in drug concentration in the blood (or plasma) after variable-length intravenous infusion of fentanyl, alfentanil, sufentanil, and remifentanil [Adapted from Egan TD, Lemmens HJ, Fiset P et al. The pharmacokinetics of the new short-acting opioid remifentanil [GI87084B] in healthy adult male volunteers. Anesthesiology. 1993;79:881–92. With permission from Wolter Kluwers Health]

References

1. Kiani J, Imam SZ. Medicinal importance of grapefruit juice and its interaction with various drugs. Nutr J. 2007;6:33.
2. Kupferschmidt HH, Ha HR, Ziegler WH, et al. Interaction between grapefruit juice and midazolam in humans. Clin Pharmacol Ther. 1995;58:20–8.
3. Product Information: COUMADIN(R) oral tablets, intravenous injection, warfarin sodium oral tablets, intravenous injection. Princeton: Bristol-Myers Squibb Company; 2007.
4. Maron BA, Rocco TP. Pharmacotherapy of congestive heart failure. In: Brunton LL, Chabner BA, Knollmann BC, editors. Goodman & Gilman's The Pharmacological Basis of Therapeutics. 12th ed. New York: McGraw-Hill Medical; 2011.
5. Tatro DS. Drug Interaction Facts: The Authority on Drug Interactions. Wolters Kluwer Health: St. Louis, MO; 2007.
6. Badyal DK, Dadhich AP. Cytochrome P450 and drug interactions. Indian J Pharmacol. 2001;33:248–59.
7. Leucuta SE, Vlase L. Pharmacokinetics and metabolic drug interactions. Curr Clin Pharmacol. 2006;1:5–20.
8. Williams JA, Ring BJ, Cantrell VE, et al. Comparative metabolic capabilities of CYP3A4, CYP3A5, and CYP3A7. Drug Metab Dispos. 2002;30:883–91.
9. Granfors MT, Wang JS, Kajosaari LI, et al. Differential inhibition of cytochrome P450 3A4, 3A5 and 3A7 by five human immunodeficiency virus (HIV) protease inhibitors in vitro. Basic Clin Pharmacol Toxicol. 2006;98:79–85.
10. May T, Rambeck B. Serum concentrations of valproic acid: influence of dose and comedication. Ther Drug Monit. 1985;7:387–90.
11. Perucca E. Clinically relevant drug interactions with antiepileptic drugs. Br J Clin Pharmacol. 2006;61:246–55.
12. Sideras K, Ingle JN, Ames MM, et al. Coprescription of tamoxifen and medications that inhibit CYP2D6. J Clin Oncol. 2010;28:2768–76.

A Brief Treatise on the Area Under the Curve

4

Michael J. Sikora MD and Barbara Jericho MD

Abstract

This chapter briefly discusses the pharmacologic parameter, commonly referred to as the Area Under the Curve, that describes the distribution and elimination of drugs from the body.

The "area under the curve" graph classically describes the plasma concentration of a drug as a function of time after an intravenous (IV) bolus of a medication plotted on x and y coordinates. Although an oversimplification, this visualization assists in estimating plasma medication levels.

In a one-compartment model, one must assume that all medication remains within the plasma compartment and does not redistribute to other body partitions. With an IV injection, the concentration of the drug is very elevated immediately after injection; however, the concentration drops exponentially as a constant fraction undergoes metabolism (Fig. 4.1). After four elimination half-lives, the level of medication approaches zero and changes minimally as time progresses.

In a two-compartment model, there is the presumption that all the drug does not remain within the plasma. It is assumed that medication distributes between the central plasma compartment and a "peripheral" partition. This imagery becomes clinically informative in relation to highly lipophilic drugs such as propofol. After a

M.J. Sikora MD (✉)
Department of Anesthesiology, Cincinnati Children's Hospital Medical Center, Cincinnati, OH, USA
e-mail: Michael.Sikora@cchmc.org

B. Jericho MD
Department of Anesthesiology, University of Illinois Hospital and Health Sciences System, University of Illinois-Chicago, Chicago, IL, USA

C. Marcucci et al. (eds.), *A Case Approach to Perioperative Drug-Drug Interactions*, DOI 10.1007/978-1-4614-7495-1_4

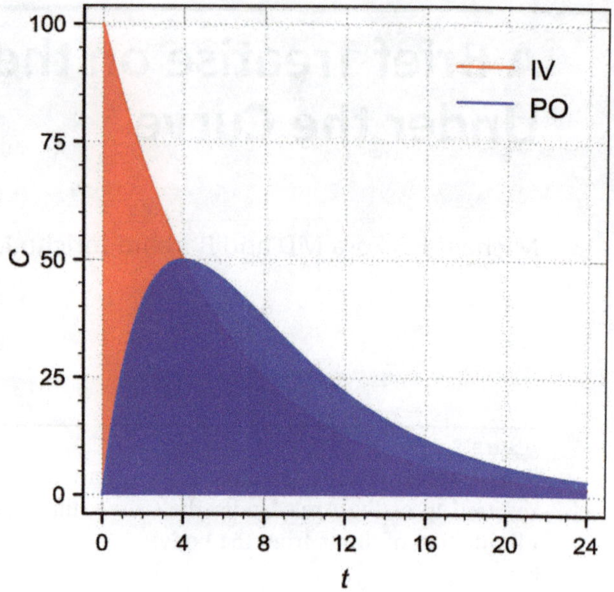

Fig. 4.1 Area Under the Curve, concentration vs. time: One-compartment model for bolus IV and PO administration [Reprinted from http://en.wikipedia.org/wiki/Bioavailability Last accessed on July 20, 2012. With permission from the Creative Commons License]

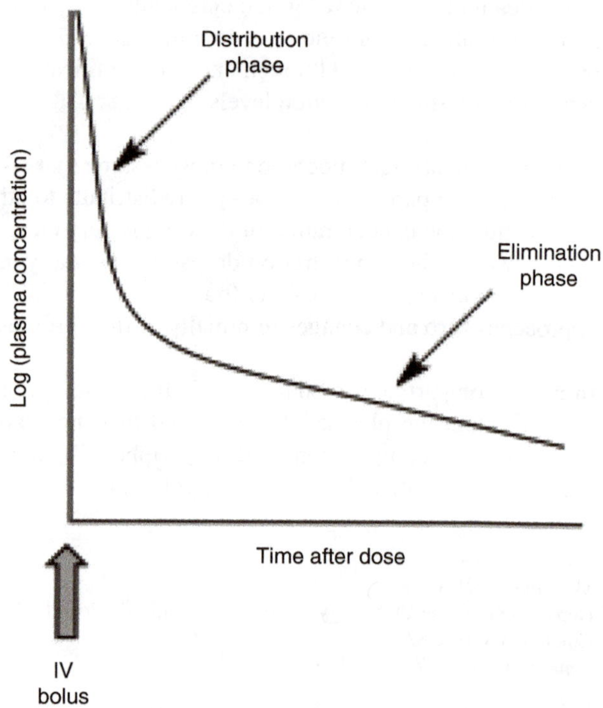

Fig. 4.2 Area Under the Curve, concentration vs. time: Two-compartment model for bolus IV administration [Reprinted from http://en.wikipedia.org/wiki/Pharmacokinetics Last accessed on July 20, 2012. With permission from the Creative Commons License]

single bolus, the concentration exponentially decreases as medication redistributes to the peripheral compartment (Fig. 4.2). With time, the concentration between the two compartments equalizes, and drug diffusion reverses. In other words, medication now moves from the peripheral to the central compartment. The concentration of medication gradually decreases within the central partition secondary to metabolism, highlighting another important assumption of the two-compartment model. Drug can only be metabolized from the central compartment; medication within the periphery is not subject to degradation. Graphically, this pharmacokinetic phenomenon is characterized by two curves. An initial distribution phase reflects diffusion of medication to the periphery. The second curve, or elimination phase, describes gradual metabolism from the central compartment. The slope of the distribution phase is much steeper than the slope of the elimination phase, indicating that drug concentration drops precipitously after injection, then more slowly due to elimination.

II

Introduction to Drug–Drug Interactions: Brief Review of Cytochrome P450 (CYP450) Enzymes, Uridine 5'-diphospho-glucuronoslytransferases (UGTs), and Transporters

CYP2D6: Where It All Began

5

John C. Sanders MBBS, FRCA, Rachel Koll MD, and Randal O. Dull MD, PhD

Abstract
This chapter discusses the genetics, metabolic actions, substrates, and inhibitors of cytochrome P450 2D6.

Cytochrome P450 (CYP) 2D6 is a member of the cytochrome P450 family of hemoproteins, which are responsible for Phase I metabolism of the majority of xenobiotics in the body. CYP2D6 accounts for about 2% to 5% of the body's P450 enzymes, but metabolizes about 25% of current drugs.[1] Most commonly, a monooxygenase reaction is catalyzed; that is the insertion of one atom of oxygen into an organic substrate – $RH + O^2 + 2H^+ + 2e^- \rightarrow ROH + H_2O$. In humans, 2D6 is expressed almost exclusively in the liver, with a small amount of activity in the intestinal wall. It is a membrane bound protein located on the cellular endoplasmic reticulum. The gene coding CYP2D6 is located on chromosome 22. Typically, substrates for the 2D6 isoenzyme are lipophilic bases.

CYP2D6 shows great phenotypic variability due to genetic polymorphism. More than 100 allelic variants with different properties have been discovered but 87% of genotypes are accounted for by five variants.[2,3] The wild-type reference is designated CYP2D6*1. Expression of the allelic variants in heterozygous or homozygous forms results in different enzyme activity levels, which are classified as: 1) poor metabolizer with little or no CYP2D6 function, 2) intermediate metabolizer with reduced function, 3) extensive metabolizer with normal function, or 4) ultrarapid metabolizer with increased CYP2D6 function. A person with two nonfunc-

J.C. Sanders MBBS, FRCA (✉)
Department of Anesthesiology, Shriners Hospitals for Children, Salt Lake City, UT, USA
e-mail: jcsanders@shrinenet.org

R. Koll MD
Department of Anesthesiology, Cincinnati Children's Hospital Medical Center, Cincinnati, OH, USA

R.O. Dull MD, PhD
Department of Anesthesiology, University of Illinois at Chicago, Chicago, IL, USA

C. Marcucci et al. (eds.), *A Case Approach to Perioperative Drug-Drug Interactions*, DOI 10.1007/978-1-4614-7495-1_5

tional alleles is phenotypically a poor metabolizer. More than two functional alleles results in an ultra-rapid metabolizer. Someone with one functional copy is either an intermediate or extensive metabolizer depending on the activity of the allele. Clinical effects of drugs that are metabolized by CYP2D6 in addition to other pathways, such as oxycodone and ß-blockers, may not be impacted by genetic variability or drug interaction involving CYP2D6 unless it is the dominant metabolic path. The biological effect of a specific allele may be substrate-dependent. For example, CYP2D6*17 is usually an allele with reduced function, but it produces variable clinical outcomes when catalyzing the metabolism of substrates such as dextromethorphan, fluoxetine, codeine, and tramadol.[4] Laboratory tests can be used to distinguish genotypes (AmpliChip, Roche Diagnostics, Indianapolis, IN), or clinical activity can be evaluated by measuring the metabolism of debrisoquine, a selective CYP2D6 substrate that may be used to predict drug interactions and patients' metabolism of drugs. An extensive review of the CYP2D6 polymorphisms has been published.[1]

Ethnicity is a factor in CYP2D6 variability. About 5% to 10% of Caucasians and 2% of Chinese are poor metabolizers of 2D6 substrates.[5,6] The incidence of poor metabolizers in African populations is highly variable (0% to 34%).[7] The incidence of persons with genotypes resulting in reduced metabolism reaches 50% in Asians and 47% of children in London.[8,9] Ultra-rapid metabolizers have not been reported in Asians, but reach 9% to 30% in Africans and 1% to 7% in Caucasians.[7]

Clinically important drug–drug interactions involving 2D6 occur because of different allelic expression and/or co-administration of substances which may be inhibitors of the 2D6 enzyme. There are actually no known inducers of 2D6, which is unique among the "common" CYP450 enzymes.[10] Biological effects depend on whether the substrate is an active drug or a prodrug like codeine. The biological effect of an active drug is enhanced in poor metabolizers or by co-administration of inhibitors and reduced in ultra-rapid metabolizers or by co-administration of inducers. The biological effect of codeine, which requires 2D6 conversion to its active form morphine, is enhanced in ultra-rapid metabolizers and reduced in poor metabolizers or by co-administration of inhibitors.

Common drugs that are 2D6 substrates and may be taken by patients presenting for anesthesia are: ß-blockers, several antiarrhythmics, some selective serotonin reuptake inhibitors (SSRIs), tricyclic antidepressants, and several antipsychotics. Some 2D6 inhibitors include: several SSRIs, 3,4-methylenedioxy-N-methylamphetamine (MDMA), ritonavir, bupropion, goldenseal, and quinidine. Medications used in the perioperative period that are 2D6 substrates include: opioids (including codeine, hydrocodone, dihydrocodone and tramadol), ondansetron, ß-blockers, and metoclopramide. Perioperative medications that are 2D6 inhibitors include celecoxib, diphenhydramine, metoclopramide, ropivacaine, cimetidine, methadone, and amiodarone.

Clinical relevance has been demonstrated. Apnea has occurred after administration of codeine to a child whose 2D6 ultra-rapid metabolizer phenotype resulted in a higher than expected conversion of codeine to morphine.[11] Ultra-rapid metabolizers may have a higher incidence of failure of ondansetron prophylaxis of postoperative vomiting.[12] Granisetron is the only 5-HT_3 antagonist that is not metabolized by CYP2D6, and thus would confer effective anti-emetic prophylaxis to an ultra-rapid metabolizer for whom ondansetron had failed.[13] Poor and intermediate metabolizers have well-documented reduced analgesic efficacy of codeine, hydrocodone, and tramadol, each of which relies on metabolism by 2D6 to an active form to have clinical effect.[7] Patients who fail to respond to prodrug opioids metabolized by 2D6 may respond better to oxycodone, which is already an active analgesic in its "parent" form and does not require conversion via CYP2D6 to become an effective analgesic (ie, it is not a prodrug). Ropivacaine infusion has been shown to be a potent inhibitor of 2D6.[14] Patients on common selective serotonin reuptake inhibitor drugs, such as fluoxetine or paroxetine, could be predicted to experience less analgesic efficacy from opioid prodrugs. The combination of paroxetine and tramadol has resulted in development of central serotonin syndrome and seizures due to overaccumulation of tramadol, which lowers seizure threshold.[15]

Dosing and efficacy of medications that are CYP2D6 substrates may be affected by age. Liver enzymes reach maturity between the ages of 2 months and 6 months. Before that age, medications that rely on conversion to active forms, such as tramadol and codeine, may not be effective and active substrates may accumulate. Although with most drugs metabolized by CYP450, pediatric dosing correlates best with body surface area, for those drugs metabolized primarily by CYP2D6, dosing should be based on body weight.[16]

Take-Home Points

- CYP2D6 substrates and inhibitors include a broad array of commonly prescribed drugs. There are no known CYP2D6 inducers, which is unique among the "common" CYP450 enzymes.

- Coadministration of CYP2D6 substrates and inhibitors will usually produce increases in the blood levels of those substrates.

- There is great variability in the genotypic and resulting phenotypic expression of CYP2D6. At standard dosages, 2D6 poor metabolizers will generate much higher-than-expected blood levels of CYP2D6 substrates, whereas ultrarapid metabolizers will generate much lower-than-expected levels.

- Many of the commonly used analgesic agents (codeine, hydrocodone, and tramadol) are prodrugs for CYP2D6, so administering these agents to 2D6 poor metabolizers, or coadministration of potent CYP2D6 inhibitors, will result in poor efficacy. Conversely, administration of these agents to ultrarapid metabolizers can result in toxicity.

References

1. Zhou SF. Polymorphism of human cytochrome P4502D6 and its clinical significance: part 1. Clin Pharmacokinet. 2009;48(11):689–723.
2. Kosarac B, Fox AA, Collard CD. Effect of genetic factors on opioid action. Curr Opin Anaesthesiol. 2009;22(4):476–82.
3. Sachse C, Brockmöller J, Hildebrand M, et al. Correctness of prediction of the CYP2D6 phenotype confirmed by genotyping 47 intermediate and poor metabolizers of debrisoquine. Pharmacogenetics. 1998;8(2):181–5.
4. Shen H, He MM, Liu H, et al. Comparative metabolic capabilities and inhibitory profiles of CYP2D6.1, CYP2D6.10 and CYP2D6.17. Drug Metab Dispos. 2007;35(8):1292–300.
5. Stamer UM, Stüber F. Genetic factors in pain and its treatment. Curr Opin Anaesthesiol. 2007;20(5):478–84.
6. Sohn DR, Shin SG, Park CW, et al. Metoprolol oxidation polymorphism in a Korean population: comparison with native Japanese and Chinese populations. Br J Clin Pharmacol. 1991;32(4):504–7.
7. Smith HS. Opioid metabolism. Mayo Clin Proc. 2009;84(7):613–24.
8. Droll K, Bruce-Mensah K, Otton SV, et al. Comparison of three CYP2D6 probe substrates and genotype in Ghanaians, Chinese and Caucasians. Pharmacogenetics. 1998;8(4):325–33.
9. Williams DG, Patel A, Howard RF. Pharmacogenetics of codeine metabolism in an urban population of children and its implications for analgesic reliability. Br J Anaesth. 2002;89(6): 839–45.
10. Voronov P, Przybylo HJ, Jagannathan N. Apnea in a child after oral codeine: a genetic variant - an ultra-rapid metabolizer. Paediatr Anaesth. 2007;17(7):684–7.
11. Madan A, Graham R, Carroll K, et al. Effects of prototypical microsomal enzyme inducers on cytochrome P450 expression in cultured human hepatocytes. Drug Metab Dispos. 2003;31: 421–31.
12. Candiotti KA, Birnbach DJ, Lubarsky DA, et al. The impact of pharmacogenomics on postoperative nausea and vomiting: do CYP2D6 allele copy number and polymorphisms affect the success or failure of ondansetron prophylaxis? Anesthesiology. 2005;102(3):543–9.
13. Janicki PK. Cytochrome P450 2D6 metabolism and 5-hydroxytryptamine type 3 receptor antagonists for postoperative nausea and vomiting. Med Sci Monit. 2005;11(10):RA322–8.
14. Wink J, Veering BT, Kruit M, et al. The effect of a long term epidural infusion of ropivacaine on CYP2D6 activity. Anesth Analg. 2008;106(1):143–6.
15. Lantz MS, Buchalter EN, Giambanco V. Serotonin syndrome following the administration of tramadol with paroxetine. Int J Geriatr Psychiatry. 1998;13(5):343–5.
16. Bartelink IH, Rademaker CM, Schobben AF, et al. Guidelines on paediatric dosing on the basis of developmental physiology and pharmacokinetic considerations. Clin Pharmacokinet. 2006;45(11):1077–97.

CYP2E1: The Anesthesia Enzyme

6

Benjamin S. Gmelch MD and Randal O. Dull MD, PhD

Abstract
This chapter discusses the genetics, metabolic actions, substrates, inducers, and inhibitors of cytochrome P450 2E1.

The metabolic function of the cytochrome P450 (CYP) 2E1 isoenzyme in oxidative and reductive reactions was first elucidated in the early1980s. It was first discovered in rabbits exposed to ethanol.[1,2] This early work in animals foreshadowed the most well-known effects of CYP2E1 in humans: principally, its function in creating toxic metabolites leading to liver injury. The most notable examples of alcohol-induced liver injury in humans are the CYP2E1 metabolism of acetaminophen to NAPQI, a reactive hepatotoxic metabolite, and lipid peroxidation by 2E1 producing hepatotoxic reactive oxygen species. CYP2E1 is found primarily within liver microsomes in cell layers near the terminal hepatic vein, and it metabolizes small hydrophobic compounds. CYP2E1 functions primarily as an oxidative enzyme, with more than 50 known environmental and pharmacologic substrates.[2] CYP2E1 activity has been the focus of many toxicology investigations, implicating the induction of this enzyme in the toxicity and carcinogenicity of many workplace-related substances, including aniline, ethylene glycol, nitrosamines, carbon tetrachloride, and benzene.[2]

The most important pharmacologic 2E1 substrates are ethanol, isoniazid, and the halogenated anesthetics enflurane, halothane, methoxyflurane, isoflurane, sevoflurane and desflurane. CYP2E1 oxidation represents an alternate pathway to alcohol dehydrogenase for the metabolism of ethanol, while it is the principal enzyme

B.S. Gmelch MD (✉)
Department of Anesthesiology, University of Utah School of Medicine, Salt Lake City, UT, USA
e-mail: Ben.gmelch@hsc.utah.edu

R.O. Dull MD, PhD
Department of Anesthesiology, University of Illinois at Chicago, Chicago, IL, USA

C. Marcucci et al. (eds.), *A Case Approach to Perioperative Drug-Drug Interactions*, DOI 10.1007/978-1-4614-7495-1_6

responsible for biotransformation of all halogenated anesthetics.[3] Isoniazid is also metabolized by glutathione transferase and *N*-acetyl transferase, with CYP2E1 metabolism as an alternative pathway.[4] Acetaminophen is a minor substrate under normal circumstances; it is primarily metabolized by glutathione reductase. However, in cases of acetaminophen overdose or induction of CYP2E1 by ethanol, the hepatotoxic metabolite NAPQI is created.[5] The calcium channel blocker verapamil is another minor substrate of 2E1, although CYP3A4 and CYP2C8 are more clinically important metabolic pathways for this drug.[5]

Chlorzoxazone, a medication used clinically to treat muscle spasms, is a CYP2E1 substrate of special importance. It is used primarily as a probe, or assay, for 2E1 activity. Its metabolite, 6-hydroxy chlorzoxazone, is easily measured in serum and used as a marker for induction or inhibition of 2E1 activity, or to assess interindividual variability of 2E1 activity.[6]

Isoniazid, tobacco smoke, and ethanol are well-described inducers of CYP2E1 activity, of particular concern in patients treated for tuberculosis, smokers, and chronic alcoholics.[5] Of recent interest is the induction of 2E1 in commonly encountered medical conditions, such as obesity and uncontrolled diabetes. Obesity increases two- to threefold the hepatic content and catalytic activity of CYP2E1, as evidenced by the increased fluoride concentrations in obese patients after exposure to halogenated anesthetics.[7] In fact, some recent investigations have shown a link between CYP2E1 activity and oxidative liver injury in nonalcoholic steatohepatitis.[8]

The only clinically potent inhibitor of CYP2E1 is disulfiram. *In vivo*, disulfiram is reduced to diethyldithiocarbamate, a specific NADPH-specific inhibitor of 2E1. Propofol has been shown to be a CYP2E1 inhibitor *in vitro*, which suggests the potential for this anesthetic drug to protect the liver from toxic CYP2E1 metabolites.[9,10] However, propofol's significance as an *in vivo* inhibitor has yet to be clearly demonstrated. Another less active inhibitor is phenethyl isocyanate, which is found in such vegetables as cabbage, brussels sprouts, and watercress.[2,5]

Of historical importance in anesthesia, enflurane, methoxyflurane, and halothane all undergo significant P450 metabolism (8%, 46%, and 75% biotransformation, respectively). Halothane in particular is oxidatively defluorinated by 2E1, producing trifluoroacetate, bromide, and a reactive intermediate. The intermediate byproduct binds to liver proteins to create a trifluoroacetylated "neoantigen," which can trigger an autoimmune response in susceptible patients, causing acute hepatic necrosis, or "halothane hepatitis." Although isoflurane is also oxidized to a reactive acyl halide metabolite capable of creating this neoantigen, the incidence of hepatitis related to isoflurane is relatively insignificant owing to its minimal CYP2E1 metabolism in humans. Although halothane is no longer used clinically in the United States, it is still commonly used in some developing countries, underscoring the importance of recognizing this potential toxicity for anesthesia providers working abroad.

The currently used halogenated anesthetics desflurane, sevoflurane, and isoflurane undergo significantly less hepatic metabolism. Of the three, sevoflurane undergoes the most 2E1 oxidation (5%), followed by isoflurane (1%) and desflurane (<0.1%).[3] The duration of anesthetic exposure does not appear to affect the degree of anesthetic metabolism, nor is the duration or potency of these halogenated anesthetics significantly influenced by CYP2E1 induction or inhibition. CYP2E1 oxidation of sevoflurane to fluoride and hexafluoroisopropanol has been linked to a fluoride-induced decrease in renal concentrating ability (not to be confused with compound A-induced nephrotoxicity), although its clinical significance has not been firmly established.

Recent investigations have focused on the genetic polymorphisms of CYP2E1, particularly with respect to preventing 2E1-mediated oxidative liver injury. For example, patients with expression of homozygous wild-type 2E1 treated with isoniazid (INH) have been shown to have an increased risk for antituberculosis drug-induced liver injury.[4] The risk for hepatotoxicity is even more pronounced in patients who are also slow acetylators (low N-acetyl transferase activity), illustrating the interplay between these metabolic pathways. This finding has important implications in isoniazid drug dosing adjustment, drug–drug interactions, and the influence of alcohol intake on drug metabolism. Other studies have investigated the impact of CYP2E1 polymorphisms on ethanol-induced liver injury.[8] This exciting new avenue of pharmacogenetics may shed more light on the role of 2E1 inducers and inhibitors in certain patient populations.

Take-Home Points

- Halogenated anesthetics are the most significant pharmacologic substrates of CYP2E1. CYP2E1 metabolism of halothane is implicated in halothane hepatitis.
- CYP2E1 is induced by common medical conditions such as obesity, diabetes, smoking, and chronic alcohol use.
- Hepatotoxicity of acetaminophen, isoniazid, and many organic industrial solvents is linked to increased activity of CYP2E1.
- Genetic polymorphisms of CYP2E1 may explain predisposition to ethanol- and drug-induced hepatotoxicity in certain populations.

References

1. Koop DR, Morgan ET, et al. Purification and characterization of a unique isozyme of cytochrome P-450 from liver microsomes of ethanol-treated rabbits. Chemistry. 1982;257:8472–80.
2. Koop DR. Oxidative and reductive metabolism by cytochrome P450 2E1. FASEB J. 1992;6:724–30.
3. Kharasch ED, Thummel KE. Identification of cytochrome P450 2E1 as the predominant enzyme catalyzing human liver microsomal defluorination of sevoflurane, isoflurane, and methoxyflurane. Anesthesiology. 1993;79:795–807.
4. Sun F, Chen Y. Drug-metabolising enzyme polymorphisms and predisposition to anti-tuberculosis drug-induced liver injury: a meta-analysis. Int J Tuberc Lung Dis. 2008;12(9): 994–1002.
5. Sandson NB. Drug-Drug Interaction Primer: A Compendium of Case Vignettes for the Practicing Clinician. Arlington: American Psychiatric Publishing, Inc; 2007. p. 359–60.
6. Peter R, Baker R. Hydroxylation of chlorzoxazone as a specific probe for human liver CYP2E1. Chem Res Toxicol. 1990;3:566–73.
7. Raucy JL, Lasker JM, et al. Induction of cytochrome P450IIE1 in the obese overfed rat. Molecul Pharmacol. 1991;39:275–80.
8. Lu Y, Cederbaum AI. CYP 2E1 and oxidative liver injury by alcohol. Free Radic Biol Med. 2008;44(5):723–38.
9. Chen TL, Uen TH, et al. Human cytochrome P450 mono-oxygenase system is suppressed by propofol. Br J Anaesth. 1995;74:558–62.
10. Lejus C, Fautrel A, et al. Inhibition of cytochrome P450 2E1 by propofol in human and porcine liver microsomes. Biochem Pharmacol. 2002;64:1151–6.

CYP3A4: The Workhorse

7

Jennifer DeCou MD, Nathaniel Birgenheier MD,
and Randal O. Dull MD, PhD

Abstract
This chapter discusses the genetics, metabolic actions, substrates, inducers, and inhibitors of cytochrome P450 3A4.

Cytochrome P450 (CYP) 3A4 is the predominant member of the P450 family, a group of mixed-function oxidases that account for the majority of Phase I biotransformation of endogenous biochemicals and xenobiotics.[1] The functional workhorse and most versatile of the P450 family, 3A4 comprises 30% of the hepatic P450 complement and accounts for 70% of the intestinal CYP activity.[2] CYP3A4 is located primarily in hepatocytes and apical enterocytes in the intestines[1]; the jejunum has the highest concentration of 3A4-expressing enterocytes.[3,4] More importantly, the 3A4 isoenzyme is estimated to take part in the metabolism of 50% to 70% of currently administered medications and supplements.[1,2] CYP3A4 also functions as a sort of "backup" enzyme; when other P450 family members that would normally biotransform a substance are unavailable due to potent exogenous inhibition or genetic polymorphism, 3A4 carries out the necessary oxidation/reduction reactions.[5]

The CYP3A4 gene locus is *7q21.3-7q22.1*. Of important note, the MDR (multi-drug resistance) gene, which codes for a P-glycoprotein that extrudes drug into the intestinal lumen, is located nearby at *7q21.1*. Their chromosomal proximity, expression in mature enterocytes, and similar substrates seem to indicate that these two proteins may work in unison to form an intestinal barrier to ingested substances.[2] Control of 3A4 gene transcription is quite complex, but recent investigations have shed some light on the molecular mechanism.[2] The pregname X receptor (PXR) and the

J. DeCou MD (✉) • N. Birgenheier MD
Department of Anesthesiology, University of Utah School of Medicine,
Salt Lake City, UT, USA
e-mail: Danielle.roussel@hsc.utah.edu

R.O. Dull MD, PhD
Department of Anesthesiology, University of Illinois at Chicago, Chicago, IL, USA

C. Marcucci et al. (eds.), *A Case Approach to Perioperative Drug-Drug Interactions*, DOI 10.1007/978-1-4614-7495-1_7

constitutive androstane receptor (CAR) have recently been discovered.[2] Members of the nuclear receptor superfamily of transcription factors, these proteins act as sensors for drugs and xenobiotics. That is, these proteins detect the presence of ingested or injected drugs and xenobiotics and increase the production of CYP3A4 in both the liver and intestine. In addition, transcription of the 3A4 gene can be induced by vitamin D via the vitamin D response (VDR) element primarily in the intestine.[2] PXR plays the primary role in determining hepatic 3A4 levels.[2]

CYP3A4 metabolizing activity varies widely amongst individuals.[1,5] Although there are no known poor metabolizers for this family, a 10-fold to 30-fold variability in enzymatic efficiency has been reported.[6] Interestingly, unlike other CYP450 family members (2D6, 2C9, 2C19) no polymorphism in the 3A4 gene has been identified.[1,3] The marked inter-individual variability is therefore thought to be related to ethnic, cultural, and dietary differences.[1,3] Additionally, age, gender, presence of liver or intestinal disease, and complex molecular mechanisms account for the wide variability in enzyme function.[1–3] Lastly, hepatic 3A4 content has been shown to vary 20-fold among individuals whereas enteric content varies 11-fold. Hepatic and enteric enzyme levels are independently regulated; nevertheless, the complex interaction between hepatic and intestinal enzyme levels and activity helps to account for such wide individual variability.[1]

CYP3A4 can catalyze many metabolic reactions. Most substrates are large, lipophilic, neutral to basic molecules.[3] Reactions carried out by 3A4 include aliphatic oxidation, aromatic hydroxylation, *N*-dealkylation, *O*-demethylation, oxidative deamination, sulfoxide formation, and *N*-hydroxylation in addition to many others.[3] Because of the significant amount of CYP3A4 located in the intestine, it plays a very important role in first-pass (also known as presystemic) drug metabolism.[3] This is best illustrated by specific dihydropyridine calcium channel blockers such as felodipine. When administered orally, felodipine undergoes 3A4 metabolism in apical enterocytes after which only 30% of it remains unchanged. Further 3A4 metabolism in hepatocytes results in only 15% bioavailability for oral felodipine.[3]

The list of substrates, inducers, and inhibitors for CYP3A4 is extensive. Substrates most commonly encountered include tertiary amine tricyclic antidepressants, antipsychotics, macrolide antibiotics, dihydropyridine calcium channel blockers, HMG-CoA reductase inhibitors (statins), carbamazepine, and steroid compounds. Clinically relevant inducers include protease inhibitors such as ritonavir, anticonvulsants, rifampin, and St. John's wort. Inhibitors of CYP3A4 include some selective serotonin reuptake inhibitors (SSRIs), several quinolone antibiotics, "azole" antifungals, and grapefruit juice. Notably, grapefruit juice (specifically bergamottin and dihydroxybergamottin) is a potent inhibitor of intestinal CYP3A4.[1,5]

With specific regard to the practice of anesthesiology, many commonly used analgesics and sedatives are CYP3A4 substrates. Specifically, midazolam, ketamine, fentanyl, alfentanil, sufentanil, methadone, and most local anesthetics are extensively metabolized by 3A4.

Because 3A4 is so heavily involved in drug metabolism, a fundamental awareness of the potential for drug–drug interactions is critical. And because CYP3A4 is so ubiquitous, its clinical relevance can be easily demonstrated in patients taking common medications. For instance, coadministration of the CYP3A4 inhibitor grapefruit juice in a patient on a calcium channel blocker (felodipine) allowed supratherapeutic levels of felodipine to result in profound refractory hypotension.[1] Case reports of torsades de pointes in patients on antihistamines or antifungals, or rhabdomyolysis in patients on statins and a quinolone antibiotic, are all too easy to find.[7–12] Midazolam levels measured by area under the curve varied by 800% depending on co-administered drugs—rifampin (an inducer) vs itraconazole (an inhibitor)![1] To be certain, as the predominant member of the CYP450 family, 3A4 is implicated in countless drug–drug interactions.

Take-Home Points

- CYP3A4 makes up the largest complement of the cytochrome P450 system, accounting for 30% of hepatic cytochrome activity and 70% of intestinal activity.
- CYP3A4 plays a role in the metabolism of 50% to 70% of currently administered medications or supplements.
- Although no known poor metabolizers exist, 3A4 activity varies 10-fold to 30-fold between individuals and is affected by age, culture, ethnicity, and diet.
- The genetics of 3A4 are complex: Recent discoveries in gene location and proximity have yielded information that suggests CYP3A4 and MDR genes play an important role in forming an intestinal barrier to ingested substances.
- The list of substrates, inducers, and inhibitors for 3A4 is extensive! Clinicians need to be aware of the many potential drug–drug interactions that may arise due to the wide ranging role of 3A4 in drug metabolism.

References

1. Dresser GK, Spence JD, et al. Pharmacokinetic-pharmacodynamic consequences and clinical relevance of cytochrome P450 3A4 inhibition. Clin Pharmacokinet. 2000;38(1):41–57.
2. Pal D, Mitra AK. MDR- and CYP3A4-mediated drug-herbal interactions. Life Sci. 2006; 78(18):2131–45.
3. Ohno Y, Hisaka A, et al. General framework for the quantitative prediction of CYP3A4-mediated oral drug interactions based on the AUC increase by coadministration of standard drugs. Clin Pharmacokinet. 2007;46(8):681–96.

4. Paine MF, Khalighi M, Fisher JM, et al. Characterization of interintestinal and intraintestinal variations in human CYP3A-dependent metabolism. J Phamacol Exp Ther. 1997;283:1552–62.
5. Sandson NB. Drug-Drug Interaction Primer: A Compendium of Case Vignettes for the Practicing Clinician. Washington DC: American Psychiatric Publishing, Inc; 2007.
6. Ketter TA, Flockhart DA, Post RM, et al. The emerging role of cytochrome P4503A in psychopharmacology. J Clin Psychopharmacol. 1995;15:387–8.
7. Monahan BP, Ferguson CL, Killeavy ES, et al. Torsades de pointes occurring in association with terfenadine use. JAMA. 1990;264:2788–90.
8. Tsai WC, Tsai LM, Chen JH. Combined use of astemizole and ketoconazole resulting in Torsades de pointes. J Formos Med Assoc. 1997;96:144–6.
9. Ayanian JZ, Fuchs CS, Stone RM. Lovastatin and rhabdomyolysis (letter). Ann Intern Med. 1988;109:682–3.
10. Corpier CL, Jones PH, Suki WN, et al. Rhabdomyolysis and renal injury with lovastatin use: report of two cases in cardiac transplant recipients. JAMA. 1988;260:239–41.
11. Biesenbach G, Janko O, Stuby U, et al. Myoglobinuric renal failure due to long-standing lovastatin therapy in a patient with pre-existing chronic renal insufficiency. Nephrol Dial Transplant. 1996;11:2059–60.
12. Hino I, Akama H, Furuya T, et al. Pravastatin-induced rhabdomyolysis in a patient with mixed connective tissue disease. Arthritis Rheum. 1996;39:1259–60.

CYP1A2: The Switch-hitter

8

Danielle Roussel MD, Emily Hagn MD,
and Randal O. Dull MD, PhD

Abstract
This chapter discusses the genetics, metabolic actions, substrates, inducers, and inhibitors of cytochrome P450 1A2

Cytochrome P450 (CYP) 1A2 is a monooxygenase that is found almost exclusively in the liver.[1] It accounts for 10% to 15% of major cytochrome p450 enzymes.[1,2] By means of hydroxylation or de-alkylation reactions, CYP1A2 metabolizes endogenous compounds such as steroids, retinols, melatonin, and arachidonic acids; it also metabolizes approximately 4% to 20% of commonly prescribed medications, and contributes to bioactivation of many procarcinogens.[1,2]

The genetic sequencing for CYP1A2 is located on chromosome 15. 1A2 is a highly polymorphic enzyme with greater than fifteen 1A2 alleles identified to date.[3] Single-point mutations in the 1A2 allele can cause changes in enzyme expression. For example, the wild-type allele *CYP1A2 *1A* exhibits normal enzyme inducibility, the *CYP1A2*1C* allele exhibits decreased enzyme inducibility, and the *CYP1A2*1 F* allele exhibits increased enzyme inducibility.[3] Allelic frequencies may vary with ethnicity. For example, four distinct single-nucleotide mutations of 1A2 were screened in 459 Caucasians and found to be significantly different from distributions seen in other ethnicities.[4] Predicting clinically significant drug–drug interactions (DDIs) or adverse drug events related to 1A2 may be complicated by the fact that 1A2 enzyme expression may vary up to 40-fold from individual to individual.[5]

D. Roussel MD (✉)
Department of Anesthesiology, University of Utah, Salt Lake City, UT, USA
e-mail: Danielle.roussel@hsc.utah.edu

E. Hagn MD
Department of Pain Management, University of Utah School of Medicine,
Salt Lake City, UT, USA

R.O. Dull MD, PhD
Department of Anesthesiology, University of Illinois at Chicago, Chicago, IL, USA

C. Marcucci et al. (eds.), *A Case Approach to Perioperative Drug-Drug Interactions*, DOI 10.1007/978-1-4614-7495-1_8

This interindividual variability is attributable to genetic and ethnic factors, as well as enzyme induction or inhibition by foods, environmental toxins like tobacco smoke, and medications.

Dietary effects on 1A2 include enzyme induction by brassica vegetables, char-grilled meats, and grape juice. Apiaceous vegetables, caffeine, and grapefruit juice inhibit 1A2 enzyme activity.[6] The degree of dietary 1A2 induction or inhibition may vary considerably from individual to individual; clinically relevant drug interactions may only occur with drugs having narrow therapeutic windows.[6] Cigarette smoking is a potent inducer of 1A2.[7] Human CYP1A2 has the ability to activate heterocyclic amines to carcinogenic and mutagenic products.[8] In multiple studies, 1A2 function was shown to be strongly induced by polycyclic aromatic hydrocarbons, some of which are found in tobacco smoke.[7,9,10] Plasma levels of the 1A2 substrates olanzapine, and clozapine have been shown to decrease in the presence of cigarette smoking.[9,11] Some investigators suggest that practitioners consider 1A2 substrate dosage reduction for persons who quit smoking and dosage increases for persons who commence smoking.[12]

Commonly prescribed medications that induce 1A2 include carbamazepine and (in persons with the *CYP1A2*1 F* allele variant) omeprazole.[13] Fluvoxamine, quinolone antibiotics (eg, norfloxacin, enoxacin, and ciprofloxacin), and oral contraceptives inhibit 1A2 enzyme activity.[13] Drugs that are preferentially metabolized by 1A2 include caffeine, clozapine, olanzapine, tacrine, and theophylline.[13] Drugs that are to a lesser degree metabolized by 1A2 include clomipramine, duloxetine, imipramine, naproxen, ondansetron, propafenone, R-warfarin, and verapamil.[13]

Concomitant use of CYP1A2 substrates, inhibitors and/or inducers has been shown to produce significant pharmacokinetic interactions.[7,11,12,14] However, medication dose adjustments may not be uniformly necessary, particularly if the drugs in question have high therapeutic indices. For example, one study showed that although plasma concentration of duloxetine significantly increased with concurrent administration of fluvoxamine, these combinations were generally well tolerated by the human research subjects.[14]

Take-Home Points

- CYP1A2 accounts for approximately 10% to 15% of major cytochrome P450 enzymes and metabolizes 4% to 20% of commonly prescribed medications.
- Interindividual variability in enzyme expression of CYP1A2 can be related to genetic, dietary, environmental, and medication effects and this variability in enzyme expression may affect drug metabolism and clinical effects.

- Concomitant use of CYP1A2 substrates, inhibitors, and inducers may necessitate medication dosage adjustments for drugs with narrow therapeutic windows or low therapeutic indices.

References

1. Wang B, Zhou SF. Synthetic and natural compounds that interact with human cytochrome P450 1A2 and implications in drug development. Curr Med Chem. 2009;16(31):4066–218.
2. Zhou SF, et al. Insights into the structure, function, and regulation of human cytochrome P450 1A2. Curr Drug Metab. 2009;10(7):713–29.
3. Zhou SF, et al. Insights into the substrate specificity, inhibitors, regulation, and polymorphisms and the clinical impact of human cytochrome P450 1A2. AAPS J. 2009;11(3):481–94.
4. Skarke C, et al. Rapid genotyping for relevant CYP1A2 alleles by pyrosequencing. Eur J Clin Pharmacol. 2005;61(12):887–92.
5. Schweikl H, et al. Expression of CYP1A1 and CYP1A2 genes in human liver. Pharmacogenetics. 1993;3(5):239–49.
6. Harris R, Jang G, Tsunoda S. Dietary effects on drug metabolism and tranport. Clin Pharmacokinet. 2003;42(13):1071–88.
7. Zevin S, Benowitz NL. Drug interactions with tobacco smoking. An update. Clin Pharmacokinet. 1999;36(6):425–38.
8. Parikh A, Josephy PD, Guengerich FP. Selection and characterization of human cytochrome P450 1A2 mutants with altered catalytic properties. Biochemistry. 1999;38(17):5283–9.
9. Desai HD, Seabolt J, Jann MW. Smoking in patients receiving psychotropic medications: a pharmacokinetic perspective. CNS Drugs. 2001;15(6):469–94.
10. Hoffmann D, Djordjevic M, Hoffmann I. The changing cigarette. Prev Med. 1997;26(4):427–34.
11. Callaghan JT, et al. Olanzapine. Pharmacokinetic and pharmacodynamic profile. Clin Pharmacokinet. 1999;37(3):177–93.
12. Kroon LA. Drug interactions with smoking. Am J Health Syst Pharm. 2007;64(18):1917–21.
13. Faber M, Jetter A, Fuhr U. Assessment of CYP1A2 activity in clinical practice: why, how, and when? Basic Clin Pharmacol Toxicol. 2005;97:125–34.
14. Lobo ED, et al. In vitro and in vivo evaluations of cytochrome P450 1A2 interactions with duloxetine. Clin Pharmacokinet. 2008;47(3):191–202.

CYP2B: 2B or Not 2B?

9

Dustin Coyle MD and Randal O. Dull MD, PhD

Abstract
This chapter discusses the genetics, metabolic actions, substrates, inducers, and inhibitors of cytochrome P450 2B6.

The functions of the cytochrome P450 (CYP) 2B family of enzymes have not been, until relatively recently, well characterized in humans. Located on chromosome 19, CYP2B6 is the only known isoform present in humans, and comprises between 1% and 10% of the P450 enzyme system.[1,2] Although CYP2B6 was originally thought to be negligible in importance in humans, it is becoming more evident that the presence of CYP2B6 is ubiquitous, but expression and inducibility are highly variable among individuals, depending on age and ethnicity.[3]

Expression of CYP2B6 is closely regulated by the constitutive androstane receptor (CAR), the pregnane X receptor, and glucocorticoid receptor.[4] CYP2B6 has been detected not only in liver, but also lung, kidney, and intestine, where it participates mostly in *N*-demethylation and hydroxylation of its substrates.[5] This has important implications for many anesthetic drugs that are metabolized by CYP2B6.

There are more than 40 substrates for CYP2B6, and the list is growing.[3] Some well-known substrates are the antidepressant bupropion, the antineoplastic agents cyclophosphamide and ifosfamide, and the antiretroviral efavirenz.[2] Clinically important inhibitors include the selective serotonin reuptake inhibitors (SSRIs) paroxetine and sertraline, estradiol, thiotepa, ticlopidine, and clopidogrel.[2,6,7]

D. Coyle MD (✉)
Department of Anesthesiology, University of Utah, Salt Lake City, UT, USA
e-mail: dustin.coyle@hsc.utah.edu

R.O. Dull MD, PhD
Department of Anesthesiology, University of Illinois at Chicago, Chicago, IL, USA

C. Marcucci et al. (eds.), *A Case Approach to Perioperative Drug-Drug Interactions*, DOI 10.1007/978-1-4614-7495-1_9

Inducers of CYP2B6 include the anticonvulsants phenobarbital, phenytoin, and carbamazepine, as well as rifampin, ritonavir, and some glucocorticoids such as dexamethasone.[8]

A profoundly important role for CYP2B6 is evolving in anesthesia. For instance, CYP2B6 is a high-affinity, high-capacity enzyme for propofol, and appears to be the major cytochrome P450 enzyme for propofol metabolism.[9] Presence of CYP2B6 in other major organs appears to be a significant factor in the extrahepatic metabolism that occurs with propofol.

Ketamine metabolism to its analgesic metabolite, norketamine, is mostly mediated via CYP3A4 at higher concentrations. However, at lower, subanesthetic doses, CYP2B6 plays a relatively larger role, since it appears to have a higher affinity for ketamine than 3A4.[10]

CYP2B6 is responsible for about 57% of the conversion of meperidine to its neurotoxic metabolite, normeperidine.[11] Thus, great caution is warranted when giving meperidine to individuals also taking CYP2B6 inducers.

CYP2B6 has recently been shown to be the main mediator in P450 metabolism of methadone.[12] It preferentially dealkylates the S enantiomer of methadone, increasing the R/S ratio. Since the R enantiomer is responsible for the analgesic effects of methadone, interindividual variation of the drug's effects can be remarkable based on the relative activity of CYP2B6.

It is clear that the importance of CYP2B6 within the cytochrome P450 system has been relatively underestimated in the past. We are now beginning to learn how much of a major player it is, especially in the realm of anesthesiology.

Take-Home Points

- The importance of the CYP2B6 enzyme is only starting to be fully elucidated.
- Important substrates of CYP2B6 include propofol, ketamine, meperidine, and methadone.
- Important inducers of CYP2B6 are phenobarbital, phenytoin, carbamazepine and dexamethasone.
- Interindividual variations in CYP2B6 expression and inducibility can produce variable effects.

References

1. Yamano S, Nhamburo PT, Aoyama T, et al. cDNA cloning and sequence and cDNA-directed expression of human P-450 IIB1: identification on chromosome 19 and differential expression of the IIB mRNAs in human liver. Biochemistry. 1989;28:7340–8.
2. Turpeinen M, Raunio H, Pelkonen O, et al. The functional role of CYP2B6 in human drug metabolism: substrates and inhibitors in vitro, in vivo, and in silico. Curr Drug Metab. 2006;7(7):705–14.
3. Stresser D, Kupfer D. Monospecific antipeptide antibody to cytochrome P-450 2B6. Drug Met Disp. 1999;27(4):517–25.
4. Mo SL, Liu YH, Duan W, et al. Substrate specificity, regulation, and polymorphism of human cytochrome P450 2B6. Curr Drug Metab. 2009;10(7):730–53.
5. Geryot L, Rochat B, Gautier JC, et al. Human CYP2B6: expression, inducibility, and catalytic activities. Pharmacogenetics. 2001;9(3):295–306.
6. Palovaara S, Pelkonen O, Uusitalo J, et al. Inhibition of cytochrome P450 2B6 activity by hormone replacement therapy and oral contraceptive as measured by bupropion hydroxylation. Clin Pharmacol Ther. 2003;74(4):326–33.
7. Turpeinen M, Tolonen A, Uusitalo J, et al. Effect of clopidogrel and ticlopidine on cytochrome P450 2B6 activity as measured by bupropion hydroxylation. Clin Pharmacol Ther. 2005;77(6):553–9.
8. Faucette SR, Wang H, Hamilton GA, et al. Regulation of CYP2B6 in primary human hepatocytes by prototypical inducers. Drug Metab Dispos. 2004;32(3):348–58.
9. Court MH, Duan SX, Hesse LM, et al. Cytochrome P-450 2B6 is responsible for interindividual variability of propofol hydroxylation by human liver microsomes. Anesthesiology. 2001;94(1):110–9.
10. Youssef H, Boulieu R. Contribution of CYP3A4, CYP2B6, and CYP2C9 isoforms to N-demethylation of ketamine in human liver microsomes. Drug Metab Dispos. 2002;30(7): 853–8.
11. Ramirez J, Innocenti F, Schuetz EG, et al. CYP2B6, CYP3A4, and CYP2C19 are responsible for the in vitro N-demethylation of meperidine in human liver microsomes. Drug Metab Dispos. 2004;32(9):930–6.
12. Totah RA, Sheffels P, Roberts T, et al. Role of CYP2B6 in stereoselective human methadone metabolism. Anesthesiology. 2008;108(3):363–74.

CYP2C9: The Support Crew I 10

Byron Douglas Fergerson MD, Crystal B. Wallentine MD, and Randal O. Dull MD, PhD

Abstract
This chapter discusses the genetics, metabolic actions, substrates, inducers, and inhibitors of P450 CYP2C9.

Cytochrome P450 2C9 is an important member of the cytochrome P450 (CYP) enzyme superfamily. It accounts for approximately 20% of the hepatic P450 enzymes and metabolizes approximately 15% of current therapeutic drugs.[1] Included in these are several commonly used drugs in the perioperative period, some of which have a low therapeutic index (such as warfarin and phenytoin). In addition, commonly used pain medications, including certain nonsteroidal anti-inflammatory drugs (NSAIDs), opioids, and several anesthetics and anesthetic adjuncts, are substrates of the 2C9 enzyme.

The gene coding for CYP2C9 is located on chromosome 10 and is expressed primarily in the liver. CYP2C9 shows selectivity for the oxidation of small, lipophilic anions that tend to be weak acids with pKa values ranging from 3.8 to 8.1.[2] CYP2C9 is highly polymorphic, with 33 variants and several subvariants.[1] *CYP2C9*1* is the wild-type allele. One of the most common variants is the *CYP2C9*2*, which was the first polymorphism identified. This gene variant codes for the intermediate metabolizer phenotype in individuals homozygous for this allele. The *CYP2C9*3* allele codes for the poor metabolizer phenotype.[3] Both of these variants typically produce reduced enzyme activity. Drugs metabolized by an individual with an intermediate or poor metabolizer phenotype may be oxidized inadequately or not at all, causing

B.D. Fergerson MD (✉)
Department of Anesthesiology, University of California, San Diego, San Diego, CA, USA
e-mail: byronfergerson@gmail.com

C.B. Wallentine MD
Department of Anesthesiology, University of Utah School of Medicine, Salt Lake City, UT, USA

R.O. Dull MD, PhD
Department of Anesthesiology, University of Illinois at Chicago, Chicago, IL, USA

C. Marcucci et al. (eds.), *A Case Approach to Perioperative Drug-Drug Interactions*, DOI 10.1007/978-1-4614-7495-1_10

an increase in plasma concentrations and thus increasing the risk for untoward effects. These pharmacogenetic polymorphisms cause significant interindividual variability in drug response. There can be a 10-fold difference in the pharmacokinetic parameters of 2C9 between individuals, which has led to genotyping as a method of ascertaining dosage parameters of drugs such as irbesartan.[4]

In addition to interindividual variability, there are significant ethnic variations in the allelic polymorphisms of CYP2C9. Approximately 1% of Caucasians are homozygotes and 22% are heterozygotes for *CYP2C9*2*. *CYP2C9*3* homozygosity in Caucasians is approximately 0.5% and heterozygosity is approximately 12%. In contrast, homozygosity in either variant is rare in the African-American and Asian populations. Heterozygosity for *CYP2C9*2* in the African-American population ~~is~~ roughly 9% and almost nonexistent in the Asian population; heterozygosity for the *CYP2C9*3* variant is roughly 4% for both populations.[5,6] Of course, the currently recognized polymorphisms only partially account for the ethnic variations. Despite a lack of *CYP2C9*2* in the Asian population, therapeutic warfarin dosing is much lower than in Caucasians.[3]

There are many drugs used in the perioperative period that are substrates of 2C9. In addition to warfarin and phenytoin, a number of these drugs are commonly found in the medication lists of preoperative patients, including carvedilol, clopidogrel, the sulfonylureas (glyburide and glipizide), angiotensin receptor II antagonists (irbesartan and losartan), sertraline, and fluvastatin. Pain medications, including celecoxib, hydromorphone, and several NSAIDs (ibuprofen, indomethacin, naproxen, and diclofenac), are also substrates for 2C9. Several agents commonly used for induction and maintenance are significantly influenced by alterations in the 2C9 enzyme, including propofol (a 30% to 50% metabolic contribution by 2C9), ketamine (30% to 40%), phenobarbital (30% to 40%), diazepam (5% to 10%), and halothane (10% to 20%).[1]

CYP2C9 activity is both induced and inhibited by several common perioperative drugs. In addition to being a substrate, barbiturates act as 2C9 inducers. There is a significant decrease in steady-state plasma concentration of warfarin with barbiturate administration. Unfortunately, the magnitude of the effect of barbiturate induction of 2C9 is unpredictable. A review of the literature suggests that in most instances, phenobarbitone administration produces inconsistent changes in the plasma concentration of phenytoin.[7,8] Amiodarone acts as an inhibitor of the 2C9 enzyme and is particularly significant because of its long half-life. Inhibition of the enzyme persists for several weeks following withdrawal of this drug leading to significantly elevated levels of both warfarin and phenytoin.[2] Antibiotics including fluconazole and several from the sulfa class are also inhibitors of 2C9. The inhibitors listed here are in addition to the competitive inhibition that may occur between substrates.

CYP2C9 is an important enzyme in the metabolism of numerous drugs. Genetic polymorphisms, ethnic variability, and interindividual expression of the gene significantly affect the plasma levels of drugs metabolized by this enzyme. CYP2C9 is, and will continue to be, an important factor to consider in the perioperative arena.

Take-Home Points

- CYP2C9 plays a major role in the metabolism of approximately 15% of drugs, many of which can be found in the perioperative period.
- CYP2C9 genetic polymorphisms and interindividual expression of these genes can affect the metabolism of certain drugs.
- There are significant ethnic variations in the allelic polymorphisms.
- CYP2C9 activity can be significantly enhanced or decreased by several common perioperative medications.

References

1. Zhou SF, Zhou ZW, Huang M. Polymorphisms of human cytochrome P450 2C9 and the functional relevance. Toxicology. 2010;278(2):165–88.
2. Miners JO, Birkett DJ. Cytochrome P4502C9: an enzyme of major importance in human drug metabolism. Br J Clin Pharmacol. 1998;45(6):525–38.
3. Muszkat M. Interethnic differences in drug response: the contribution of genetic variability in ß adrenergic receptor and cytochrome P4502C9. Clin Pharmacol Ther. 2007;82(2):215–8.
4. Hallberg P, Karlsson J, Kurland L, et al. The CYP2C9 genotype predicts the blood pressure response to irbesartan: results from the Swedish Irbesartan Left Ventricular Hypertrophy Investigation vs Atenolol (SILVHIA) trial. J Hypertens. 2002;20(10):2089–93.
5. Adcock DM, Koftan C, Crisan D, et al. Effect of polymorphisms in the cytochrome P450 CYP2C9 gene on coumadin anticoagulation. Arch Pathol Lab Med. 2004;128(12):1360–3.
6. Kirchheiner J, Brockmoller J, et al. Clinical consequences of cytochrome P450 2C9 polymorphisms. Clin Pharmacol Ther. 2005;77(1):1–16.
7. Nation RL, Evans AM, Milne RW. Pharmacokinetic drug interactions with phenytoin (part I). Clin Pharmacokinet. 1990;18:37–60.
8. Nation RL, Evans AM, Milne RW. Pharmacokinetic drug interactions with phenytoin (part II). Clin Pharmacokinet. 1990;18:131–50.

CYP2C19: The Support Crew II

11

Barbara Jericho MD, Alfredo Aguiar MD, and Randal O. Dull MD, PhD

Abstract
This chapter discusses the genetics, metabolic actions, substrates, inducers, and inhibitors of cytochrome P450 2C9.

Cytochrome P450 (CYP) 2C19 is member of the family of CYP enzymes involved in the Phase I metabolism of a number of clinically significant substrates, including the hydroxylation of mephenytoin.[1] There are numerous alleles CYP2C19 alleles (eg, *CYP 2C19*1* to *CYP 2C19*8* and *CYP2C9*17*), which accounts for the great variability in the pharmacokinetics and efficacy of commonly used CYP2C19 substrate drugs.[2,3]

The phenotypic expression of poor and extensive metabolizers is due to the number and type of alleles present for this enzyme. There is great variation in terms of which alleles are found among varying ethnic groups–5% of Caucasians, 5% of African Americans, and 20% of persons with Asian ethnicity have been found to have deficient CYP2C19 activity. Two alleles, *CYP2C19*2* and *CYP2C19*3*, cause the majority of these poor metabolizing phenotypes. The ultra-rapid metabolizer phenotype is seen in approximately 18% of Ethiopians, 18% of Swedes, and 4% of Chinese, likely due to the allele *CYP2C19*17*.[2,3]

B. Jericho MD (✉)
Department of Anesthesiology, University of Illinois Hospital and Health Sciences System, University of Illinois-Chicago, Chicago, IL, USA
e-mail: Jericho@uic.edu

A. Aguiar MD
Department of Anesthesiology, University of Utah SOM, Salt Lake City, UT, USA

R.O. Dull MD, PhD
Department of Anesthesiology, University of Illinois at Chicago, Chicago, IL, USA

C. Marcucci et al. (eds.), *A Case Approach to Perioperative Drug-Drug Interactions*, DOI 10.1007/978-1-4614-7495-1_11

Substrates of CYP2C19 include mephenytoin, proton pump inhibitors (eg, omeprazole, lansoprazole, pantoprazole), several antidepressants and anticonvulsants (phenobarbital, hexobarbital, mephobarbital, citalopram, amitriptyline, diazepam, imipramine, and clomipramine), as well as clopidogrel and R-warfarin. The HIV drug nelfinavir and the antimalarial drug chloroguanide are also substrates of 2C19. This enzyme is also responsible for at least 80% of the metabolism of the proton pump inhibitors as well as mephobarbital, hexobarbital, and carisoprodol. Approximately 30% to 65% of the following drugs are metabolized by CYP2C19: citalopram, sertraline, fluoxetine, imipramine, clomipramine, diazepam, flunitrazepam, proguanil, and moclobemide. Inhibitors of 2C19 include omeprazole, cimetidine, fluvoxamine, ritonavir, and isoniazid (INH). Inducers of 2C19 include phenytoin, carbamazepine, and rifampin.[2,4]

Prodrugs that rely on CYP2C19 to form active metabolites include proguanil and clopidogrel. Deficiency of CYP2C19 activity therefore causes these drugs to lose pharmacodynamic effectiveness. Clopidogrel resistance has been recognized and has been associated with the poor metabolizer phenotype that corresponds to the *CYP2C19*2* allele.[5–7] This has been directly correlated with recurrent ischemic events and poor outcomes in those with acute coronary syndromes and in those requiring percutaneous coronary interventions.[7] Stent re-stenosis is a common problem and perhaps genetic testing will help identify those individuals at higher risk, or at least identify those in which clopidogrel would not be efficacious. Because several of the proton pump inhibitors (PPIs) are meaningful 2C19 inhibitors, they can produce the same difficulties as are seen in poor 2C19 metabolizers. Sim and colleagues showed that *CYP2C*17* homozygotes have approximately 30% to 40% less area under the plasma-concentration time curve of omeprazole compared to *CYP2C19*1* homozygotes.[3]

As competitive inhibitors of 2C19, PPIs are also substrates of this enzyme, and thus are also susceptible to genotypic and phenotypic differences. Pantoprazole appears to have less of this effect with clopidogrel than other PPIs.[8] Shimatani and colleagues showed that homozygous extensive metabolizers attained significantly less acid suppression for initial treatment of gastroesophageal reflux disease when treated with omeprazole, lansoprazole, and rabeprazole.[9] Failure at treating *Helicobacter pylori* and healing related gastric ulcers has been shown with all three of these PPIs in extensive metabolizers.[10,11]

The wide use and clinical importance of 2C19 substrates, and the great ethnic variability of this member of the cytochrome P450 family, suggests potential clinical utility for genetic testing. The failure of clinical effects of a variety of antidepressants and PPIs in a number of populations may be explained by genetic polymorphisms.[2] The recognition of clopidogrel resistance and the sequelae of adverse cardiovascular consequences also suggests an area where morbidity and mortality may be reduced in the future through genetic testing.

Take-Home Points

1. CYP2C19 acts on a number of clinically significant substrates including antidepressants, anticonvulsants, proton pump inhibitors, and antiplatelet/anticoagulant drugs.
2. There is great ethnic variability with respect to both poor and extensive metabolizers, and genetic testing could play an important role.
3. Prodrugs, such as clopidogrel and proguanil, need to be metabolized to become biologically active. Thus poor metabolizers show increased concentration of the prodrug, but little active metabolite and pharmacodynamic effect.
4. Substrates of CYP2C19, such as antidepressants and proton pump inhibitors, may be metabolized very rapidly in homozygous extensive and ultrarapid metabolizers and patients may not have the anticipated clinical outcome.
5. The presence of both inhibitors and prodrugs, such as in the case of omeprazole and clopidogrel, could lead to decreased effect of the prodrug. In the case of clopidogrel, this can lead to adverse cardiovascular outcomes.

References

1. Kupfer A, Desmond PV, Schenker S, et al. Family study of a genetically determined deficiency of mephenytoin hydroxylation in man [letter]. Pharmacologist. 1979;21:173.
2. Desta Z, Zhao X, Shin JG, et al. Clinical significance of the cytochrome P450 2C19 genetic polymorphism. Clin Pharmacokinet. 2002;41:12.
3. Sim S, Risinger C, Dahl ML, et al. A common novel *CYP2C19* gene variant causes ultrarapid drug metabolism relevant for the drug response to proton pump inhibitors and antidepressants. Clin Pharmacol Ther. 2006;79:103–13.
4. Wedlund PJ. The CYP2C19 enzyme polymorphism. Pharmacology. 2000;61(3):174–83.
5. Ford N. Clopidogrel resistance: pharmacokinetic or pharmacogenetic? J Clin Pharmacol. 2009;49(5):506–12.
6. Hulot JS, Bura A, Villard E, et al. Cytochrome P450 2C19 loss-of function polymorphism is a major determinant of clopidogrel responsiveness in healthy subjects. Blood. 2006;108(7):2244–7.
7. Shuldiner A, O'Connell J, Bliden K, et al. Association of cytochrome P450 2C19 genotype with the antiplatelet effect and clinical efficacy of clopidogrel therapy. JAMA. 2009;302(8): 849–57.
8. Norgard N, Mathews K, Wall G. Drug-drug interactions between clopidogrel and the proton pump inhibitors. Ann Pharmacother. 2009;43:1266–74.
9. Shimatani T, Inoue M, Kuroiwa T, et al. Acid-suppressive effects of rabeprazole, omeprazole, and lansoprazole at reduced and standard doses: A crossover comparative study in homozygous extensive metabolizers of cytochrome P450 2C19. Clin Pharmacol Ther. 2006;79:144–52.
10. Furuta T, Shirai N, Takashima M, et al. Effects of genotypic differences in CYP2C19 status on cure rates for Helicobacter pylori infection by dual therapy with rabeprazole plus amoxicillin. Pharmacogenetics. 2001;11:341–8.
11. Furuta T, Shirai N, Takashima M, et al. Effect of genotypic differences in CYP2C19 on cure rates for *Helicobacter pylori* infection by triple therapy with a proton pump inhibitor, amoxicillin, and clarithromycin. Clin Pharmacol Ther. 2001;69:158–68.

Uridine 5′-diphospho-glucuronoslytransferases (UGTs): Conjugating Cousins

12

Neil B. Sandson MD

Abstract

This chapter discusses the chemical pathways, metabolic actions, substrates, inducers, and inhibitors of the uridine 5′-diphosphate glucuronosyltransferases, also known as UGTs.

Uridine 5′-diphosphate glucuronosyltransferases (UGTs) are a family of enzymes that perform Phase II conjugative metabolism (glucuronidation), which usually follows the Phase I oxidative metabolism performed by cytochrome P450 (CYP) enzymes or other oxidative metabolic steps. This system functions analogously to the P450 system, with several enzymes that also have alpha-numeric labels (1A4, 2B15, etc.) and with each enzyme having its own substrates, inhibitors, and inducers. Just as the P450 system is the "workhouse" of Phase I metabolism, UGTs play a similar role in relation to Phase II metabolism.

Phase I metabolic contributions will generally be both more important and more implicated in clinically meaningful drug–drug interactions (DDIs) than Phase II metabolism. Phase I oxidation is a potent process that tends to inactivate most pharmacologically active compounds (with prodrugs being the major exception). However, there are a few specific drugs, such as lamotrigine, haloperidol, olanzapine, valproate, and possibly morphine, for which the UGTs are the main metabolic contributors.[1–5]

N.B. Sandson MD
Department of Psychiatry, University of Maryland Medical System, Baltimore, MD, USA

Department of Psychiatry, VA Maryland Health Care System, Baltimore, MD, USA
e-mail: sandson.marcucci@comcast.net

C. Marcucci et al. (eds.), *A Case Approach to Perioperative Drug-Drug Interactions*, DOI 10.1007/978-1-4614-7495-1_12

Table 12.1 Uridine 5′-diphosphate glucuronosyltransferases (UGTs) Substrates and Inhibitors

	1A1	1A3	1A4	1A6	1A9	2B7	2B15
Substrates	*Bilirubin*	Atorvastatin	Clozapine	*Serotonin*	*Thyroxine*	Codeine	Phenytoin metabolites
	Acetaminophen	Buprenorphine	Doxepin	Acetaminophen	Acetaminophen	Cyclosporine	
	Atorvastatin	Diclofenac	Imipramine	Ketoprofen	Diclofenac	Diclofenac	
	Buprenorphine	Fenoprofen	Lamotrigine		Flavonoids	Hydromorphone	
	Ethinyl estradiol	Gemfibrozil	Meperidine		Labetalol	Ketoprofen	
	Gemfibrozil	Ibuprofen	Olanzapine		Propofol	Lorazepam	
	Simvastatin	Losartan			Propranolol	Losartan	
		Morphine				Morphine	
		Simvastatin				Naproxen	
						Oxycodone	
						Tacrolimus	
						Temazepam	
						Valproate	
Inhibitors	Tacrolimus		Diclofenac	Silymarin (milk thistle)	Cyclosporine A	Amitriptyline	
			Probenecid		Diflunisal	Clofibrate	
			Sertraline		Silymarin (milk thistle)	Codeine	
			Valproate		Tacrolimus	Diazepam	
						Diclofenac	
						Fenoprofen	
						Fluconazole	
						Guanfacine	
						Ibuprofen	
						Ketoprofen	

						Methadone	
						Morphine	
						Naproxen	
						Oxazepam	
						Probenecid	
						Propofol	
						Ranitidine	
						Temazepam	
						Trimethoprim	
						Valproate	
Inducers	Clofibrate		Carbamazepine	Dexamethasone	Polyaromatic hydrocarbons	Ganciclovir	
	Dexamethasone		Ethinyl estradiol	Polyaromatic hydrocarbons		Phenobarbital	
	Flavonoids		Methsuximide			Rifampin	
	Phenobarbital		Oxcarbazepine			Tobacco smoking	
	Phenytoin		Phenobarbital				
	Ritonavir		Phenytoin				
			Primidone				
			Rifampin				

With regard to these drugs and a few others, metabolic DDIs will generally occur when they are coadministered with UGT inhibitors and inducers (see Table 12.1).

As a form of chemical "conjugation" (combining compounds), it may seem odd that glucuronidation would be considered a form of metabolism, insofar as we superficially think of metabolic events as "breaking down" compounds. However, glucuronide groups are generally quite polar, so when these groups are added to pharmacologic agents or their post-oxidation metabolites, the resulting compounds are more water soluble, and thus much more readily excretable in urine, bile, and feces.

Take-Home Points

- The UGT family of enzymes are the "conjugating cousins" of the cytochrome P450 enzyme family. P450 enzymes are concerned with Phase I (oxidative) metabolism and UGTs are concerned with Phase II (conjugative) metabolism by glucuronidation.
- Glucuronidation by UGTs generally adds polar groups to compounds to make them more water soluble and excretable.
- UGTs have substrates, inducers, and inhibitors, just as the cytochrome P450 enzymes do.
- UGTs are the main metabolic pathway for lamotrigine, haloperidol, olanzapine, valproate, and possibly morphine.

References

1. Hiller A, Nguyen N, Strassburg CP. Retigabine N-glucuronidation and its potential role in enterohepatic circulation. Drug Metab Dispos. 1999;27(5):605–12.
2. Kudo S, Ishizaki T. Pharmacokinetics of haloperidol: an update. Clin Pharmacokinet. 1999;37(6):435–56.
3. Linnet K. Glucuronidation of olanzapine by cDNA-expressed human UDP-glucuronosyltransferases and human liver microsomes. Hum Psychopharmacol. 2002;17(5):233–8.
4. Ethell BT, Anderson GD, Burchell B. The effect of valproic acid on drug and steroid glucuronidation by expressed human UDP-glucuronosyltransferases. Biochem Pharmacol. 2003;65(9):1441–9.
5. Chau N, Elliot DJ, Lewis BC, et al. Morphine glucuronidation and glucosidation represent complementary metabolic pathways that are both catalyzed by UDP-glucuronosyltransferase 2B7: kinetic, inhibtion, and molecular modeling studies. J Pharmacol Exp Ther. 2014;349(1):126–37.

The Cytochrome P450 System in Disease States—A Brief Review

13

Catherine Marcucci MD

Abstract

This chapter briefly discusses the cytochrome P450 system in several disease states, including heart, liver, and kidney failure.

The effects of acute, severe illness as well as prolonged organ failure on the body's ability to metabolize drugs is not completely characterized at this time. However, as the sciences of solid organ transplantation, clinical pharmacology, and pharmacogenomics advance, it is clear that the competent clinician will have an increasing need for a thorough knowledge of the cytochrome P450 (CYP) system. It is very clear that diseases, from mild to frank organ failure, affect drug metabolism, but it seems as if this process varies considerably based on the organ.

Renal failure has long been associated with changes in the excretion of many drugs. What has recently been shown, however, is a possible effect of acute kidney injury on CYP-mediated drug metabolism in humans. Kirwan et al. have reported in several studies that acute kidney failure decreases metabolism of midazolam and that increasing severity and duration of renal failure are associate d with decreased midazolam elimination. They proposed a CYP3A-based etiology for these changes in drug metabolism.[1,2]

Heart failure is also associated with changes in drug metabolism and the cardiac and hepatic CYP enzymes, although the mechanisms have not been fully established and appear complicated. Zordoky et al. have suggested that heart failure may be associated with an upregulation of cardiac CYP enzymes, with the production of both protective and deleterious metabolites, and a downregulation of hepatic CYP

C. Marcucci MD
Anesthesia Services Department, Philadelphia Veterans Affairs Medical Center, Philadelphia, PA, USA
e-mail: sandson.marcucci@comcast.net

C. Marcucci et al. (eds.), *A Case Approach to Perioperative Drug-Drug Interactions*, DOI 10.1007/978-1-4614-7495-1_13

enzymes due to decreased hepatic perfusion, hepatocellular damage, and release of proinflammatory cytokines.[3]

Orthotopic liver transplantation provides a set of unique clinical events with respect to drug metabolism. It is expected that hepatic failure, ranging from mild inflammatory disease to severe, chronic liver disease, would affect the body's ability to metabolize drugs. What is interesting is that the limited data show that the effect is not uniform. Adedoyin et al. studied patients with mild to moderate liver disease by using single drug probes for CYP2C19 and CYP2D6 and found selectivity in the effect of liver disease on these enzymes, with 2C19 being more sensitive than 2D6.[4] Frye et al. employed a cocktail of drugs as *in vivo* probes of the cytochrome P450 enzymes 1A2, 2C19, 2D6, and 2E1 in patients with varying severity of liver disease.[5] Again, it was determined that CYP enzyme activity is differentially affected by the presence of liver disease, with the metabolism of mephenytoin (the 2C19 probe), significantly decreased, indicating greater sensitivity of that enzyme to the perturbations of the disease state.

There is now considerable research and clinical interest in both donor and recipient 2C19 genotype and phenotype as a predictor, and marker of hepatic function, graft survival, and clinical recovery from orthotopic liver transplant.[6,7]

Finally, pregnancy is not a disease state, of course. However, there are significant physiologic changes in the gravid patient, including increased plasma volume and increased hepatic and renal flow. Obstetricians and maternal-fetal health specialists see patients who take a variety of drugs that are metabolized via the cytochrome P450 system or commonly interact with other drugs, such as psychiatric drugs, anticonvulsants, antibiotics, street drugs including cocaine, methadone, and buprenorphine, as well as HIV medications including protease inhibitors.[8] There is the growing recognition for a rigorous and science-based approach to prescribing for pregnant patients and anticipating drug–drug interactions that may occur through the choices patients make. Early studies are intriguing, such as a suggestion of induction of 2D6 during pregnancy with changes in the metabolism and response to opioids.[9] There is still a paucity of human data, especially in humans, and much work remains to be done.

Take-Home Points

- Changes in drug metabolism are possible and even probable in disease states involving the kidneys, heart, and (especially) liver.
- It has been suggested that both upregulation and downregulation of cytochrome P450 enzymes occurs in disease states.

- Both donor and recipient CYP2C19 genotype and phenotype are of clinical interest and relevancy in the situation of orthotopic liver transplant.
- Pregnancy is associated with significant physiologic changes, including possible changes in the metabolism of drugs by the cytochrome P450 system.

References

1. Kirwan CJ, Lee T, Holt DW, et al. Using midazolam to monitor changes in hepatic drug metabolism in critically ill patients. Intensive Care Med. 2009;35(7):1271–5. Epub 2009 Feb 7.
2. Kirwan CJ, MacPhee IA, Lee T, et al. Acute kidney injury reduces the hepatic metabolism of midazolam in critically ill patients. Intensive Care Med. 2012;38(1):76–84. Epub 2011 Oct 18.
3. Zordoky BN, El-Kadi AO. Modulation of cardiac and hepatic cytochrome P450 enzymes during heart failure. Curr Drug Metab. 2008;9(2):122–8.
4. Adedoyin A, Arns PA, Richards WO, et al. Selective effect of liver disease on the activities of specific metabolizing enzymes: investigation of cytochromes P450 2C19 and 2D6. Clin Pharmacol Ther. 1998;64(1):8–17.
5. Frye RF, Zgheib NK, Matzke GR, et al. Liver disease selectively modulates cytochrome P450–mediated metabolism. Clin Pharmacol Ther. 2006;80(3):235–45.
6. Chiu KW, Nakano T, Hu TH, et al. Influence of CYP2C19 genotypes on graft pathological findings and postoperative liver function in recipients after living-donor liver transplantation. Ann Transplant. 2010;15(4):38–43.
7. Chiu KW, Nakano T, Tseng HP, et al. Western blotting analysis for quantitative detection of CYP2C19 expression in liver tissues in the setting of living donor liver transplantation. Hepatogastroenterology. 2012;59(115):805–8.
8. McCance-Katz EF. Drug interactions associated with methadone, buprenorphine, cocaine, and HIV medications: implications for pregnant women. Life Sci. 2011;88(21–22):953–8.
9. Madadi P, Avard D, Koren G. Pharmacogenetics of opioids for the treatment of acute maternal pain during pregnancy and lactation. Curr Drug Metab. 2012;13(6):721–7.

III
Drug–Drug Interactions: Paradigms and Core Concepts

P-glycoprotein and Organic Anion-transporting Polypeptide (OATP) Transporters

14

Dustin Coyle MD, Erica D. Wittwer MD, PhD, and Juraj Sprung MD, PhD

Abstract
This chapter discusses the genetics, metabolic pathways, substrates, inducers, and inhibitors of the P-glycoprotein and OATP transporters.

The uptake and elimination of drugs in the human body is not always one of simple diffusion. Several elaborate systems of proteins, known collectively as the transporters, line the lumen of the gut, the kidney, and the blood–brain barrier and stand guard. These energy-dependent transporters are coded by the human genome to transport specific substances and will also act as transporters for certain molecules created by humans via the miracle of modern pharmacology. Other drugs and substances ingested by humans act as inhibitors and inducers of these proteins—much as drugs can act as inhibitors and inducers of the cytochrome P450 (CYP) metabolic enzymes in the liver. This creates a substrate–inhibitor–inducer paradigm for the transporters that allows us to evaluate and understand drug interactions that happen "at the doorway" of the human body and the subsequent effect on bioavailability and clinical efficacy.

These transport systems move drugs both into and out of the physiological milieu. Thus induction of a transporter that extrudes substances back into the gut lumen will have the same effect as induction of a metabolic enzyme, to decrease bioavailability and eliminate the drug from the body.

D. Coyle MD (✉)
Department of Anesthesiology, University of Utah, Salt Lake City, UT, USA
e-mail: dustin.coyle@hsc.utah.edu

E.D. Wittwer MD, PhD • J. Sprung MD, PhD
Department of Anesthesiology, Mayo Clinic, Rochester, MN, USA

C. Marcucci et al. (eds.), *A Case Approach to Perioperative Drug-Drug Interactions*, DOI 10.1007/978-1-4614-7495-1_14

P-glycoprotein. Human P-glycoprotein (P-gp) is a transmembrane efflux transporter protein that lines the gastrointestinal, urinary, and biliary tracts, as well as the blood–brain barrier. It belongs to the superfamily of ATP-binding cassette (ABC) transporters, and is encoded by the Multiple Drug Resistance (*MDR1*) gene, located on chromosome 7.[1,2]

The major role of P-gp is to regulate the amount of substances that are absorbed or excreted from the gut, cerebral vasculature, and the urinary and biliary tracts. In general, P-gp increases the excretion of drugs from organs (Fig. 14.1). It does this in an energy-dependent manner, using ATP.[1,2] P-gp has been demonstrated on the apical side of enterocytes, where it actively transports substrates absorbed into those cells from the gut lumen back into the luminal space for excretion.[1,2] During this process, some of the substrate inevitably gets reabsorbed, and re-exposed to intracellular metabolizing enzymes. P-gp performs a similar function in the blood–brain barrier, pumping substrate absorbed by astrocytes and capillary endothelial cells back into the bloodstream.[4] P-gp located on the apical surfaces of hepatic bile canalicular cells and renal tubular epithelial cells helps eliminate drugs from the body by excreting them from the bloodstream into bile and urine, respectively.[1] Substrates are absorbed from the bloodstream at the basolateral side of these cells, metabolized mainly by CYP3A4 enzymes, then excreted into the bile and urine for elimination.

Since P-gp prevents the systemic absorption of many substances from the gut lumen, it is considered part of the "first-pass effect" seen by many orally ingested medications.[3] P-glycoprotein shares a broad range of substrates with CYP3A4, and they act in conjunction with one another to metabolize many orally administered drugs.[1,2] Substrates that are passively absorbed into the enterocytes are metabolized by CYP3A4. P-gp can pump unmetabolized drug back into the intestinal lumen

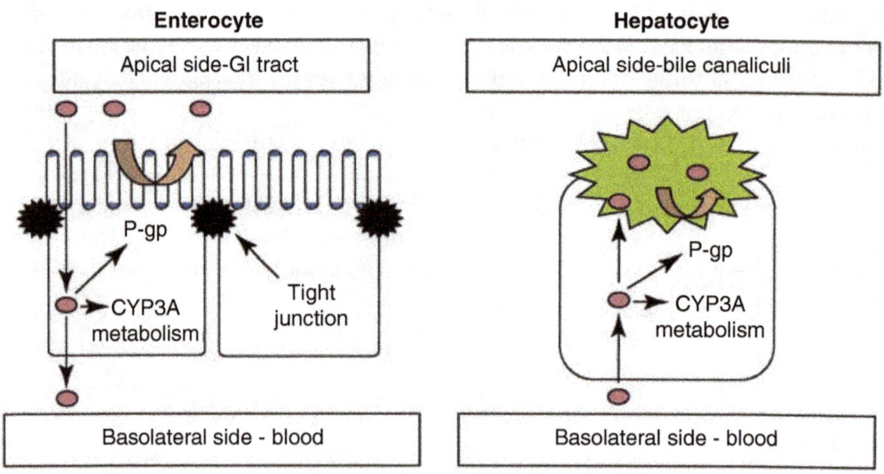

Fig. 14.1 Barriers to drug absorption in the intestine (left) and liver (right): apical and basolateral membranes, tight junctions between cells, P-glycoprotein–mediated, and CYP3A-mediated metabolism

where it can then be passively reabsorbed, and re-exposed to CYP3A4.[1,2] This repetitive process limits the oral bioavailability of drugs that are P-gp and CYP3A4 substrates. However, P-gp activity is easily saturable in the gut, and can be overcome by high dosages of orally administered substrate. Saturation of blood–brain barrier P-gp is less likely after orally administered substrate because the plasma concentration after oral absorption of most drugs is generally significantly low enough as to not overcome the transport rate by P-gp. Intravenous administration of drugs, especially small, lipophilic ones, are more likely to achieve significant concentrations in the brain due to passive diffusion and active transport into neural tissue overcoming the ability of P-gp to pump out the substrate.[1]

Common substrates of P-gp of interest to anesthesiologists include antiarrhythmics like digoxin, quinidine, verapamil, and diltiazem; several fluoroquinolone antibiotics; anticonvulsants like phenobarbital and phenytoin, ondansetron, ranitidine, dexamethasone, and morphine.[3] Vecuronium excretion into bile is profoundly reduced in mice that are P-gp deficient.[1]

Inhibition of P-glycoprotein occurs in three main ways: non-competitive inhibition on the transporter itself, inhibition of ATP hydrolysis at the ATP-binding site, or inhibition of protein kinase C, which is involved in ATP coupling to the transporter.[2] Inhibition will effectively increase the systemic absorption of a co-administered P-gp substrate (Fig. 14.2). In humans, it has been shown that

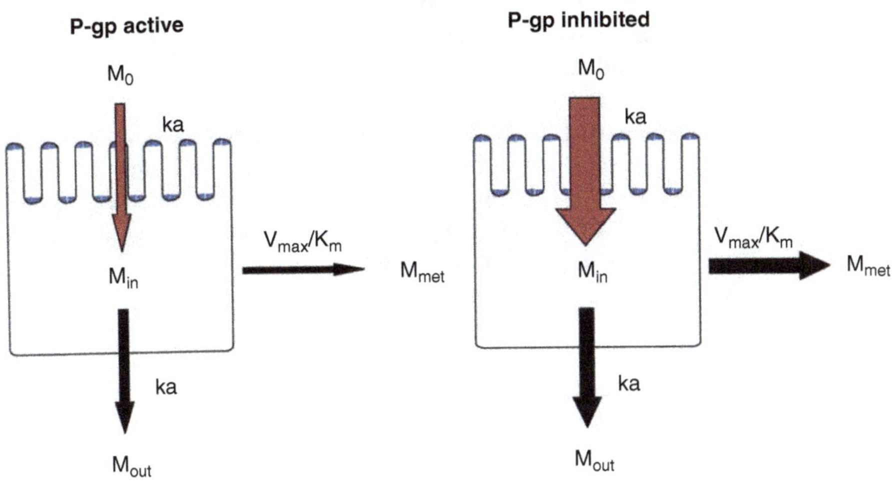

Fig. 14.2 Metabolism and transport in the presence (left) or absence (right) of P-gp efflux. P-gp affects the rate of drug entering the cell through the apical membrane (ka). Width of arrow indicates rate of transport/metabolism. M_0, dose applied; M_{in}, amount of parent in the cell that is available to be cleared; M_{met}, mass of metabolites formed from parent; Mout, mass of parent in basolateral chamber; V_{max}/K_m, rate of CYP3A-mediated metabolism [Reprinted from Beverly Knight, Matthew Troutman and Dhiren R Thakker. Deconvoluting the effects of P-glycoprotein on intestinal CYP3A: a major challenge. Current Opinions in Pharmacology 2006;6:528-532. With permission from Elsevier]

co-administration of a P-gp inhibitor along with morphine, a P-gp substrate, increased the plasma levels of morphine by twofold.[2] Furthermore, administration of loperamide, a potent opioid that is a P-gp substrate with extremely low oral bioavailability and almost no penetration across the blood-brain barrier, along with quinidine, a potent P-gp inhibitor, will increase plasma and brain loperamide levels enough to cause respiratory depression.[3] Co-administration of oral digoxin, a high binding P-gp substrate, with verapamil, a potent P-gp inhibitor, causes significantly increased oral absorption, and decreased renal excretion of digoxin.[1] Common inhibitors of P-gp include verapamil, cyclosporine, ritonavir, amiodarone, proton pump inhibitors, several selective serotonin reuptake inhibitors (SSRIs), and grapefruit juice.[3] Of particular interest to anesthesiologists is the observation that midazolam may be a P-gp substrate, and appears to inhibit P-gp transport of other substrates.[5] The opioids fentanyl, sufentanil, and alfentanil do not appear to be P-gp–substrates, but were shown to inhibit P-gp mediated digoxin transport.[6]

Induction of P-gp does not occur via direct drug binding, but instead is regulated by nuclear factors, most importantly the YB-1 protein, at the transcriptional level.[2] P-gp induction by an inducer will decrease the systemic absorption of a co-administered P-gp substrate by increasing efflux out of absorptive cells. High-dose dexamethasone has been shown to increase liver and intestinal P-gp protein levels.[1,7] Clinically achievable plasma levels of aspirin have been shown to induce P-gp in some cancer cell lines, but the clinical relevance of this finding in other cells that express P-gp is not well characterized.[8,9] St. John's wort, a commonly used over-the-counter herbal antidepressant, has been studied extensively due to its ability to induce P-gp. It has been shown to reduce steady-state plasma levels of many drugs, including cyclosporine and tacrolimus.[2]

Organic Anion Transporting Polypeptides (OATP): OATPs are a subfamily of 11 influx transporter proteins that are encoded by the *SLCO* family of genes located on several chromosomes. Like P-gp, OATPs are found on intestinal enterocytes, cells lining the blood–brain barrier, renal tubular epithelial cells, and hepatic bile canalicular cells, and transport a broad array of substances. Unlike P-gp, OATPs are located on both the apical and basolateral sides of these cells, providing transport of substrates into the cytosol.[10]

OATPs provide ATP-mediated transport of many organic compounds like bile acids, conjugated steroids, glucuronides, eicosanoids, and thyroid hormone.[10,11] OATP1B1, which is located mostly in the liver, has been shown, in vitro, to transport several drug types including HMG-CoA reductase inhibitors, angiotensin converting enzyme (ACE) inhibitors, and angiotensin receptor blockers.[10] Mutations of this protein are associated with simvastatin-induced myopathy. OATP1A2, found in brain, liver, kidney, and intestine, has been shown to transport rocuronium, and is inhibited by verapamil, dexamethasone, and naloxone, among others.[10] Apple, orange, and grapefruit juices all inhibited the intestinal uptake of fexofenadine, a histamine antagonist that is a substrate of OATP.[11]

While our current understanding of specific perioperative drug interactions involving P-gp and OATP is limited, it appears that they are likely significantly involved in this arena. It seems prudent for anesthesiologists to understand the pharmacokinetics of these transporters, and constantly be aware of their potential role in hazardous drug–drug interactions.

Take-Home Points

- P-gp and OATP are drug transporters that have a broad array of substrates, inhibitors, and inducers.
- P-gp is an efflux transporter present in the gut, the kidneys, and the blood–brain barrier.
- P-gp shares many substrates with CYP3A4 and is physiologically linked with CYP3A4 in drug elimination processes.
- There are many important substrates of P-gp that are of interest to anesthesiologists, including digoxin, verapamil, ondansetron, dexamethasone, vecuronium, and possibly midazolam. (A list of P-gp substrates and inhibitors may be found at www.mhc.com/Cytochromes).
- OATP is an influx transporter found in the gut, kidneys, and blood–brain barrier.
- Important substrates of OATP include statins, ACEIs, angiotensin receptor blockers (ARBs), rocuronium, verapamil, dexamethasone, and naloxone.
- Grapefruit juice, apple juice, and orange juice are strong inhibitors of both P-gp and OATP.

References

1. Lin JH. Drug-drug interaction mediated by inhibition and induction of p-glycoprotein. Adv Drug Deliv Rev. 2003;55:53–81.
2. Zhou SF. Structure, function, and regulation of P-glycoprotein, and its clinical relevance in drug disposition. Xenobiotica. 2008;38(7–8):802–32.
3. Oesterheld JR. P-glycoprotein drug interactions. http://www.mhc.com//Cytochromes//PGP//index.html. Last Accessed on July 27 2012.
4. Miller DS, Bauer B, Hartz AM. Modulation of p-glycoprotein at the blood-brain barrier: opportunities to improve central nervous system pharmacotherapy. Pharmacol Rev. 2008; 60(2):196–209.
5. Tolle-Sander S, Rautio J, Wring S, et al. Midazolam exhibits characteristics of a highly permeable p-glycoprotein substrate. Pharm Res. 2003;20(5):757–64.
6. Wandel C, Kim R, Wood M, et al. Interaction of morphine, fentanyl, sufentanil, alfentanil, and loperamide with the efflux drug transporter p-glycoprotein. Anesthesiology. 2002;96(4): 913–20.

7. Shimada T, Tereda A, Yokogawa K, et al. Lowered blood concentration of tacrolimus and its recovery with changes in expression of CYP3A and P-glycoprotein after high-dose steroid therapy. Transplantation. 2002;74(10):1419–24.
8. Flescher E, Rotem R, Kwon P, et al. Aspirin enhances multidrug resistance gene 1 expression in human Molt-4 T lymphoma cells. Anticancer Res. 2000;20(6B):4441–4.
9. Rotem R, Tzivony Y, Flescher E. Contrasting effects of aspirin on prostate cancer induction of drug resistance. Prostate. 2000;42(3):172–80.
10. Kalliokoski A, Niemi M. Impact of OATP transporters on pharmacokinetics. Br J Pharmacol. 2009;158(3):693–705.
11. Hansten P, Levy RH. Role of P-glycoprotein and organic anion transporting polypeptides in drug absorption and distribution: focus on H1-Receptor antagonists. Clin Drug Invest. 2001;21(8):587–96.

The "Fatal Forty" 15

Neil B. Sandson MD, Michael P. Hutchens MD,
F. Jacob Seagull PhD, and Catherine Marcucci MD

Abstract
This chapter discusses the "**Fatal Forty.**" These **forty drugs** or drug classes are involved in drug–drug interactions that are the basis for this book and are "must know" for the perioperative clinician.

The *sine qua non* for mastery of pharmacokinetic drug–drug interactions (DDIs) is mastery of both the cytochrome P450 (CYP) enzyme system and the associated transporter systems. These two marvels of the human body are integral to all four of the processes of pharmacokinetic drug handling—absorption, distribution, metabolism, and excretion. Part and parcel of mastering pharmacokinetic DDIs is understanding how drugs, foods, herbs, spices, and other important compounds interact with the individual enzymes and transporters as substrates, inhibitors, and inducers. These interactions are fascinating when connected with their clinical consequences, but their complexity makes it challenging for the beginner to make these essential connections.

Thus, to the beginning reader (and even to the more advanced DDI student), making these critical connections can seem daunting. In our experience, most learners who

N.B. Sandson MD (✉)
Department of Psychiatry, University of Maryland Medical System, Baltimore, MD, USA

Department of Psychiatry, Baltimore VA Medical Center VA Maryland Health Care System
Baltimore, MD, USA
e-mail: sandson.marcucci@comcast.net

M.P. Hutchens MD
Department of Anesthesiology and Perioperative Medicine,
Oregon Health and Science University
Portland, OR, USA

F.J. Seagull PhD
Department of Learning Health Sciences, University of Michigan Medical School,
Ann Arbor, MI, USA

C. Marcucci MD
Anesthesia Services Department, Philadelphia Veterans Affairs Medical Center,
Philadelphia, PA, USA

C. Marcucci et al. (eds.), *A Case Approach to Perioperative Drug-Drug Interactions*, DOI 10.1007/978-1-4614-7495-1_15

are left to their own devices will abandon the subject. The various enzymes and drugs are initially approached with enthusiasm, but good intentions are quickly lost in a fog of letters, numbers, and seemingly endless random and disconnected facts. The frustration and temptation to quit the subject is especially great if the student attempts to conquer the material by rote memory.

Fortunately, there is a better way. In our thinking and teaching about DDIs, we always think and speak of the enzymes and transporters, substrates, inhibitors, and inducers as families or groups. It is really no different than meeting a large, crazy family for the first time or joining a large, diverse club and figuring out who runs in which crowd.

We therefore introduce the reader to the **"Fatal Forty."**[1] This group of **forty drugs** and other substances interact significantly with the cytochrome P450 enzyme system and the transporters that encompass the fundamentals of pharmacokinetic DDIs. Master these drugs and their interactions, and you will have mastered a framework to which the details of other drugs and other DDIs can be added as corresponding clinical situations arise or time and energy permit.

Five Approaches to Learning the Fatal Forty: To further aid the reader and provide additional pathways into the realm of these forty drugs and associated drug classes, we suggest five separate approaches to the **Fatal Forty:** the Card Catalogue Approach, the Pharmacology Approach, the Clinician's Approach, the "Perpetrators and Victims (of DDIs)" Approach, and the **"Top Ten"** Approach.

I The Card Catalogue Approach: This is a simple alphabetical list of the drugs and substances comprising the **Fatal Forty**. We recommend that you clip or copy this list and review it often, perhaps when you sit down to look at your posted cases or preoperative evaluations. In addition, each appearance of a DDI involving a **Fatal Forty** drug in the table of contents or individual scenarios is in bold font.

Amiodarone	*Fluoxetine*	*Quinolones*
Azole antifungals	*Fluvoxamine*	*Rifampin*
Bupropion	*Grapefruit juice*	*Ritonavir*
Calcium channel blockers	*Ketoconazole*	*Statins*
Carbamazepine	*Lamotrigine*	*St. John's wort*
Cimetidine	*Lithium*	*Sulfonylureas*
Clopidogrel	*Macrolides*	*Tamoxifen*
Clozapine	*Methadone*	*Theophylline*
Codeine	*NSAIDs*	*Thioridazine*
Cyclobenzaprine	*Paroxetine*	*Tobacco*
Digoxin	*Phenobarbital*	*Tramadol*
(Es)Omeprazole	*Phenytoin*	*Tricyclic antidepressants*
Ethinylestradiol	*Pimozide*	*Warfarin*
	Quinidine	

[1] The term **"Fatal Forty"** is merely a catchy alliteration that is used for educational purposes only! Use of this term is in no way intended to suggest or imply that appropriate use of any of so-cited medication would prove likely or immediately fatal.

<u>**II The Pharmacology Approach**</u>: This is the one the editors tend to use. Each of these **forty drugs** has certain defining pharmacologic characteristics that make them of particular value when learning DDIs. We remember the **Fatal Forty drugs by organizing them into six pharmacological classifications or "families."**

A. ***Drugs that have a low therapeutic index***: There are a number of **Fatal Forty** drugs that have low therapeutic index (LD50/ED50) ratios. In less headachy terms, low therapeutic index drugs are those drugs for which small changes in blood levels, possibly due to inhibition of metabolism, can have big clinical effects. And remember that a DDI that inhibits metabolism of a drug can easily cause changes in the blood level of that drug. Low therapeutic index drugs on the **Fatal Forty** list and their clinical uses and/or toxic consequences are:

Clozapine—seizures and oversedation

Cyclobenzaprine—common drug in pain clinics, 1A2 substrate

Digoxin—arrhythmias

Lamotrigine—toxic dermatologic syndromes

Lithium—nephrotoxicity

Methadone—arrhythmias and central nervous system (CNS)/cardiopulmonary depression

Pimozide—malignant QT prolonger

Thioridazine—malignant QT prolonger

Tricyclic antidepressants—QT prolongation

Warfarin—changes in coagulability

B. ***Drugs that are pan-inhibitors or pan-inducers:*** These **Fatal Forty** drugs are classified together because they are very "busy" DDI drugs, in that they inhibit and induce many enzymes. They are busy, busy, busy, and there is always the potential for a DDI when they appear in a drug list.

Amiodarone—pan-inhibitor of cytochrome P450 enzymes (CYP450)

Cimetidine—pan-inhibitor of CYP450

Fluoxetine—pan-inhibitor of CYP450

Fluvoxamine—less common than fluoxetine, but still a CYP450 pan-inhibitor

Ritonavir—pan-inhibitor and pan-inducer of CYP450

Phenobarbital—pan-inducer of CYP450

Carbamazepine — pan-inducer of CYP450, P-glycoprotein substrate, and CYP3A4 substrate

Phenytoin—CYP2C9 greater than 2C19 substrate, P-glycoprotein substrate, CYP450 pan-inducer (except for 1A2), and high plasma protein binding

Rifampin—pan-inducer of CYP450 and P-glycoprotein inducer

C. ***Drugs that are CYP3A4 inhibitors:*** Remember that 3A4 is the workhorse P450 enzyme. Although there are individual genetic variations that lead to absent functioning of other P450 enzymes (eg, 2D6), a "poor metabolizer" genotype and corresponding phenotype for 3A4 is nonexistent— this is because it is likely that this genotype is lethal in the embryonic state. We recommend that you get your dander up when you see a drug that is a 3A4 inhibitor on a med list. Start surveying the drug list for possible DDIs and don't forget to *always* ask outpatients about grapefruit juice.

Ketoconazole—most potent 3A4 inhibitor, especially important because 3A4 is the "sink" enzyme, or in other words, it is the "high-capacity" enzyme. In fact, a reason that fluconazole was developed was that the ketoconazole inhibition of 3A4 metabolism of endogenous cortisol by ketoconazole was so significant that patients actually got Cushingoid.

Diltiazem and verapamil—potent and ubiquitous 3A4 inhibitors.

Grapefruit juice—a sufficiently potent 3A4 inhibitor that most hospitals don't allow it on patient food trays.

Macrolides—except for azithromycin, common and potent 3A4 inhibitors.

Keep in mind that the pan-inhibitors listed above also inhibit 3A4.

D. Prodrugs: These are drugs that must be converted to a biologically active form for clinical efficacy. The DDIs associated with these drugs are troublesome and dangerous because few clinicians or patients understand or recognize the prodrug conversion, much less the DDIs that prevent this necessary pharmacological step. Many prodrugs are metabolized to active compounds by CYP2D6, so mastering prodrug DDIs is also a starting point for learning the 2D6 inhibitors (see also "Perpetrators and Victims").

Codeine—prodrug at CYP2D6

Tamoxifen—prodrug at 2D6

Tramadol—2D6 prodrug, common medications

Clopidogrel—prodrug at 3A4 and 2C19

E. Common drugs: These are drugs that are commonly mixed up with DDIs and also in such common clinical use that everyone needs to know them.

Calcium-channel blockers—these drugs in general are CYP3A4 substrates; diltiazem and verapamil are also 3A4 and P-glycoprotein inhibitors

Clopidogrel— prodrug at CYP3A4 and 2C19

Omeprazole—CYP2C19 substrate and inhibitor; P-glycoprotein inhibitor

Ethinylestradiol—CYP3A4 substrate, 2C19 and 1A2 inhibitor, and uridine 5′-diphosphoglucuronoslytransferase 1A4 (UGT1A4) inducer

Grapefruit juice—3A4 and 1A2 inhibitor

Macrolides—except for azithromycin, all are 3A4 and P-glycoprotein inhibitors

Statins—lovastatin, simvastatin, and atorvastatin are all CYP3A4; simvastatin is also a 2D6 substrate; fluvastatin is a 2C9 substrate and inhibitor; all seem to be P-glycoprotein inhibitors

Sulfonylureas—2C9 substrates

Smoked tobacco—1A2 and 2E1 inducer

***F. Drugs for which there is a rare but serious complication of a DD*I** or a very unusual pharmacological profile.

Statins—very common drugs. High blood levels are associated with rhabdomyolysis, which is unusual but very serious. Somewhat complicated metabolic profile—atorvastatin, simvastatin, and lovastatin are CYP3A4 substrates. Simvastatin is also a 2D6 substrate. Fluvastatin is a 2C9 substrate and inhibitor. Most statins are P-glycoprotein inhibitors and have variable effects on warfarin.

Smoked tobacco— unlike most P450 inducers, smoked tobacco acts as a 1A2 inducer in a very shortened time frame (1–3 days instead of 1–3 weeks).

III The Clinician Approach: This approach to the **Fatal Forty** is based on the idea that it will be easiest to first learn what you most need to know in your own practice. For example, if you take care of pain patients— here are some of the drugs you need to know and why you need to know them:

Codeine—prodrug at 2D6 (converts to morphine).

Methadone—2D6 inhibitor, low Ti, QT prolongation, and 3A4 and 2B6 substrate.

Cyclobenzaprine—common drug in pain clinics, 1A2 substrate.

Tramadol—2D6 prodrug, common medication.

Tricyclic antidepressants—these drugs have a low therapeutic index. They are substrates of 2D6. Tertiary amine tricyclic antidepressants (TCAs) are also substrates of 2C19, 1A2, and 3A4.

IV The Perpetrators and Victims Approach: This approach is based on the notion that some of the **Fatal Forty** drugs are known for being "perpetrators" of drug interaction mischief while other **Fatal Forty** drugs are "victims"—in other words, the trashers and the trashed. But *remember*, individual drugs can also be in either role, depending on the specific circumstances.

"Perpetrators" of DDIs

Amiodarone
Azoles
Bupropion
Diltiazem/Verapamil
Carbamazepine
Cimetidine
(Es)Omeprazole
Ethinylestradiol
Fluoxetine
Fluvoxamine
Grapefruit juice
Macrolides
Methadone
NSAIDs
Paroxetine
Phenobarbital
Phenytoin
Quinidine
Quinolones
Rifampin
Ritonavir
St. John's wort
Smoked tobacco

"Victims" of DDIs

Carbamazepine
CCBs
Ethinylestradiol
Hydrocodone
Lamotrigine
Lithium
Methadone
Phenytoin
Pimozide
Quinidine
Statins
Sulfonylureas
Tamoxifen
Thioridazine
Tramadol
Tricyclic antidepressants
Warfarin

V The **"Can't do 40! Can only do 10!" Approach:** If you are a busy resident or fellow or a somewhat fearful or tentative student of pharmacology, then start low and go slow. Take a look at our **Terrible Ten** list of drugs and work on gaining mastery of the associated DDIs for these drugs. This will give you a solid foundation in the key concepts, as well as a solid start on drugs with the most dangerous and common interactions. We've chosen these particular drugs based on frequency of use, frequency of interaction, and "badness" of interaction.

Calcium channel blockers	*Quinolones*
Ethinylestradiol	*Ritonavir*
Fluoxetine	*Tobacco*
Methadone	*TCAs*
Phenytoin	*Warfarin*

Take-Home Points

- While the entire domain of DDIs is vast, mastering those associated with the **Fatal Forty** will enable clinicians to anticipate the most important DDIs likely to befall their patients.
- Read this chapter often!

The Six Patterns of Pharmacokinetic Drug–Drug Interactions

16

Neil B. Sandson MD and Catherine Marcucci MD

Abstract
This chapter discusses the six patterns of cytochrome P450-mediated drug–drug interactions.

Drugs and other substances involved in pharmacokinetic drug–drug interactions (DDIs) mediated by the cytochrome P450 (CYP) enzymes can act as substrates, inhibitors, or inducers of the one or more of the specific enzymes. In addition, there are six recognized patterns of DDIs. Mastery of these basic terms and patterns is well worth the effort for the beginning DDI student. Even clinicians who are knowledgeable about DDIs in general and the cytochrome P450 enzymes specifically will find some benefit in reviewing the basics presented below.

Substrate

A compound that is metabolized by an enzyme into a metabolic end product. Usually this results in eventual deactivation of the agent in preparation for elimination from the body. In the rare case of "prodrugs," these agents are initially inactive and rely on enzymes to be metabolized into active compounds.

N.B. Sandson MD (✉)
Department of Psychiatry, University of Maryland Medical System, Baltimore, MD, USA

Department of Psychiatry, Baltimore VA Medical Center, VA Maryland Health Care System, Baltimore, MD, USA
e-mail: sandson.marcucci@comcast.net

C. Marcucci MD
Anesthesia Services Department, Philadelphia Veterans Affairs Medical Center, Philadelphia, PA, USA

C. Marcucci et al. (eds.), *A Case Approach to Perioperative Drug-Drug Interactions*, DOI 10.1007/978-1-4614-7495-1_16

Inhibitor

An agent that interferes with, or inhibits, the functioning of the enzyme or enzymes that metabolize substrates. Enzymatic inhibition comes in two main varieties. The first, ***competitive inhibition***, is when two substrates compete for the same substrate binding site(s) on an enzyme. The competitive inhibitor binds so avidly to this substrate binding site that it effectively displaces the other substrate(s), but the enzyme otherwise functions normally. The second type of inhibition, ***noncompetitive, or allosteric, inhibition,*** occurs when an agent binds to a nonsubstrate binding site on an enzyme. In so doing, the allosteric inhibitor renders the enzyme less efficient in metabolizing all substrates of that enzyme. The introduction of inhibitors leads to *substrate accumulation* and *decreased metabolite formation.* Inhibitors of cytochrome P450 enzymes generally act within hours to days, as a function of their half-lives, which determine when they are able to gain access to, and then inhibit, the enzymes in question.

Inducer

An agent that causes the liver (or other target organ) to produce more of an enzyme, leading to increased metabolism of the substrates of the induced enzyme. This is a purely quantitative concept. The produced enzyme is no more intrinsically active than otherwise; there is just more of it. In the concept of *enzymatic stimulation,* which is being considered for CYP3A4, the enzyme is rendered more efficient, aside from its quantity in the liver and/or gut. The introduction of inducers leads to ***increased metabolite formation*** and ***more rapid depletion of substrate(s).*** Induction of P450 enzymes can be evident within several days but generally takes 2 to 3 weeks to reach full effect.

Variability

There is vast interindividual variability in enzymatic efficiency (10-fold to 30-fold differences in 3A4 function, for example) across the world population, with some trends within specific ethnic groups.[1] This does not even consider those individuals who lack copies of the genes that code for various P450 enzymes, who are referred to as "poor metabolizers" or "polymorphic" for the specific P450 enzymes in question. By contrast, individuals who have extra copies of P450 genes are referred to as "ultrarapid metabolizers." In general, metabolically normal individuals (called "extensive metabolizers") who are exposed to an agent that strongly inhibits a given P450 enzyme are functionally converted to "poor metabolizers" with regard to that specific P450 enzyme, as long as they are exposed to that agent. Conversely, individuals exposed to an inducer may function as ultrarapid metabolizers for that P450 enzyme. Poor metabolizers/polymorphic individuals will generally have much higher blood levels of a substrate at a given dose than will extensive metabolizers. Although this is counterintuitive, the rate at which poor metabolizers/polymorphic individuals metabolize a substrate of that enzyme is *not* influenced by introducing an inhibitor of that enzyme. There is no way to become an "ultrapoor metabolizer." The inhibitor is redundant.

There are six basic patterns of cytochrome P450 drug–drug interactions.

Pattern 1: An Inhibitor Is Added to a Substrate

This pattern generally results in increases in substrate levels. If the substrate has a low therapeutic index, toxicity may result unless care is exercised (such as closely checking blood levels or lowering substrate doses in anticipation of the interaction).

> Example: *Paroxetine is added to nortriptyline* (see "**Pining for Pete in the Pain Clinic**")

Nortriptyline is a commonly prescribed pain drug that is metabolized by CYP2D6. Paroxetine is a common depression, anxiety, and post-traumatic stress disorder drug. It is a strong 2D6 inhibitor. Adding paroxetine to a medication panel that contains nortriptyline will increase blood levels of nortriptyline and put the patient at risk to tricyclic antidepressant toxicity.

Pattern 2: A Substrate Is Added to an Inhibitor

This pattern may cause increased bioavailability and prolonged action of the substrate. It may also cause difficulties if the substrate has a low therapeutic index and is titrated according to preset guidelines that do not take into account the presence of an inhibitor. If the substrate is titrated to specific blood levels or to therapeutic effect, or with an appreciation that an inhibitor is present, then toxicity is less likely to arise.

> Example: *Fentanyl is added to ritonavir* (see "**Sleeping Beauty**")

Fentanyl, a widely used synthetic opioid, is metabolized mainly by the hepatic CYP3A4 isozyme to its major oxidative metabolite, norfentanyl. Ritonavir, a protease inhibitor commonly used in the treatment of HIV infection, is one of the most potent inhibitors of 3A4. It can markedly prolong the action of fentanyl.

Pattern 3: An Inducer Is Added to a Substrate

This pattern generally results in decreases in substrate levels. A decrease in levels of the substrate may result in a loss of efficacy of the substrate, unless blood levels are followed and/or the substrate doses are increased in anticipation of the interaction.

> Example: *Phenytoin added to cyclosporine* (see "**No Fits At Uffizi**")

Cyclosporine is metabolized by CYP3A4. Phenytoin is a paninducer, it induces 3A4 as well as CYP2C9 and 2C19. The addition of an inducer to a drug with a narrow therapeutic index will lower the blood levels of the substrate drug, in this case cyclosporine, and can have serious clinical sequelae.

Pattern 4: A Substrate Is Added to an Inducer

This pattern may lead to ineffective dosing if preset dosing guidelines are followed that do not take into account the presence of an inducer. If the substrate is titrated to specific blood levels or to clinical effect, or with an appreciation that an inducer is present, then dosing is more likely to be effective.

> *Example: Midazolam added to carbamazepine* (see "**Lack of Sedation**")

Carbamazepine is a CYP1A2 and CYP3A4 inducer (as well as an inducer of Phase II glucuronidation). Midazolam is a 3A4 substrate. A patient on chronic carbamazepine will not have equal bioavailability and sedative effect with a given midazolam dose that a patient who is not taking carbamazepine.

Pattern 5: Reversal of Inhibition

A substrate and an inhibitor have been co-administered and equilibria have been achieved, and then the inhibitor is discontinued. This leads to a resumption of normal enzyme activity and generally results in decreases in levels of substrate and increased metabolite formation. This may result in loss of efficacy of the substrate unless blood levels are followed and/or substrate doses are increased in anticipation of the reversal of inhibition.

> *Example: Fluconazole is discontinued in the presence of prednisone* (see "**Addisonian Adjustment**")

Prednisone is a CYP3A4 substrate. Fluconazole is a moderate 3A4 inhibitor. When fluconazole is discontinued after a period of coadministration with prednisone, 3A4 resumes its higher baseline level of activity, so at the same dosage of prednisone, levels of prednisone will decrease.

Pattern 6: Reversal of Induction

A substrate and an inducer have been co-administered and equilibria have been achieved, and then the inducer is discontinued. This gradually (over 1–3 weeks) results in decreased amounts of available enzyme, leading to increased levels of substrate and decreased metabolite formation. This may result in substrate toxicity if the substrate has a low therapeutic index, unless blood levels are followed and/or substrate doses are decreased in anticipation of the reversal of induction.

<u>*Example:*</u> *Smoking is discontinued in the presence of theophylline* (see **"Induction Crashes: Are There Clues In The Ashes?"**)

A smoker had been stably maintained on theophylline. Smoked tobacco is a CYP1A2 inducer and theophylline is a 1A2 substrate. Sudden cessation of smoking during an admission to the ICU after a motor vehicle accident caused an abrupt removal of the inducer leading to increased levels of theophylline, a drug with a narrow therapeutic index. This caused hemodynamic instability on induction of anesthesia.

The Exception

When prodrugs (hydrocodone, tramadol, cyclophosphamide, etc.) are the substrates in question, the clinical concerns are reversed. An inhibitor added to a prodrug substrate concern will cause loss of efficacy, not toxicity (*see* **"Ultimate Ultram Primer I: My Mood Is Better But Boy Do I Hurt**). And when an inducer added to a prodrug substrate, the concern is toxicity, not loss of efficacy, and so forth.

Take-Home Points

- A substrate is a compound that is metabolized into an end product.
- An inhibitor is an agent or compound that interferes with, or inhibits, the functioning of the enzyme or enzymes that metabolize substrates.
- An inducer is an agent or compound that causes the liver (or other target organ) to produce more of an enzyme, leading to increased metabolism of the substrates of the induced enzyme.
- There are six basic patterns of cytochrome P450 drug–drug interactions: **inhibitor added to substrate; substrate added to an inhibitor; inducer added to a substrate; substrate added to an inducer; reversal of inhibition; reversal of induction.**
- When prodrugs are the substrates, the clinical concerns of efficacy and toxicity are reversed.

Reference

1. Ketter TA, Flockhart DA, Post RM, et al. The emerging role of cytochrome P450 3A in psychopharmacology. J Clin Psychopharmacol. 1995;15(6):387–98.

17 The Problem with the Drug–Drug Interaction Software: A Procrustean Dilemma

Neil B. Sandson MD, F. Jacob Seagull PhD,
Wayne T. Nicholson MD, PharmD, MSc,
and Catherine Marcucci MD

Abstract
This chapter discusses the risks of relying exclusively on drug–drug interaction software.

When the ancient Greek hero, Theseus, travelled to Crete, he encountered and vanquished several formidable foes. One of these was Procrustes. Procrustes's modus operandi was to invite guests into his home and, after lavishly feeding them, insist that they sleep in one of his beds. But there was a catch. If the guest was tall, Procrustes would take him to a short bed and insist on cutting off his legs so he would fit. Alternatively, if the guest was short, he would take them to a long bed and stretch them on a rack until they fit. Procrustes's guests were a uniformly unhappy lot, until Theseus turned the tables and subjected Procrustes to his own hospitality.

N.B. Sandson MD (✉)
Department of Psychiatry, University of Maryland Medical System, Baltimore, MD, USA

Department of Psychiatry, VA Maryland Health Care System, Baltimore, MD, USA
e-mail: sandson.marcucci@comcast.net

F.J. Seagull PhD
Department of Learning Health Sciences, University of Michigan Medical School, Ann Arbor, MI, USA

W.T. Nicholson MD, PharmD, MSc
Department of Anesthesiology, Mayo Clinic, Rochester, MN, USA

C. Marcucci MD
Anesthesia Services Department, Philadelphia Veterans Affairs Medical Center, Philadelphia, PA, USA

C. Marcucci et al. (eds.), *A Case Approach to Perioperative Drug-Drug Interactions*, DOI 10.1007/978-1-4614-7495-1_17

Physicians and other health care providers who have acknowledged and undertaken the need to incorporate a knowledge and mastery of perioperative drug–drug interactions (DDIs) in their daily practice face a crucial question. It is a given that the information imparted in a few lectures in medical school and a few more in training is simply not enough to maintain excellence and currency in clinical practice. How then and by what means do responsible clinicians augment and sustain their working knowledge base? Can a clinician rely solely on the widely available commercial and institutional software for the identification and avoidance of the DDIs that will keep her patients safe and free from undue clinical events?

We believe the answer is no.

In spite of diligent efforts, the designers of DDI computer programs are in a quandary that would be familiar to the guests of the mythical Procrustes. For that reason, we do not recommend either an overconfidence or overreliance on DDI computer software.

Of course, we do not mean to imply that DDI software programs can or should be ignored or even significantly discounted. They can be helpful and they are here to stay. But the evidence base on DDI software programs, and e-prescribing in general, although still young and fairly scant, is not entirely favorable. Weingart et al. performed a survey of ambulatory care physicians to characterize assessments of an e-prescribing system with allergy and drug interaction alerts.[1] Although physicians indicated that e-prescribing improved the quality of care and prevented medical errors overall, they were much less positive about alerts triggered by discontinued medications, alerts that failed to account for appropriate drug combinations, and an excessive number of alerts. A second paper by Weingart et al. acknowledged that ambulatory care clinicians override as many of 91% of drug interaction alerts and reported the development of an empirical model to estimate the potential impact of medication safety alerts.[2] They concluded, in part, that preventing drug interactions saves lives and health care dollars, however, 331 alerts were required to prevent one adverse drug event. A third paper by Isaac et al. concluded "Clinicians override most medication alerts, suggesting that current medication safety alerts may be inadequate to protect patent safety."[3]

Why and what situations does this happen? The problem is evident when considering the situation of a hypothetical clinician who wants to add a potential drug to the regimen of a medically complex patient. She searches her memory of the subject and finds nothing. She types the new prospective regimen into an internet drug interaction program, and is then faced with a lengthy collection of potential interactions. The vagueness of these designations and the breadth of the list makes it difficult to judge. She asks the person next to her what they would do. They shrug. She gazes at the list of DDIs again. She then is tempted to just shut the thing off, go for it, and hope for the best. Finally, she picks up the phone and calls the surgical pharmacy. Fortunately, the ICU PharmD is in. He straightens out her medication list and answers her questions.

So, to further understand the problems at the crux of the DDI software conundrum faced by this hypothetical young doctor, one must first look at the nature of DDIs. Of course, many DDIs are unambiguously and uniformly important. For instance, DDIs that produce drastic blood level increases in narrow therapeutic index agents (tricyclic antidepressants, lithium, digoxin, etc.) will almost invariably pose grave toxicity concerns. Additionally, DDIs that cause a significant decrease in drug concentrations lead to subtherapeutic levels and can be expected to produce therapeutic failures with potentially catastrophic outcomes. However, for the majority of DDIs, the situation is not so clear-cut. Some DDIs are situational, dependent on several factors to come into alignment. Most DDIs produce potential and/or actual suboptimal outcomes, but not frank toxicity or complete loss of efficacy. Indeed, some DDIs can be beneficial, whether by accident or the deliberate mobilization of mechanistic synergies. The question of how to address this majority of DDIs poses the first daunting challenge for the designers of DDI programs.

Secondly, most of the time, the mere fact that a DDI results from concomitant administration of two drugs does not establish that a particular DDI has any real clinical significance. Within the human species, there is great variability of both pharmacodynamic and pharmacokinetic profiles. This variability can be due to several factors including age, genetics, and pathology. This results in a spectrum of clinical responses to a given DDI, ranging from no discernible change to outright toxicity/therapeutic failure. And again, some DDIs are helpful, whether by serendipity or design. This intra-patient variability of clinical consequences arising from most DDIs makes it difficult to create a DDI program that provides consistently useful output. After all, who wants a DDI program whose most frequent result to most queries is, "anything could happen"? One might regard this as a simplistic criticism but let us examine the consequences arising from different "DDI priorities."

Intuitively, to avoid the unhelpful "anything could happen" message, the designers and programmers might design a DDI program that prioritizes probable events and de-emphasizes the merely possible. In epidemiologic language, this involves increasing *specificity* at the cost of *sensitivity*. The fewer false alarms, the more missed important interactions. While many practitioners might regard such a lack of "false alarm" alerts in the program as "user-friendly," this is small consolation to the persons who avoidably suffer from consequences of predictable and preventable DDIs that are missed by this program.

On the other hand, programs and software can be made more sensitive, to greatly minimize the risk of ever missing an important DDI. However, the price now paid is lack of specificity. In other words, the more sensitive the program, the more trivial and even frankly irrelevant "false alarm" alerts.

As noted in the papers cited above, the false alarm phenomenon is one of the biggest issues faced when using a DDI software program. An ongoing series of false and nuisance alarms caused by overly sensitive DDI programs can and will lead to "alert fatigue." The human factors consequences of false alarms and alert fatigue are well-recognized and have been quantified. For example, it has been determined that people have a tendency to "probability match" their responses to the perceived value to the alert. That is, alerts that are 'false alarms" 90% of the time will be ignored 90% of the time.[4] More fundamentally, technologies like DDI programs act like a member of the medical team—they can provide valuable information that is useful, or they can become a burden on the team by not contributing added value. Humans have an innate and inbred ability to understand who is a good team member. People learn who to listen to on their team and who to trust. DDI programs that often "cry wolf," and who are unreliable or untrustworthy team members teach people to develop feelings of frustration and dislike, and to mistrust the program itself.

Another problem with computerized DDI programs arises due to certain inherent structural shortcomings that decrease the effectiveness of the programs. It is becoming clear that DDI databases need to take into account more patient-specific information.[5] However, most programs have not progressed to this extent; they can't supply the critical weighing of mitigating and/or exacerbating patient factors that are essential for sound clinical decision making. More simply put, clinical context is everything for both the provider and the patient, and the programs aren't very good at that. The programs don't know you, they don't know what you consider obvious, and they don't know what you would find usefully informative. Similarly, they don't know your patient. DDI programs don't "understand" the patient and context in which you operate. Few programs consider the individualized characteristics of a patient when generating warnings. As examples, hypertension as a side effect may be much more dangerous to a 92-year-old with diabetes than a healthy 27-year-old, but few DDI programs change the severity rating of a side-effect based on patient characteristics like age. The threshold for accepting risk for a given drug-drug interaction may be different if the drug therapy is contemplated for a patient with difficult to manage pain in the clinical setting of significant psychiatric disease. And of course, at this time, most DDI programs do not take into account whether a patient is a poor metabolizer at the CYP2D6 enzyme. This leads to information that is not properly prioritized, and further increases the difficulties of an efficient working relationship with a DDI program.

Interaction with DDI programs can also be a problem. On handheld devices, the process of inputting drugs into the DDI program can be inelegant, tedious, or even frustrating. For a clinician working with a DDI program imbedded in a patient's records, it can be difficult and slow for a clinician to make her way through her chart tasks in the face of repeated warnings that may be technically true, but have limited clinical relevance.

Lastly, it's not good to be too dependent on technology. Give a man a fish and you feed him for the day. Teach him to fish and you feed him for a lifetime (as well as getting the whole weekend to yourself). DDI programs "give you a fish" by providing a list of interactions. Even if they do it correctly and meaningfully (which we know they don't), this teaches you primarily one thing: to depend on DDI programs. Learning the fundamentals of DDIs can "teach you to fish," so that you can work with confidence even when the technology is not available. Learning about DDIs can free you from depending on the program, and help you work more with patients, not computer programs.

What does the future hold for DDI software programs? The issues described above are still prevalent and the clinician must remain ever-vigilant. One possible solution is to implement more nuance and gradation into DDI programs rather than the binary choice of expressing or suppressing a given DDI. However, even simple attempts in software modification need to be done with caution, since interactions that cause patient harm may be suppressed.[6] Some programs employ a graded alert system that shows the severity of the interaction or probability of an alert's validity (red-yellow-green light symbols and other such maneuvers). However, these programs require cognitive burden on the provider. One can no longer rely on the program to provide simple "safe" vs. "unsafe" output and be guided by such unambiguous determinations. But most programs have not progressed to this extent; they can't supply the critical weighing of mitigating and/or exacerbating patient factors that are essential for sound clinical decision making. The genetic revolution has led to the new paradigm of "individualized medicine" in patient care. True individualization in therapy however, will occur only when genetics are fully integrated with all the factors, like active pathology, that currently cause variability, including DDIs. Unfortunately, we are still a long distance from that goal.

We feel the best approach to the current state of drug event and drug interaction software is to consider that acquiring fluency about drug–drug interactions is like urgently needing to learn a second language because one finds oneself suddenly living in an increasingly bilingual world. It is far better to immerse oneself in the culture of France in order to learn to speak French than it is to try to learn the language by having conversations in French that are hampered by laboriously looking up each word, one at a time. This book is designed to be a critical tool in your DDI "language immersion" process.

In summary, for better or worse, our best defense against the silent epidemic of DDIs is a well-trained, aware, and conscientious clinician who devotes specific attention to the issue of DDIs on behalf of every single patient they treat, and general attention to the subject at large. So review the vignettes, scan the tables, immerse yourself in the **Fatal Forty**, and ownership of this domain will come your way. Your patients may never know the difference, but your thanks will come in the form of decreased morbidity and mortality, and improved outcomes as well.

Take-Home Points

- Software drug–drug interaction programs are generally a necessary but not sufficient component in the mastery of DDIs.
- The sensitivity and specificity of the commercial and chart DDI software programs are often inversely proportional.
- Clinicians using these programs must be aware of, and guard against, alert fatigue.
- The editors recommend that you use commercial DDI programs much as you would use a foreign language dictionary—as a reference source, but not the sole resource for living in a foreign country. In other words, take time to actually learn and work towards fluency in the DDI language!

References

1. Weingart SN, Simchowitz B, Shiman L, et al. Clinicians' assessments of electronic medication safety alerts in ambulatory care. Arch Intern Med. 2009;169(17):1627–32.
2. Weingart SN, Simchowitz B, Padolsky H, et al. An empirical model to estimate the potential impact of medication safety alerts on patient safety, health care utilization, and cost in ambulatory care. Arch Intern Med. 2009;169(16):1465–73.
3. Isaac T, Weissman JS, Davis RB, et al. Overrides of medication alerts in ambulatory care. Arch Intern Med. 2009;169(3):305–11.
4. Bliss JP, Gilson RD, Deaton JE. Human probability matching behaviour in response to alarms of varying reliability. Ergonomics. 1995;38(11):2300–12.
5. Smithburger PL, Buckley MS, Bejian S, et al. A critical evaluation of clinical decision support for the detection of drug-drug interactions. Expert Opin Drug Saf. 2011;10(6):871–82.
6. Horn JH, Hansten, PD. Customization of drug interaction software: caution is warranted. Pharmacy Times; 2011. http://www.pharmacytimes.com/publications/issue/2011/August2011/Customization-of-Drug-Interaction-Software. Last Accessed on 17 Sept 2012.

Pharmacogenomics 18

Chad D. Moore PhD, William Hartman MD, PhD,
Michael P. Hutchens MD, and Randal O. Dull MD, PhD

Abstract
This chapter discusses the essential terms and concepts of drug–gene interactions or how genetics affect pharmacology. This subset of pharmacology is also known as pharmacogenomics.

Since the inception of pharmacology, it has been acknowledged that different patients respond differently to the same medication. While many non-genetic factors (i.e., age, weight, organ function, concomitant therapy, etc.) can influence how a patient reacts to medication, the existence of large population variability is consistent with genetic factors as the major determinant of drug response. In fact, it is estimated that genetics are responsible for 20% to 95% of the variability observed in a drug's pharmacokinetics and pharmacodynamics.[1] Consideration of this inter-patient variability in drug response is critical in the clinical setting, as pharmaceuticals are one of the most common causes of adverse events, resulting in morbidity, mortality, and increased cost of treatment. In 1994, it was estimated that even when drugs were appropriately administered, over 2.2 million hospitalized patients suffered severe adverse drug reactions (ADRs), and over 100,000 had fatal ADRs, making ADRs between the fourth and sixth leading cause of death in the United States.[2]

C.D. Moore PhD (✉)
Department of Pharmacology and Toxicology, University of Utah,
Salt Lake City, UT, USA
e-mail: chad.moore@pharm.utah.edu

W. Hartman MD, PhD
Department of Anesthesiology, Mayo Clinic, Rochester, MN, USA

M.P. Hutchens MD
Department of Anesthesiology & Perioperative Medicine,
Oregon Health & Science University, Portland, OR, USA

R.O. Dull MD, PhD
Department of Anesthesiology, University of Illinois at Chicago, Chicago, IL, USA

C. Marcucci et al. (eds.), *A Case Approach to Perioperative Drug-Drug Interactions*, DOI 10.1007/978-1-4614-7495-1_18

Recognition that specific genetic variants were responsible for differences in drug effects began as early as the 1950s, giving rise to the field of pharmacogenetics.[3,4] However, today the field has evolved into a genome-wide approach that explores inherited variations in genes that dictate drug response and investigates the ways these variations can be used to predict patient's drug response. This genome-wide approach is what is now referred to as pharmacogenomics (although the two terms are currently used synonymously). The development of this field has challenged the previous notion of one drug and dose fits all, with the promise of a more individualized approach to drug therapy. The essential clinical benefit of pharmacogenomics is the ability to predict a patient's drug response prior to administration, thereby preventing possible ADRs, improving drug therapy and improving overall therapeutic outcome.

How Genetics Affect Pharmacology

To understand the utility of pharmacogenomics, it is important to understand how genetics can affect the therapeutic action of a drug. A drug's pharmacokinetic action is dependent on the absorption, distribution, metabolism, and elimination (ADME) of the compound. Proteins such as membrane transporters and metabolizing enzymes control the ADME of every drug, determining the concentrations of drug at the site of action at different points in time. Once at the target, the interaction of the drug with the receptor results in the pharmacodynamic action of the compound. This combination of pharmacokinetics and pharmacodynamics controls the therapeutic outcome for all drugs, and the proteins that ultimately determine these factors are regulated by a patient's genome.

Every human is born with a unique DNA sequence inherited from our parents, which encodes that person's genome. This sequence is comprised of the four nucleotides adenosine (A), thymine (T), guanine (G), and cytosine (C), which carry the messages to construct specific proteins in the following process. Select portions of a DNA sequence, that encode information for specific genes, are transcribed into pre-messenger RNA (pre-mRNA). The pre-mRNA is further processed by splicing-out non-coding regions of RNA (introns), leaving only the coding regions of RNA (exons), which are spliced together to form mature mRNA. The structures of proteins are encoded in mRNA by three nucleotide units (codons), which correlate to specific amino acids. Specialized protein aggregations, called ribosomes, translate these codons to form chains of amino acids that ultimately form proteins. This highly organized and controlled process results in the production of every protein found in an individual's body.

With the completion of the Human Genome Project, it was discovered that despite the human genome containing roughly three million base pairs, only 1.1% of the DNA was comprised of exons, while introns accounted for 24% and inter-genic

DNA spanned the remaining 75% of the genome.[5] Furthermore, despite the size of the genome, interpersonal variation in DNA sequences are relatively rare, with only one nucleotide differing for every 1000 to 2000 bases.[6] When these variations occur in more than 1% of the population, they are classified as "polymorphisms," while less common variations are classified as "mutations" or "rare inborn errors." The most common variations result from single nucleotide polymorphisms (SNPs, pronounced "snips"), which are single-base variants in a DNA sequence. Over 1.4 million SNPs have been identified in the human genome. The vast majority of these SNPs are found in the non-coding and intronic regions of DNA and they usually have no functional consequences; they are therefore known as "silent" SNPs. However, non-coding segments of DNA can contain promoter regions that control the expression of various genes. SNPs found within these promoter regions can result in increased or decreased protein expression. Similarly, SNPs found within intronic DNA can produce changes in the splicing of pre-mRNA, resulting in truncated, nonfunctioning proteins. Relatively fewer SNPs (approximately 60,000) are found within the coding regions of DNA. SNPs within an exon result in an altered codon, which encodes for a specific amino acid. In some cases these altered codons will still encode for the proper amino acid, known a "synonymous substitution," resulting in a normal protein. Conversely, "non-synonymous" SNPs results in codons that change an amino acid; with the outcome of this substitution being a change in protein structure or function.

Despite SNPs being a relatively small change, they have been associated with clinically relevant changes in the pharmacological action of various drugs. Consequences of SNPs have been linked to 1) decreased clearance of drugs, leading to "functional overdose"; 2) rapid clearance of drugs, resulting in loss of efficacy; 3) failure to convert prodrugs to active compounds; 4) altered pharmacodynamics; and 5) idiosyncratic toxicities. In this chapter, we focus on therapeutic consequences of various SNPs. This chapter is not meant to be a comprehensive review, but rather to provide relevant examples to illustrate the utility of pharmacogenomics as a molecular diagnostic method to improve drug therapy.

Metabolism

One of the first examples of the utility of pharmacogenetics involves a protein well known to anesthesiologists, butyrylcholinesterase (BCHE).[7] This enzyme is responsible for the hydrolysis of ester-containing compounds such as the neuromuscular blocking drugs (succinylcholine and mivacurium) and local anesthetics (procaine, chloroprocaine, and cocaine). Succinylcholine is rapidly metabolized and inactivated by BCHE, which accounts for its short half-life of approximately 1 to 3 minutes. However, it has been well documented that in some individuals a typical dose of succinylcholine results in prolonged muscle paralysis. Various polymorphisms in the coding region of the BCHE gene have since been identified, and account for this prolonged paralysis. The most frequent SNPs of BCHE are the atypical and Kalow variants, which describe the nucleotide substitution of A with G at position 209, and of G with A at position 1615, respectively. These substitutions result in amino acid changes from aspartic acid to glycine at codon 70, and from alanine to threonine at codon 539, respectively. Both variants are associated with BCHE enzymes that have decreased ability to hydrolyze succinylcholine, producing prolonged muscle relaxation.[8]

Cytochrome P450 (CYP) enzymes are a superfamily of microsomal drug-metabolizing enzymes that catalyze the vast majority of Phase I drug metabolism. As the primary metabolizers of clinically relevant drugs, polymorphisms found within the genes of CYPs can have profound effects on drug therapy and potential ADRs. A specific enzyme in this family, CYP2D6, is one of the most extensively studied and classic examples of pharmacogenetics in drug metabolism.[9] CYP2D6 is of particular interest because it metabolizes numerous drugs as diverse as codeine, dextromethorphan, propranolol, nortriptyline, and tramadol. Furthermore, to date, 85 different variants have been described for this one gene (www.cypalleles.ki.se). These polymorphisms greatly influence the enzyme's metabolic efficiency, resulting in patients being classified into four major phenotypes: 1) poor metabolizers, subjects with little to no enzyme activity; 2) intermediate metabolizers, subjects with decreased enzyme activity; 3) extensive metabolizers, subjects with a normal range of 2D6 activity; and 4) ultra-rapid metabolizers, subjects with multiple copies of the *CYP2D6* gene, resulting in greater than normal enzyme activity. Identification of a patient's 2D6 genotype would greatly enhance the ability to predict the metabolism of various drugs used in the pre-, intra-, and postoperative setting.

With the high incident rate of cardiovascular disease in America, patients undergoing ß-blocker therapy are commonly encountered in the clinical setting. Patients with the 2D6 poor metabolizer genotype demonstrate decreased clearance of ß blockers, such as metoprolol and propranolol, leading to an increase in their pharmacodynamic effects, and potential ADRs.[10] In the case of metoprolol, patients with the CYP2D6 ultrarapid metabolizer genotype have approximately 100% greater clearance of metoprolol compared to rapid metabolizers (see Chap. 127, "**Too Slow To Flow**").

CYP2D6 poor metabolizers demonstrate poorer clearance of the R-enantiomer of carvedilol (an α-receptor antagonist and ß-receptor antagonist), leading to a much greater alpha-blockade than would otherwise be predicted.[11] As this is becoming a popular adjunct in the treatment of heart failure, the implications of 2D6 isozyme variation in patients treated with carvedilol undergoing anesthesia could be dramatic. Ondansetron is also at least partly metabolized by 2D6 and 2D6 ultrarapid metabolizers are thought to metabolize the medication too quickly to gain a therapeutic benefit from the drug. In these cases, the appropriate response is not to administer more ondansetron, but to change the therapeutic approach altogether (see also Chap. 162, "**Bounce Back**").[12]

The ultra-rapid metabolizer genotype and phenotype can have a profound effect on the efficacy of normally benign prodrugs. Codeine and tramadol are both prodrugs that are converted via CYP2D6 to the active analgesic opioid receptor agonists morphine and *O*-desmethyltramadol, respectively. While standard dosages of these compound usually result in mild analgesia and central nervous system depression, 2D6 ultrarapid metabolizers have been shown to have serious ADRs, such as respiratory depression, with even small dosages (see also Chap. 63, "**Too Much of a Good Thing**").[13,14] Conversely, patients who are 2D6 poor metabolizers exhibit limited conversion of codeine and tramadol to their active metabolites, and they will therefore be more likely to provide beneficial analgesia. Prior knowledge of a patient's 2D6 genotype would allow alteration of dosage or substitution of medication to prevent ADRs and optimize therapy.

The commonly prescribed vitamin K antagonist warfarin is a CYP2C9 substrate. At least two CYP2C9 variants exist, with alleles designated as *CYP2C9*2* and *CYP2C9*3* respectively. The presence of either of those alleles in an individual can greatly decrease warfarin clearance, and patients with these polymorphisms are much more likely to experience excessive anticoagulation and bleeding.[15] Warfarin's genomics are complex however, as the activity of the drug is also dependent on the effectiveness of vitamin K epoxide reductase (VKORC1).[16] Studies have demonstrated that approximately 25% of the coumadin variability can be attributed to the presence of a single nucleotide polymorphism (SNP) present in this gene. Together, variations of CYP2C9 and VKORC1 have significant implications for perioperative care and complications. 2C9 is also an important metabolizer of the popular nonsteroidal anti-inflammatory drug (NSAID) celecoxib (Celebrex®), a cyclooxygenase-2 inhibitor. Known genetic polymorphisms in the *CYP2C9* gene lead to an inability of this enzyme to effectively metabolize this drug. The result is a dramatic increase in drug plasma levels, and has lead to a manufacturer drug information warning to use caution when administering celecoxib to "poor metabolizers of CYP2C9 substrates."[17]

A final example in which the pharmacokinetics of a drug commonly used to anesthetize patients is influenced by an individual's genome is that of propofol. For some individuals, a very small propofol dose can produce profound sedation. These patients likely have a "functional polymorphism" in the gene for the propofol metabolizing enzyme, CYP2B6.[18] This polymorphism, which carries a frequency of homozygous carriers in the Caucasian population of approximately 2%, leads to reduced CYP2B6 activity, and thus enhanced propofol action.

Transporters

Transport proteins play an important role in the pharmacokinetics of drugs because they regulate the absorption, distribution, and excretion of drugs and their metabolites. Because these transporters are one of the major factors controlling the duration and concentrations of drugs at their sites of action, polymorphisms that alter the functioning of these proteins can have profound effects on a compound's therapeutic outcome. The ATP-binding cassette (ABC) family of membrane transporters is one of the most important families of transporters involved in drug distribution. Of the 49 known human ABC transporters, P-glycoprotein (encoded by the *ABCB1* gene, also called *MDR1*) is the most recognized, due to its wide tissue distribution throughout the body, and its role in transporting a wide array of compounds, including digoxin, quinine, vinblastine, dexamethasone, cyclosporine, and loperamide. One of the most important functions of P-glycoprotein is to prevent the accumulation of xenobiotics in the brain through efflux of compound across the blood–brain barrier. Of importance to anesthesiologists, P-glycoprotein is a major determinant of opioid bioavailability in the brain, thereby affecting systemic analgesia. A SNP in the *ABCB1* gene (substitution of C with T at position 3435) has been associated with decreased expression of P-glycoprotein. Patients with this polymorphism have demonstrated increase concentrations of P-glycoprotein substrates, such as digoxin and morphine, in their cerebrospinal fluid.[9,14] Although clinical significance of this polymorphism remains uncertain, it demonstrates the ability of transporter polymorphisms to effect the ADME of relevant compounds.

Receptors

While polymorphisms of drug metabolizing enzymes and transporters affect the concentration of drug at the target, genetic variation within the targets (i.e., receptors) can have profound effects on drug efficacy. Severe pain can be therapeutically addressed with opioid analgesics that act through the opioid receptors. The majority of clinically relevant opioid analgesics work through the μ_1-opioid receptor (encoded by the *OPRM1* gene). The *OPRM1* gene has been shown to have several polymorphisms that result in meaningful functional consequences.[19,20] One of the most common *OPRM1* SNPs (10.5%-18.8% allelic frequency) is the nucleotide substitution of A with G at position 118, resulting in an amino acid change from asparagine to aspartate at codon 40.[21] Patients who are carriers (heterozygous) for this polymorphism were found to require higher dosages of analgesics (i.e., alfentanil and morphine) to obtain pain relief than non-carriers of this SNP. Interestingly, carriers of this SNP were also found to tolerate the higher plasma levels of opioids, without increases in opioid toxicities or side effects, such as nausea and vomiting. Therefore, while this SNP requires an increase in opioid demand to achieve therapeutic analgesia, it may also broaden the therapeutic index of opioid analgesics.[22]

The β_2-receptor, a site of action for some ß-agonist drugs, is coded by the gene *ADBR2*, a gene associated with significant variability. Polymorphisms in the *ADBR2* gene produce a β_2-receptor that can be more or less sensitive to therapy leading to differences in bronchodilation.[23] Oddly, however, the same polymorphism associated with bronchoconstriction is associated with increased survival in trauma patients.[24] Both factors may be of use to future anesthesia providers attempting to tailor care to individual patients.

Although we have discussed a few significant pharmacogenomically influenced anesthesia agents, it is important to remember that this field is relatively new, and additional data should be expected. Additional anesthetic/pharmacogenetic data are emerging regarding metabolism of midazolam (extensive metabolism via variant CYP3A5), local anesthetics (sodium channel variations and metabolism via CYP3A4) and volatile agents (variation in GABA receptors and melanocortin receptor 1).[25,26] The latter variation in volatile agent effect correlated with the same melanocortin-1 variant that produces red hair has received extensive press coverage.[27] It should be expected that public interest in the potential of pharmacogenomics will only increase; thus our attention to this field is vital.

Take-Home Points

- It has long been recognized that variations of specific genes can affect the pharmacology of a drug, giving rise to the field of pharmacogenetics. However, because the therapeutic effects of drugs are determined by the interplay of various genes (i.e., those coding for transporters, receptors, and metabolizing enzymes), the ability to characterize the polygenic determinants is advantageous in predicting a drug's therapeutic outcome.

- With the advances in human genomics and completion of the Human Genome Project, the ability to use a genome-wide approach to individualize a patient's drug therapy is rapidly becoming more realistic.

- Currently, individualization of therapy based on genomics is only reasonable for very few drugs, due to the costs of genetic mapping and our limited knowledge of functionally important polymorphisms. Currently, genotyping is done most commonly for the CYP2D6 and CYP2C19 isozymes.

- However, genotyping techniques are rapidly improving to the point where it is possible to screen for a panel of thousands of SNPs in genes that affect ADME and pharmacodynamics.

- As our knowledge of functionally relevant polymorphisms continues to advance through research, the practicality of pharmacogenomics in widespread clinical practice will only continue to increase.

References

1. Kalow W, Tang BK, Endrenyi L. Hypothesis: comparisons of inter- and intra-individual variations can substitute for twin studies in drug research. Pharmacogenetics. 1998;8:283–9.
2. Lazarou J, Pomeranz BH, Corey PN. Incidence of adverse drug reactions in hospitalized patients: a meta-analysis of prospective studies. JAMA. 1998;279:1200–5.
3. Kalow W. Familial incidence of low pseudocholinesterase level. Lancet. 1956;268:576–7.
4. Evans DA, Manley KA, McKusick VA. Genetic control of isoniazid metabolism in man. Br Med J. 1960;2:485–91.
5. Venter JC, Adams MD, Myers EW, et al. The sequence of the human genome. Science. 2001;291:1304–51.
6. Sachidanandam R, Weissman D, Schmidt SC, et al. A map of human genome sequence variation containing 1.42 million single nucleotide polymorphisms. Nature. 2001;409: 928–33.
7. Kalow W, Maykut MO. The interaction between cholinesterases and a series of local anesthetics. J Pharmacol Exp Ther. 1956;116:418–32.
8. Levano S, Ginz H, Siegemund M, et al. Genotyping the butyrylcholinesterase in patients with prolonged neuromuscular block after succinylcholine. Anesthesiology. 2005;102:531–5.
9. Johansson I, Ingelman-Sundberg M. Genetic polymorphism and toxicology–with emphasis on cytochrome p450. Toxicol Sci. 2011;120:1–13.
10. Zhou SF. Polymorphism of human cytochrome P450 2D6 and its clinical significance: part II. Clin Pharmacokinet. 2009;48:761–804.
11. Zhou HH, Wood AJ. Stereoselective disposition of carvedilol is determined by CYP2D6. Clin Pharmacol Ther. 1995;57:518–24.
12. Candiotti KA, Birnbach DJ, Lubarsky DA, et al. The impact of pharmacogenomics on postoperative nausea and vomiting: do CYP2D6 allele copy number and polymorphisms affect the success or failure of ondansetron prophylaxis? Anesthesiology. 2005;102:543–9.
13. Gasche Y, Daali Y, Fathi M, et al. Codeine intoxication associated with ultrarapid CYP2D6 metabolism. N Engl J Med. 2004;351:2827–31.
14. Stamer UM, Stuber F, Muders T, et al. Respiratory depression with tramadol in a patient with renal impairment and CYP2D6 gene duplication. Anesth Analg. 2008;107:926–9.
15. Joffe HV, Xu R, Johnson FB, Longtine J, Kucher N, Goldhaber SZ. Warfarin dosing and cytochrome P450 2C9 polymorphisms. Thromb Haemost. 2004;91(6):1123–8.
16. Sconce EA, Khan TI, Wynne HA, et al. The impact of CYP2C9 and VKORC1 genetic polymorphism and patient characteristics upon warfarin dose requirements: proposal for a new dosing regimen. Blood. 2005;106:2329–33.
17. Pfizer: Celebrex Drug Information. Chicago
18. Court MH, Duan SX, Hesse LM, Venkatakrishnan K, Greenblatt DJ. Cytochrome P-450 2B6 is responsible for interindividual variability of propofol hydroxylation by human liver microsomes. Anesthesiology. 2001;94:110–9.
19. Hoffmeyer S, Burk O, von Richter O, et al. Functional polymorphisms of the human multidrug-resistance gene: multiple sequence variations and correlation of one allele with P-glycoprotein expression and activity in vivo. Proc Natl Acad Sci U S A. 2000;97:3473–8.
20. Meineke I, Freudenthaler S, Hofmann U, et al. Pharmacokinetic modelling of morphine, morphine-3-glucuronide and morphine-6-glucuronide in plasma and cerebrospinal fluid of neurosurgical patients after short-term infusion of morphine. Br J Clin Pharmacol. 2002;54: 592–603.
21. Skarke C, Kirchhof A, Geisslinger G, et al. Comprehensive mu-opioid-receptor genotyping by pyrosequencing. Clin Chem. 2004;50:640–4.
22. Lotsch J, Geisslinger G. Are mu-opioid receptor polymorphisms important for clinical opioid therapy? Trends Mol Med. 2005;11:82–9.
23. Taylor DR, Hall IP. ADRB2 polymorphisms and beta2 agonists. Lancet. 2007;370:2075–6.
24. Morris Jr JA, Norris PR, Moore JH, et al. Genetic variation in the autonomic nervous system affects mortality: a study of 1,095 trauma patients. J Am Coll Surg. 2009;208(5):663–8.

25. Cohen M, Sadhasivam S, Vinks AA. Pharmacogenetics in perioperative medicine. Curr Opin Anaesthesiol. 2012;25(4):419–27.
26. Chidambaran V, Ngamprasertwong P, Vinks AA, et al. Pharmacogenetics and anesthetic drugs. Curr Clin Pharmacol. 2012;7(2):78–101.
27. Liem EB, Lin CM, Suleman MI, et al. Anesthetic requirement is increased in redheads. Anesthesiology. 2004;101(2):279–83.

The Pharmacoepidemiology of Drug Interactions: Why and How They Are Important

19

Joseph A. Lovely PharmD, BCPS, Stephen Esper MD, MBA, Michael P. Hutchens MD, Wayne T. Nicholson MD, PharmD, MSc, and Catherine Marcucci MD

Abstract
This chapter discusses the pharmacoepidemiology of drug–drug interactions—how, why, and when clinicians encounter DDIs.

When contemplating the drug-drug interaction (DDI) universe, four questions naturally arise: Are DDIs important? Is this something I actually need to worry about? In what ways might I encounter DDIs in my practice? How do I begin to identify and deal with them?

J.A. Lovely PharmD, BCPS (✉)
Department of Pharmacy Services, St. Marys Hospital, Mayo Clinic, Rochester, MN, USA
e-mail: Lovely.Joseph@mayo.edu

S. Esper MD, MBA
Department of Anesthesiology, University of Pittsburgh Medical Center, Pittsburgh, PA, USA

M.P. Hutchens MD
Department of Anesthesiology & Perioperative Medicine, Oregon Health & Science University, Portland, OR, USA

W.T. Nicholson MD, PharmD, MSc
Department of Anesthesiology, Mayo Clinic, Rochester, MN, USA

C. Marcucci MD
Anesthesia Services Department, Philadelphia Veterans Affairs Medical Center, Philadelphia, PA, USA

C. Marcucci et al. (eds.), *A Case Approach to Perioperative Drug-Drug Interactions*, DOI 10.1007/978-1-4614-7495-1_19

The answers to the first two questions are easy: Yes, you **do** have to worry about this and yes, DDIs **are** important because they are part and parcel of a major public health initiative—the enhancement of patient safety and welfare by the elimination of medical errors.

Drug safety is a significant component of the overall patient safety movement. This in turn is based on the science of pharmacoepidemiology—the study of the use and effects of drugs in large numbers of people. One focus of pharmacoepidemiology is the study of adverse effects suffered by patients when they use therapeutic drugs.[1] These adverse effects can result from medication errors, adverse drug reactions, and adverse drug events. None of these terms precisely defines a DDI in the sense we are using it in this book. DDIs are not a subset of adverse drug reactions, rather if DDIs are severe enough and/or go unremedied, they become the *cause* of them.

For a number of reasons, the epidemiology of DDIs is complex and the true incidence of DDIs remains unknown.[2–5] Fortunately, we are learning about the incidence of adverse drug reactions and adverse drug events and it is often possible to infer what proportion of these are DDI-related.[6]

Adverse drug reactions and adverse drug events are common, costly, and cause a significant morbidity and mortality.[7,8] For example, in 2007, the Institute of Medicine estimated that between 380,000 and 450,000 preventable adverse drug reactions occur annually.[9] It has been reported that an estimated 5.3% of hospital admissions were due to an adverse drug reaction.[10,20] Adverse drug reactions are also costly: A 1997 study reported that an adverse drug reaction increased the cost of a hospitalization by $5,857. Assuming 400,000 preventable adverse drug reactions occurred in 2006 in the United States, the total cost of adverse drug reactions for that year was $3.5 billion.[9] Unfortunately, patients admitted to hospitals for reasons other than drug or medication events incur adverse drug reaction-related injuries as well. In hospitalized patients, drug complications were the most common type of adverse event (19%) in a review of disabling injuries caused by medical treatment.[11] Also, a recent study of community hospital patients found an incidence of adverse drug events of 1.1% of hospitalized patients.[12] Tragically, adverse drug reactions are a significant cause of mortality, and may rank as high as fourth among the leading causes of in-hospital death.[12] A meta-analysis of 39 studies revealed the incidence of serious adverse drug reactions at 6.7%, with more than 2 million US patients affected in 1994.[13] Of those patients, 106,000 (0.32%) had fatal adverse drug reactions.

Using these data, we can make some sobering inferences about DDIs. For example, DDIs account for at least 3% to 5% of in-hospital medication errors.[14] Since a 1995 study found that 3% of 264 studied adverse drug events were caused by DDIs and there are 36 million hospital discharges per year in the US, a conservative estimate of the incidence of DDI-linked adverse drug reactions suggests there are at least 110,000 per year in the US that reach the level of detection of harm and are elucidated as true DDIs.[14,15] Since DDIs are often unrecognized, the incidence is surely higher.

Anesthesiologists encounter DDIs in two ways—those they "inherit" due to patients' preexisting medical conditions and medications, and those that are potentially caused in the perioperative period due to several unique aspects of our practice.

As for DDIs that are unwittingly passed on to us from the outpatient prescribers, the data are sobering. For example, a study of retail pharmacies in Norway showed that, for 15% to 20% of patients, commonly prescribed medications that inhibit CYP3A4 and C2D6 were co-prescribed with medications metabolized by those enzymes.[16] Specific DDIs are also associated with identified patient cohorts. For instance, patients with hepatic cirrhosis are known to have a high incidence of potential DDIs (21%), and 13% of these DDIs resulted in harm to the patient (adverse drug reaction). Use of agents with primary hepatic clearance, as well as impaired renal function, increased the risk for adverse drug reactions, and the drugs most commonly associated with DDIs were angiotensin-converting enzyme inhibitors, nonsteroidal anti-inflammatory drugs, diuretics, and anticoagulants. In another study at a US Veterans hospital, researchers identified at least one clinically significant drug interaction in 83% of younger patients and 89% of older patients at an HIV-specialty clinic where most patients have both antiretroviral and nonantiretroviral DDIs.[17] Perhaps predictably, younger patients had more DDIs involving antihistamine, corticosteroid, hormonal, and erectile dysfunction agents, whereas older patients had DDIs involving antihypertensive and antidiabetic agents. Similarly, Miller et al. found that 42% of HIV clinic patients had at least one DDI requiring dosage adjustment, discontinuation of a medication, or both.[18] Independent risk factors for clinically significant DDIs were 1) age older than 42 years; 2) more than three comorbid conditions; 3) more than three antiretroviral agents; and 4) treatment with a protease inhibitor.

There is also abundant evidence of the presence of potential DDIs in inpatient settings of all types. A large review of adverse drug reactions in hospital patients found that 17% were due to DDIs, thus suggesting that the huge number of adverse drug reactions in hospital patients is significantly driven by DDIs.[19] Reimche et al. evaluated all adult admissions to a Canadian teaching hospital and found potential DDIs in 19% of patients, with increased risk ratio for DDIs of approximately 1.5 associated with admission to a medical or surgical service.[20]

A review of DDIs leading to adverse drug reactions in oncology patients, many of whom are also perioperative patients, found that 2% of unplanned admissions were due to DDIs and that one-third of oncology patients had documentary evidence of a potential DDI, with the most likely DDI combinations involving warfarin, antihypertensives, and anticonvulsants.[21] Clearly, these data demonstrate that DDIs are neither uncommon nor insignificant. Even if our personal practices were flawless and we ourselves never undertook any action that resulted in a clinically significant DDI, we would need to exercise continuous vigilance to identify and treat the consequences of the DDIs visited upon us when we undertake the care of referred patients.

How do patients entering the perioperative period incur the risk for potential "new" DDIs? We believe there are four significant factors.

First, drugs and other therapies are stopped and started in the perioperative period. It is pretty easy to understand how this happens. For example, well-meaning primary care providers adjust hypertensive and diabetic medications (both classes of drugs are members of the **Fatal Forty**) when patients go in for preoperative evaluations and "medical optimization." Surgeons prescribe preoperative courses of antibiotics. Analgesic use, both prescription and over-the-counter, increases as patients try to deal with illnesses and injuries. Bowel preps are undertaken. Patients get on the Internet to research dietary and naturopathic strategies to strengthen immune systems, mitigate symptoms, and then start taking herbs and supplements they have read or heard about. Coagulation modifiers such as aspirin, clopidogrel, and warfarin are stopped. Stringent diets of all types are started. And, of course, patterns of smoking, alcohol, and recreational drug use does not stay constant—patients either use less in an attempt to quit before surgery or use more due to anxiety or fear of the upcoming lack of access.

Second, there is acute-on-chronic administration of drugs in the perioperative period. Look for a moment at the Table of Contents of this book. The array of drugs and drug classes we work with every day is truly impressive. Yes, the psychiatrists and the neurologists work with amitriptyline and phenytoin, and the cardiologists work with amiodarone and metoprolol. But these clinicians do not also work with lidocaine, isoflurane, and rocuronium.

Third, there is a veritable "witch's brew" of medications given in the intensive care unit (ICU). ICU physicians practice at a special and rare location on the pharmacological spectrum. The ICU drugs are all potent and most are given intravenously—antibiotics, amiodarone, digoxin, vasopressors, vasodilators, total parenteral nutrition, sedatives, opioids, immunosuppressants, neuromuscular blockers, IV anesthetics, calcium channel blockers, and the list goes on. The potential for DDIs is enormous and will surely trip up the inattentive or unprepared provider. And of course, remember that the debilitated nature of ICU patients almost certainly is an additional risk factor facing providers trying to keep patients safe from the effects of unintended DDIs.

Fourth, the chronic pain practice setting provides many opportunities to encounter and commit DDIs. There is a robust overlap between the chronic pain, addiction, psychiatric, and neurology patient cohorts. The physicians for these very deserving patients utilize a common medication panel that is heavily represented on the **Fatal Forty**—amitriptyline and other tricyclic antidepressants, methadone, buprenorphine, phenytoin, carbamazepine, cyclobenzaprine, phenobarbital, and methadone. Add to this pharmacologic mix ritonavir and smoking tobacco (both members of the ***Fatal Forty***), and it is not surprising that one study found that patients with non cancer chronic pain were found to have a 26% incidence for potential DDIs (in this population, surprisingly, *younger* patients had a slightly higher risk of potential DDIs than those older than 65 years of age, and middle-age patients (35 to 44 years of age) had the highest risk).[22]

How should we begin to identify and deal with perioperative DDIs? The answer is to know our drugs, look for and anticipate the interactions instead of waiting for them to find you, think about potential DDIs in every situation, and above all, ask questions, if you don't know or aren't sure. All practitioners have had the experience of taking care of a patient that doesn't do as well as expected and nobody can figure out why. Keep suspicions and vigilance for DDIs high in your assessments and differential diagnoses.

In the preceding chapters, we have presented our lists of the **Fatal Forty** and **Top Ten**, as well as reading lists for junior and senior anesthesia trainees. We also believe that dedicating time to learning how the core anesthetic drugs are metabolized, and further how each drug acts as a substrate and/or inhibitor, will amply repay the provider's efforts. This is really no different than learning the minimum alveolar concentration (MAC) of each volatile anesthetic or the equipotent dosages of the various opioids—tasks that are set and accepted by all anesthesia trainees and practitioners. To this end, we have created an appendix containing the editors' personal compilations of the enzymes where a number of the most common anesthetic drugs take action. These are the files on our personal desktops—each entry does not necessarily denote a proven or reported DDI, but rather represents the possibility of an interaction that may as yet be unreported or for which the pharmacogenomics are still being elucidated. We have also included below a short list of sources and resources, again from our personal files, which we believe are high in both accuracy and accessibility.

As we have noted elsewhere, we are on the crest of a wave of new information concerning both drug–drug interactions and drug–gene interactions. Of course, the interactions themselves are not new—they have been there all along. But we have now switched on the flashlight. Welcome to the club.

Recommended Sources for the Study of DDIs

Drug Interaction Principles for Medical Practice: Cytochrome P450s, UGTs, P-Glycoproteins. Kelly Cozza MD, Scott Armstrong MD, Jessica Oesterheld MD; American Psychiatric Publishing, Inc. 2003.

Principles of Drug Biotransformation by Evan Kharasch MD PhD in Anesthetic Pharmacology: Physiologic Principles and Clinical Practice. Alex Evers, Mervyn Maze, editors, Churchill Livingstone, 2004.

Drug Interactions Casebook: The Cytochrome P450 System and Beyond. Neil B. Sandson MD; American Psychiatric Publishing Inc. 2003.

Dr. Oesterheld's site is at: **http://www.mhc.com/Cytochromes**

Dr. Flockhart's site is at: **www.drug-interactions.com**

PubMed is at: www.ncbi.nlm.nih.gov/pubmed

The Physicians' Desk Reference online is at: www.pdr.net

Dr. Sandson's website is at: **www.druginteractionworld.com**

References

1. Strom BL, Kimmel SE. Textbook of Pharmacoepidemiology. West Sussex, UK: John Wiley & Sons; 2006.
2. Friedman MA, Woodcock J, Lumpkin MM, et al. The safety of newly approved medicines: do recent market removals mean there is a problem? JAMA. 1999;81:1728–34.
3. Figueiras A, Tato F, Fontaiñas J, et al. Influence of physicians' attitudes on reporting adverse drug events: a case-control study. Med Care. 1999;37:809–14.
4. Eland IA, Belton KJ, van Grootheest AC, et al. Attitudinal survey of voluntary reporting of adverse drug reactions. Br J Clin Pharmacol. 1999;48:623–7.
5. Chyka PA, McCommon SW. Reporting of adverse drug reactions by poison control centers in the US. Drug Saf. 2000;23:87–93.
6. Harmark L, van Grootheest AC. Pharmacovigilance: methods, recent developments and future perspectives. Eur J Clin Pharmacol. 2008;64:743–52.
7. Classen DC, Pestotnik SL, Evans RS, et al. Adverse drug events in hospitalized patients. Excess length of stay, extra costs, and attributable mortality. JAMA. 1997;277:301–6.
8. Phillips DP, Christenfeld N, Glynn LM. Increase in US medication-error deaths between 1983 and 1993. Lancet. 1998;351:643–4.
9. Committee on Identifying and Preventing Medication Errors, Board on Health Care Services; Aspden P, Wolcott JA, Bootman JL, Cronenwett LR, editors. Preventing medication errors: quality chasm series. Washington, DC, The National Academies Press, 2007. Available from: http://www.nap.edu/catalog/11623.html. Last accessed on 13 Sept 2012.
10. Raschetti R, Morgutti M, Menniti-Ippolito F, et al. Suspected adverse drug events requiring emergency department visits or hospital admissions. Eur J Clin Pharmacol. 1999;54:959–63.
11. Leape LL, Brennan TA, Laird N, et al. The nature of adverse events in hospitalized patients: results of the Harvard Medical Practice Study II. N Engl J Med. 1991;324:377–84.
12. Hug BL, Keohane C, Seger DL, et al. The costs of adverse drug events in community hospitals. Jt Comm J Qual Patient Saf. 2012;38(3):120–6.
13. Lazarou J, Pomeranz BH, Corey PN. Incidence of adverse drug reactions in hospitalized patients: a meta-analysis of prospective studies. JAMA. 1998;279:1200–5.
14. Leape LL, Bates DW, Cullen DJ, et al. Systems analysis of adverse drug events. JAMA. 1995;274:35–43.
15. Hospital Utilization in non-Federal Short Stay Hospitals. Centers for Disease Control Prevention. http://www.cdc.gov/nchs/fastats/hospital.htm. Last accessed 14 July 2012.
16. Molden E, Garcia BH, Braathen P. Co-prescription of cytochrome P450 2D6/3A4 inhibitor-substrate pairs in clinical practice: a retrospective analysis of data from Norwegian primary pharmacies. Eur J Clin Pharmacol. 2005;61:119–25.
17. Yiu P, Nguyen NN, Holodniy M. Clinically significant drug interactions in younger and older human immunodeficiency virus-positive patients receiving antiretroviral therapy. Pharmacotherapy. 2011;31(5):480–9.
18. Miller CD, El-Kholi R, Faragon JJ, Lodise TP. Prevalence and risk factors for clinically significant drug interactions with antiretroviral therapy. Pharmacotherapy. 2007;27(10):1379–86.
19. Krahenbuhl-Melcher A, Schlienger R, Lampert M, et al. Drug-related problems in hospitals: a review of the recent literature. Drug Saf. 2007;30:379–407.
20. Reimche L, Forster AJ, van Walraven C. Incidence and contributors to potential drug-drug interactions in hospitalized patients. J Clin Pharmacol. 2011;51(7):1043–50. Epub 2010 Oct 6.
21. Riechelmann RP, Del Giglio A. Drug interactions in oncology: how common are they? Ann Oncol. 2009;20(12):1907–12. Epub 2009 Aug 27.
22. Pergolizzi JV. Quantifying the impact of drug-drug interactions associated with opioids. Am J Manag Care. 2011;17 Suppl 11:S288–92.

The Lawyers Can Read, Too: Cases from the Courtroom

20

Jessica Voge MD and David K. Miller JD

Abstract
This chapter discusses three actual cases of serious patient injury and/or death resulting from drug–drug interactions and the outcome of the subsequent tort action.

Introduction

Lawyers and physicians often disagree—sometimes with fervor—about medical malpractice, but there can be no argument about the fact that medication errors occur often and can have catastrophic consequences. From stories in the common press[1] to studies published in the medical literature, commentators have correctly described the issue as one of global concern[1] *(see both footnote and reference, below)*. While the true incidence of medication errors is often disputed, and just as often a function of how "errors" are defined, there is no question that the incidence of true errors is much greater than the public expects. Therefore, the area is a prime one for malpractice claims and resulting payments by medical liability insurance carriers.

[1] Most notable examples: Actor Heath Ledger's death from the mixing of prescription drugs; actor Dennis Quaid's newborn twins receiving an adult dose of heparin; singer Michael Jackson's death from the ill-advised use of propofol).

J. Voge MD (✉)
Department of Obstetrics & Gynecology, Oregon Health and Science University, Portland, OR, USA
e-mail: voge@ohsu.edu

D.K. Miller JD
Miller & Wagner, LLP, Portland, OR, USA

C. Marcucci et al. (eds.), *A Case Approach to Perioperative Drug-Drug Interactions*, DOI 10.1007/978-1-4614-7495-1_20

There is very little dispute about why claims arising from medication errors often result in very high jury verdicts or favorable settlements for patients. Inherent in these claims is "system error" or simple inattention to detail. Malpractice claims involving the "second-guessing" of considered, informed physician judgments are generally unsuccessful before juries, but claims involving medication errors do not, by definition, involve one or more physicians engaging in considered judgment about whether to treat a patient this way or that way; whether to operate or not operate. Contrary to the claims of those who advocate stringent "tort reform," juries are exceptionally forgiving to physicians in such cases. However, the opposite is generally true when either an incorrect medication, a medication incompatible with other medications being taken by the patient, or an erroneous dose is administered. Juries will often "take out their frustrations" on a system that permits obvious errors that produce catastrophic results.

The following cases are examples of claims/lawsuits that involved medications used in combination with others either by mistake or ignorance. All of the cases resulted in awards to the patient or their family. Although damaging to the patient, such cases can also be devastating to providers. It is hoped these cases demonstrate situations from which the reader can learn, thus lessening the chance of similar mistakes occurring in the future.

Case #1: Really Tragic

This case involved the interaction of intraoperative Toradol® (ketorolac) with other nonsteroidal anti-inflammatory drugs (NSAIDs) in a spine surgery case.

A 32-year-old man, otherwise in good health and enjoying a very active lifestyle, was appropriately evaluated and determined to be in need of an anterior cervical diskectomy and fusion at C6-7. The patient was admitted by his neurosurgeon to a large, regional medical center. The record was in conflict as to the patient's preadmission use of NSAIDs for control of arm pain caused by his cervical disk; however, it later became very clear the patient had used a variety of NSAIDs for pain relief for months prior to his hospitalization. Intraoperatively, the neurosurgeon ordered Toradol® (30 mg IV) for postoperative analgesia. The surgery was uncomplicated and lasted 2 hours. The patient was admitted to the postanesthesia care unit (PACU). Over the course of an hour in the PACU the patient developed quadriplegia. The anesthesiologist was called first to the PACU and immediately notified the neurosurgeon, who arrived to the PACU shortly thereafter. The patient was evaluated, imaged, and returned to surgery. A large epidural hematoma was discovered to be compressing the patient's spinal cord. After evacuation of the hematoma, the patient recovered but with significant permanent neurological impairment of his left upper extremity.

Legal Issues/Result

There were numerous issues that gave rise to the litigation brought by the patient against the hospital and the anesthesiologist. Because the neurosurgeon was significantly critical of the PACU nurse for not summoning him to the unit sooner, he was not named as a defendant in the case. The central issue in the case involved the delay on the part of the PACU nurse in summoning the surgeon to the PACU when the patient showed signs of neurologic deficits while recovering. The cause of the hematoma and the role played by the patient's NSAID use preadmission, and the inconsistency in the record relating to the patient's history of NSAID use were key causation issues in the case.

The patient had been referred by his primary care physician to the neurosurgeon for consultation. After imaging and exam, the neurosurgeon recommended surgery. The patient had been taking NSAID medications for months prior to admission to the hospital. The surgeon's history and physical was silent as to the patient's NSAID use. The anesthesiologist's preoperative history form made only cursory mention of NSAID use. Depositions revealed conflicting testimony as to which physician bore responsibility for determining an accurate preoperative history of NSAID use and the degree to which that would have affected the choice to use intraoperative Toradol®. After the patient suffered his severe neurologic complication, however, the hematologist who consulted on the case took a very detailed history and documented enough NSAID use to raise serious questions about whether ketorolac should have been administered in the face of preoperative NSAID use. While the medical literature was replete with references to the potential for epidural bleeding from ketorolac alone, or in combination with other NSAIDs, it was less than clear whether the amounts and timing of the preoperative NSAIDs in combination with the Toradol® was a substantial cause of the epidural hematoma.

The case was settled short of trial for a substantial sum. The surgeon's criticism of the PACU nurse's delay in summoning him back to the PACU when the patient demonstrated neurological deficits was likely the key factor prompting settlement. The anesthesiologist was dismissed from the case without payment. The inaccuracies in the record relating to the patient's NSAID use, coupled with the dramatic nature of the postoperative hematoma, raised serious questions about whether "the left hand knew what the right hand was doing," a suspicion that can often cause a jury to be suspicious of the entire medical "team."

After the case was resolved, it was learned that the hospital and its surgery departments investigated the potential dangers of using ketorolac in spine cases, particularly when there was a history of use of other NSAID use by patients.

Case #2: Disaster After Day Surgery—Hydrocodone and Prednisone

A 40-year-old woman, somewhat overweight (BMI of 37.8), with known sleep apnea but otherwise healthy and active was referred by her primary care physician to an otolaryngologist for consultation regarding snoring, nasal obstruction, and obstructive sleep apnea. A sleep study had been performed and revealed significant apneic events (an AHI score of 77). The study was known by the otolaryngologist at the time of the consultation. On the day of the examination, the patient was suffering from an upper respiratory infection (the patient's primary care physician had previously prescribed a narcotic cough suppressant, which the patient had used). After examination, the surgeon recommended a nasoseptal reconstruction, a bilateral submucous reduction of the inferior turbinates, a tonsillectomy and an uvulectomy, in part because the patient had "failed CPAP." The surgery was recommended and approved by the patient's health insurer to be performed as a "day surgery." The surgery was uneventful, produced minimal bleeding, and considered successful. The patient was given one tablet/dose of prednisone following the surgery to help reduce postoperative inflammation and instructed to take another tablet the following morning at home. The patient was placed in a recovery suite to await discharge the evening of the surgery. Prior to discharge, the patient was given a prescription for hydrocodone/acetaminophen (Norco®, 325 mg capsules, one to two tablets to be taken every 3 hours, as needed for pain). The patient was discharged home in the care of her husband, who was a radiology technician at a neighboring hospital. The patient took—and the husband recorded—the hydrocodone/acetaminophen and prednisone as directed but, nonetheless, was in considerable pain. During the middle of the second night following discharge, the patient was found deceased by her husband while reclined in a semi-upright position. Autopsy revealed extensive swelling of the pharynx and toxicology revealed a level of hydrocodone within the reported "fatal range," albeit on the low end of the range (0.17 mg/L). The patient was otherwise opioid naive.

Legal Issues/Result

The patient's husband commenced a wrongful death action against the surgeon, which was settled for a substantial sum. A consulting forensic pathologist concluded the cause of death was related to the patient's loss of her airway due to narcotic suppression and swelling. The central issue in the case involved the combined use of hydrocodone with prednisone in a patient with known sleep apnea. A secondary issue was the decision on the part of the surgeon to perform an extensive, painful surgery on this patient without monitoring her oxygen level as an in-patient for at least 48 hours after surgery. Consulting experts criticized the surgeon's apparent lack of awareness of the "rebound effect" produced by steroids (swelling of tissues following an initial period of swelling reduction). Concern was also expressed about the choice of Norco® as a postoperative pain medication, given its relatively high concentration of hydrocodone. An issue underlying the case was the role of the health insurer in approving and, in fact, encouraging the surgical procedure to be performed as a "day surgery," thus contributing to the patient's lack of monitoring postoperatively, a process that would have likely saved her life.

Case #3: A Truly Awful Fentanyl Patch Outcome

A very healthy, active, and high wage-earning 38-year-old father of four young children was involved in a late-night single-car motor vehicle accident following a competitive soccer game. The patient was taken by ambulance to a local hospital at approximately midnight on the evening of the accident and found to have two rib fractures and a small scapular fracture. The patient was admitted by the hospital's "trauma service" and came under the care of a local surgeon. The decision was made to admit the patient for the balance of the night, treat his pain, and discharge him the following day. While in the hospital, the patient received two standard doses (4 mg IV) of morphine sulfate in the emergency department and hydromorphone (Dilaudid®) by PCA while in his hospital room. After consultation with an orthopedist, the surgeon ordered nursing staff to place a fentanyl patch (75 mcg) on the patient to help him control postinjury pain. A prescription was written for three more patches. The patient was opioid naive with absolutely no history of narcotic use prior to his one night admission to the hospital. It was later learned that the patient had a sleep study performed 2 years before this admission and had been found to have "mild sleep apnea" and prescribed continuous positive airway pressure (CPAP), which he rarely used. Prior to discharge, the patient was given two tablets of oxycodone/acetaminophen (Percocet®) by mouth and was discharged from the hospital at approximately 4:30 p.m. on the day following his admission. He traveled with his wife to the wrecking yard to view his vehicle, went home for a small meal, and retired on the couch in a semi-reclined position at approximately 9:00 p.m. The patient's wife was awakened by their barking dog at approximately 2:30 a.m. and found her husband deceased on the couch in the same position she had left him. The cause of death was "fentanyl intoxication." Toxicology revealed an amount of fentanyl in the patient's system nearly two times greater than he should have had with use of a 75-mcg patch. (The defense contended "post-mortem redistribution" was the cause, which plaintiff disputed.)

Legal Issues/Result

The patient's wife commenced a wrongful death action against the hospital, the physician who prescribed the fentanyl patch, and the patch manufacturer. All defendants contributed to a very substantial settlement in favor of the patient's surviving family. The thrust of the case against the surgeon was the decision to use a fentanyl patch in an obviously "opioid naive" patient, contrary to the manufacturer's recommendation. The claim against the hospital was that it failed to have systems in place that would alert—and prevent—the administration of a contraindicated drug to an inpatient. The claim against the manufacturer was that the warnings about the danger of the product were insufficient and that the patch delivered more fentanyl than it was supposed to, thus was defective.

The case demonstrated the importance of a hospital's independent duty to have safeguards in place to prevent—or at least provide another level of warning against—the administration of a contraindicated medication. The case also raised serious questions about the ordering of the so-called "pain patches" in circumstances that might be considered "off-label." The surgeon's defense was that the patient was going to be in long-term pain and would, therefore, ultimately be a patient who was not opioid naive, thus ordering the patch was consistent with the manufacturer's instructions. The manufacturer, of course, disagreed. The "finger-pointing" between the various defendants clearly contributed to the favorable result for the plaintiff.

Take-Home Points

- Medication interactions that are unanticipated can lead to disastrous and tragic outcomes for patients and their families.
- Medication errors and interactions can lead to malpractice litigation, which can be devastating and embarrassing to providers and the hospitals where they work.
- Although responsibility for patient care is sometimes shared (e.g., between the anesthesiologist, PACU nurse, and neurosurgeon) legal responsibility for errors is assigned during litigation.

Reference

1. Wheeler SJ, Wheeler DS. Medication errors in anesthesia and critical care. Anesthesia. 2005;60:257–73.

Drug–Drug Interactions Involving Inhalational Anesthetic Agents

IV

Introduction 21

Catherine Marcucci MD

Abstract
This introduces drug–drug interactions involving inhalational anesthetics.

The inhalational anesthetics are such a part and parcel of anesthesia practice that we take for granted that we have mastered their pharmacology. Right at the beginning of training, we learn the minimum alveolar concentration (MAC) of each anesthetic. We learn the effects of altitude on the delivery of the anesthetics and other facts regarding the use and maintenance of vaporizers. We listen to but don't concentrate on the folklore and historical anecdotes about each inhalational anesthetic. We listen to and do concentrate on the inhalational anesthetic preferences of our teachers and mentors. And then, confident we have achieved competency with these drugs, we become complacent in our use of them. Too often, as we are busy with the other many pressing aspects of learning and doing anesthesia, we are in serious risk of regarding the inhalational anesthetics simply as agents that we turn on and off or turn up and down. But this complacency is something of a mistake. Collectively, the editors have frequently seen problems occur in the operating room because of clinicians' failure to keep in mind that inhalational anesthetics are among the most potent drugs given in the perioperative period—and that they are often administered to patients on a panoply of other potent medications.

With this in mind, this section presents case scenarios covering a number of clinical situations. We have included the basics such the additive nature of MACs as well as discussing in more detail the interactions of inhalational anesthetics with several of the ubiquitous antihypertensive drugs and the interactions of inhalational anesthetics in patients having somatosensory evoked potential monitoring.

C. Marcucci MD
Anesthesia Services Department, Philadelphia Veterans Affairs Medical Center, Philadelphia, PA, USA
e-mail: sandson.marcucci@comcast.net

C. Marcucci et al. (eds.), *A Case Approach to Perioperative Drug-Drug Interactions*, DOI 10.1007/978-1-4614-7495-1_21

That Sums It Up

22

Inhalational anesthetics, additive minimum alveolar concentration (MAC)

James A. Jernigan MD and James W. Ibinson MD, PhD

Abstract
This case discusses the additive nature of the minimum alveolar concentration (MAC) for volatile anesthetics.

Case

On Monday, at 6:25 AM, an anesthesia resident was running late with his room setup for his 7 AM start for an elective surgical case under general anesthesia for an otherwise healthy college student. He performed an appropriate machine check-out, set up his airway equipment, and drew up his drugs, but did not have time to go back to the anesthesia workroom.

After an uncomplicated induction and intubation, the patient was started on isoflurane. Approximately 1 hour into the case, the anesthesia machine indicated "Low Isoflurane: Refill Reservoir." There was no additional isoflurane in the room. The resident called the anesthesia technician to request more isoflurane but the support personnel were all called to two simultaneous traumas and forgot about the request for isoflurane. The isoflurane became depleted.

J.A. Jernigan MD (✉)
Department of Anesthesia - PGY3, University of Pittsburgh Medical Center, Pittsburgh, PA, USA
e-mail: jerniganja@upmc.edu

J.W. Ibinson MD, PhD
Department of Anesthesiology, University of Pittsburgh School of Medicine, Pittsburgh, PA, USA

C. Marcucci et al. (eds.), *A Case Approach to Perioperative Drug-Drug Interactions*, DOI 10.1007/978-1-4614-7495-1_22

Instinctively, the resident changed to the sevoflurane vaporizer. After a few minutes, the sevoflurane end-tidal concentration was 1% and the isoflurane end-tidal concentration was still 1.1%. The gas analyzer displayed a minimum alveolar concentration (MAC) of 1.5%.

Discussion

This is an example of additive synergistic pharmacodynamic drug effects.

MACs of inhalational gases are additive.[1,2]

One MAC is the percent volume of expired inhalational anesthetic that prevents movement in 50% of patients to surgical stimulus. The MACs for desflurane, sevoflurane, isoflurane, and nitrous oxide are roughly 6%, 2%, 1.2%, and 105% respectively. Other MACs have been defined and determined as well. "MAC-awake" is the end-tidal anesthetic concentration at which 50% of patients respond to commands. It is widely believed that an end-tidal anesthetic concentration greater than the MAC-awake value will prevent patients from remembering intraoperative events. This value varies for each agent, but is approximately one-third of MAC for isoflurane, desflurane, and sevoflurane.[3] Like MAC, this value decreases with age, but not with opioids (at lower doses). Additionally, "MAC-BAR" is the concentration that blocks autonomic response to any surgical stimulation. This is approximately 1.3 (for isoflurane and desflurane) to 2.2 (sevoflurane) times their respective MAC concentrations.[3]

The MACs of inhalational anesthetics are additive. Gas analyzers sample the end-tidal gas mixture to determine the MAC of each inhalational gas present during exhalation. For example, adding 0.5 MAC of desflurane (3%) and 0.5 MAC of nitrous oxide (52%) results in approximately 1 MAC.

Based on this, combining desflurane, sevoflurane, or isoflurane with nitrous oxide may be beneficial for patients without contraindications who are having inhalational agent-induced intraoperative hypotension, but for whom reducing the depth of anesthesia is not an option. Nitrous oxide tends to stimulate the sympathetic nervous system causing minimal or slight increase in arterial blood pressure, heart rate, and cardiac output. Other anesthetic agents like inhalational gases, opioids, and propofol can cause hypotension; adding nitrous oxide can decrease the percentage of other inhalational anesthetics required and may decrease their side effects while keeping the MAC the same.[3] This is not meant to imply that nitrous oxide is free from side effects; indeed nitrous oxide can cause nausea and vomiting, myocardial depression, and decreased tidal volumes just as the other inhalational agents can.

Additionally, nitrous oxide can cause the rapid (and potentially dangerous) expansion of closed air spaces.

Inhalational MACs are decreased with the addition of opioids.

MACs of anesthetic inhalational agents are reduced when used in conjunction with opioids. For example, a 50% reduction in the MAC of isoflurane can be achieved by reaching a fentanyl blood level of 1.7 ng/mL.[4] Studies have verified that other opioids such as alfentanil, sufentanil, and remifentanil also decrease the MAC of isoflurane, albeit at different respective plasma concentrations.[5–7]

Table 22.1 lists common opioids used during anesthesia. The target plasma concentration of opioids used to reduce inhalation anesthetics to their respective MAC concentrations has been studied. The opioid bolus and infusion rates to achieve these plasma levels are also listed but must be used with clinical discretion for each patient.

The use of multiple agents relies on the principle of MAC addition to decrease the dose-dependent side effects of each specific agent.

In general, the inhalational agents cause decreases in the cerebral metabolic rate of oxygen utilization ($CMRO_2$), an increase in cerebral blood flow (CBF) and intracranial pressure (ICP), and a decrease in the amplitude of sensory evoked potentials. These occur in a dose-dependent manner, so the addition of other agents, such as remifentanil, allows for a reduction in the inhaled agent's concentration and creates a more favorable monitoring situation. For example, it is recommended that isoflurane be limited to 0.5 MAC when evoked potentials are to be monitored[1].

Table 22.1 Target Plasma Concentration Parameters for Common Opioids

Opioid	Target Plasma Concentration to Reduce Inhalation Agents to MAC Awake	Bolus and Infusion Rate to Achieve Target Plasma Concentration
Fentanyl	1–4 ng/mL	Bolus: 3–10 μg/kg Infuse: 0.02–0.07 μg/kg/min
Alfentanil *	40–160 ng/mL	Bolus: 20–80 μg/kg Infuse: 0.25–1 μg/kg/min
Sufentanil	0.15–0.5 ng/mL	Bolus: 0.15–0.5 μg/kg Infuse: 0.003–0.01 μg/kg/min
Remifentanil[a]	1–(5–15) ng/mL	Bolus: 0.25–1 μg/kg Infuse: 0.025–(0.2–1.0) μg/kg/min

[Based on data from Ref. [8]]

[a]Remifentanil and alfentanil bolus should be given as a rapid infusion over 1 to 2 minutes

Take-Home Points

- The minimum alveolar concentration (MAC) of inhalational gases can be summed together.
- The MAC requirement can be decreased by the concurrent use of opioids.
- Using adjunctive therapy can decrease the MAC requirement while also decreasing the side effects of anesthetic gases.

Summary

Interaction: pharmacodynamic
Substrates: inhalational anesthetics, opioids
Mechanism/site of action: various
Clinical effect: anesthetic depth is increased by additive fractional dosing

References

1. Morgan GE, Mikhail MS, Murray MJ. Clinical anesthesiology. 4th ed. New York: McGraw-Hill; 2006.
2. Eger 2nd EI, Saidman LJ, Brandstater B. Minimum alveolar anesthetic concentration: a standard of anesthetic potency. Anesthesiology. 1965;26:756–63.
3. Eger EI, Eisenkraft JB, Weiskopf RB, editors. The pharmacology of inhaled anesthetics. Sponsored by the Dannemiller Memorial Educational Foundation. San Antonio, TX; 2002.
4. McEwan AI, Smith C, Dyar O, Goodman D, Smith LR, Glass PS. Isoflurane minimum alveolar concentration reduction by fentanyl. Anesthesiology. 1993;78:864–9.
5. Westmoreland CL, Sebel PS, Gropper A. Fentanyl or alfentanil decreases the minimum alveolar anesthetic concentration of isoflurane in surgical patients. Anesth Analg. 1994;78:23–8.
6. Brunner MD, Braithwaite P, Jhaveri R, et al. MAC reduction of isoflurane by sufentanil. Br J Anaesth. 1994;72:42–6.
7. Lang E, Kapila A, Shlugman D, Hoke JF, Sebel PS, Glass PS. Reduction of isoflurane minimum alveolar concentration by remifentanil. Anesthesiology. 1996;85:721–8.
8. Glass PS, Gan TJ, Howell S, et al. Drug interactions: volatile anesthetics and opioids. J Clin Anesth. 1997;9(6 Suppl): 185–225.

1 + 1 + 1 + 1 = ?

23

Variable effects of combined substances

Anthony T. Silipo DO, Raymond M. Planinsic MD,
Erica D. Wittwer MD, PhD, Juraj Sprung MD, PhD,
and Wayne T. Nicholson MD, PharmD, MSc

Abstract
This case discusses the ubiquitous but poorly understood pharmacodynamic interactions between multiple anesthetic, sedative, and opioid agents.

Case

On a Saturday evening, a 62-year-old intoxicated man was brought to the emergency department after sustaining a right femur fracture in a motor vehicle accident.

His only outpatient medication was alprazolam 0.5 mg as needed for anxiety attacks. His wife gave a history that the patient had become very nervous before delivering a "father of the bride" speech earlier that day, so he took a dose of alprazolam. Although not a habitual drinker, he also drank many glasses of champagne at the reception. A head computed tomography was normal and his blood alcohol concentration was 0.14%. He received a total of 8 mg of morphine in the prehospital and preoperative period.

A.T. Silipo DO (✉)
Department of Anesthesiology, University of Pittsburgh Medical Center, Magee Women's Hospital and Presbyterian Medical Center, Pittsburgh, PA, USA
e-mail: silipoat@upmc.edu

R.M. Planinsic MD
Department of Anesthesiology, University of Pittsburgh School of Medicine, Pittsburgh, PA, USA

E.D. Wittwer MD, PhD • J. Sprung MD, PhD • W.T. Nicholson MD, PharmD, MSc
Department of Anesthesiology, Mayo Clinic, Rochester, MN, USA

C. Marcucci et al. (eds.), *A Case Approach to Perioperative Drug-Drug Interactions*, DOI 10.1007/978-1-4614-7495-1_23

The patient underwent an uneventful open reduction and internal fixation of the right femur under general anesthesia. He received a total of 250 mcg of fentanyl and hydromorphone (1.0 mg) intraoperatively. He was extubated at the end of the operative case with stable vital signs, normothermia, no signs of residual muscles weakness, and resumption of spontaneous ventilation. He tolerated extubation for a short time but soon became somnolent with oxyhemoglobin saturation values decreasing to around 80% to 82%, even with constant stimulation. Naloxone was administered in 0.04 mg increments until he became more alert and his respirations were regular. He was transferred to the postanesthesia care unit where he spent 3 hours, during which nursing staff monitored him closely for recurring sedation before admission to a monitored care unit overnight.

Discussion

This is an example of several ubiquitous but poorly understood pharmacodynamic interactions between multiple agents.

Although this total opioid dose given over a period of 6 hours may be appropriate for a patient with a very painful injury such as a femur fracture, the addition of alcohol and other sedative medications should always be considered when administering these drugs. Alcohol itself was used as a sole anesthetic dating back to the 1800s.[1] Although alcohol is frequently consumed, there is a lack of reliable information about the interaction of alcohol and anesthetic agents. Many drugs with sedative properties contain warnings about combining the medication with alcohol, but the specific pharmacokinetic or pharmacodynamic interactions are not well described.

Pharmacologic interactions can be described as synergistic (effect greater than the sum of each drug), additive (effect equal to the sum of each drug), or infra-additive (effect less than expected sum of each agent) (Figs. 23.1 and 23.2). Interacting drugs that demonstrate synergistic interactions suggest different sites of action.[2] Increased hypoxemia and apnea caused by fentanyl (μ-opioid receptor) in combination with midazolam or alprazolam (γ-amino butyric acid or "GABA" receptor) is an example of different receptor systems resulting in synergism.[3] However, interactions of drugs on similar receptors are more likely to result in additive interactions. Alcohol is a central nervous system depressant, which in part targets $GABA_A$ receptors increasing neuronal chloride conductance resulting in cell hyperpolarization.[4] Benzodiazepines, propofol, barbiturates, etomidate, and inhaled anesthetics also facilitate GABA-mediated mechanisms and neuronal hyperpolarization. These sedative interactions usually result in synergistic or additive outcomes depending on the combination.[2]

Additive or synergistic effects are not always the rule with sedative combinations (Fig. 23.2).[9] For example, infra-additive effects were described by Johnstone and

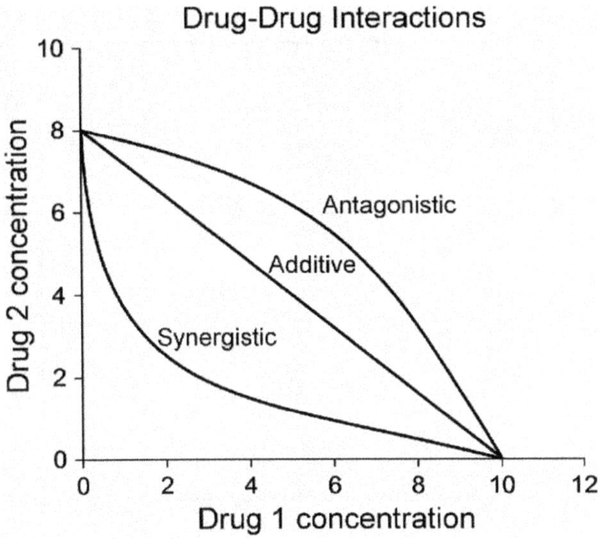

Fig. 23.1 Isobolographic cartoon of the various types of drug interactions. Drug interactions can be antagonistic (infra-additive), additive, or synergistic (supra-additive). The concentrations depicted on the graph axes are arbitrary values and not representative of any particular drugs. [Modified from Krejcie TC, Avram MJ: When Duzitol does not do it all: The two sides of drug synergy. *Anesth Analg*. 2011;113(3):441–3. With permission from Wolter Kluwers Health].

colleagues in a mouse study of isoflurane in the setting of acute ethanol use.[5] Although anesthetic effects were greater with the combination of two, they were less than the expected sum.[5] Another consideration is the impact of acute versus chronic alcohol consumption on adverse effects. Wolfson and Freed demonstrated that acute and chronic alcohol intoxication should be viewed as separate entities with respect to their influence on halothane anesthesia in a rat model.[6] Specifically, acute administration of alcohol reduced anesthetic requirements (such as minimum alveolar concentration), and chronic alcohol consumption increased tolerance to halothane.

The interaction of alcohol and intravenous anesthetics has been studied in a similarly limited fashion. Garfield and Bukusoglu used a mouse model to study the effect of alcohol administration on the anesthetic effects of propofol.[7] The interaction was additive for the hypnotic property of propofol as well as propofol induced anesthesia. The influence of chronic alcohol administration on barbiturate effect has been studied using a rat model and it was found that cross-tolerance to the anesthetic effects of barbiturates in ethanol-tolerant rats is not consistent with all barbiturates.[8]

Taken together, the interaction between alcohol and anesthetic agents is quite complicated and the lack of human data contributes to the difficulty of applying the available information to clinical care. At this time, an understanding of the similar mechanisms of action of alcohol and anesthetics in addition to the limited animal data must be used with clinical experience to guide patient care. Unpredictable responses to anesthetics in the presence of acute or chronic alcohol intoxication as well as withdrawal should be anticipated. Anesthetic agents should be titrated to effect and special consideration of airway protection should be given to such

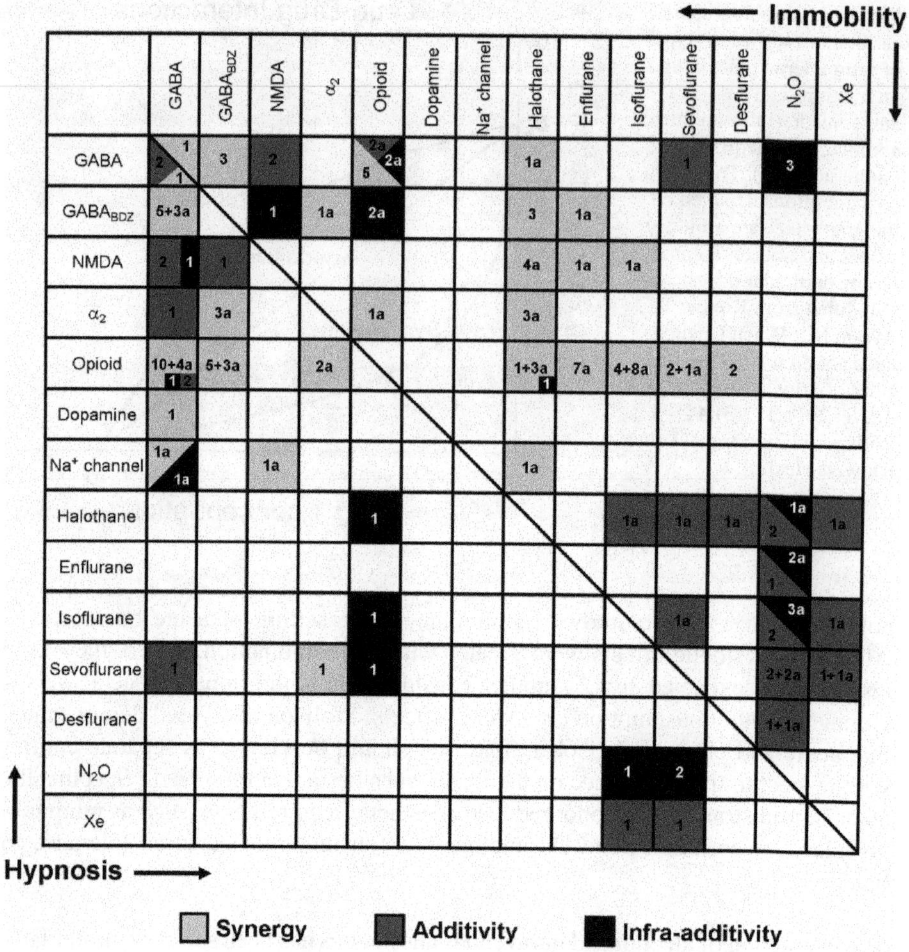

Fig. 23.2 Interaction grid summarizing the data on drug interactions in humans and animals for hypnosis and immobility by pharmacological class; **GABA** (γ-aminobutyric acid): GABA acting drugs (propofol, thiopental, and etomidate); **GABABDZ**: agents acting at the benzodiazepine binding site (midazolam, diazepam); **NMDA** (*N*-methyl-D-aspartate): NMDA receptor antagonist (ketamine); **α2**: α2 adrenergic agonists (dexmedetomidine, clonidine); **Opioid**: drugs acting at μ-opioid receptor (morphine, fentanyl, and remifentanil); **Dopamine**: dopamine antagonists (droperidol, metoclopramide); **Na + channel**: sodium channel blockers (lidocaine, bupivacaine)
The right upper half of the grid (above the thick diagonal) summarizes interactions for the end point of immobility; the left lower half (below the thick diagonal) summarizes interactions for the end point of hypnosis. Synergy is coded as light gray, additivity as dark gray, and infra-additivity as black. The number refers to the number of studies attesting to a particular interaction with animal data carrying the suffix "a" [Modified from Hendrickx JF. Eger EI 2nd. Sonner JM. Shafer SL. Is synergy the rule? A review of anesthetic interactions producing hypnosis and immobility. Anesth Analg. 2008;107(2):494–506. With permission from Wolter Kluwers Health]

patients. The combination of alcohol + benzodiazepine + opioid + inhaled and/or intravenous anesthetic agents = an unpredictable situation requiring vigilant clinical monitoring and careful perioperative decision making.

Take-Home Points

- Pharmacologically, sedative mixtures can result in synergistic, additive, or infra-additive interactions depending on the combination.
- Although greater sedative effects are expected, administration of anesthesia to a patient with acute alcohol intoxication creates a situation that is not always predictable.
- Anesthesia providers should consider the impact of acute versus chronic alcohol consumption on anesthesia requirements and adverse effects.

Summary

Interactions: pharmacodynamic
Substrates: anesthetics, propofol, benzodiazepines, opioids, fentanyl
Sites of Action: multiple, including μ-opioid and GABA receptors
Clinical effects: variable

References

1. Barash PG, Cullen BF, Stoelting RK. Clinical anesthesia. 5th ed. Philadelphia: Lippincott Williams & Wilkins; 2006. p. 118–9.
2. Hendrickx JF, Eger 2nd EI, Sonner JM, Shafer SL. Is synergy the rule? A review of anesthetic interactions producing hypnosis and immobility. Anesth Analg. 2008;107(2):494–506.
3. Bailey PL, Pace NL, Ashburn MA, Moll JW, East KA, Stanley TH. Frequent hypoxemia and apnea after sedation with midazolam and fentanyl. Anesthesiology. 1990;73(5):826–30.
4. Brunton L, Chabner B, Knollman B. Goodman and Gilman's the pharmacological basis of therapeutics. 12th ed. New York: McGraw-Hill; 2011. p. 629–47.
5. Wolfson B, Freed B. Influence of alcohol on anesthetic requirements and acute toxicity. Anesth Analg. 1980;59:826–30.
6. Johnstone RE, Kulp RA, Smith TC. Effects of acute and chronic ethanol administration on isoflurane requirement in mice. Anesth Analg. 1975;54:277–81.
7. Garfield JM, Bukusoglu C. Propofol and ethanol produce additive hypnotic and anesthetic effects in the mouse. Anesth Analg. 1996;83:156–61.
8. Curran MA, Newman LM, Becker GL. Barbiturate anesthesia and alcohol tolerance in a rat model. Anesth Analg. 1988;67:868–71.
9. Krejcie TC, Avram MJ. When Duzitol does not do it all: the two sides of drug synergy. Anesth Analg. 2011;113(3):441–3.

A Delayed Surgeon Is a Dismayed Surgeon

24

Nitrous oxide, dexmedetomidine, somatosensory evoked potentials

Jonathan Anson MD

Abstract
This case discusses a pharmacodynamic interaction between dexmedetomidine and nitrous oxide, resulting in decreased amplitude signals of somatosensory evoked potential measurements.

Case

A resident on the second day of her neuroanesthesia rotation was posted on a case involving general anesthesia with somatosensory evoked potential (SSEP) monitoring for a C4-C6 fusion on an elderly female. The patient had a history of hypertension and coronary artery disease (CAD).

Induction of anesthesia with propofol, fentanyl, and succinylcholine was uneventful. Anesthesia was maintained with a dexmedetomidine infusion and 0.5 minimum alveolar concentration (MAC) sevoflurane. The pins were placed and the patient was positioned prone. Good-quality baseline SSEP signals were obtained. Two hours into the case, the neuromonitoring technician reported "we've lost the SSEPs," which was confirmed by the covering neurologist. Physiologic and hemodynamic causes of SSEP loss were ruled out and retractors were removed without improvement in the SSEP signals. The surgeon feared spinal cord compromise and decided to perform a "wake up test" with the patient still prone in pins to rule out a true neurologic deficit.

J. Anson MD
Department of Anesthesiology, Penn State Milton S. Hershey Medical Center,
Penn State Hershey Medical Center, Hershey, PA, USA
e-mail: janson@hmc.psu.edu

C. Marcucci et al. (eds.), *A Case Approach to Perioperative Drug-Drug Interactions*, DOI 10.1007/978-1-4614-7495-1_24

The anesthesia resident turned off the sevoflurane and decreased the dexmedetomidine infusion rate to allow the patient to be awake for a neurologic exam. The patient still had not emerged enough to follow commands 30 minutes later despite an undetectable level of end-tidal sevoflurane. The anesthesia attending was paged and quickly noticed the nitrous oxide flowmeter showed a 2:1 nitrous oxide-to-oxygen ratio. The embarrassed anesthesia resident admitted that he had turned on the nitrous oxide because he was afraid 0.5 MAC of an inhalational agent wasn't enough to prevent awareness and had forgotten it was on. He had also used nitrous oxide because he was concerned that using other inhalational anesthetics would decrease the blood pressure significantly below the baseline mean arterial blood pressure and he was worried about the patient's history of CAD and the risk for visual loss due to the prone position. The nitrous oxide was discontinued, the patient woke up and moved all extremities on command, and then was reanesthetized with sevoflurane. The surgical procedure resumed with an irate surgeon complaining loudly and at length. That evening the attending called the crestfallen resident to review the effect of inhalational anesthetics on evoked potentials (EPs) and reassure him that all anesthesiologists have been in the situation of wondering why the patient won't wake up and then realizing that the nitrous oxide is still on.

Discussion

SSEP monitoring is a noninvasive technique used to assess the integrity of the somatosensory system intraoperatively without having to perform a "wake up test." Continuous SSEP monitoring can warn a surgeon about impending neurologic injury and allow intervention before a permanent injury occurs. Common procedures that utilize SSEP monitoring includes spinal surgery, scoliosis repair, spinal fractures, intracranial procedures (aneurysms), and carotid endarterectomy. SSEPs monitor pathways supplied by the posterior spinal artery, thus it is still possible to miss motor tract injuries if SSEP alone are monitored.[1] For this reason, SSEPs are usually combined with motor evoked potentials (MEPs) to monitory anterior spinal artery pathways. Needles are placed in peripheral nerves and repeated electrical stimulations of 1 to 2 HZ are given. These electrical stimulations travel from the periphery to the central nervous system in a stepwise fashion via dorsal root ganglia, first order neurons (ipsilateral posterior column), second-order neurons (cross to contralateral side), medial lemniscus, thalamus, third-order neurons and sensory cortex. The electrical impulses can be monitored at several points along this circuit, with the potential sites generally classified as cortical or subcortical potentials.

The latency and amplitude of neuromonitoring signals are the most commonly utilized data. Signal latency is defined as the time from peripheral electrical stimulation to peak voltage at the measurement site. Amplitude is the voltage measurement from the peak apex to the next trough. Changes in baseline amplitude and latency intraoperatively may be indicative of compromised sensory pathways. By definition, a decrease in amplitude of >50% or an increase in latency of >15% is considered a significant change. SSEP amplitude and latency changes lasting for >15 minutes may lead to permanent neurologic changes. Typically, interventions in response to decreased amplitude or increased latency are aimed at improving spinal cord perfusion. Surgical retractors are often removed to improve blood flow. Physiologically, blood pressure and oxygen delivery are optimized. Often SSEP signal changes are a result of anesthetic drugs, therefore, anesthesia-related signal changes must be considered in the differential diagnosis.

Unfortunately for anesthesia providers, many drugs that are commonly used intraoperatively can negatively impact SSEP monitoring (see Table 24.1). Inhalational anesthetic agents all have a dose-dependent decrease in amplitude and increase in latency.[2] However, up to 0.5 MAC isoflurane is compatible with satisfactory SSEP signals.[2] Nitrous oxide decreases SSEP cortical amplitude with little or no effect on latency. At equipotent concentrations, nitrous oxide results in more profound changes in cortical SSEPs than any other inhalational anesthetic agent.[1] In the scenario above, it was the resident's use of nitrous oxide that lead to the SSEP signal changes and subsequent "wake up test."

Intravenous anesthetic agents can impact SSEP signals as well. Propofol minimally decreases SSEP signals and is often the anesthetic drug of choice in these types of cases. Etomidate has been shown to increase amplitude and latency, therefore, infusions of etomidate may help augment SSEP signals.[3] Similarly, ketamine has been demonstrated to significantly increase signal amplitude (no change in latency) and can be utilized to improve SSEP recordings.[4] Intravenous opioids such as fentanyl, remifentanil, and sufentanil cause minimal changes in latency and amplitude, making them attractive choices as part of a balanced anesthetic.[1] Because many anesthetic drugs can alter SSEP signals, maintenance of anesthesia should be kept as consistent as possible intraoperatively. Large changes in anesthetic management or boluses of drugs that effect SSEP should be avoided to prevent creating a delayed and dismayed surgeon.

Table 24.1 Effect of Anesthetic Drugs on Somatosensory Evoked Potential Parameters

Drug	Latency	Amplitude
Isoflurane	Increased	Decreased
Sevoflurane	Increased	Decreased
Desflurane	Increased	Decreased
Nitrous oxide	No change	Decreased (significant)
Etomidate	Increased	Increased
Ketamine	No change	Increased
Midazolam	No change	Decreased
Fentanyl/remifentanil	Increased (minimal)	Decreased (minimal)
Propofol	None	Decreased (minimal)

Take-Home Points

- SSEP monitoring is a minimally invasive technique for assessing the integrity of sensory patients in anesthetized patients.
- SSEP signals are affected by many drugs used perioperatively and care must be taken to avoid significant changes in anesthetic management intraoperatively.
- Administration of nitrous oxide will significantly decrease the amplitude of SSEP signals.
- Changes in SSEP amplitude and/or latency can be cumulative with coadministration of certain additional anesthetic agents.
- It is very easy to turn on the nitrous oxide and forget that it is on!

Summary

Interaction: pharmacodynamic
Substrates: dexmedetomidine and nitrous oxide
Site of action: sensory pathways involving dorsal root ganglia, first-order neurons (ipsilateral posterior column), second-order neurons (cross to contralateral side), medial lemniscus, thalamus, third-order neurons, sensory cortex
Clinical effect: additive decrease in amplitude of somatosensory evoked potentials

References

1. Sloan TB, Heyer EJ. Anesthesia for intraoperative neurophysiologic monitoring of the spinal cord. J Clin Neurophysiol. 2002;19(5):440–3.
2. Peterson DO, Drummond JC, Todd MM. Effects of halothane, enflurane, isoflurane, and nitrous oxide on somatosensory evoked potentials in humans. Anesthesiology. 1986;65:35–40.
3. Koht A, Schutz W, Schmidt G, et al. Effects of etomidate, midazolam, and thiopental on median nerve somatosensory evoked potentials and the additive effects of fentanyl and nitrous oxide. Anesth Anal. 1988;67:435–41.
4. Schubert A, Licina MG, Lineberry PG. The effect of ketamine on human somatosensory evoked potentials and its modification by nitrous oxide. Anesthesiology. 1990;72(6):1104.

Relax, It's Only Gentamicin

25

Inhalational anesthetics, aminoglycoside antibiotics, neuromuscular junction

Brian Gierl MD and Ferenc E. Gyulai MD

Abstract
Aminoglycoside antibiotics and inhalational anesthetics can profoundly impair neuromuscular function in patients with underlying disease.

Case

A 43-year-old man with a history of penicillin anaphylaxis and end-stage myasthenia gravis complicated by recurrent pneumonia and dysphagia presented for elective gastric feeding tube placement. The patient took his usual dose of pyridostigmine and was at baseline with respect to myasthenia gravis symptoms. He was breathing comfortably with reduced breath sounds bilaterally. The preoperative chest x-ray showed decreased lung volumes but no signs of infection.

The patient underwent an uncomplicated propofol, fentanyl, and desflurane anesthetic with a reduced dose of rocuronium. Gentamicin (100 mg) intravenously was dosed at the surgeon's request because of the history of penicillin anaphylaxis. At the conclusion of the case, the patient received a full dose of sugammadex but had no response to train-of-four (TOF) stimulation in the presence of an end-tidal desflurane concentration of 6.0%. The patient was transported to the intensive care unit (ICU) with propofol sedation where he began to make an effort to breath. Several hours later he was able to maintain his own oxygenation with an FiO2 of 40% and minimal ventilator support. He was eventually extubated and remained stable until his discharge the next day.

B. Gierl MD (✉)
Department of Anesthesiology, University of California San Diego, San Diego, CA, USA
e-mail: gierl.brian@gmail.com

F.E. Gyulai MD
Department of Anesthesiology, University of Pittsburgh Medical Center, Pittsburgh, PA, USA

C. Marcucci et al. (eds.), *A Case Approach to Perioperative Drug-Drug Interactions*, DOI 10.1007/978-1-4614-7495-1_25

Discussion

This is a complex synergistic pharmacodynamic interaction at both the receptor and transmitter levels.

When an electrical impulse reaches the axon terminal of a motor neuron, voltage-gated calcium channels open and allow calcium to enter the neuron. Intracellular calcium interacts with proteins to mobilize acetylcholine (ACh) vesicles and fuse them with the cell membrane. The vesicles exocytose the ACh, which traverses the neuromuscular junction (NMJ), binds acetylcholine receptors (AChRs), and depolarizes the target myocyte. The calcium concentration strongly influences ACh release—such that doubling extracellular calcium concentration increases ACh release 16-fold. Conversely, limiting calcium entry into the neuron decreases ACh release such that some muscle fascicles do not depolarize and contract. This can cause weakness that may lead to respiratory failure in a patient with an underlying neuromuscular or respiratory disease.

Postoperative weakness carries a broad differential diagnosis. After assessing and treating airway, breathing, and circulation, a TOF monitor should be used to assess muscle strength. In the presence of a reduced TOF, evaluate neuromuscular blockade drug (NMBD) and NMBD reversal agent dosing throughout the case. If this is normal, search for other causes such as residual anesthetic, an electrolyte disturbance, or an underlying neuromuscular syndrome.

Aminoglycoside antibiotics inhibit calcium ion entry into the cell through the T-type voltage-gated calcium channels in a dose-dependent manner. The reduction in intracellular calcium decreases ACh release, resulting in weakness. The weakness can be so severe in patients with neuromuscular disorders to require intubation.[1] In healthy patients, high doses of aminoglycosides (eg, gentamicin 4 mg/kg versus the standard 1–2 mg/kg) have been shown to reduce the neuromuscular blocker dose required for muscle relaxation and delay the return of muscle function.[2] Calcium administration can reduce but not eliminate the weakness induced by aminoglycosides. Although aminoglycosides are classically associated with weakness, the quinine moiety in fluoroquinolone antibiotics can precipitate myasthenic crisis in patients with myasthenia gravis.

Inhalational anesthetics reduce muscle strength in the perioperative period by binding AChRs and inhibiting motor end-plate depolarization, even in the absence of neuromuscular blockade.[3] Volatile anesthetics also enhance the effectiveness of NMBDs by increasing the affinity of NMBDs for the AChR.[4] The effect of the inhalational anesthetic manifests itself as a sigmoidal dose–response curve that is more proportional to the blood concentration than lipid solubility. Therefore, desflurane's higher minimum alveolar concentration (MAC) alters the action more so than the other volatile anesthetics at equi-MAC dosages.

Take-Home Points

- Aminoglycoside antibiotics limit calcium entry into the presynaptic axon terminal of spinal motor neurons.
- This reduces ACh release after endogenous neuromuscular transmission of electrocutaneous stimulation and diminishes the subsequent muscle response.
- Volatile anesthetics act postsynaptically by binding to myocyte AChRs and inhibiting motor end-plate depolarization.
- Inhalational anesthetics reduce NMBD requirements in comparison to total intravenous anesthesia (TIVA) techniques.
- Thus, TIVA may be preferred for patients with underlying neuromuscular pathology so that residual weakness does not compromise postoperative respiratory function.
- The effect of the volatile anesthetic manifests itself as a sigmoidal dose–response curve that is more proportional to the blood concentration than lipid solubility.

Summary

Interaction: pharmacodynamic
Substrates: aminoglycoside antibiotics, inhalational anesthetics
Mechanism/site of action: T-type–gated calcium channels on axon terminals of motor neurons, acetylcholine receptors on neuromuscular junction motor endplates, acetylcholine receptors
Clinical effect: decreased release of acetylcholine as well as decreased binding of acetylcholine to motor neuron acetylcholine receptors leads to neuromuscular weakness

References

1. Barrons RW. Drug-induced neuromuscular blockade and myasthenia gravis. Pharmacotherapy. 1997;17(6):1220–32.
2. Dotan ZA, Hana R, Simon D, et al. The effect of vecuronium is enhanced by a large rather than a modest dose of gentamicin as compared with no preoperative gentamicin. Anesth Analg. 2003;96(3):750–4.
3. Waud BE, Waud DR. Comparison of the effects of general anesthethics on the end-plate of skeletal muscle. Anesthesiology. 1975;43(5):540–7.
4. Paul M, Fokt RM, Kindler CH, et al. Characterization of the interactions between volatile anesthetics and neuromuscular blockers at the muscle nicotinic acetylcholine receptor. Anesth Analg. 2002;95(2):362–7.

Jaundice After Surgery

26

Halothane hepatitis, CYP2E1

Jonathon E. Kivela MD, Toby N. Weingarten MD,
and Juraj Sprung MD, PhD

Abstract
This case discusses possible pharmacokinetic interactions involving halothane and possible cytochrome P450 2E1 inhibitors including isoniazid, disulfiram, and watercress.

Case

A 60-year-old woman with a history only of obesity and recent appendectomy presented to the operating room for a total abdominal hysterectomy and bilateral salpingo-oophorectomy for the treatment of papillary adenocarcinoma of the uterus. The anesthetic for the appendectomy had been unremarkable. Anesthetic and sedative agents included intravenous (IV) fentanyl, midazolam, sodium thiopental, and halothane. Neuromuscular agents included succinylcholine and vecuronium.

Similar anesthetic and neuromuscular agents were used for the hysterectomy. The procedure lasted 100 minutes and the intraoperative and immediate postoperative course was unremarkable.

The patient was discharged from the hospital on postoperative day 4.

However, the patient presented to her primary care doctor on postoperative day 8 reporting fevers as high as 38.3 °C and jaundice. She denied abdominal pain, nausea, or vomiting. Her primary care doctor elected to admit her to the hospital for further evaluation and management of her fever.

J.E. Kivela MD (✉) • T.N. Weingarten MD • J. Sprung MD, PhD
Department of Anesthesiology, Mayo Clinic, Rochester, MN, USA
e-mail: Kivela.jonathon@gmail.com

C. Marcucci et al. (eds.), *A Case Approach to Perioperative Drug-Drug Interactions*, DOI 10.1007/978-1-4614-7495-1_26

A complete blood cell count was normal except for a mild eosinophilia, serum electrolytes were normal, and international normalized ratio (INR), alanine aminotransferase, and aspartate aminotransferase were slightly elevated. Over the next 7 days, the patient became more jaundiced, and her INR, alanine aminotransferase and aspartate aminotransferase values continued to increase. Despite aggressive medical management, she died on postoperative day 15. Histologic examination at autopsy showed centrilobular necrosis of the hepatic cells.

Discussion

This is an example of hepatotoxicity arising from halothane metabolites.

Halothane was first introduced in England in 1956 and in the United States in 1958.[1] Its use has almost been eliminated in developed countries, but it still continues to be the main anesthetic in such countries as Iran, South Africa, Tunisia, Kenya, and India because of its low cost.[2]

The first case report of halothane hepatitis appeared in 1958. By 1963, more than 350 cases had been reported.[3] The National Halothane Study reported that the incidence of halothane hepatitis was 1 in 35,000 anesthesia cases.[1] Risk factors for halothane hepatitis are 1) repeat exposures, especially when repeat exposures occur within 28 days; 2) middle age, with the peak between 50 and 60 years; 3) obesity; 4) female sex; and 5) a family history of halothane hepatitis. Signs and symptoms include fever (which is usually the first sign), malaise, anorexia, gastrointestinal problems, jaundice, eosinophilia, and transaminitis with normal or slightly elevated alkaline phosphatase. Histologic examination of the liver shows centrilobular necrosis.[1] The mortality of halothane hepatitis is 75%.[4]

Halothane hepatitis is an immunologic response to halothane metabolites. After halothane is inhaled, 50% of it is metabolized by pathways of both oxidation and reduction in the liver. The main enzyme involved in its metabolism is cytochrome P450 2E1, but P450 2A6 also has a minor role.[5] Halothane is first oxidized to bromide and an unstable intermediate, trifluoroacetyl chloride. This intermediate compound binds to liver proteins, which form trifluoroacetylated protein neoantigens. Susceptible patients can then generate anti–trifluoroacetylated protein antibodies. These antibodies mediate hepatic necrosis on reexposure to halothane (Fig. 26.1).[6] Research is underway to look at possible medications that can be used before halothane exposure to inhibit 2E1 (known inhibitors of 2E1 include isoniazid, disulfiram, and watercress). This inhibition would prevent the formation of trifluoroacetyl chloride and thus prevent the formation of autoantibodies, ultimately preventing halothane hepatitis.

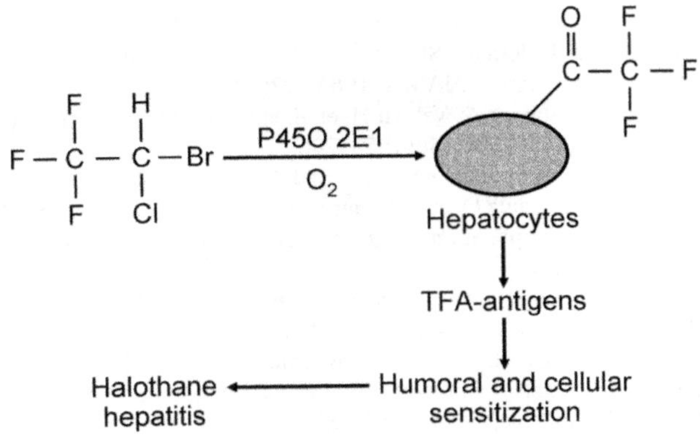

Fig. 26.1 Pathway for the generation of the immune response after halothane exposure in susceptible patients. Halothane is metabolized to a trifluoracetylated adduct, which binds to proteins in hepatocytes. The body recognizes the altered liver proteins as non-self and generates an immune response that, on subsequent exposure, leads to toxicity and cellular death. A similar process may occur after anesthetic exposure to other fluorinated drugs that generate a trifluoroacetylated or similar adduct. Abbreviation: TFA, trifluoroacetyl [Adapted from Njoku D, Laster MJ, Gong DH, et al. Biotransformation of halothane, enflurane, isoflurane, and desflurane to trifluoroacetylated liver proteins: association between protein acylation and hepatic injury. Anesth Analg. 1997;84(1):173–8. With permission from Wolter Kluwers Health]

Take-Home Points

- Halothane is the main volatile anesthetic agent used in developing countries.
- Halothane hepatitis is rare and occurs in 1 in 35,000 anesthesia cases.
- Risk factors for halothane hepatitis include frequent repeated exposures, middle age, obesity, female sex, and family history.
- P450 2E1 is the main enzyme involved in the metabolism of halothane.
- Research is underway to inhibit 2E1, thus preventing halothane hepatitis.

Summary

Interaction: pharmacokinetic
Substrate: halothane
Enzyme: 2E1
Inhibitor: undetermined, possibilities include isoniazid, disulfiram, and watercress
Clinical effect: possible decreased conversion of halothane to hepatotoxic metabolites

References

1. Summary of the national Halothane Study: possible association between halothane anesthesia and postoperative hepatic necrosis. JAMA. 1966;197(10):775–88.
2. Eghtesadi-Araghi P, Sohrabpour A, Vahedi H, et al. Halothane hepatitis in Iran: a review of 59 cases. World J Gastroenterol. 2008;14(34):5322–6.
3. Ray DC, Drummond GB. Halothane hepatitis. Br J Anaesth. 1991;67(1):84–99.
4. Kharasch ED, Hankins D, Mautz D, et al. Identification of the enzyme responsible for oxidative halothane metabolism: implications for prevention of halothane hepatitis. Lancet. 1996;347(9012):1367–71.
5. Spracklin DK, Hankins DC, Fisher JM, et al. Cytochrome P450 2E1 is the principal catalyst of human oxidative halothane metabolism in vitro. J Pharmacol Exp Ther. 1997;281(1):400–11.
6. Njoku D, Laster MJ, Gong DH, et al. Biotransformation of halothane, enflurane, isoflurane, and desflurane to trifluoroacetylated liver proteins: association between protein acylation and hepatic injury. Anesth Analg. 1997;84(1):173–8.

Everybody Clear?

27

Halothane, epinephrine, arrhythmia

Nikhli Patel MD, Barbara Jericho MD, and Randal O. Dull MD, PhD

Abstract

The case discusses a pharmacodynamic reaction between halothane and epinephrine resulting in arrhythmias.

Case

A 3-year-old, 14-kg girl without significant past medical history or known drug allergies underwent a tonsillectomy/adenoidectomy for known tonsillar and adenoid hypertrophy. She was premedicated with oral midazolam and brought to the operating room. The patient underwent an inhalational induction with 70% nitrous oxide, oxygen, and a slow titration up to 3% halothane. The intubation was uncomplicated. Anesthesia was maintained with nitrous oxide, oxygen, and 2% halothane. The surgical procedure began with the infiltration of peritonsillar tissue with 2% lidocaine 4 cc with 1:100,000 epinephrine. Within minutes of infiltration, the patient developed multifocal premature ventricular contractions followed by ventricular fibrillation. The surgical procedure was immediately stopped and manual ventilation with 100% oxygen was initiated with discontinuation of all anesthetic gases. Defibrillation with 2 joules/kg was successful with the return to normal sinus rhythm.

N. Patel MD (✉) • R.O. Dull MD, PhD
Department of Anesthesiology, University of Illinois at Chicago, Chicago, IL, USA
e-mail: Itsnikhilpatel@gmail.com

B. Jericho MD
Department of Anesthesiology, University of Illinois-Chicago, University of Illinois Hospital and Health Sciences System, Chicago, IL, USA

C. Marcucci et al. (eds.), *A Case Approach to Perioperative Drug-Drug Interactions*, DOI 10.1007/978-1-4614-7495-1_27

Discussion

This is an example of a pharmacodynamic interaction.

Several decades ago, the occurrence of cardiac arrhythmias when adrenergic drugs, especially epinephrine, were coadministered with halogenated anesthetic agents, especially halothane, was reported in a wide range of clinical scenarios and has been the subject of extensive research.[1–14]

Is this relevant to today's practitioner? The answer is yes! Drug–drug interactions concerning halothane and epinephrine are far from being only of historical interest. It is certainly true that sevoflurane and desflurane have replaced halothane for use in adults in the United States (US) and the developed world. However, halothane is still used at times by pediatric anesthesiologists, even in the US, for bronchoscopies and similar procedures as it provides a smooth and reliable induction and emergence. It is also very inexpensive compared to sevoflurane and desflurane and is in widespread, if not universal use, in the developing world. Western practitioners would almost certainly encounter it on medical missions. Furthermore, published reports in the emerging field of nanotechnology and nanomedicine have suggested that "new tricks for the halothane old dog" may be possible. In a 2011 report in the *British Journal of Anaesthesia* entitled, "Nanomedicine: Is Really the Future of Anaesthesia" the authors stated, "Introducing nanocarriers inside the halothane molecule can increase its benefits as an anesthetic in the lungs and cardiovascular system and prevent exposure to the liver."[15]

The exact mechanisms by which interactions between halogenated anesthetics and sympathomimetics result in increased arrhythmogenicity is not known. However, it is thought that the halogenated anesthetics produce conduction changes that increase impulse re-entry into the myocardial tissue.

Catecholamines, like epinephrine, independently induce arrhythmias by increasing spontaneous depolarization (phase 4) of automatic cells, which more quickly reach the threshold potential for depolarization and therefore increases the overall rate of depolarization of these cells. The enhanced rate of depolarization of these cells exceeds the rate of the sino-atrial (SA) or atrio-ventricular node and can thereby suppress or override them.

The occurrence of arrhythmias is further increased in situations of increased mean arterial pressure, tachycardia, hypoxia, and hypercapnia, all of which are associated with increased circulating endogenous catecholamines.[16] Furthermore, cardiac stretch decreases the threshold of epinephrine-induced automaticity thereby producing multifocal pacemaker activity.

Multiple studies have compared the effect of current day volatiles and epinephrine-induced arrhythmias.[17,18] These studies indicate that significantly higher levels of plasma epinephrine were needed to observe premature ventricular contractions with newer age inhalational anesthetics such as sevoflurane and isoflurane.

Take-Home Points

- Halothane is in extremely widespread use in developing and undeveloped nations due to its low cost. Halothane continues to be in limited use in the developed countries for its anesthetic advantages. It has been suggested that the application of nanotechnology might play a role in the clinical reemergence of halothane.
- Halothane has long been recognized to "sensitize" the myocardium and to be associated with cardiac irritability and intraoperative arrhythmias when coadministered with sympathomimetics.
- The suggested mechanism is the involvement of the increased automaticity of latent cardiac pacemakers.
- Halothane and epinephrine can be used in conjunction with appropriate attention to doses and monitoring that are patient and case specific.
- Modern day inhalational anesthetics (sevoflurane, desflurane, isoflurane) are relatively safe to use when local anesthetics with epinephrine are used.

Summary

Interaction: pharmacodynamic
Substrates: halothane and epinephrine
Mechanism/site of action: exact mechanism unknown, conduction changes induced by halothane that permit increased re-entry into myocardial cells occurs in the situation of epinephrine-induced delayed phase 4 depolarization and decreased automaticity of the SA node, ultimately resulting in the escape of latent pacemakers
Clinical effects: manifestations of ectopic pacemaker foci in the heart with arrhythmias

References

1. Katz RL, Epstein RA. The interaction of anesthetic agents and adrenergic drugs to produce cardiac arrhythmias. Anesthesiology. 1968;29:763–84.

2. Imamura S, Ikeda K. Comparison of the epinephrine induced arrhythmogenic effect of sevoflurane with isoflurane and halothane. J Anesth. 1987;1(1):62–8.
3. Katz RL, Matteo RS, Papper EM. The injection of epinephrine during general anesthesia with halogenated hydrocarbons and cyclopropane in man. Anesthesiology. 1962;23(5):597–600.
4. Johnstone M. Adrenaline and noradrenaline during anaesthesia. Anaesthesia. 1953;8:32–42.
5. Hirshom WI, Taylor RG, Sheehan JC. Arrhythmias produced by combinations of halothane and small amounts of vasopressor. Br J Oral Surg. 1965;2:131–6.
6. Andersen N, Johansen SH. Incidence of catechol-amine-induced arrhythmias during halothane anesthesia. Anesthesiology. 1963;24(1):51–6.
7. Forbes AM. Halothane, adrenaline and cardiac arrest. Anaesthesia. 1966;21(1):22–7.
8. Reisner LS, Lippmann M. Ventricular arrhythmias after epinephrine injection in enflurane and in halothane anesthesia. Anesth Analg. 1975;54(4):468–70.
9. Ikezono E, Yasuda K, Hattori Y. Effects of propranolol on epinephrine-induced arrhythmias during halothane anesthesia in man and cats. Anesth Analg. 1969;48(4):598–604.
10. Ueda W, Hirakawa M, Mae O. Appraisal of epinephrine administration to patients under halothane anesthesia for closure of cleft palate. Anesthesiology. 1983;58(6):574–6.
11. Kaufman L. Unforeseen complications encountered during dental anaesthesia. Cardiac arrhythmias during dental anaesthesia. Proc R Soc Med. 1966;59(8):731–4.
12. Alexander JP. Dysrhythmia and oral surgery. Br J Anaesth. 1971;43(8):773–8.
13. Fletcher E. Dysrhythmia and oral surgery. II. Junctional rhythms. Br J Anaesth. 1972;44(11):1179–82.
14. Katz RL, Katz GJ. Surgical infiltration of pressor drugs and their interaction with volatile anaesthetics. Br J Anaesth. 1966;38(9):712–8.
15. Gupta AK, Mehta A, Ommid M. Nanomedicine: is really the future of anaesthesia. Brit J Anaes. Out of the blue E-letters. 2011. http://bja.oxfordjournals.org/forum/topic/brjana_el%3B7944. Last Accessed 22 June 2012.
16. Moore MA, Weiskopf RB, Eger 2nd EI, Wilson C, Lu G. Arrhythmogenic doses of epinephrine are similar during desflurane or isoflurane in humans. Anesthesiology. 1993;79(5):943–7.
17. Navarro R, Weiskopf RB, Moore MA, et al. Humans anesthetized with sevoflurane or isoflurane have similar arrhythymic response to epinephrine. Anesthesiology. 1994;80(3):545–9.
18. Weiner N. Norepinephrine, epinephrine, and the sympathomimetic amines. In: Gilman AG, Goodman LS, Rall TW, Murad F, editors. Goodman and Gilman's the pharmacological basis of therapeutics. 7th ed. New York: MacMillan Publishing Company; 1985.

The Hemodynamic Hole

28

General anesthetics, angiotension-converting enzyme inhibitors (ACE-Is), angiotensin II receptor blockers (ARBs)

Arun L. Jayaraman MD, PhD and Theresa A. Gelzinis MD

Abstract

This case discusses multiple cumulative pharmacodynamic interactions between general and neuraxial anesthetics, angiotensin converting enzyme inhibitors and angiotensin receptor blockers, resulting in significant intraoperative hypotension.

Case

A 56-year-old Caucasian man with history of a right inguinal hernia presented for laparoscopic herniorrhaphy. His past medical history included hypertension and non-insulin–dependent diabetes mellitus, for which he was prescribed lisinopril 10 mg and glyburide 2.5 mg, respectively. He denied any medication allergies. During the preoperative assessment, the patient stated that he took lisinopril but not glyburide on the morning of surgery. Following induction of general anesthesia, the patient became profoundly hypotensive, with a blood pressure of 70/30 mm Hg that did not improve despite administration of fluid boluses and significant doses of ephedrine and phenylephrine. A vasopressin infusion was initiated at a rate of 0.03 units/minute, which resulted in prompt normalization of the patient's blood pressure. The surgery proceeded without further complications and the patient emerged from general anesthesia uneventfully.

A.L. Jayaraman MD, PhD (✉)
Department of Anesthesiology, Columbia University Medical Center, New York, NY, USA
e-mail: aljayaraman@gmail.com

T.A. Gelzinis MD
Department of Anesthesiology, University of Pittsburgh Medical Center, Pittsburgh, PA, USA

C. Marcucci et al. (eds.), *A Case Approach to Perioperative Drug-Drug Interactions*, DOI 10.1007/978-1-4614-7495-1_28

Discussion

This is an example of multiple cumulative pharmacodynamic interactions.

Angiotensin-converting enzyme inhibitors (ACE-Is) and angiotensin receptor blockers (ARBs) are commonly used to treat a number of medical conditions, including hypertension and congestive heart failure, and they also administered to limit progression of diabetic nephropathy. In patients with congestive heart failure, ACE-Is are considered first-line therapy due to their beneficial effects on left ventricular remodeling. ARBs are frequently prescribed to patients intolerant of ACE-Is. In patients with severe congestive heart failure or hypertension, both an ACE-I and ARB may be prescribed, as this is thought to result in additive renin-angiotensin-aldosterone system (RAAS) suppression. The benefits of such combined therapy have been called into question due to an increased risk for proteinuria and renal dysfunction seen with dual therapy.

These medications target RAAS. Specifically, ACE-Is block angiotensin II production, whereas ARBs inhibit the effects of angiotensin II at the angiotensin receptor. This results in reduced arterial blood pressure via several mechanisms, including antagonizing the synthesis or effects of the vasoconstrictor angiotensin II, blunting aldosterone secretion, and increasing levels of the vasodilator bradykinin. In the perioperative setting, this results in dampening of the normal, physiological, renin-mediated response to hemorrhage, hypotension, and sympathetic stimulation.

Severe hypotension following induction of general anesthesia in patients taking ACE-Is was first described in 1989.[1] Since then, numerous case reports and prospective studies have replicated these findings, although a few have not. This post-induction hypotension is largely attributed to a cumulative sympatholysis–that of general/neuraxial anesthesia combined with the effects of ACE-I/ARB medications which, in addition to the effects detailed previously, impede angiotensin II-induced catecholamine release. Of note, it has been reported that such hypotension is exacerbated by hypovolemia.[2] Also, heed must be paid to the nature of the antihypertensive agent itself, as data indicate that ARBs produce more profound hypotension than other antihypertensive agents, including ACE-Is.[3]

As with hypotension of any etiology, ACE-I/ARB-associated hypotension should be promptly recognized and addressed. Initial treatment includes standard therapy with intravenous fluid boluses and sympathomimetic agents such as phenylephrine and ephedrine. Of note, this hypotension seems to be relatively refractory to alpha one adrenergic receptor stimulation.[3] If hypotension persists, a vasopressin infusion at 0.03 units/minute is the preferred means of managing refractory hypotension secondary to RAAS antagonism.[4] Alternatively, a 1-mg intravenous bolus of terlipressin, a synthetic vasopressin analogue, can be administered.[5,6] Although more efficacious than norepinephrine in this setting, terlipressin may decrease splanchnic blood flow.[7,8] Bradycardia, due to the inhibition of RAAS-mediated release of catecholamines, can be prevented or treated with glycopyrrolate administration.[9]

There are certain perioperative situations where ACEI/ARB-associated hypotension may be particularly problematic, including surgery in the sitting/beach chair and prone positions, due to increased potential for hypotensive neurologic injury. Additionally, vasoplegia is of significant concern in procedures requiring cardiopulmonary bypass (CPB). There have been multiple studies showing that patients undergoing CPB while taking ACE-Is have a greater incidence of hypotension than those in whom ACE-I therapy was suspended preoperatively and that the degree of hypotension is correlated with ACE-I dosage.[10–13]

Although there is no clear consensus regarding withholding ACE-I/ARB therapy preoperatively, it is important to balance the risk for poorly controlled hypertension or decompensated heart failure with those of profound perioperative hypotension. Some advocate continuing ACE-I/ARB therapy preoperatively, whereas others adopt a more nuanced approach, holding ACE-I/ARB therapy in those taking it for mild to moderate hypertension and continuing it in those patients with severe hypertension or left ventricular dysfunction. Complicating this decision is a recent retrospective study involving over 60,000 patients undergoing noncardiac surgery that found chronic ACE-I therapy to be associated with a significant decrease in 30-day mortality, although preoperative cessation of ACE-Is was not specifically addressed.[13] Given their variable pharmacokinetics, if the decision is made to hold these medications preoperatively, they should be stopped 12 to 24 hours prior to surgery. It remains to be seen if similar hemodynamic effects are observed with direct renin inhibitors, such as aliskiren (Novartis®), which represent a rather novel class of medications that target RAAS.

Take-Home Points

- ACE-I and/or ARB therapy may result in significant hypotension following induction of general or neuraxial anesthesia.
- If refractory to more conventional therapies, this hypotension may be effectively treated with either a vasopressin infusion or a bolus of terlipressin.
- There are insufficient data to support routinely discontinuing these medications preoperatively.
- Deliberate and individualized decisions regarding continuing or discontinuing ACE-Is/ARBs must be made in light of each patient's medical comorbidities and the anticipated hemodynamic changes/requirements of the anesthetic/surgery that they are to undergo.

Summary

Interaction: pharmacodynamic
Substrates: general and neuraxial anesthetics, angiotensin converting enzyme inhibitors and angiotensin receptor blockers
Mechanism/site of action: renin-angiotensin-aldosterone system, sympathetic nervous system
Clinical effect: significant or profound hypotension

References

1. McConachie I, Healy TEJ. ACE inhibitors and anaesthesia. Postgrad Med J. 1989;65:273–4.
2. Coriat P, Richer C, Douraki T, et al. Influence of chronic angiotensin-converting enzyme inhibition on anesthetic induction. Anesthesiology. 1994;81:299–307.
3. Brabant SM, Bertrand M, Eyraud D, et al. The hemodynamic effects of anesthetic induction in vascular surgery patients chronically treated with angiotensin II receptor antagonists. Anesth Analg. 1999;89:1388–92.
4. Papadopoulos G, Sintou E, Siminelakis S, et al. Perioperative infusion of low-dose vasopressin for prevention and management of vasodilatory vasoplegic syndrome in patients undergoing coronary artery bypass grafting–a double blind randomized study. J Cardiothorac Surg. 2010;5:17.
5. Eyraud D, Mouren S, Teugels K, et al. Treating anesthesia-induced hypotension by angiotensin II in patients chronically treated with angiotensin converting enzyme inhibitors. Anesth Analg. 1998;86:259–63.
6. Eyraud D, Brabant S, Mathalie D, et al. Treatment of intraoperative refractory hypotension with terlipressin in patients chronically treated with an antagonist of the renin-angiotensin system. Anesth Analg. 1999;88:980–4.
7. Boccara G, Ouattara A, Godet G, et al. Terlipressin versus norepinephrine to correct refractory arterial hypotension after general anesthesia in patients chronically treated with renin-angiotensin system inhibitors. Anesthesiology. 2003;98:1338–44.
8. Morelli A, Tritapepe L, Rocco M, et al. Terlipressin versus norepinephrine to counteract anesthesia-induced hypotension in patient treated with renin-angiotensin system inhibitors: effects on systemic and regional hemodynamics. Anesthesiology. 2005;102:12–9.
9. Prys-Roberts C. Withdrawal of antihypertensive drugs before anesthesia. Anesth Analg. 2002;94:767–8.
10. Hasija S, Makhija N, Choudhury M, et al. Prophylactic vasopressin in patients receiving the angiotensin converting enzyme inhibitor ramipril undergoing coronary artery bypass graft surgery. J Cardiothorac Vasc Anesth. 2010;24(2):230–8.
11. Tuman KJ, McCarthy RJ, O'Connor CJ, et al. Angiotensin converting enzyme inhibitors increase vasoconstrictor requirements after cardiopulmonary bypass. Anesth Analg. 1995;80(3):473–9.
12. Shahzamani M, Yousefi Z, Frootaghe AN, et al. The effect of angiotensin converting enzyme inhibitor on hemodynamic instability in patients undergoing cardiopulmonary bypass: results of a dose comparison study. J Cardiovasc Pharmacol Ther. 2009;14(3):185–91.
13. Tippin J, Naughton F, Wijeysundera D, et al. ACE inhibitors reduce 30-day mortality after non-cardiac surgery. Society of Cardiovascular Anesthesiologists annual meeting. 2011.

Alpha-2 to the Rescue but Beware Bradycardia

29

Inhalational anesthetics, α_2-agents

Phillip Adams DO and Nashaant N. Rizk MD

Abstract
This case discusses multiple pharmacodynamic interactions between dexmedetomidine and desflurane, resulting in sedation, analgesia, and possible bradycardia and hypotension.

Case

A 52-year-old man with a body mass index (BMI) of 47 kg/m^2 presented for a laparoscopic roux-en-Y gastric bypass surgery. He had a moderately decreased functional status with easy fatigability. He was currently taking hydrochlorothiazide for hypertension and metformin for type 2 diabetes mellitus. In addition, he had obstructive sleep apnea for which he intermittently wore his continuous positive airway pressure (CPAP) machine while sleeping. Preoperative electrocardiogram and laboratory values were within normal limits aside from a blood glucose level of 148 mg/dL.

The anesthesia team was concerned about the use of opioid analgesics and the increased risk for postoperative respiratory depression and mechanical ventilation, given the patient's body habitus and preoperative functional status. It was determined that dexmedetomidine would be used in place of opioid analgesics. The attending anesthesiologist cautioned the resident to be vigilant for bradycardia.

During the procedure, mean blood pressures were maintained around 70 mm Hg and heart rate was maintained at approximately 75 beats per minute. Only 0.6 MAC desflurane was needed to maintain bispectral index (BIS) values 45 to 50.[1] After the

P. Adams DO (✉) • N.N. Rizk MD
Department of Anesthesiology, University of Pittsburgh Medical Center, Pittsburgh, PA, USA
e-mail: adamsp@upmc.edu

C. Marcucci et al. (eds.), *A Case Approach to Perioperative Drug-Drug Interactions*, DOI 10.1007/978-1-4614-7495-1_29

surgery was complete, the desflurane was discontinued and the patient was awakened and extubated in about 10 minutes. In the recovery room, he had stable vital signs, no signs of hypoxemia or respiratory depression, and did not require much use of his patient-controlled analgesia (PCA).[1]

After being observed in the postanesthesia care unit (PACU) for 70 minutes, the patient remained comfortable and was transferred to floor in stable condition.

Discussion

This is an example of multiple and complex pharmacodynamic interactions.

Alpha-2 adrenergic agonists (α_2 agonists) have been used for years for several different reasons. Uses of α_2 agonists include treatment of hypertension, analgesic adjuncts for both acute and chronic pain, regional and neuraxial anesthetic adjuncts, analgesics for diabetic neuropathy, surgical premedication and anxiolysis, treatment of postoperative shivering, and aids in overcoming alcohol and narcotic withdrawal, to name a few.[2]

Commonly used α_2 agonists include clonidine, dexmedetomidine, and tizanidine. There are several other agents that are commonly used in veterinary medicine and still more that are currently under development. The routes of administration are variable. Clonidine and tizanidine are common oral medications, whereas dexmedetomidine is traditionally administered intravenously. Clonidine is also available in a transdermal patch and has been approved for epidural administration for the treatment of chronic pain associated with malignancy. Intrathecal administration of these medications has also been performed.

Alpha-2 agonists exert their action via binding to guanine nucleotide-binding regulatory proteins (G proteins), in particular central inhibitory G proteins, which decrease intracellular adenylate cyclase.[3] By contrast, α_1-adrenergic receptor activation is most notable postsynaptically in the periphery. Agonism of peripheral α_1-adrenergic receptors elicits an excitatory effect on the cell and manifestations, such as vasoconstriction, are clinically observed. Clonidine has a selectivity ratio for α_2:α_1 of 220:1, whereas dexmedetomidine is much more selective for α_2 receptors with a selectivity ratio of 1,620:1.[3] Alpha-2 agonists bind presynaptically on the central α_{2A} receptor subtype on afferent nociceptive C fibers and also postsynaptically on the central α_{2C} receptor subtype on spinal dorsal horn neurons (Fig. 29.1).[4,5] By binding presynaptically to nociceptive afferent fibers, α_2 agonists prevent the release of neuroexcitatory glutamate.[5] Postsynaptic binding to dorsal horn neurons hyperpolarizes these cells and halts further transmission of the nociceptive stimulus.[5] The sedative and analgesic effects are thought to be further mediated by the central action on the locus coeruleus (a major noradrenergic center of the brain), amygdala, and the descending inhibitory pathways of the spinal cord.[2,3]

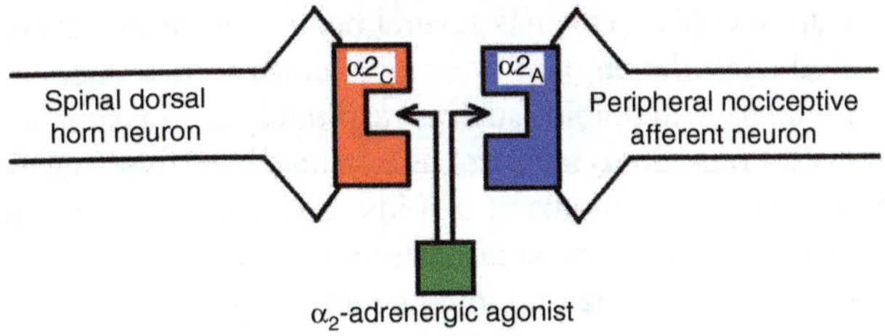

Fig. 29.1 Figure illustrating the central pre- and postsynaptic binding of α_2-adrenoreceptor agonists. Presynaptic binding to nociceptive afferent nerves prevents neuroexcitatory glutamate release. Postsynaptic binding to spinal dorsal horn neurons hyperpolarizes the neuron and prevents conductance of the noxious stimulus [Based on data from refs[4,5]]

The use of α_2 agonists does not come without the possibility of adverse effects. Most commonly, patients can experience bradycardia and hypotension associated with the use of α_2 agonists due to the sympatholytic effects. Furthermore, patients on chronic clonidine therapy as part of an antihypertensive regimen should not have their clonidine suddenly discontinued, as this could result in sympathetic overactivity and rebound hypertension.[6]

Minimum Alveolar Concentration (MAC) Effect

Alpha-2 agonists have been shown to reduce the MAC of inhalational anesthetics. Even single doses of intravenous dexmedetomidine (2 μg/kg) or oral clonidine (5 μg/kg) can reduce the MAC of inhalational anesthetics and provide cardiovascular stability.[7,8] Continuous infusion of dexmedetomidine throughout the operative procedure has been shown to decrease the MAC of sevoflurane by as much as 17% in cases where sevoflurane and dexmedetomidine were the only agents used.[9] Higher doses of dexmedetomidine can reduce isoflurane MAC by as much as 47%.[10]

Furthermore, α_2 agonists have been shown to not only decrease inhalational anesthetic requirements, but intravenous anesthetic requirements as well. When clonidine is administered during intravenous anesthesia with propofol, BIS values decrease and there can be up to a 20% reduction in the amount of propofol required.[11]

Analgesic Effects

In addition to their ability to lower the MAC of inhalational anesthetics, α_2 agonists have opioid-sparing, analgesic effects. Alpha-2 agonists can also augment the analgesic effects of opioids when given concurrently. A single preoperative dose of oral clonidine can reduce postoperative morphine PCA use by as much as 37%.[12] Dexmedetomidine infusions in the postoperative period can reduce morphine requirements by up to 66%.[13] This has several beneficial implications in the perioperative period. Reducing the amount of opioids consumed reduces the side effects commonly encountered with opioids such as respiratory depression, nausea, pruritus, and constipation. Not only do α_2 agonists reduce postoperative nausea and vomiting (PONV) due to the reduced amounts of opioids consumed, but some research shows that norepinephrine binding in the area postrema can result in emesis.[12] Therefore, reduced levels of norepinephrine due to α_2 agonists could have a more direct antiemetic effect.[12]

Furthermore, intravenous and epidural administration of clonidine has been shown to be effective as the sole analgesic in the postoperative period.[14] Epidural clonidine administration was associated with less sedation with equal analgesia when compared to intravenous clonidine.[14]

Take-Home Points

- Alpha-2 agonists can reduce the MAC of inhalational anesthetics when given as a premedication or administered as an infusion throughout the procedure. Using less inhalational agent can have beneficial effects on a patient's cardiovascular status (although hypotension and bradycardia are possible adverse effects of α_2 agonists) as well as reduce the incidence or severity of PONV.[15]

- Alpha-2 agonists have analgesic properties that can permit a reduction in the amount of perioperative opioid that is needed. By reducing the amount of opioids that are administered, there can be less of a risk for opioid-induced respiratory depression and also a decrease in opioid-induced PONV.[15,16]

Summary

Interactions: pharmacodynamic (multiple)
Substrates: dexmedetomidine, desflurane
Mechanism of action/sites: pre- and post-synaptic central α_2 receptors in multiple locations
Clinical effect: sedation, analgesia (bradycardia and hypotension are also possible)

References

1. Feld JM, Hoffman WE, Stechert MM, et al. Fentanyl or dexmedetomidine combined with desflurane for bariatric surgery. J Clin Anesth. 2006;18:24–8.
2. Wallace AW. Clonidine and modification of perioperative outcome. Curr Opin Anaesthesiol. 2006;19:411–7.
3. Giovannoni MP, Ghelardini C, Vergelli C, Dal Piaz V. α_2-agonists as analgesic agents. Med Res Rev. 2009;29(2):339–68.
4. Pan YZ, Li DP, Pan HL. Inhibition of glutamatergic synaptic input to spinal lamina II_o neurons by presynaptic α_2-adrenergic receptors. J Neurophysiol. 2002;87:1938–47.
5. Chen SR, Chen H, Yuan WX, Pan HL. Increased presynaptic and postsynaptic α_2-adrenoceptor activity in the spinal dorsal horn in painful diabetic neuropathy. J Pharmacol Exp Ther. 2011;337:285–92.
6. Vongpatanasin W, Kario K, Atlas SA, et al. Central sympatholytic drugs. J Clin Hypertens. 2011;13:658–61.
7. Katoh T, Ikeda K. The effect of clonidine on sevoflurane requirements for anaesthesia and hypnosis. Anaesthesia. 1997;52:377–81.
8. Lawrence CJ, De Lange S. Effects of single pre-operative dexmedetomidine dose on isoflurane requirements and peri-operative haemodynamic stability. Anaesthesia. 1997;52:736–44.
9. Fragen RJ, Fitzgerald PC. Effect of dexmedetomidine on the minimum alveolar concentration (MAC) of sevoflurane in adults age 55 to 70 years. J Clin Anesth. 1999;11:466–70.
10. Aantaa R, Jaakola ML, Kallio A, et al. Reduction of the minimum alveolar concentration of isoflurane by dexmedetomidine. Anesthesiology. 1997;86:1055–60.
11. Fehr SB, Zalunardo MP, Seifert B, et al. Clonidine decreases propofol requirements during anaesthesia: effect on bispectral index. Br J Anaesth. 2001;86:627–32.
12. Park J, Forrest J, Kolesar R, et al. Oral clonidine reduces postoperative PCA morphine requirements. Can J Anaesth. 1996;43:900–6.
13. Arain SR, Ruehlow RM, Uhrich TD, et al. The efficacy of dexmedetomidine versus morphine for postoperative analgesia after major inpatient surgery. Anesth Analg. 2004;98:153–8.
14. Bernard JM, Kick O, Bonnet F. Comparison of intravenous and epidural clonidine for postoperative patient-controlled analgesia. Anesth Analg. 1995;81:706–12.
15. Gan TJ. Risk factors for postoperative nausea and vomiting. Anesth Analg. 2006;102:1884–98.
16. Carollo DS, Nossaman BD, Ramadhyani U. Dexmedetomidine: a review of clinical applications. Curr Opin Anaesthesiol. 2008;21(4):457–61.

Hot Stuff!

30

Triggering drugs, ryanodine receptor, malignant hyperthermia

Cornelius B. Groenewald MD, ChB
and Juraj Sprung MD, PhD

Abstract
This case discusses a drug–gene interaction. Administration of the triggering drugs isoflurane and succinylcholine interacted with a genetic variation of the ryanodine receptor causing malignant hyperthermia during general anesthesia.

Case

A 23-year-old man with no significant previous medical history and no known drug allergies presented to the emergency department with an open left tibial fracture after a motorcycle crash. It was determined that he needed an emergent débridement and washout of the fracture. He had never undergone general anesthesia and was not aware of any anesthetic-related complications in his family.

The patient had an uncomplicated rapid-sequence induction and intubation with propofol and succinylcholine chloride. After induction, his blood pressure was 135/70 mm Hg; heart rate was 75 beats per minute (bpm), and body temperature was 36.7 °C. Anesthesia was maintained with isoflurane in air and oxygen, and he received intravenous hydromorphone for pain control. He was stable during the first hour of anesthesia.

C.B. Groenewald MD, ChB (✉)
Department of Anesthesiology & Pain Medicine,
Seattle Children's Hospital and the University of Washington,
Seattle, WA, USA
e-mail: neelsgroenewald@gmail.com

J. Sprung MD, PhD
Department of Anesthesiology, Mayo Clinic, Rochester, MN, USA

C. Marcucci et al. (eds.), *A Case Approach to Perioperative Drug-Drug Interactions*, DOI 10.1007/978-1-4614-7495-1_30

One hour after anesthetic induction, the patient's end-tidal CO_2 concentration increased from 32 mm Hg to 50 mm Hg, despite repeated adjustments of mechanical ventilation. His heart rate and blood pressure increased to 165/95 mm Hg and 110 bpm, and the anesthesiologist administered additional pain medication. The patient's temperature increased to 38.5 °C. Efforts to control hypercapnia proved difficult, and the resident suspected that malignant hyperthermia (MH) might be developing.

The anesthesiology attending was paged to the operating room and decided to initiate the MH protocol. Arterial blood gas testing showed respiratory and metabolic acidosis ($PaCO_2$,75 mm Hg; serum bicarbonate, 15 mEq/L). Serum potassium concentration was 6.4 mEq/L, and an electrocardiogram showed widening of the QRS complex and tall, peaked T waves.

Before the MH protocol was initiated, the patient's temperature reached 41.2 °C. The surgeons quickly packed the wound and completed the operation. Isoflurane was discontinued, the patient's endotracheal tube was connected to a fresh breathing circuit and a new CO_2 canister was placed, and his lungs were hyperventilated with 100% oxygen. Anesthesia was continued with propofol infusion. Simultaneously, the pharmacist prepared dantrolene sodium with sterile water, which was administered intravenously. An infusion of glucose and insulin also was administered to treat hyperkalemia. Soon, the patient's temperature and end-tidal carbon dioxide level started to decrease. The anesthesiologist called the Malignant Hyperthermia Association of the United States hotline (1-800-MHHYPER) to speak with an MH expert, who agreed that the case might be MH. The patient was transferred to the intensive care unit for an overnight stay, where he was extubated the following morning. The rest of his hospital stay was uneventful.

Six months after this episode, the patient had a muscle biopsy and a contracture test result was positive for caffeine and halothane, confirming MH.

Discussion

This is an example of a drug–gene interaction.

More specifically, this is a genetic variation (of the ryanodine receptor) influencing the toxicity (malignant hyperthermia) with triggering drugs (isoflurane and succinylcholine) during general anesthesia.

MH is a potentially fatal pharmacogenetic syndrome of skeletal muscle that develops after exposure to halogenated volatile anesthetics (ie, enflurane, methoxyflurane, isoflurane, sevoflurane, desflurane, and halothane) and the depolarizing muscle relaxant succinylcholine.[1]

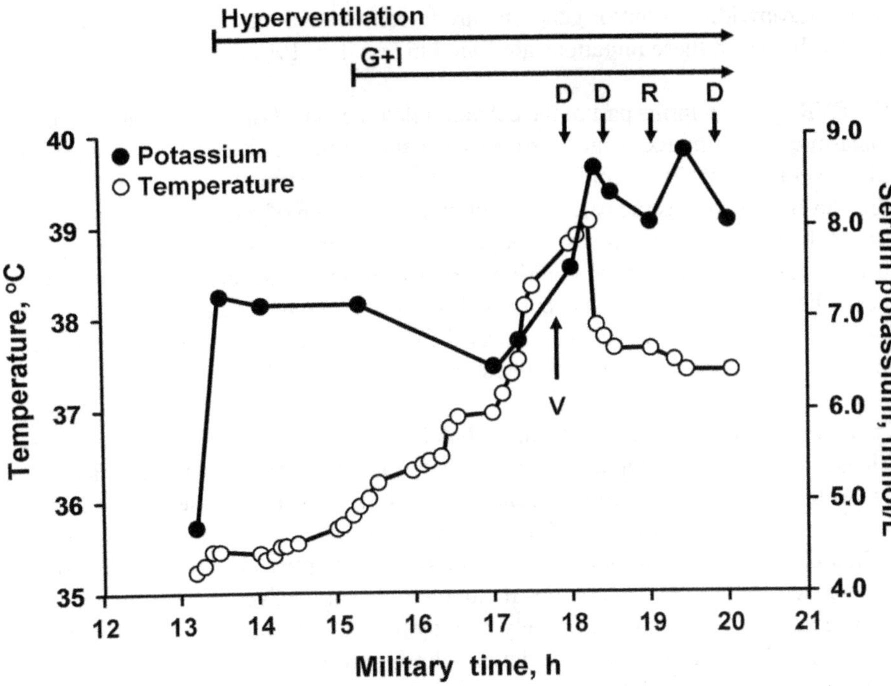

Fig. 30.1 Changes in body temperature and serum potassium concentration over time during anesthesia of a patient with diabetes mellitus and end-stage renal disease who had malignant hyperthermia. Treatments consisted of D, dantrolene; G+I, glucose and insulin infusion; R, successful cardiopulmonary resuscitation; and V, verapamil. Clearly, temperature increase is gradual and a late sign of malignant hyperthermia [Adapted from Sprung J, DeBoer G, Zanettin G et al: Intraoperative hyperkalemia as a triggering mechanism or presenting sign of malignant hyperthermia in two patients with chronic renal failure. Anesthesiology. 1995;82:1518–22. With permission from Wolter Kluwers Health]

Signs and symptoms of MH are those of a hypermetabolic state and generally present with continuously increasing hypercapnia, despite adjustment of mechanical ventilation. This response is associated with metabolic acidosis, hyperkalemia (Fig. 30.1), hypercalcemia, and elevated serum creatine phosphokinase levels, as well as increased heart rate and blood pressure. Elevated temperature develops later, and eventually the patient becomes rigid.[2]

Genetic inheritance of MH is autosomal dominant; however, its expression is variable and up to 50% of individuals with the genetic inheritance may give a history of a previous uneventful general inhalational anesthesia.[3] During the past 15 years, more than 100 families with MH susceptibility have been identified in Europe, the United States, and Japan. For 50% to 80% of these individuals, the disorder is linked to the type 1 ryanodine receptor gene (*RYR1*) located on chromosome 19.[4,5] Most *RYR1* mutations occur in the area of amino acid residues 35 to 614 (N-terminal region), 2117 to 2458 (central region), and 3916 to 4973 (C-terminal region). Other areas identified include the dihydropyridine receptor gene on chromosome 7 and the α_1 subunit on chromosome 1; however, these mutations are found in less than 1% of patients.

The RYR1 protein forms part of the calcium release channel of the skeletal muscle sarcoplasmic reticulum. Exposure to triggering agents causes excessive release of intracellular calcium from the sarcoplasmic reticulum in the presence of an abnormal *RYR1*. High levels of myoplasmic calcium result in the activation of pumps and exchangers to drive calcium back to its reservoirs (ie, mitochondria and the sarcoplasmic reticulum), in an energy-intensive process requiring adenosine triphosphate and resulting in a hypermetabolic state. Hyperthermia occurs, and the accompanying increased metabolic rate causes tachycardia, hypertension, increased CO_2 production, and acidosis. Eventually, calcium levels reach the contractile threshold and the patient becomes rigid.[1]

Treatment is aimed at removing the inhalational anesthetic and reducing calcium release from the sarcoplasmic reticulum through dantrolene administration. Dantrolene is the skeletal muscle relaxant that inhibits Ca^{++} release from the sarcoplasmic reticulum during excitation-contraction coupling and suppresses the uncontrolled Ca^{++} release that underlies the skeletal muscle pharmacogenetic disorder in persons with MH.[6] Other strategies include giving supportive ventilation, maintaining adequate hemodynamics, actively cooling the patient, and treating the metabolic (acidosis) and electrolyte (hyperkalemia) abnormalities.

Genetic testing identifies only about 30% of MH-susceptible patients through sequencing of the abnormal *RYR1* and is not widely used currently. The gold standard for diagnosis continues to be muscle biopsy with the caffeine-halothane contracture test, which is administered at only five locations in North America.[7]

Take-Home Points

- MH is an autosomal-dominant pharmacogenetic disorder with variable expression. Triggering agents include enflurane, methoxyflurane, isoflurane, sevoflurane, desflurane, halothane, and succinylcholine.
- The abnormally functioning *RYR1* causes increased intracellular calcium concentration, which in turn leads to markedly increased metabolism and heat production.
- Treatment involves stopping all triggering agents and administering dantrolene.
- The Malignant Hyperthermia Association of the United States provides 24-hour coverage to medical personnel with questions regarding MH and can be reached at 1-800-MHHYPER.

Summary

Interaction: pharmacogenomic

Substrates: enflurane, methoxyflurane, isoflurane, sevoflurane, desflurane, halothane, and succinylcholine

Gene(s): type 1 ryanodine receptor gene (*RYR1*) located on chromosome 19 (50%–80% of patients) and the dihydropyridine receptor gene on chromosome 7, and α_1 subunit on chromosome 1; however, these mutations are found in less than 1% of patients (less common)

Mechanism/site of action: *RYR1* mutation results in excessive release of intracellular calcium from the sarcoplasmic reticulum with activation of pumps and exchangers to drive calcium back to its reservoirs in an energy-intensive process requiring adenosine triphosphate and resulting in a hypermetabolic state

Clinical effect: constellation of malignant hyperthermia symptoms, including hypercapnia, metabolic acidosis, hyperkalemia, hypercalcemia, tachycardia, hypertension, hyperthermia (late effect), and rigidity (late effect)

References

1. Zhou J, Allen PD, Pessah IN, et al. Neuromuscular disorders and malignant hyperthermia. In: Miller RD, editor. Miller's anesthesia, vol. 1. 7th ed. Philadelphia: Churchill Livingstone; 2010. p. 1171–96.
2. Larach MG, Localio AR, Allen GC, et al. A clinical grading scale to predict malignant hyperthermia susceptibility. Anesthesiology. 1994;80:771–9.
3. Brandom BW. The genetics of malignant hyperthermia. Anesthesiol Clin North America. 2005;23:615–9.
4. Carpenter D, Robinson RL, Quinnell RJ, et al. Genetic variation in RYR1 and malignant hyperthermia phenotypes. Br J Anaesth. 2009;103:538–48.
5. Sambuughin N, Holley H, Muldoon S, et al. Screening of the entire ryanodine receptor type 1 coding region for sequence variants associated with malignant hyperthermia susceptibility in the North American population. Anesthesiology. 2005;102:515–21.
6. Fruen BR, Mickelson JR, Louis CF. Dantrolene inhibition of sarcoplasmic reticulum Ca2+ release by direct and specific action at skeletal muscle ryanodine receptors. J Biol Chem. 1997;272:26965–71.
7. Malignant Hyperthermia Association of the United States [Internet]. Guideline: testing for malignant hyperthermia susceptibility [cited 14 Sep 2009]. Available from: http://medical.mhaus.org/PubData/PDFs/treatmentposter.pdf.

Part V
Drug–Drug Interactions Involving Intravenous Anesthetic Agents

31 Introduction

Catherine Marcucci MD

Abstract
This section introduces drug–drug interactions involving intravenous anesthetic agents.

Because the intravenous anesthetic agents are given essentially as unit doses, drug–drug interactions (DDIs) in this drug class have not generally been determined to involve induction or inhibition of the cytochrome P450 system. Remember that inhibition of P450 enzymes generally happens on the order of days and induction on the order of weeks—this requires sustained dosing of the drug.

Nonetheless, significant and clinically relevant DDIs do occur with these drugs as anyone can attest who has ever looked in dismay at the precipitate that formed in an intravenous line just as induction was taking place.

Another interesting DDI that occurs in this drug class is the interaction between dexmedetomidine and spinal bupivacaine (see **Dexy's Midnight Spinal**). The phenomenon of prolongation of the block has been reported, but the mechanism is still not fully elucidated. It is a good illustration, however, of the need to remain vigilant and motivated to educate oneself about attendant DDIs whenever a new anesthetic drug comes on the market. The drug is introduced and then, usually in fairly short order, the case reports start appearing.

C. Marcucci MD
Anesthesia Services Department, Philadelphia Veterans Affairs Medical Center, Philadelphia, PA, USA
e-mail: sandson.marcucci@comcast.net

C. Marcucci et al. (eds.), *A Case Approach to Perioperative Drug-Drug Interactions*, DOI 10.1007/978-1-4614-7495-1_31

How to Successfully Occlude an Intravenous Line

32

Thiopental, rocuronium, line precipitation

Helga Komen MD, Juraj Sprung MD, PhD
and Toby N. Weingarten MD

Abstract
This case discusses the chemical interaction of thiopental sodium and rocuronium resulting in precipitation.

Case

A 34-year-old man presented to the emergency department with fever, severe abdominal pain, vomiting, and clinical signs of peritonitis. A computed tomographic scan revealed acute appendicitis, and immediate emergent open appendectomy was planned. With some difficulty, a 22-gauge (22-g) intravenous (IV) line was placed on the dorsum of his left hand. The anesthesia team intended to place larger IV access after induction.

A rapid-sequence induction with cricoid pressure to minimize the risk for aspiration was planned. After the patient received adequate preoxygenation, the anesthesiologist rapidly administered thiopental (500 mg), followed by rocuronium (70 mg).

However, immediately after administration of rocuronium, the IV line ceased to flow. Inspection of the tubing revealed a white precipitate. The nurse anesthetist began to gently and slowly mask-ventilate (allowing the end-tidal carbon dioxide to rise while preserving arterial oxygen saturation above 90%, balancing the

H. Komen MD (✉)
Department of Anesthesiology and Critical Care Medicine,
University Hospital Rijeka, Rijeka, Croatia
e-mail: helga.komen@ri.t-com.hr

J. Sprung MD, PhD • T.N. Weingarten MD
Department of Anesthesiology, Mayo Clinic, Rochester, MN, USA

C. Marcucci et al. (eds.), *A Case Approach to Perioperative Drug-Drug Interactions*, DOI 10.1007/978-1-4614-7495-1_32

risk for gastric insufflation with that of hypoxemia) with a mixture of sevoflurane and 100% oxygen while the surgical nurse continued to apply cricoid pressure. The anesthesiologist successfully placed a 20-g IV line in the right hand and, because the patient showed respiratory efforts, also administered succinylcholine (80 mg). Fortunately, the patient did not have oxyhemoglobin desaturation or vomit while the second IV line was placed, and his trachea was successfully intubated.

Discussion

This is an example of a physicochemical (acid–base) interaction.

Thiopental is a commonly used anesthetic induction drug. Thiopental is unstable in water or normal saline and is stored as a salt with sodium. Before use, it is reconstituted in water or normal saline. The reconstituted form is alkaline (pH >10).[1] Acidification of the reconstituted solution results in formation of a precipitate of thiopental as a free acid.[1]

Numerous drugs used in the practice of anesthesia are in acidic solutions and may cause thiopental to precipitate (Table 32.1). A mixture of these medications with thiopental, or their administration in conjunction with or immediately after the administration of thiopental, can cause the formation of fine crystalline particles that may block an IV catheter or needle, especially one that has a small bore (≤20 g).[1–4]

In the case of rapid-sequence induction, when rocuronium bromide is given in close temporal sequence with thiopental, precipitation can occur. The precipitation is immediate and firm, and frequently the IV line cannot be flushed to overcome the blockage. Similar incompatibility with thiopental is found with other muscle relaxants, such as succinylcholine and vecuronium.[2,4]

Human plasma is effective in dissolving thiopental particles, and therefore it is unlikely that clinically significant particles of thiopental will stay intact on entering the bloodstream. However, mixing thiopental with pancuronium, vecuronium, or rocuronium has the potential to disrupt IV access because of occlusion with particles.[4,5] So, when thiopental is used in conjunction with a muscle relaxant, the anesthesiologist must flush the IV tubing adequately before subsequent administration of the muscle relaxant. This step is especially important to keep in mind during rapid-sequence anesthetic induction, when succinylcholine or rocuronium typically are administered in close temporal sequence with thiopental.

Table 32.1 Incompatibility of thiopental with commonly used anesthetic drugs

Muscle relaxants
Atracurium
Pancuronium
Rocuronium
Succinylcholine
Vecuronium
Vasoactive medications
Diltiazem
Dobutamine
Dopamine
Ephedrine
Labetalol
Nicardipine
Phenylephrine
Anticholinergic medications
Atropine
Glycopyrrolate
Benzodiazepines
Midazolam
Opioids
Alfentanil
Morphine
Sufentanil

[Based on Data from refs.[1–4]]

Take-Home Points

- Thiopental is an alkaline solution and is unstable in water and in normal saline. When mixed with an acidic solution, the thiopental precipitates.
- Rocuronium is an acidic solution and can cause thiopental precipitation when given simultaneously through the same needle with or immediately after thiopental sodium.
- The precipitate, particularly in a small-bore needle or IV line, may result in blockage of the catheter.
- Succinylcholine, vecuronium, and pancuronium have similar characteristics regarding interaction with thiopental sodium, and care must be taken to avoid precipitation when this combination is used.

Summary

Interaction: physicochemical (acid–base)
Precipitants: thiopental (alkaline or base compound) and rocuronium (acidic solution)
Clinical effect: formation of precipitate with occlusion of line

References

1. Reves JG, Glass PSA, Lubarsky DA, et al. Intravenous anesthetics. In: Miller RD, editor. Miller's anesthesia, vol. 1. 7th ed. Philadelphia: Churchill Livingstone; 2010. p. 728.
2. Trissel LA. Handbook on injectable drugs. 15th ed. Bethesda: American Society of Health-System Pharmacists; 2008. p. 1493–9.
3. Trissel LA. Handbook on injectable drugs. 15th ed. Bethesda: American Society of Health-System Pharmacists; 2008. p. 1463–5.
4. Mahisekar UL, Callan CM, Derasari M, et al. Infusion of large particles of thiopental sodium during anesthesia induction. J Clin Anesth. 1994;6:55–8.
5. Molbegott L. The precipitation of rocuronium in a needleless intravenous injection adaptor. Anesthesiology. 1995;83:223.

A Curious Cause of Seizures

33

Fatal Forty DDI: ketamine, theophylline

Charles Galaviz MD and Randal O. Dull MD, PhD

Abstract
This case discusses a ketamine/theophylline interaction of unknown etiology resulting in decreased seizure threshold.

Case

A 24-year-old, 65 kg woman presented to the hospital for diagnostic abdominal laparoscopy. Because she had a history of severe asthma requiring hospitalization and intubation, she was admitted to the hospital on the night before her surgery for optimization of her asthma before planned general anesthesia.

She was given a loading dose of aminophylline (5.9 mg/kg), followed by an aminophylline maintenance infusion (1 mg/kg/hr). The following morning, she was taken to the operating room, anesthesia was induced with ketamine (100 mg) over 2 minutes. Within minutes, ventilation became impossible due to jaw rigidity, and her upper extremities developed extensor posturing. The patient's heart rate also increased from 80 to 120 beats per minute. Succinylcholine (80 mg) was given, and ventilation via mask became easy. The patient was intubated, and the rest of the intraoperative course was uneventful.

C. Galaviz MD (✉)
Department of Anesthesiology, University of Utah, Salt Lake City, UT, USA
e-mail: Charles.galaviz@hsc.utah.edu

R.O. Dull MD, PhD
Department of Anesthesiology, University of Illinois at Chicago, Chicago, IL, USA

C. Marcucci et al. (eds.), *A Case Approach to Perioperative Drug-Drug Interactions*, DOI 10.1007/978-1-4614-7495-1_33

Discussion

This is an example of a drug–drug interaction of undetermined mechanism.

Drug–drug interactions between ketamine and theophylline resulting in seizures have been reported.[4,5] The mechanism is not known. Aminophylline is a combined preparation of theophylline and ethylenediamine. Theophylline is a substrate for cytochrome P450 1A2 (primarily), and is secondarily a substrate for cytochromes 2E1 and 3A4, (it is important to note that some studies have shown that 3A4 does not contribute to theophylline metabolism.)[1,2] Ketamine has been thought of as primarily a substrate for cytochrome 2B6 and a minor substrate for 3A4 and 2C9 (although recent research suggests that at clinical concentrations 3A4 may be the principal enzyme responsible for ketamine metabolism in the liver).[1,3] Neither drug is an inducer or inhibitor of P450 enzymes.

There are several case reports of seizures with this drug combination.[4,5] Theophylline is rarely used in the United States, however, the drug is still commonly used in Africa, Asia, South America, and parts of Eastern Europe. In the cases that have been reported, ketamine was always given to someone who was already receiving theophylline, and the seizure began shortly after the ketamine was administered. A laboratory study in mice demonstrated that the combination of ketamine and theophylline did, in fact, lower the seizure threshold though no mechanism for this decrease in the threshold was postulated.

High concentrations of theophylline are associated with multiple deleterious side effects, one of which is seizures. Because ketamine was administered to a patient who was already getting theophylline, and the seizure occurred shortly after the ketamine was administered; the inference is raised that the addition of ketamine resulted in an increase of the fraction of theophylline available in the bloodstream. If so, the possible mechanisms could involve either displacement of theophylline by ketamine on the transport proteins in the bloodstream, or a change in the profile of which drug between the two is preferentially metabolized by 3A4.

Take-Home Points

- Ketamine and theophylline are both metabolized by more than one cytochrome P450 enzyme.
- Ketamine administration to someone who is already receiving aminophylline (theophylline) has been reported to result in seizures.
- The mechanism for such seizures is unknown. Thus, it is prudent to avoid this combination of drugs.

Summary

Interaction: unknown
Substrates: theophylline and ketamine
Mechanism/site of action/enzyme: unknown, possibly displacement of protein binding or differential metabolism at cytochrome 3A4
Clinical effect: decreased seizure threshold

References

1. Flockhart DA. Drug interactions: cytochrome P450 drug interaction table. Indiana University School of Medicine (2007). http://medicine.iupui.edu/clinpharm/ddis/table.asp. Accessed 16 Nov 2009.
2. Ha HR, Chen J, Frieburghaus AU, et al. Metabolism of theophylline by cDNA-expressed human cytochromes P-450. Br J Clin Pharmacol. 1995;39:321–6.
3. Hijazi Y, Boulieu R. Contribution of CYP3A4, CYP2B6, and CYP2C9 isoforms to *N*-demethylation of ketamine in human liver microsomes. Drug Metab Dispos. 2002;30: 853–8.
4. Hirshman CA, Krieger W, Littlejohn G, et al. Ketamine-aminophylline-induced decrease in seizure threshold. Anesthesiology. 1982;56:464–7.
5. Shannon M. Life-threatening events after theophylline overdose a 10-year prospective analysis. Arch Intern Med. 1999;159:989–94.

Magnesium Mama and the Mad Dad

34

Magnesium sulfate, propofol, remifentanil, vecuronium

Ana Maria Manrique MD, Catherine Marcucci MD, and Kathirvel Subramaniam MD

Abstract
This case discusses pharmacodynamic drug–drug interactions between magnesium sulfate and intravenous anesthetics and between magnesium sulfate and vecuronium. Additional information regarding the use of magnesium for perioperative patients is presented.

Case

A 36-year-old woman with four previous pregnancies and severe preeclampsia underwent emergency Cesarean section (C-section) due to fetal bradycardia in her 31st week of pregnancy.

She had been admitted the day before with complaints of severe headache, dizziness, and blurred vision. She reported allergies to penicillin, morphine, and codeine. She had generalized edema and a blood pressure of 160/110 mm Hg on admission. Initial laboratory tests showed 2+proteinuria, hematocrit 35.2%, platelet count

A.M. Manrique MD (✉)
Department of Anesthesiology, Children's Hospital of Pittsburgh, Pittsburgh, PA, USA
e-mail: Ana.Manrique@chp.edu

C. Marcucci MD
Anesthesia Services Department, Philadelphia Veterans Affairs Medical Center, Philadelphia, PA, USA

K. Subramaniam MD
Department of Anesthesiology, University of Pittsburgh Medical Center, Presbyterian Hospital, Pittsburgh, PA, USA

C. Marcucci et al. (eds.), *A Case Approach to Perioperative Drug-Drug Interactions*, DOI 10.1007/978-1-4614-7495-1_34

110,000 and creatinine 1.8 g/dL. Serum electrolytes, liver function, and coagulation tests were within normal limits. Fetal ultrasound showed a fetus in breech position, consistent with 30 weeks gestation. The estimated fetal weight was 1430 g.

The patient was transported to the obstetrical intensive care unit (ICU) and magnesium sulfate ($MgSO_4$) was started (6 g loading dose, 2 g/h maintenance). Intravenous (IV) fluid administration including $MgSO_4$ was restricted to 125 cc/h. Central venous and arterial lines were inserted and a urinary catheter was placed. A uterine stress test showed fetal bradycardia (90/minute) and the patient was rushed to the operating room.

In the operating room, the patient was tachycardic and her blood pressure was 170/110 mm Hg. Clindamycin (600 mg) was administered and $MgSO_4$ infusion was continued at 2 g/hr. It was decided to administer general anesthesia for C-section because of the emergent nature of the procedure. The patient was induced with propofol and intubated easily after muscle relaxation with succinylcholine. The baby was delivered with Apgar scores of 7/9 and had a strong and vigorous cry. Anesthesia was maintained with desflurane 3.0% after delivery of the baby and muscle relaxation was obtained with vecuronium. No bispectral index (BIS) monitor was used. The mother developed two episodes of hypotension requiring fluid bolus and ephedrine boluses (total 15 mg). The abdominal wall was severely edematous and the surgeons advised the anesthesia team that surgical closure would be difficult and prolonged. The surgeons asked for "maximum relaxation" to facilitate closure. The patient received a total of 10 mg of vecuronium and a remifentanil infusion was started. The closure lasted over an hour and the train-of-four (TOF) was 0/4 at the end of surgery and after 30 minutes into recovery. Temperature, glucose, and electrolytes were within normal range. The patient was transported to ICU and placed on mechanical ventilation with a propofol infusion for sedation and amnesia.

When he first visited his wife at her bedside in the ICU, the exhausted new father grew increasingly agitated and angry and had to be escorted to the lounge to talk to the teams. After 4 hours in the ICU, two twitches appeared on the TOF monitor, the patient was reversed, and the propofol infusion was discontinued. However, the patient did not meet criteria for extubation at that time as she was not sufficiently arousable. The anesthesia and ICU teams met again with the new father to explain the situation and reassure him. With some difficulty the nursing staff persuaded her husband to get some sleep and he found the patient fully alert and extubated by the morning.

Discussion

This is an example of two pharmacodynamic drug–drug interactions involving magnesium sulfate.

Magnesium is an active ion with important function in most of the cellular process. Magnesium is involved in the activation of membrane calcium ATPase and sodium-potassium (Na-K) ATPase and has an important role in transmembrane ion exchanges during depolarization and repolarization. Therefore, magnesium is critical in the maintenance of calcium and potassium equilibrium and membrane stabilization.[1]

Magnesium sulfate ($MgSO_4$) is widely used as coadjuvant therapy in the treatment of preeclampsia for the prevention of seizures. $MgSO_4$ is a tocolytic agent as well.[2] There is a general consensus that magnesium works by maintaining membrane stabilization though it is debatable.[3] The MAGPIE study performed in United Kingdom compared $MgSO_4$ with placebo in preeclamptic women and demonstrated that $MgSO_4$ reduces the risk of eclampsia by almost half (relative risk 0.42), and 95% confidence interval (CI) 0.29–0.60).[4] $MgSO_4$ is found to be useful for the prevention of arrhythmias in cardiac surgery and intensive care unit.[5] Magnesium is useful in the prevention of hemodynamic responses to intubation and during pheochromocytoma resection.[2,6]

Magnesium's molecular action includes competitive calcium channel block thus decreasing the calcium conductance of presynaptic voltage-dependent calcium channels. Magnesium also limits the outflow of calcium from the sarcoplasmic reticulum. Magnesium has also been shown to be a noncompetitive *N*-methyl-D-aspartate (NMDA) receptor antagonist, which may contribute to its role as a useful adjuvant pain drug.[21,22]

Although the findings are not universal across all studies and all doses, a number of authors report that administration of magnesium sulfate, particularly intraoperatively and in repeated doses, decreases requirements of intravenous anesthetics and opioid narcotics in both obstetrical and nonobstetrical patients.[13–20] Gupta et al. demonstrated decreased requirements for fentanyl and propofol with magnesium infusion during total intravenous anesthesia.[13] A study by Schultz-Stubner et al. demonstrated reduction of remifentanil requirements of over 30% with a post-induction dose of 50 mg/kg.[14] Similarly, Telci et al. showed a reduction of 38% in propofol requirements and a reduction of over 50% in remifentanil requirements with the administration of 30 mg/kg of magnesium.[15] Kwon and Lee studied the use of IV magnesium in women undergoing C-section and found that preoperative magnesium attenuated BIS readings in the pre-delivery period and decreased use of both midazolam and fentanyl.[19] They further suggested that the antagonism of NMDA receptors and calcium channel blockade could be responsible for the modification of perioperative sedation and analgesia in their study. No BIS monitor was used in this case, thus the empirical use of propofol and remifentanil drips to an estimated level of anesthetic and amnestic depth, both intraoperatively and postoperatively, may have rendered BIS readings significantly below those normally thought to insure adequate sedation and amnesia.

The need to ensure ongoing sedation and amnesia was of course mandated by the prolonged neuromuscular block, a factor which the clinician must always consider with the use of magnesium. The calcium channel-blocking actions described above collectively result in decreased release of acetylcholine from the end plate of the presynaptic motor neuron. Therefore, administration of $MgSO_4$ increases the sensitivity to nondepolarizing muscle relaxants (NDMRs).[7] Czarnetzki et al. performed a randomized and double-blinded study that compared the onset and duration of rocuronium between patients who received $MgSO_4$ infusion (60 mg/kg over 15 minutes) and a control group.[7] They found a rapid onset and longer duration for rocuronium in $MgSO_4$ group. However, Kussman et al. could not demonstrate any difference in onset but showed prolonged duration of action of rocuronium in patients receiving $MgSO_4$; the difference in results could be explained by the fact that patients in the Kussman study received magnesium as bolus instead of 15 minutes infusion before rocuronium.[8] Several other authors noticed shortened onset (35% to 50%) and prolonged duration (25% + 90%) of NDMRs with magnesium administration.[9–11] Na et al. demonstrated a reduction in the requirement for muscle relaxants when $MgSO_4$ infusion was administered for postoperative analgesia in patients with cerebral palsy.[12] Pregnant patients have an increased susceptibility to inhalation agents that may amplify the duration of muscle relaxants. In addition, antibiotics administered (clindamycin in this patient) may interact with muscle relaxants. $MgSO_4$ elimination was decreased as well in these patients if the kidneys are involved in preeclampsia. Small, incremental doses of NDMRs are used and it is important to monitor the neuromuscular junction and magnesium levels in these patients to avoid adverse interactions. Succinylcholine is not affected and a normal dose is recommended for intubation in $MgSO_4$ treated patients. Because magnesium has been shown to have preventive effects against succinylcholine fasciculations and myalgia, it is not necessary to administer defasciculating dose of NMDRs in $MgSO_4$ treated patients.

Magnesium is a physiologic antagonist at dihydropyridine calcium receptors and produces smooth muscle relaxation. Excessive $MgSO_4$ can produce progressive inhibition of catecholamine release from adrenergic nerve endings, adrenal medulla, and postganglionic sympathetic fibers, which results in decreased systemic vascular resistance. $MgSO_4$ worsens the hypotensive response of epidural blocks especially with the extensive blockade required for C-section. Experimental studies showed that ephedrine is preferred over phenylephrine to restore blood pressure and uterine blood flow after epidural block in hypermagnesemic conditions. During induction of anesthesia, it may be beneficial to continue $MgSO_4$ infusion because this may prevent hemodynamic response to intubation. Since calcium is integral to hemostasis, the effect of $MgSO_4$ on perioperative bleeding and coagulation is not clear at this point and merits further investigation.

Take-Home Points

- Homeostasis of magnesium in the intracellular environment is important to maintain the balance between calcium and potassium. Imbalance of this ion causes alteration in the cellular activation of enzymatic process and unbalanced action of the membrane potential.

- Magnesium is known to decrease the requirement for intravenous anesthetics, and narcotic analgesics by central nervous system depressant effects. Studies have found that the need for both propofol and remifentanil is decreased with the administration of magnesium sulfate. Antagonism of the NMDA receptor has been suggested as a possible mechanism.

- Magnesium sulfate administration causes faster onset and prolonged duration of nondepolarizing muscle relaxants. Clinically significant prolongation of muscle relaxation can occur by the interaction between the drugs administered during anesthesia such as muscle relaxants, antibiotics, and inhalational anesthetics. Careful monitoring of neuromuscular junction is recommended.

- Significant hypotension can occur with α -receptor antagonists and regional blockade in patients receiving magnesium.

- Since magnesium has wide therapeutic applications in anesthesia and critical care, anesthesiologists should be aware of its potential interactions with other commonly used drugs in the perioperative period.

Summary

Interaction 1: pharmacodynamic
Substrates: magnesium sulfate, propofol, and remifentanil
Mechanism/site of action: NMDA receptor antagonism
Clinical effects: augmentation of effects of intravenous anesthetics and pain medications

Interaction 2: pharmacodynamic
Substrates: magnesium sulfate and vecuronium
Mechanism/site of action: decreased release of acetylcholine from the presynaptic neuron at the neuromuscular junction end plate, increasing the sensitivity to non-depolarizing neuromuscular blockers
Clinical effect: prolonged neuromuscular weakness

References

1. James MF. Magnesium: an emerging drug in anaesthesia. Br J Anaesth. 2009;103:465–7.
2. Greene MF. Magnesium sulfate for preeclampsia. N Engl J Med. 2003;348:275–6.
3. Soave PM, Conti G, Costa R, et al. Magnesium and anaesthesia. Curr Drug Targets. 2009;10: 734–43.
4. Magpie Trial Collaborative Group. Do women with pre-eclampsia, and their babies, benefit from magnesium sulphate? The Magpie Trial: a randomised placebo-controlled trial. Lancet. 2002;359:1877–90.

5. Fawcett WJ, Haxby EJ, Male DA. Magnesium: physiology and pharmacology. Br J Anaesth. 1999;83:302–20.
6. Lysakowski C, Dumont L, Czarnetzki C, et al. Magnesium as an adjuvant to postoperative analgesia: a systematic review of randomized trials. Anesth Analg. 2007;104:1532–9.
7. Czarnetzki C, Lysakowski C, Elia N, et al. Time course of rocuronium-induced neuromuscular block after pre-treatment with magnesium sulphate: a randomised study. Acta Anaesthesiol Scand. 2009;11:1–8.
8. Kussman B, Shorten G, Uppington J, et al. Administration of magnesium sulphate before rocuronium: effects on speed of onset and duration of neuromuscular block. Br J Anaesth. 1997;79(1):122–4.
9. James MF, Schenk PA, Van der Veen BW. Priming of pancuronium with magnesium. Br J Anaesth. 1991;66:247–9.
10. Lampl E, Dandoy M. Priming of atracurium with magnesium. Br J Anaesth. 1993;70:A139.
11. Fuchs-Buder T, Wilder-Smith OH, Borgeat A, et al. Interaction of magnesium sulphate with vecuronium induced neuromuscular block. Br J Anaesth. 1995;74:405–9.
12. Na HS, Lee JH, Hwang JY, et al. Effects of magnesium sulphate on intraoperative neuromuscular blocking agent requirements and postoperative analgesia in children with cerebral palsy. Br J Anaesth. 2010;104:344–50.
13. Gupta K, Vohra V, Sood J. The role of magnesium as an adjuvant during general anesthesia. Anaesthesia. 2006;61:1058–63.
14. Schultz-Stubner S, Wettmann G, Reyle-Hahn SM, et al. Magnesium as part of balanced general anesthesia with propofol, remifentanil, and mivacurium: a double-blind, randomized prospective study in 50 patients. Eur J Anaesthesiol. 2001;18(11):723–9.
15. Telci L, Esen F, Akcora D, et al. Evaluation of effects of magnesium sulphate in reducing intraoperative anaesthetic requirements. Br J Anaesth. 2002;89:594.
16. Khafagy HF, Osman ES, Naguib AF. Effects of different dose regimens of magnesium on pharmacodynamics and anesthetic requirements of balanced general anesthesia. J Egypt Soc Parasitol. 2007;37(2):469–82.
17. Dabbagh A, Elyasi H, Razavi SS, et al. Intravenous magnesium sulfate for post-operative pain in patients undergoing lower limb orthopedic surgery. Acta Anaesthesiol Scand. 2009;53(8):1088–91.
18. Lysakowki C, Dumont L, Czarnetzki C, et al. Magnesium as an adjuvant to postoperative analgesia: a systematic review of randomized trials. Anesth Analg. 2007;104(6):1532–9.
19. Lee DH, Kwon IC. Magnesium sulphate has beneficial effects as an adjuvant during general anaesthesia for Caesarean section. Br J Anaesth. 2009;103(6):861–6.
20. Altan A, Turgut N, Yildiz F, et al. Effects of magnesium sulphate and clonidine on propofol consumption, haemodynamics and postoperative recovery. Br J Anaesth. 2005;94:438–41.
21. Mayer ML, Westbrook GL, Guthrie PB. Voltage-dependent block by Mg^{2+} of NMDA responses in spinal cord neurons. Nature. 1984;309:261–3.
22. Woolf CJ, Thompson SW. The induction and maintenance of central sensitization is dependent on N-methyl-D-aspartatic acid receptor activation: implications for treatment of post-injury pain hypersensitivity states. Pain. 1991;44:293–9.

Dexy's Midnight Spinal

35

Dexmedetomidine, bupivacaine spinal, multiple mechanisms, CYP3A4, CYP2D6

Michael P. Hutchens MD, Edward A. Kahl MD, and Matthias J. Merkel MD, PhD

Abstract
This case discusses a possible pharmacokinetic interaction between bupivacaine and dexmedetomidine. Bupivacaine is a cytochrome P450 2D6 and cytochrome 3A4 substrate. Dexmedetomidine has been shown, in vitro, to inhibit both enzymes.

Case

A 68-year-old obese man with right knee osteoarthritis presented to the operating room for right knee arthroplasty under spinal anesthesia. His body mass index was 39.1 and he was known to have chronic renal insufficiency (creatinine 1.8 mg/dL). A spinal anesthetic of 15 mg of hyperbaric intrathecal bupivacaine was placed and a dexmedetomidine infusion was started at 1mcg/kg/h for 15 minutes followed by 0.5 mcg/kg/h. Thirty minutes into the procedure, the dexmedetomidine infusion was reduced to 0.3 mcg/kg/h due to excessive sedation. This dose was maintained until the start of skin closure, at which time dexmedetomidine was discontinued. The total time elapsed since intrathecal injection was 150 minutes. At that time, the patient had bilateral dense motor block of the lower extremities and a sensory block to cold at T12.

Sixty minutes after arrival to postanesthesia care unit (PACU) or 3.5 hours following spinal injection, Eileen, the PACU nurse, paged the anesthesia provider because the patient's spinal block had shown no signs of fade, and the patient was still

M.P. Hutchens MD (✉) • E.A. Kahl MD • M.J. Merkel MD, PhD
Department of Anesthesiology & Perioperative Medicine,
Oregon Health & Science University, Portland, OR, USA
e-mail: hutchenm@ohsu.edu

C. Marcucci et al. (eds.), *A Case Approach to Perioperative Drug-Drug Interactions*, DOI 10.1007/978-1-4614-7495-1_35

somnolent. The busy anesthesia provider's initial response was "Come on, Eileen!" However, her exam confirmed Eileen's finding. The injection site of the spinal was examined and appeared normal. Radiology was called for emergent magnetic resonance imaging (MRI) to rule out spinal hematoma. Over the course of the ensuing fifty minutes, while arrangements were being made for MRI, his spinal block faded and he had complete return of motor and sensory function. Pain score was 3/10. The patient did well postoperatively and was discharged from the hospital 3 days later.

Discussion

This is an example of a possible interaction of an inhibitor added to a substrate.

Bupivacaine, an amide local anesthetic, is metabolized primarily by hepatic cytochrome 3A4 and partially by cytochromes 2D6 and 2C19.[1]

Dexmedetomidine is a selective α_2 agonist used for sedation. It is an imidazole derivative and the active S-isomer of medetomidine. Dexmedetomidine is cleared by both hepatic metabolism and renal excretion, with an elimination half-life of 2 to 2.67 hours in healthy adults. Hepatic metabolism of dexmedetomidine occurs primarily via cytochrome 2A6.[2]

Dexmedetomidine has also been shown, in vitro, to be an inhibitor of 3A4 and 2D6. It is a weak competitor inhibitor of 3A4 and binds reversibly to the heme (ferric) ion of 2D6.[3,4] The clinical significance of the *in vitro* inhibitory effect of dexmedetomidine on 3A4 and 2D6 has not yet been fully elucidated.

The coadministration of intravenous dexmedetomidine with intrathecal bupivacaine has been reported to prolong both spinal motor block and sensory block.[5–7] In the patient in the case presented here, the delay in regression of the block was significant enough to raise fears of the rare, but devastating, complication of spinal hematoma.

Although the exact mechanism of the interaction remains unclear, there certainly is the potential for clinically significant interactions involving inhibition of the 3A4 and 2D6 isoforms (responsible for the metabolism of bupivacaine) as hinted at by the *in vitro* data. There is also the possibility of dexmedetomidine-mediated vasoconstriction resulting in reduced effector site clearance of bupivacaine.

In our clinical scenario, the patient experienced deeper sedation than was anticipated. In patients with renal impairment, the elimination half-life of dexmedetomidine is shortened, but the fraction of free, non–protein-bound drug increases.[8]

The renal impairment (patient's estimated glomerular filtration rate using the Modification of Diet in Renal Disease (MDRD) formula is 38 mL/min/1.73 m^2, chronic kidney disease stage 3) of the patient, most likely increased the amount of free, unbound dexmedetomidine in plasma, resulting in prolonged sedation.

Take-Home Points

- Dexmedetomidine has been shown to have deeper sedative effects in patients with impaired renal function due to the increased fraction of unbound dexmedetomidine in plasma.
- The combination of intravenous dexmedetomidine and intrathecal bupivacaine increases the duration of bupivacaine neuraxial blockade. This may be used to advantage during surgeries under spinal anesthesia but, as in our case vignette, can also result delays in the regression of the spinal block, triggering work up for more devastating complications.
- Dose adjustment, such as omission of initial bolus infusion and reduction of infusion rate of dexmedetomidine, may need to be taken into account for patients with renal and/or hepatic impairment.
- The drug effect cannot only be prolonged due to reduced clearance of the medication, but also enhanced due to lower protein binding.

Summary

Interaction: pharmacokinetic (possible)
Substrate: bupivacaine
Enzyme: 2D6 and 3A4
Inhibitor: intravenous dexmedetomidine
Clinical effect: prolonged motor and sensory block

References

1. Gantenbein M, Attolini L, Bruguerolle B, et al. Oxidative metabolism of bupivacaine into pipecolylxylidine in humans is mainly catalyzed by CYP3A. Drug Metab Dispos. 2000;28:383–5.
2. Product information: Precedex(R) IV injection, dexmedetomidine hydrochloride IV injection. Lake Forest: Hospira Inc; 2008.
3. Tie Y, McPhail B, Hong H, et al. Modeling chemical interaction profiles: II. molecular docking, spectral data-activity relationship, and structure-activity relationship models for potent and weak inhibitors of cytochrome P450 CYP3A4 isozyme. Molecules. 2012;17(3):3407–60.

4. Rodrigues AD, Roberts EM. The in vitro interaction of dexmedetomidine with human liver microsomal cytochrome P4502D6 (CYP2D6). Drug Metab Dispos. 1997;25(5):651–5.
5. Saadawy I, Boker A, Elshahawy MA, et al. Effect of dexmedetomidine on the characteristics of bupivacaine in a caudal block in pediatrics. Acta Anaesthesiol Scand. 2009;53(2):251–6.
6. Al-Mustafa MM, Badran IZ, Abu-Ali HM, et al. Intravenous dexmedetomidine prolongs bupivacaine spinal analgesia. Middle East J Anesthesiol. 2009;20(2):225–31.
7. Kaya FN, Yavascaoglu B, Turker G, et al. Intravenous dexmedetomidine, but not midazolam, prolongs bupivacaine spinal anesthesia. Can J Anaesth. 2010;57(1):39–45.
8. De Wolf AM, Fragen RJ, Avram MJ. The pharmacokinetics of dexmedetomidine in volunteers with severe renal impairment. Anesth Analg. 2001;93(5):1205–9.

Drug–Drug Interactions Involving Local Anesthetics

VI

Introduction 36

Catherine Marcucci MD

Abstract
This section introduces drug–drug interactions involving local anesthetics.

Interestingly, the dental community has been very proactive in raising awareness of drug–drug interactions (DDIs) including those involving the local anesthetics. Reports, summaries, and clinical guidelines were published as early as the early 1990s and have continued to this day.[1–4] And this makes sense in a certain way. The dentists and their allied practitioners have a compelling need for anesthetics that are both reliable and safe. The dental extraction or repair doesn't go forward if the block doesn't set up or the patient is bleeding profusely and, the recent development of "sedation dentistry" aside, the dentists don't have what we have to get them through—the intravenous lines, the propofol, the ketamine, etc. Similarly, they are not equipped, on a routine basis, to handle clinically significant local anesthetic toxicity.

And this is the issue with local anesthetic DDIs that we would like to highlight for the reader. It is generally not a question of a little dizziness—these DDIs either result in blocks that don't work, blocks that last too long and distress the patient and provider both, or toxicity, all of which are clinical events to be avoided. Local anesthetic toxicity due to DDIs is an especially important consideration. One is taught of the thresholds between bupivacaine neurological toxicity and cardiovascular toxicity, but as every experienced anesthesia practitioner can tell you, this threshold can and is broached more quickly than you think while you are still trying to diagnose and manage the initial presentation.

DDIs involving local anesthetics are a particular interest of the editors and, in 2006, we published a case report on a patient who suffered cardiac arrest and needed cardiac pacing for an extended period of time after an apparently uncomplicated

C. Marcucci MD
Anesthesia Services Department, Philadelphia Veterans Affairs Medical Center, Philadelphia, PA, USA
e-mail: sandson.marcucci@comcast.net

C. Marcucci et al. (eds.), *A Case Approach to Perioperative Drug-Drug Interactions*, DOI 10.1007/978-1-4614-7495-1_36

axillary block.[5] Elements of the complicated DDI we believe this patient suffered are presented in this book in the cases "Smoking Guns I and II." There was a little bit of pushback, if memory serves correct, in the form of letters to the editor from readers who didn't buy the DDI story and felt certain that frank overdose or intravascular injection was the cause. Because we ourselves had not done the block and did not have bupivacaine blood levels, we could not prove that the DDI had happened, but were confident in our reasoning and pharmacology. And, slowly but surely, the anesthesia community seems to have become more aware of this potentially serious, but often unrecognized clinical situation. Recently, we read a report on convulsions after normal dosing of lidocaine which the authors felt were caused by a probable drug interaction.[6]

As you go through these chapters, keep in mind that the local anesthetics are substrates of cytochromes (CYP) 1A2 and 3A4—and a lot of other drugs and substrates also interact with these particular isoenzymes. Bupivacaine is the outlier, as it is a substrate of cytochromes 3A4, 2D6, and 2C19. Of course, as these drugs also have potent effects on the sympathetic nervous system, as such they are involved in their share of pharmacodynamic DDIs as well.

A careful perusal of local anesthetic DDIs will make you both a safer and more precise practitioner of regional anesthesia as well as give you something to chat about the next time you are at a reception over at the dental school.

References

1. Moore PA, Gage TW, Hersh EV, et al. Adverse drug interactions in dental practice. Professional and educational implications. J Am Dent Assoc. 1999;130(1):47–54.
2. Pyle MA, Faddoul FF, Terezhalmy GT. Clinical implications of drugs taken by our patients. Dent Clin North Am. 1993;37(1):73–90.
3. Girndt M. Dental care with local anesthesia: should the patient first discontinue ACE inhibitors? MMW Fortschr Med. 2011;153(9):20.
4. Henderson S. Drug interactions with local anesthetics preparations used by primary care dental practitioners. Dent Update. 2010;37(4):236–8, 241.
5. Marcucci C, Sandson NB, Thorn EM, et al. Unrecognized drug-drug interactions: a cause of intraoperative cardiac arrest? Anesth Analg. 2006;102(5):1569–72.
6. Landy C, Schaeffer E, Raynaud L, et al. Convulsions after normal dose of lidocaine: a probable drug interaction. Br J Anaesth. 2012;108(4):701.

Comfortably Numb

37

Local anesthetics

Joseph J. Yurigan DO and Todd M. Oravitz MD

Abstract
This case discusses the additive effects of local anesthetics.

Case

A 65-year-old 70 kg man presented to the operating room for open surgical repair of a left wrist fracture sustained in a motor vehicle accident after leaving a local bar the prior evening. He had a history of congestive heart failure, type 2 diabetes mellitus, well-controlled hypertension, and chronic obstructive pulmonary disease (COPD). He smoked a pack of cigarettes daily and drank on a daily basis and used intravenous recreational drugs. Preoperatively, the anesthesia team noted a recent echocardiogram (ECG) showing mild left ventricular dilation with an estimated ejection fraction of 40% and mild left ventricular hypertrophy, electrocardiogram showing normal sinus rhythm with moderate voltage criteria for left ventricular hypertrophy. He was also noted to have mildly icteric sclerae, and a slightly enlarged liver. Laboratory data were within normal limits except for aspartate aminotransferase/aluminic aminotransferase (AST/ALT) 60/31 IU/L.

An uncomplicated ultrasound guided infraclavicular block with a mixture of 20 mL each of bupivacaine 0.75% and mepivacaine 1.5% was performed without signs of intravascular injection. Twenty minutes after removing the needle, the patient had a generalized tonic-clonic seizure. Midazolam (3 mg) and propofol (100 mg) were given and the airway was secured. The patient's ECG changed to ventricular

J.J. Yurigan DO (✉)
Department of Anesthesiology, University of Pittsburgh Medical Center, Pittsburgh, PA, USA
e-mail: yuriganjj@upmc.edu

T.M. Oravitz MD
Department of Anesthesiology, University of Pittsburgh School of Medicine, Pittsburgh, PA, USA

C. Marcucci et al. (eds.), *A Case Approach to Perioperative Drug-Drug Interactions*, DOI 10.1007/978-1-4614-7495-1_37

tachycardia. A pulse was not palpable and the Advanced Cardiac Life Support (ACLS) protocol was initiated. A rapid bolus of 100 mL of intralipid 20% was administered, followed by an infusion of 0.25 mL/kg/min for the next 10 minutes. After the bolus of intralipid the patient became hemodynamically stable, surgery was postponed, and he was transferred to the ICU.

Discussion

This is an example of a mixed additive pharmacodynamic and pharmacokinetic (distribution) interaction.

Mixtures of local anesthetics for regional anesthesia are used to compensate for long latency of longer acting agents like bupivacaine with agents that are rapidly acting, but shorter in duration such as mepivacaine or lidocaine.[1] The systemic effects from combining local anesthetics correlates to the principle of summation (drug A + drug B = 2A or 2B). When following the dosage limits of local anesthetics, guidelines are presumed additive and toxicities are dependent on each other.[2] In this scenario, 20 cc of 0.75% bupivacaine and 20 cc of 1.5% mepivacaine were used. When local anesthetics are mixed in equal volume the original concentration is reduced by half. Therefore, a total of 40 cc of 0.375% bupivacaine and 0.75% of mepivacaine was used. A 150 mg total dose of bupivacaine was determined by calculating 3.75 mg/cc multiplied by 40 cc. The total dose of mepivacaine was 300 mg (7.5 mg/cc multiplied by 40 cc). The maximum dose for bupivacaine is 3 mg/kg and for mepivacaine it is 4.5 mg/kg. In our 70 kg patient, that equates to total maximum doses of 210 mg bupivacaine and 315 mg mepivacaine. The percentage of the maximum dose of bupivacaine is calculated as 150 mg/210 mg, or 71%. Similarly, for mepivacaine, it is 300 mg/315 mg, or 95%. Both local anesthetics are individually under the maximum threshold, however, when both percentages are added together (71% bupivacaine + 95% mepivacaine = 166%), the toxic dose threshold is exceeded by 66%. A study done by Hartrick demonstrated that when mepivacaine and bupivacaine are added together, both amide local anesthetics competitively bind to α_1-glycoprotein and albumin. This results in increased free fraction of plasma concentrations, with the potential for increased systemic toxicity.[3]

When large amounts or repeated doses are required, hepatic clearance should be considered for aminoamide local anesthetics. Both liver and kidney function decline 50% by the age of 65.[4] The half-life of lidocaine in patients with normal hepatic function is 1.5 hours; however, in patients with liver disease, it may be as long as 5 hours. Congestive heart failure patients demonstrated a prolonged rate of metabolism of lidocaine or other amide local anesthetics from the blood. Medications such as ß-blockers present a concern for clinicians due to its function of reducing hepatic blood flow, therefore prolonging the elimination of local anesthetics.[5]

Systemic reactions can occur by placement of intrathecal, intravascular, or excessive dosing of local anesthetics. The central nervous and cardiovascular systems have a direct correlation with the potency of the local anesthetic utilized.[6] When large amounts or repeated doses are required, hepatic clearance should be considered for aminoamide local anesthetics.[2]

During the initial symptoms of central nervous system (CNS) toxicity, patients may experience dizziness, auditory, or visual disturbances. Patients may also experience drowsiness or disorientation, followed by convulsions and CNS excitation. When a significantly large dose or intravenous injection is administered, seizures may progress to respiratory depression or respiratory arrest. If patients received CNS depressant drugs with local anesthetics the excitatory phase of CNS toxicity may be bypassed directly to respiratory depression or respiratory arrest.[2]

The CNS excitatory phase correlates with the blockade of the inhibitory pathway in the cerebral cortex and the activation of glutamate, which functions as an excitatory neurotransmitter and may lead to seizure activity. Moreover, seizure activity produces hypoventilation which causes respiratory and metabolic acidosis. Increasing levels of $PaCO_2$ will augment cerebral blood flow, therefore providing the brain with more local anesthetic.[7] Elevated levels of carbon dioxide, which diffuse into neuronal cells, reduce intracellular pH, thus converting the base form of local anesthetics to cationic ones. Since the cationic form has limited ability to cross nerve membranes, ion trapping occurs, which exacerbates CNS toxicity.[2]

Protective measures should be employed when patients present with CNS depression or excitation. Assisted ventilation and circulatory support is used to correct the acidosis and hypercapnia. Benzodiazepines or thiopental are administered for terminating the excitation phase of CNS toxicity.[2]

Local anesthetic toxicity can also affect the heart and peripheral blood vessels. Direct cardiac effects in fast conducting tissues of Purkinje fibers and ventricular muscle result in a reduction in the rate of depolarization. This decrease in rate is caused by minimizing the availability of fast conduction sodium channels. There is also inhibition of cardiac duration and refractory period as well.

Not all local anesthetics have the same degree of potency or effect on cardiac tissue. For example, bupivacaine decreases the rapid phase of depolarization more than mepivacaine or lidocaine. High levels of local anesthetics will delay conduction time, which is demonstrated by lengthened PR intervals and durations of QRS complexes on ECG.[2] Dose-dependent effects of local anesthetics can decrease pacemaker activity to a degree that produces sinus bradycardia or arrest. Also, myocardial contractility is decreased by the negative ionotropic action of local anesthetics. The negative ionotropic effect is caused by inhibiting calcium influx and decreases in cardiac sarcolemmal calcium and sodium currents.

Direct peripheral vascular effects of local anesthetics are dose related. Lower concentrations produce vasoconstriction, while elevated concentrations cause vasodilation.[8] The only local anesthetic to produce vasoconstriction at all concentrations is cocaine.

When comparing local anesthetics, bupivacaine has the greatest effect on cardiotoxicity. There is greater difficulty in cardiac resuscitation with patients who received bupivacaine, due to its slow dissociation from the sodium ion channel. Cardiac arrest or severe ventricular tachycardia should follow ACLS protocol. Patients who experience cardiovascular collapse should also receive a rapid bolus of intralipid 20% at 1.5 mL/kg without delay. Once the bolus is completed, an infusion of 0.25 mL/kg/min intralipid should be administered for the next 10 minutes.[2]

Take-Home Points

- Systemic effect from combining local anesthetics follows the principle of summation (drug A + drug B = 2A or 2B). When following the dosage limits of local anesthetics, guidelines are presumed additive and toxicities are dependent on each other.

- When large amounts or repeated doses of aminoamide local anesthetics are required, hepatic clearance needs to be considered.

- Systemic effects on the central nervous and cardiovascular systems have a direct correlation with the potency of the local anesthetic utilized.

Summary

Interaction: pharmacodynamic
Substrates: bupivacaine and mepivacaine
Enzyme/site of action: neuronal and cardiac cell sodium channels, CNS neurotransmitters
Clinical effect: increase in anesthetic drug effect and toxicity

Interaction: pharmacokinetic (distribution)
Substrates: bupivacaine and mepivacaine
Enzyme/site of action: α_1-glycoprotein, albumin
Clinical effect: increase in free plasma fraction leading to potential for increased systemic toxicity

References

1. Gadsden J, Hadzic A, Gandhi K, et al. The effect of mixing 1.5% mepivacaine and 0.5% bupivacaine on duration of analgesia and latency of block onset in ultrasound-guided interscalene block. Anesth Analg. 2011;112(2):471–6.
2. Berde CB, Strichartz GR, Miller RD, Eriksson LI, Fleisher LA, Wiener-Kronish JP. Local anesthetics. In: Young WL, editor. Miller's anesthesia. 7th ed. Philadelphia: Elsevier/Churchill Livingstone; 2009.
3. Hartrick C, Dirkes W, Coyle D, et al. Influence of bupivacaine on mepivacaine protein binding. Clin Pharmacol Ther. 1984;36:546–50.
4. Montamat SC, Cusack BJ, Vestal RE. Management of drug therapy in the elderly. N Engl J Med. 1989;321:303–9.
5. Thomson PD, Melmon KL, Richardson JA, et al. Lidocaine pharmacokinetics in advanced heart failure, liver disease, and renal failure in humans. Ann Intern Med. 1973;78:499–508.
6. Scott DB. Evaluation of clinical tolerance of local anaesthetic agents. Br J Anaesth. 1975;47:328–31.
7. Englesson S. The influence of acid–base changes on central nervous system toxicity of local anaesthetic agents. I. An experimental study in cats. Acta Anaesthesiol Scand. 1974;18:79–87.
8. Johns RA, Difazio CA, Longnecker DE. Lidocaine constricts or dilates rat arterioles in a dose dependent manner. Anesthesiology. 1985;62:141–4.

Naturally Occurring and Nasty

38

Cocaine, propranolol

Lauren Partyka MD and Li Meng MD, MPH

Abstract
This case discusses the pharmacodynamic interaction between cocaine and propranolol, resulting in hypertension and exaggerated cocaine toxicity.

Case

The senior anesthesiology resident was called to the trauma boy of the Emergency Department to do a preoperative evaluation for a 37-year-old man with a history of asthma who presented with a left open femoral fracture after a gunshot wound to the leg, sustained at an after-hours dance club. Initially, the patient was oriented to person, place, and time, and was able to answer questions. He complained of severe leg pain, chest pressure, a "fluttering" in his chest, and dizziness, stating, "I can't get air." He was a heavy smoker and drinker but adamantly denied other drug use and stated that he did not use cocaine, "except if I have a toothache or something like that." He denied use of other medications and medication allergies.

The patient was diaphoretic and nauseated. His vital signs were elevated with a heart rate of 130 beats per minute, systolic blood pressure of 150 mm Hg, and temperature of 101 °F. The ECG confirmed sinus tachycardia. After multiple attempts to place a peripheral intravenous line, he was finally given a β-blocker. His tachycardia improved slightly, but his blood pressure escalated to a systolic of 170 mm Hg.

L. Partyka MD (✉)
Department of Anesthesiology, University of Pittsburgh Medical Center, Pittsburgh, PA, USA
e-mail: partykalm@upmc.edu

L. Meng MD, MPH
Department of Anesthesiology, University of Pittsburgh School of Medicine, Pittsburgh, PA, USA

C. Marcucci et al. (eds.), *A Case Approach to Perioperative Drug-Drug Interactions*, DOI 10.1007/978-1-4614-7495-1_38

About 20 minutes later, he suddenly became agitated and confused and started vomiting with subsequent oxygen desaturation. The anesthesia resident decided to secure the patient's airway. On direct laryngoscopy, oropharyngeal ulcers and an inflamed epiglottis were noted. Chest x-ray confirmed appropriate endotracheal tube placement and showed diffuse bilateral infiltrates and an enlarged heart. A Foley catheter was inserted, yielding red-tinged urine. The urine toxicology drug screen was positive for cocaine metabolites. Upon closer physical examination, track marks were noted bilaterally along the upper extremities. The patient was treated with lidocaine, sodium bicarbonate, and diazepam. He was transferred to the ICU for further care.

Discussion

This is an example of a pharmacodynamic interaction.

Cocaine produces a state of profound vasoconstriction via increased catecholamines at the sympathetic nerve terminals. Medications that are β-antagonists such as propranolol have been found to increase systemic vascular resistance and decrease cardiac output, thus enhancing the cardiovascular effects of cocaine toxicity.

Cocaine is benzoylmethylecgonine, an ester of benzoic acid and the nitrogen-containing base ecgonine; ecgonine is a tropine derivative related to atropine and scopolamine. It is the only naturally occurring local anesthetic.[1] Toxicity is not as profound with chewing coca leaves as with using manufactured cocaine hydrochloride that can be absorbed via any mucous membrane. Cocaine can be snorted or inhaled in the "free base" and "crack" forms or injected intravenously or intramuscularly.[1,2] It is metabolized in the plasma and liver and excreted in the urine, thus making urine drug screens ideal for detecting its presence.[3]

With its multiple means of administration and the ease of production, cocaine abuse and dependence has become a significant problem in the United States. Over 6 million Americans of all ages regularly use the drug, leading to greater than 143,000 Emergency Department visits in 2006.[1,4] While its physiologic effects are short with the chronotropic effect of IV cocaine peaking between 5 and 15 minutes, it causes intense vasoconstriction that can injure multiple organ systems.[5] Cocaine blocks the reuptake of norepinephrine, dopamine, and serotonin at the presynaptic sympathetic nerve junctions, producing an accumulation of catecholamines in the synaptic clefts and leading to a state of increased sympathetic stimulation.[1,2]

Acute cocaine ingestion causes euphoria and is associated with risky behavior resulting from the increased dopamine accumulation. Signs of toxicity include agitation, anxiety, panic, psychosis, hyperthermia, hypertension, tachycardia, mydriasis, seizures (often precipitated by increased serotonin), stupor, and respiratory and cardiac depression.[1,4] Acute hypertension can lead to hemorrhagic strokes while vasospasm and endothelial injury increase the risk for ischemic strokes.[4] Chronic cocaine use is associated with a more rapid progression of coronary artery disease thought to be associated with direct endothelial injury, which causes platelet aggregation, thromboxane production, coronary artery thrombosis, and vasospasm.[1] In the gastrointestinal system, it may lead to intestinal ischemia, infarction, perforation, or hemorrhage.[6] Cocaine is also associated with renal infarctions, acute renal failure, and rhabdomyolysis-induced acute tubular necrosis. Respiratory pathology includes thermal epiglottitis, crack lung, and pulmonary hypertension.[4]

The local anesthetic effects of cocaine produce a block of the fast sodium channels in nerve cells, leading to decreased conduction of nerve impulses.[1] In the heart, it decreases the rate of depolarization and amplitude of the action potential, slowing its rate of conduction and predisposing the user to arrhythmias and sudden death.[1] Overall, the intense sympathetic stimulation associated with cocaine toxicity increases myocardial irritability and lowers the fibrillation threshold.[3]

Therefore, use of additional pressors may have little effect on the sympathetic nervous system to elevate blood pressure during a state of cocaine toxicity. Phenylephrine, a direct-acting sympathomimetic, is used to increase venous constriction and elevate preload and afterload to increase blood pressure. In cocaine toxicity, there would be few α_1 receptors available to bind the additional pressor used because cocaine already creates a maximal sympathetic state.[7] Likewise, ephedrine, an indirect-acting sympathomimetic that stimulates release of norepinephrine, would provide little benefit in elevating blood pressure during cocaine toxicity since there would be no further norepinephrine to release into the synaptic terminals.[7]

Additionally, it is hypothesized that chronic cocaine use causes upregulation of α receptors, which results in coronary artery vasospasm if one is treated with an α-adrenergic agonist such as phenylephrine or ephedrine.[8] Using a norepinephrine drip can enhance tachycardia as it further propagates β- and α-adrenergic receptor stimulation via increases in calcium concentrations in the cardiac myocyte that lead to increased heart rate, cardiac contractility, and a greater potential for dysrhythmias.

There is no antidote for cocaine-induced hypertensive crisis and tachycardia. Treatment usually involves symptom control. Interestingly, β-blockers have been found to increase blood pressure via unopposed α-adrenergic stimulation as shown through increased peripheral and coronary vascular resistance. This leads to an increased depressant effect of cocaine on the heart and increased mortality.[2,4] One study showed that patients on β-blockers at the time of cocaine toxicity were more likely to develop a myocardial infarction.[9] Additional studies using small doses of cocaine given to patients undergoing cardiac catheterization showed coronary artery vasospasm was exacerbated by the β-blocker, propranolol, and relieved by phentolamine.[10] Finally, animal studies indicate that labetalol, an α- and β-blocker with greater β than α antagonist effects, also increases the risk for seizure and death. Instead, benzodiazepines such as diazepam have been found to be effective in treating cocaine-induced hypertension. If unsuccessful, vasodilators such as nitroprusside and nitroglycerine may be used.[4] Phentolamine, an α-blocker, has been used to block the sympathetic effect of norepinephrine.[4, 10]

Take-Home Points

- Cocaine toxicity leads to a state of increased sympathetic stimulation and resultant vasoconstriction, which can harm multiple organ systems.
- β-blockers, such as propranolol, have been found to increase blood pressure during cocaine-induced hypertension and tachycardia via unopposed α-adrenergic stimulation.
- Use of pressor support in the presence of cocaine ingestion may enhance the possibility of coronary artery vasospasm and the potential for dysrhythmias.

Summary

Interaction: pharmacodynamic
Substrates: cocaine and propranolol
Mechanism/site of action: increased sympathetic stimulation due to blockade of cathecholamine reuptake by cocaine, possible upregulation of alpha receptors by cocaine and unopposed α-receptor stimulation by propranolol
Clinical effect: acute cocaine toxicity and hypertension

References

1. Shanti C, Lucas C. Cocaine and the critical care challenge. Crit Care Med. 2003;31(6):1851–9.
2. Voigt L. Anesthetic management of the cocaine abuse patient. AANA J. 1995;63(5):438–43.
3. Torres M, Rocha S, Rebelo A, et al. Cardiovascular toxicity of cocaine of iatrogenic origin. Case report. Rev Port Cardiol. 2007;26(12):1395–404.
4. Glauser J, Queen J. Selected topics: toxicology: an overview of non-cardiac cocaine toxicity. J Emerg Med. 2007;32(2):181–6.
5. Hill G, Ogunnaike B, Johnson E. General anaesthesia for the cocaine-abusing patient. Is it safe? Br J Anaesth. 2006;97(5):654–7.
6. Lingamfelter D, Knight L. Sudden death from massive gastrointestinal hemorrhage associated with crack cocaine use. Am J Forensic Med Pathol. 2010;31(1):98–9.

7. Stoelting R, Miller R. Sympathomimetics. In: Basics of anesthesia. 5th ed. Philadelphia: Churchill Livingstone; 2007.
8. Lustik S, Chhibber A, van Vliet M, et al. Ephedrine-induced coronary artery vasospasm in a patient with prior cocaine use. Anesth Analg. 1997;84:931–3.
9. Mohamad T, Kondur A, Vaitkevicius P, et al. Cocaine-induced chest pain and [beta]-blockade: an inner city experience. Am J Ther. 2008;15(6):531–5.
10. McCord J, Jneid H, Hollander J, et al. Management of cocaine-associated chest pain and myocardial infarction: a scientific statement from the American Heart Association Acute Cardiac Care Committee of the Council on Clinical Cardiology. Circulation. 2008;117:1897–907.

LOL-LOL: Little Old Lady—Lots of Lido

39

Lidocaine, bupivacaine

Kitling M. Lum BSN, RN, CCRN-CSC
and Kelly N. Stafford BSN, RN, CCRN-CSC

Abstract
This case discusses a pharmacodynamic interaction between lidocaine and bupivacaine. Coadministration causes a synergistic anesthetic effect in the peripheral nerve system with additive cardiovascular and central nervous system toxicity.

Case

A frail 40 kg, 85-year-old woman presented for a colectomy for Crohn's disease. Her past medical history included recent, unintentional weight loss, osteoarthritis, chronic renal insufficiency, and chronic pain related to a previous hip fracture, for which she took vicodin. She stated she drank one "Old Fashion" cocktail each evening. The patient consented to patient-controlled epidural analgesia (PCEA) for postoperative pain management. A T10 epidural catheter was placed and a standard infusion of bupivacaine 0.125% and hydromorphone (10 mg/mL) was ordered with a dosing range of 1-20 mL/h. Following uneventful surgery, the patient was admitted to the intensive care unit (ICU) due to her advanced age and poor nutritional status. Early the next morning the pain service anesthesiologist noted that the patient reported 10/10 pain despite infusion of the maximum epidural dose (20 mL/h). The patient was lethargic but easily arousable, refusing to use her incentive spirometer (IS) or get out of bed. The anesthesiologist increased the concentration of the

K.M. Lum BSN, RN, CCRN-CSC (✉)
Cardiac and Surgical Intensive Care Unit, Oregon Health and Science University, Portland, OR, USA
e-mail: lumk@ohsu.edu

K.N. Stafford BSN, RN, CCRN-CSC
Cardiac & Surgical ICU, Oregon Health and Science University, Portland, OR, USA

C. Marcucci et al. (eds.), *A Case Approach to Perioperative Drug-Drug Interactions*, DOI 10.1007/978-1-4614-7495-1_39

bupivacaine to 0.25% and continued the hydromorphone at 10 mg/mL. The new PCEA infusion was started at 10 mL/h. The nurse titrated the infusion to 15 mL/h over several hours. The patient reported adequate pain control, used her IS with encouragement, and transferred to the chair several times with assistance.

On postoperative day 2, the surgical resident placed a left subclavian central venous catheter in order to deliver parenteral nutrition. The patient suffered a pneumothorax during the placement. Her oxygen requirements increased from 2L to 6L per nasal cannula and her respiratory rate increased to 24 breaths per minute but she remained hemodynamically stable. A left pleural chest tube was planned. After local infiltration of 8 mL of 2% lidocaine (20 mg/mL), most to deep tissue after a small skin wheal, the patient suffered a tonic-clonic seizure and subsequent cardiac arrest. Advanced Cardiac Life Support (ACLS) protocols were started promptly. The patient required intubation, multiple defibrillations for ventricular fibrillation, and a bolus of 20% lipid emulsion followed by an infusion.

Discussion

This is an example of a synergistic pharmacodynamic interaction.

Adequate postoperative pain management is crucial after major abdominal surgery so that normal functions such as ventilation, coughing, gastrointestinal function, and mobility are minimally impaired. Studies have shown that PCEA for postoperative analgesia after major abdominal surgery is more effective when local anesthetics are infused with narcotic medications.[1]

Bupivacaine is the most commonly used epidural anesthetic for postoperative analgesia. It is a long-acting (120-240 minutes) aminoamide that reversibly blocks the sodium channels of nerve fibers, disrupting depolarization and thereby blocking transmission of pain signals. Infusion of anesthetic into the epidural space near the nerve fibers produces relief of pain with minimal effect on peripheral sensation or muscle action. Epidural, as opposed to perineural or subcutaneous, infusions may result in greater systemic absorption that can result in peripheral vasodilation and reduced systemic blood pressure as well as increased risk for systemic toxicity.[2]

Lidocaine 1% solution (10 mg/ml) is the most common anesthetic for local infiltration prior to chest tube placement. Lidocaine has an onset of action of 2 to 5 minutes and duration of 30 to 120 minutes which is long enough to complete most procedures. Higher concentrations, such as a 2% solution (20 mg/mL), do not promote improved onset or duration of analgesia and may increase the risk for toxicity.[3] Aspiration during infiltration is recommended when the involved area is close to major blood vessels.[4] Even without inadvertent intravenous infusion, rapid infusion into the highly vascular intercostal space results in rapid systemic absorption.[5]

In this case, the total bupivacaine 0.25% dose at 15 mL/h x 2.5 mg/mL = 37.5 mg/h. Bupivacaine toxicity occurs at 2 to 2.5 mg/kg, or 80 to 90 mg for this small patient. The total dose of lidocaine 2% delivered was 8 mL x 20 mg/mL = 160 mg. The maximum dose of lidocaine is 4 to 4.5 mg/kg or 160 to 180 mg for this patient. In elderly patients with either liver or kidney disease, the total dose should be decreased by 50% or about 80 mg in this case.[3]

Bupivacaine and lidocaine can, at toxic levels, produce depressed central nervous system (CNS) effects such as decreased level of consciousness and seizures as well as cardiotoxic effects such as bradycardia and myocardial depression resulting in cardiovascular collapse.[6]

In this case, a combination of steady state 0.25% bupivacaine via the epidural space and rapidly injected lidocaine at a high dose and concentration into the highly vascular intercostal space resulted in blockade of the sodium channels in the CNS and heart resulting in seizure and cardiac arrest.

Take-Home Points

- PCEA is a great postoperative analgesia modality. Ropivacaine, although less potent, may be an alternative for PCEA in those with those at increased risk for local anesthetic toxicity (elderly, low body weight, cardiac history). Bupivacaine is a racemic mix of S(-) and R(+) enantiomers. R(+) enantiomers increase binding to the sodium channels of the neuro- and cardiac tissues. Ropivacaine is a pure S(-) enantiomer, and is less toxic to the neuro and cardiovascular systems.[1]

- Lidocaine 1% is the standard local infiltration dose for procedures. Dilution to 0.5% is recommended in elderly patients and those patients with liver or kidneys disease.

- Clinicians must evaluate all current medications prior to any procedure and keep in mind that local anesthetic toxicity is a risk when local anesthetic is used in the setting of epidural or spinal anesthesia and analgesia.

- Local anesthetics are highly lipid-soluble and protein-bound. Lipids and protein are probably not found in high quantities in this tiny, 40 kg patient, therefore increasing her risk for local anesthetic toxicity at somewhat normal infusion rates.

- In the setting of local anesthetic toxicity, standard supportive care should be instituted (intubation, mechanical ventilation, IV fluids, vasopressors for hypotension, benzodiazepines for seizures, BLS/ACLS algorithms), as well as an intravenous bolus and infusion of 20% lipid emulsion. As local anesthetics are highly lipid soluble, this will bind systemic toxic local anesthetic and reverse toxicity.

Summary

Interaction: pharmacodynamic
Substrates: lidocaine, bupivacaine
Mechanism/site of action: sodium channel (peripheral nerve)
Clinical effect: synergistic anesthetic effect in the peripheral nerve system with additive cardiovascular and central nervous system toxicity

References

1. Pouzeratte Y, Delay JM, Brunat G, et al. Patient-controlled epidural analgesia after abdominal surgery: ropivacaine versus bupivacaine. Anesth Analg. 2001;93:1587–92.
2. Stoelting RK. Pharmacology and physiology in anesthetic practice. 3rd ed. Philadelphia: Lippincott-Raven; 1999. p. 158–81.
3. McGee DL. Local and topical anesthesia. In: Roberts JR, Hedges JR, editors. Clinical procedures in emergency medicine. 5th ed. Philadelphia: Saunders Elsevier; 2010. p. 481.
4. Achar S, Kundu S. Principles of office anesthesia: part I. Infiltrative anesthesia. Am Fam Physician. 2002;66(1):91–4.
5. Morgan GE Jr., Mikhail MS, Murray MJ. Chapter 14. Local anesthetics. In: Morgan GE Jr., Mikhail MS, Murray MJ, editors. Clinical anesthesiology. 4th ed. New York: McGraw-Hill; 2006. http://www.accessmedicine.com/content.aspx?aID=887357. Accessed 27 Jan 2012.
6. Dukes MN, editor. Meyler's side effects of drugs: the international encyclopedia of adverse drug reactions and interactions. 15th ed. Amsterdam: Excerpta Medica; 2006. p. 568–71.

The Spinal Countdown

General anesthesia after spinal anesthesia

40

Audra M. Webber MD and Franklyn P. Cladis MD, FAAP

Abstract
This case discusses primary and secondary pharmacodynamic interactions between general anesthesia and spinal anesthesia resulting in hypotension and bradycardia.

Case

The anesthesiologist looked at his patient, looked at the clock, and then looked at his patient again, who was an otherwise healthy 65 kg 14-year-old boy undergoing a right patellar reconstruction with hamstring harvest. The anesthesiologist was in the dreaded position of knowing without a doubt that the surgery was going to outlast the spinal as the surgeons had decided to start over and harvest tendon from the contralateral leg and had gone to talk to the parents.

With just a bit of midazolam and fentanyl sedation, the patient had easily tolerated placement of the spinal needle at L4-L5 interspace and a spinal anesthetic of 0.75% bupivacaine at 0.3 mg/kg was given with a resulting dense surgical block (Bromage score of 3). No intravenous fluid preload had been given, as the anesthesiologist remembered that pediatric patients maintain hemodynamic stability with spinal anesthesia as opposed to adults. A propofol infusion had been started at 50 mcg/kg/min. Vital signs were stable (heart rate was 62 beats per minute) and the patient's oxygen saturation (SpO_2) was 100% on oxygen by nasal cannula.

A.M. Webber MD (✉)
Department of Anesthesiology, Kosair Children's Hospital, Louisville, KY, USA
e-mail: audra.webber@gmail.com

F.P. Cladis MD, FAAP
Department of Anesthesiology, The University of Pittsburgh School of Medicine, Children's Hospital of Pittsburgh of UPMC, Pittsburgh, PA, USA

C. Marcucci et al. (eds.), *A Case Approach to Perioperative Drug-Drug Interactions*, DOI 10.1007/978-1-4614-7495-1_40

General anesthesia was induced with 2.5 mg/kg propofol, a 4.0 laryngeal mask airway (LMA) was placed without difficulty, and sevoflurane 2.5% was started with pressure control ventilation until the patient resumed spontaneous ventilations. The anesthesiologist heard the oximeter tone deepen before he saw it. The blood pressure cuff cycled but did not display a reading. The SpO_2 continued to drop and the patient's heart rate was now 32 beats per minute. The patient had only a faint carotid pulse. The overhead call went out, the sevoflurane went off, and fluids and emergency medications including atropine (1 mg) were given. The patient's heart rate did not increase and there was still no blood pressure by cuff measurement. Epinephrine (500 mcg) was given, and after a few seconds the SpO_2 began to rise. The blood pressure cuff cycled to read a pressure of 113/69 mm Hg. A radial pulse was now palpable. The patient was further stabilized over the next ten minutes. At that point, the surgeon walked back into the operating room, clapping his hands, and said, "Okay, people, let's get this party started!"

Discussion

This is an example of a primary pharmacodynamic interaction (hypotension) combined with a secondary pharmacodynamic interaction (bradycardia).

The incident in this case stemmed from a misconception regarding spinal anesthesia in the pediatric patient. While it is true that pediatric patients have very little hemodynamic derangement with spinal anesthetics, this applies only to patients in the neonatal period to ~5 years old.[1] In this age range spinal anesthetics tend to require larger doses of local anesthetic and their effects are less prolonged. From age 6 years onward, children can exhibit signs of a sympathectomy similar to that of adults, with older children (teenagers) having cardiovascular responses almost identical to that of adults.[2] Additionally, in a patient with a functioning spinal anesthetic who has been on a propofol infusion for approximately half an hour, regular induction doses of propofol are unnecessary, especially if one is placing an LMA (which is far less stimulating than an endotracheal tube).

Propofol reduces blood pressure by decreasing sympathetic activity, which can compound any sympathectomy incurred by a spinal anesthetic. In addition, propofol is known to induce bradycardia and even asystole and the myocardial depressant effect is dose dependent.[3,4] In most patients, the bradycardia is offset by the sympathetic nervous system response. In this patient, however, the spinal anesthetic obviated this response, and the patient experienced significant bradycardia and hypotension, which translated into decreased SpO_2 due to decreased cardiac output. Additionally, induction doses of propofol attenuate the heart rate response to atropine in a dose-dependent manner and should not have been the first agent used to treat the bradycardia.[5] While spinal anesthesia has been shown to be safe and effective in pediatric patients undergoing low abdominal and lower extremity orthopedic procedures, the same precautions must be observed as in adults.[6]

Take-Home Points

- The sympathectomy incurred by a spinal anesthetic does not occur in pediatric patients only up to age 5 or 6. Older pediatric patients, while likely less effected hemodynamically than adults, should be considered to have the potential for hemodynamic derangement, and be treated accordingly.
- If inducing anesthesia after a spinal anesthetic, it is wise to remember that normal induction doses are unnecessary, especially if the patient has been receiving the same agent for sedation.
- If you are treating propofol-induced bradycardia, atropine will not be as effective and epinephrine may be a wiser first agent.

Summary

Interactions: pharmacodynamic
Substrates: bupivacaine/propofol and propofol/atropine
Sites of action: sympathetic nervous system
Clinical effect: pronounced hypotension and refractory bradycardia

References

1. Lopez T, Sanchez FJ, Garzon JC, et al. Spinal anesthesia in pediatric patients. Minerva Anestesiol. 2012;78:78–87.
2. Dalens BJ. Regional anesthesia in children. In: Miller RD, editor. Miller's anesthesia. 7th ed. New York: Churchill Livingstone Inc; 2009. p. 2519–57.
3. Tramèr MR, Moore RA, McQuay HJ. Propofol and bradycardia: causation, frequency and severity. Br J Anaesth. 1997;78(6):642–51.
4. Pagel PS, Warltier DC. Negative inotropic effects of propofol as evaluated by the regional preload recruitable stroke work relationship in chronically instrumented dogs. Anesthesiology. 1993;78(1):100–8.
5. Horiguchi T, Nishikawa T. Heart rate response to intravenous atropine during propofol anesthesia. Anesth Analg. 2002;95(2):389–92.
6. Imbelloni LE, Vieira EM, Sperni F, et al. Spinal anesthesia in children with isobaric local anesthetics: report on 307 patients under 13 years of age. Paediatr Anaesth. 2006;16(1):43–8.

Are Drug–Drug Interactions The Smoking Guns of Local Anesthetic Toxicity? Smoking Gun I

41

Fatal Forty DDI: ropivacaine, fluoxetine, CYP1A2, CYP3A4

L. Michele Noles MD

Abstract

This case discusses a pharmacokinetic interaction between ropivacaine and fluoxetine. Ropivacaine is a cytochrome P450 3A4 and cytochrome 1A2 substrate. Fluoxetine is an inhibitor of both enzymes. Coadministration may result in ropivacaine toxicity.

Case

A 68-year-old, 96 kg man with a history of hypertension, depression, and anxiety was scheduled for a total shoulder replacement. An interscalene continuous nerve block catheter was planned for postoperative pain. His outpatient medications included alprazolam (0.25 mg bid prn anxiety), temazepam (15–30 mg qhs), and fluoxetine (20 mg q day), as well as amlodipine, bupropion, meclizine, and metoprolol. The patient received midazolam (2 mg) for anxiolysis in the block area and blockade of the brachial plexus was performed via the interscalene approach with ultrasound guidance. Ropivacaine 0.5% (30 mL) was administered in divided doses with intermittent negative aspiration, and ultrasound visualization of local anesthetic spread around the brachial plexus was noted. The patient tolerated the

L.M. Noles MD
Department of Anesthesiology & Perioperative Medicine,
Oregon Health and Science University, Portland, OR, USA
e-mail: nolesl@ohsu.edu

C. Marcucci et al. (eds.), *A Case Approach to Perioperative Drug-Drug Interactions*, DOI 10.1007/978-1-4614-7495-1_41

procedure well, there were no apparent complications, and good motor and sensory block were soon established. Upon arrival in the operating room approximately 20 minutes later, the patient became agitated and confused. (*Personal communication, Catherine Marcucci MD*)

Discussion

This is an example of a substrate added to an inhibitor.

Ropivacaine is metabolized primarily by cytochrome P450 (CYP) 1A2 with cytochrome 3A4 serving as a secondary enzyme for metabolism.[1] Fluoxetine and its principal metabolite norfluoxetine are together significant inhibitors of both of these enzymes.[2] Inhibition of the action of these enzymes results in decreased rate of metabolism of ropivacaine. Thus, the presence of fluoxetine and norfluoxetine likely led to a greater serum concentration of ropivacaine at the administered dosages than would normally have been expected. In this case, the patient's resulting ropivacaine neurologic toxicity manifested as a change in mental status.

Anesthesiologists and other anesthesia providers should be aware of the cytochrome 450 enzymes that metabolize the most commonly used local anesthetics for regional blockade. Ropivacaine, lidocaine, and mepivacaine undergo primary and/or secondary metabolism by cytochromes 1A2 and 3A4, whereas bupivacaine is metabolized chiefly by 3A4, with minor contributions by 2D6 and 2C19.[3]

Unrecognized pharmacokinetic and pharmacodynamic drug–drug interactions (DDIs) may play a role in producing "unexpected" cases of local anesthetic toxicity. When regional anesthesia is planned or when confronted with apparent local anesthetic toxicity in a patient with an uncomplicated working block without excessive dosing, patients' medication lists should be reviewed for the presence of a DDI "smoking gun" in the form of significant inhibitors of these enzymes. See Tables 41.1 and 41.2.[4,5]

Table 41.1 INHIBITORS of Cytochrome P450 1A2

Fluoroquinolone Antibiotics (ciprofloxacin, enoxacin)
Selective Serotonin Reuptake Inhibitors (fluvoxamine, fluoxetine)
Other (Potent) Inhibitors: Mexiletine, Propafenone

[Based on data from Ref. [4,5]]

Table 41.2 INHIBITORS of Cytochrome P450 3A4

Antidepressants	Antimicrobials	Other (Potent) Inhibitors
Selective serotonin reuptake inhibitors	*Antibiotics*	Diltiazem
Citalopram	Ciprofloxacin	Grapefruit juice
Fluoxetine	Norfloxacin	Mibefradil
Fluvoxamine	Quinupristin/dalfopristin	Methadone
Norfluoxetine	Sparfloxacin	
Paroxetine	*Azole Antifungals*	
Sertraline	Fluconazole	
Other antidepressants	Itraconazole	
Nefazodone	Ketoconazole	
	Miconazole	
	Macrolide antibiotics	
	Clarithromycin	
	Erythromycin	
	Nonnucleoside reverse transcriptase inhibitors	
	Delavirdine	
	Efavirenz	
	Protease inhibitors	
	Amprenavir	
	Indinavir	
	Lopinavir/ritonavir	
	Nelfinavir	
	Ritonavir	
	Saquinavir	
	Antipsychotics	
	Haloperidol	
	Pimozide	

[Based on data from Ref. [4,5]]

Take-Home Points

- Ropivacaine, lidocaine, and mepivacaine undergo metabolism by P450 cytochromes 1A2 and 3A4. Bupivacaine undergoes metabolism by 3A4, 2D6, and 2C19.
- There are numerous inhibitors of these cytochrome P450 enzymes in multiple drug classes.
- Consider that you may be dealing with an unrecognized DDI when there is apparent local anesthetic toxicity without apparent intravascular or excessive dosing.

Summary

Interaction: pharmacokinetic
Substrate: ropivacaine
Enzymes: 3A4 and 1A2
Inhibitor: fluoxetine

References

1. Tatro DS. Drug interaction facts. The authority on drug interactions. St. Louis: Wolters Kluwer Heath; 2009.
2. von Moltke LL, Greenblatt DJ, Duan SX, et al. Phenacetin O-deethylation by human liver microsomes in vitro: inhibition by chemical probes, SSRI antidepressants, nefazodone and venlafaxine. Psychopharmacology (Berl). 1996;128:398–407.
3. Gantenbein M, Attolini L, Bruguerolle B, et al. Oxidative metabolism of bupivacaine into pipecolylxylidine in humans is mainly catalyzed by CYP3A. Drug Metab Dispos. 2000;28:383–5.
4. Sandson NB. Drug interactions casebook, the cytochrome P450 system and beyond. Arlington: American Psychiatric Publishing, Inc.; 2003.
5. Cozza KL, Armstrong SC. The cytochrome P450 system, drug interaction principles for medical practice. Arlington: American Psychiatric Publishing, Inc.; 2001.

Are Drug-Drug Interactions The Smoking Guns of Local Anesthetic Toxicity? Smoking Gun II

42

Bupivacaine, methocarbamol

L. Michele Noles MD

Abstract
This case discusses a possible synergistic pharmacodynamic interaction between bupivacaine and methocarbamol, leading to CNS depression and change in mental status.

Case

A 65-year-old, 110 kg woman underwent right knee videoarthroscopy under general anesthesia. Outpatient medications included methocarbamol (500 mg qid) for muscle spasms, amlodipine, atenolol, simvastatin, eplerenone, and a nicotine patch. She received infiltration of 50 mL bupivacaine 0.5% into the joint at the end of the operative case. She experienced prolonged hypotension and confusion in the postanesthesia care unit (PACU), at one point becoming nonverbal even while conscious. Her vital signs stabilized and mental status cleared over several hours. She was eventually discharged home after an extended PACU stay.

L.M. Noles MD
Department of Anesthesiology & Perioperative Medicine,
Oregon Health and Science University, Portland, OR, USA
e-mail: nolesl@ohsu.edu

C. Marcucci et al. (eds.), *A Case Approach to Perioperative Drug-Drug Interactions*, DOI 10.1007/978-1-4614-7495-1_42

Discussion

This is an example of a possible synergistic pharmacodynamic drug–drug interaction (DDI) leading to bupivacaine toxicity.

The surgical team administered a total of 250 mg bupivacaine into the intra-articular space, certainly in the higher dose range. However, the pharmacokinetics of local anesthetics administered into joint spaces is not as straightforward as local anesthetics administered intravascularly or even for peripheral nerve blockade. It has been reported that absorption into the bloodstream, and hence increases in serum levels, are slower than for other routes of administration and are somewhat dependent on both the management of the lower extremity tourniquet as well as the concomitant use of epinephrine.[1,2] While there are reports of bupivacaine toxicity at approximately 1.3 mcg/mL, other sources have stated that with "few exceptions, toxic reactions to bupivacaine do not occur at plasma levels below 4 micrograms/ml."[3–5] Because a blood level was not obtained, it is difficult to state conclusively whether this patient's bupivacaine dose alone led to a toxic serum level and the resulting clinical effects. There is, however, a known potent pharmacodynamic DDI between bupivacaine and the methocarbamol that the patient was taking regularly for muscle spasm. It has long been recognized that when administered with other potential central nervous system (CNS) depressants, methocarbamol has a strongly synergistic effect, including fatal interactions.[6] This DDI very likely potentiated the negative neurologic effects of the bupivacaine, especially if bupivacaine was present in the bloodstream at elevated or toxic levels. The synergistic effects resulting from the combination of these two agents almost certainly led to an exacerbated CNS depression that would have been less likely and less severe if the patient had received only one of these agents.

This highlights the need for anesthesiologists, in their role as perioperative consultants, to educate themselves on DDIs, not only to improve their own drug selection, but also in order to better advise their colleagues on safe local anesthetic administration.

Take-Home Points

- Intravascular absorption of bupivacaine after intra-articular administration is less predictable than after other routes of administration.
- Bupivacaine toxicity is associated with CNS signs and symptoms.
- Methocarbamol is associated with CNS depression.

- Methocarbamol is known to act synergistically with other CNS depressant drugs.
- Extra caution is advised in clinical situations involving administration of local anesthetics and methocarbamol.

Summary

Interaction: pharmacodynamic
Substrates: bupivacaine and methocarbamol
Mechanism: synergistic combination of CNS depressant effects
Clinical effects: change in mental status

References

1. Solanki DR, Enneking FK, Ivey FM, et al. Serum bupivacaine concentrations after intraarticular injection for pain relief after knee arthroscopy. Arthroscopy. 1992;8:44–7.
2. Katz JA, Kaeding CS, Hill JR, et al. The pharmacokinetics of bupivacaine when injected intra-articularly after knee arthroscopy. Anesth Analg. 1988;67:872–5.
3. Scott DB, Lee A, Fagan D. Acute toxicity of ropivacaine compared with that of bupivacaine. Anesth Analg. 1989;69:563–9.
4. Knudsen K, Beckman Suurkula M, Blomberg S, et al. Central nervous and cardiovascular effects of i.v. infusions of ropivacaine, bupivacaine and placebo in volunteers. Br J Anaesth. 1997;78:507–14.
5. Hasselstrom LJ, Mogensen T. Toxic reaction of bupivacaine at low plasma concentration. Anesthesiology. 1984;61:99–100.
6. Ferslew KE, Hagardorn AN, McCormick WF. A fatal interaction of methocarbamol and ethanol in an accidental poisoning. J Forensic Sci. 1990;35:477–82.

A Perfect Storm?

43

Fatal Forty DDI: omeprazole, nicardipine, diltiazem, bupivacaine, CYP3A4, CYP2C19, CYP2D6

J. Andrew Dziewit MD and Nabil M. Elkassabany MD

Abstract

This case discusses the pharmacokinetic interactions between bupivacaine, nicardipine, omeprazole, and diltiazem. Bupivacaine is a cytochrome P450 3A4, 2C19, and 2D6 substrate and omeprazole, nicardipine, and diltiazem inhibit these, resulting in bupivacaine toxicity.

Case

A 73-year-old, 80 kg man underwent open repair of an abdominal aortic aneurysm. His past medical history was significant for hypertension, coronary artery disease, and peripheral vascular disease. He had suffered two previous strokes with no residual sensory or motor deficits. He also had gastroesophageal reflux disease (GERD) and was taking omeprazole (20 mg) twice daily.

Prior to the surgical procedure an epidural catheter was placed at the T9-T10 level. Repair of the aneurysm was uneventful. Intraoperatively, the patient received a total of 5 mg of preservative-free morphine and 20 mL of 0.25% bupivacaine in increments of 5 mL through his epidural catheter. At the conclusion of surgery, the patient was extubated without difficulty.

In the postanesthesia care unit (PACU), the patient was confused and his gaze became disconjugate. A noncontrast computed tomography (CT) scan of the brain

J.A. Dziewit MD (✉)
Department of Anesthesia and Perioperative Medicine, Crozer Chester Medical Center, Upland, PA, USA
e-mail: jadziewit@gmail.com

N.M. Elkassabany MD
Section of Orthopedic Anesthesiology, Department of Anesthesiology and Critical Care, University of Pennsylvania, Philadelphia, PA, USA

C. Marcucci et al. (eds.), *A Case Approach to Perioperative Drug-Drug Interactions*, DOI 10.1007/978-1-4614-7495-1_43

was negative for any acute findings. Shortly after, the patient's gaze normalized and he became more oriented to time and place. An epidural infusion was started at a rate of 8 mL/hr of 0.1% bupivacaine with fentanyl (5 mcg/mL). Later that evening, the patient was started on a nicardipine infusion for control of hypertension. A *post hoc* review revealed that the patient received 48 hours of continuous nicardipine infusion and received the bupivacaine epidural infusion for 72 hours, with an average infusion rate of 8 to 10 mL/h. During this interval, the patient had signs of waxing and waning deterioration in mental status.

On postoperative day 3, the patient was again noted to be confused. Fentanyl was removed from the epidural infusion, as it was thought to be contributing to the deterioration of the patient's mental status. That same day, the patient was started on his preoperative medications, which included diltiazem (120 mg/d). About 12 hours later, the patient required intubation for "worsening mental status" and possible aspiration. Mechanical ventilation was initiated. Chest X-ray revealed bilateral lower lobe infiltrates. After reintubation, his epidural infusion was stopped and the catheter was removed. His mental status did not improve. Acute brain infarction and hemorrhage were ruled out by serial MRI studies. The patient's clinical picture was consistent with acute respiratory distress syndrome with subsequent respiratory failure. The patient underwent tracheostomy for prolonged postoperative mechanical ventilation and respiratory failure on postoperative day 10.

Discussion

This is an example of multiple inhibitors added to a substrate.

Postoperative cognitive dysfunction (POCD) and postoperative delirium (POD) are relatively common in elderly patients, especially after vascular surgery involving the aorta.[1] The pathophysiology of these derangements is still poorly understood. POD has been identified as an independent predictor of prolonged hospitalization and increased perioperative mortality. The cost incurred because of POCD and POD is a significant burden on the health care system.[2]

Drug–drug interactions (DDIs) are often cited as a possible mechanism for the occurrence of POCD. In this case, the temporal relationship between the patient's mental status deterioration and the addition of certain medications is a clue that may suggest DDIs as a possible cause.

The use of an epidural infusion of bupivacaine, with or without an opioid, for postoperative analgesia after vascular procedures is a common practice. However, central nervous system toxicity of local anesthetics is not usually very high on the list of causes of postoperative mental dysfunction.

Bupivacaine is metabolized via the cytochrome P450 (CYP) enzyme system, mainly through the 3A4 enzyme. It is N-dealkylated to form pipecolylxylidine (PPX), a less toxic metabolite.[3] Very little unchanged bupivacaine is eliminated in the urine. The CYP enzymes 2C19 and 2D6 also serve as secondary pathways for the metabolism of bupivacaine.

Both the patient's home medication (omeprazole) and newly added inpatient medications (nicardipine and diltiazem) inhibited the P450 enzymes responsible for bupivacaine metabolism. Omeprazole has been shown to be a moderate inhibitor of cytochrome 2C19. It is also a milder inhibitor of 2C9 and 3A4.[4] Nicardipine strongly inhibits 3A4 as well as 2D6 and the cytochrome 2C enzymes (especially 2C8 and 2C19).[5] Diltiazem and its N-demethylated metabolite have been shown to inhibit CYP3A4.[6]

The inhibition of all three P450 pathways involved in the metabolism of bupivacaine may have dangerously increased the bupivacaine level above its systemic toxicity threshold. This was demonstrated by the patient's progression from confusion to increased cognitive and respiratory dysfunction, to the point of requiring reintubation.

Symptoms of central nervous system toxicity from local anesthetics can be broken down into two stages. *Early or mild toxicity* includes symptoms of light-headedness, dizziness, tinnitus, circumoral numbness, abnormal taste, confusion, and drowsiness. Symptoms of *severe toxicity* can result in tonic-clonic convulsions leading to progressive loss of consciousness, coma, respiratory depression, and respiratory arrest.[7]

Take-Home Points

- Keep DDIs on your list of causes of postoperative mental dysfunction.
- Familiarize yourself with the metabolic pathways of the drugs that you are using routinely.
- DDIs can occur regardless of the route of drug administration.
- Omeprazole and other proton pump inhibitors such as lansoprazole are significant P450 inhibitors.
- Some calcium channel blockers, like nicardipine and diltiazem, are inhibitors of cytochrome P450 metabolism.

- Symptoms of mild local anesthetic systemic toxicity include: light-headedness, dizziness, tinnitus, circumoral numbness, abnormal taste, confusion and drowsiness.
- Symptoms of severe toxicity include tonic-clonic convulsions, loss of consciousness, coma, respiratory depression, and respiratory arrest.

Summary

Interaction: pharmacokinetic
Substrate: bupivacaine
Enzyme: 3A4, 2C19, and 2D6
Inhibitors: nicardipine (3A4, 2C19, 2D6), omeprazole (2C19, 3A4), and diltiazem (3A4)
Clinical effect: bupivacaine toxicity

Acknowledgment: The editors wish to thank John E. Scharf MD for his contribution to the publication of this drug–drug interaction.

References

1. Schneider F, Bohner H, Habel U, et al. Risk factors for postoperative delirium in vascular surgery. Gen Hosp Psychiatry. 2002;24:28–34.
2. Leslie DL, Marcantonio ER, Zhang Y, et al. One-year health care costs associated with delirium in the elderly population. Arch Intern Med. 2008;168:27–32.
3. Gantenbein M, Attolini L, Bruguerolle B, et al. Oxidative metabolism of bupivacaine in to pipecolyxylidine in humans is mainly catalyzed by CYP3A. Drug Metab Dispos. 2000;28: 383–5.
4. Ko J, Sukhova N, Thacker D, et al. Evaluation of omeprazole and lansoprazole as inhibitors of cytochrome P450 isoforms. Drug Metab Dispos. 1997;25:853–62.
5. Katsunori N, Noritaka A, Takafumi I, et al. Inhibitory effects of nicardipine to cytochrome P450 (CYP) in human liver microsomes. Biol Pharm Bull. 2005;28:882–5.
6. Sutton D, Butler A, Nadin L, et al. Role of CYP3A4 in human hepatic diltiazem N-demethylation: inhibition of CYP3A4 activity by oxidized diltiazem metabolites. J Pharmacol Exp Ther. 1997;282:294–300.
7. Bukbirwa H, Conn D. Toxicity from local anaesthetic drugs. Update Anesth. 1999;10:1.

Shake Rattle and Roll

44

Fatal Forty DDI: lidocaine, cimetidine, CYP3A4

Hans P. Sviggum MD and Juraj Sprung MD, PhD

Abstract

This case discusses a pharmacokinetic interaction between lidocaine and cimetidine. Lidocaine is a cytochrome P450 3A4 substrate and cimetidine is a 3A4 inhibitor. Coadministration results in lidocaine toxicity.

Case

A 52-year-old, 74 kg man was scheduled for open reduction and internal fixation of a displaced metacarpal fracture suffered while participating in a rock 'n' roll dance contest at the local county fair. He had tripped on his partner's feet and tumbled to the floor, falling on his outstretched right hand. His past medical history included occasional migraine headaches and gastroesophageal reflux disease, which was well controlled with cimetidine.

The anesthetic plan called for an axillary block. Light sedation was achieved with midazolam. Following transarterial puncture, 20 mL of 1% lidocaine with epinephrine (1:200,000) was deposited posterior to the axillary artery, 20 mL anterior to the axillary artery, 5 mL into the coracobrachialis muscle to block the musculocutaneous nerve, and 5 mL to block the intercostobrachial nerve.

As the surgical technician prepared the patient's right arm for surgery and applied sterile drapes, the patient reported feeling dizzy and lightheaded. He then became restless and agitated and tried to climb off the operating room table. As the anesthesia resident moved to keep him from falling, the patient began shaking and proceeded to exhibit violent general tonic-clonic seizure activity. Midazolam (2 mg)

H.P. Sviggum MD (✉)
Department of Anesthesiology, Mayo Clinic College of Medicine, Rochester, MN, USA
e-mail: sviggum.hans@mayo.edu

J. Sprung MD, PhD
Department of Anesthesiology, Mayo Clinic, Rochester, MN, USA

C. Marcucci et al. (eds.), *A Case Approach to Perioperative Drug-Drug Interactions*, DOI 10.1007/978-1-4614-7495-1_44

was given intravenously with propofol (60 mg). The seizure activity ceased. The patient was ventilated by mask with 100% oxygen. He resumed spontaneous respirations within 30 seconds and regained consciousness a minute later. The procedure was cancelled, and he was admitted to the intensive care unit for further observation.

Discussion

This is an example of an inhibitor added to a substrate.

Lidocaine is an amide local anesthetic that is extensively metabolized in the liver. Its metabolism occurs primarily through the cytochrome P450 (CYP) 3A4 isozyme and, to a lesser extent, the cytochrome P450 1A2 isozyme. Lidocaine is metabolized through a sequential process starting with oxidative *N*-dealkylation. The metabolites are then excreted by the kidney. Only 3% of lidocaine is excreted unchanged.

Cimetidine is a histamine$_2$-receptor antagonist that acts by inhibiting histamine action at the histamine$_2$-receptors of the parietal cells within gastric glands in the folds of the stomach, thus decreasing basal gastric acid secretion. It is also a potent inhibitor of 3A4. Treatment with cimetidine significantly affects the pharmacokinetics of lidocaine. Drugs that inhibit hepatic microsomal enzymes, such as cimetidine, may allow the accumulation of an unexpectedly high (possibly toxic) blood level of lidocaine by inhibiting its metabolism. Many sources agree that cimetidine treatment inhibits the metabolism of lidocaine by interfering with hepatic microsomal enzyme activity.[1–5] However, the overall effect of cimetidine on the disposition of lidocaine is complex and likely multifactorial.

Cimetidine not only inhibits the oxidative drug metabolism of lidocaine, but it also may impair hepatic clearance of lidocaine by other mechanisms. Reduction of hepatic blood flow by drugs or hypotension decreases the hepatic clearance of amide local anesthetics. Although the data are varied, one study reported that hepatic blood flow decreased 33% after repeated administration of cimetidine.[6] By reducing lidocaine clearance, cimetidine increases blood and tissue concentrations of lidocaine and enhances its potential toxicity. In this situation, local anesthetic toxicity is a real and potentially dangerous situation.

Feely et al. looked at the effects of oral cimetidine treatment on a short duration intravenous lidocaine infusion.[2] They found that the cimetidine-treated group showed a 25% to 30% reduction in lidocaine clearance, a decreased volume of distribution, and reduced protein binding compared with the placebo group. Cimetidine prolonged the half-life of lidocaine and also increased its peak plasma concentration. Cimetidine-induced lidocaine toxicity during the short infusion period occurred in five of the six study participants who had been treated with cimetidine. The elevated peak plasma concentration of lidocaine suggests that a cimetidine-induced increase in acute toxicity is likely due to altered distribution.[2] Any factor which decreases the volume of the distribution of lidocaine increases the plasma concentration, thus increasing the risk for toxicity.

Although there are a number of local anesthetics and histamine$_2$-receptor antagonists, neurotoxicity does not seem to be increased by any other combination of these drugs than lidocaine and cimetidine. The interaction between cimetidine and lidocaine has been well described; however, cimetidine did not alter the pharmacokinetics or metabolism of another type of amide local anesthetic, bupivacaine hydrochloride.[7] Similarly, the histamine$_2$-receptor antagonist ranitidine hydrochloride was not found to substantially impair the systemic clearance of lidocaine.[5] The absence of ranitidine effects on the disposition of lidocaine suggests that histamine$_2$-receptor blockade may not decrease hepatic blood flow and that cimetidine impairs drug elimination only by inhibition of hepatic microsomal enzymes.

Take-Home Points

- Lidocaine is extensively metabolized by the cytochrome P450 system, specifically the 3A4 isozyme.
- Cimetidine, a histamine$_2$-receptor blocker, increases the risk for lidocaine toxicity by decreasing its clearance and increasing its peak plasma concentration. This response is likely a multifactorial phenomenon. Cimetidine has been found to be a potent inhibitor of the 3A4 isozyme, which is primarily responsible for the metabolism of lidocaine.
- Patients taking cimetidine acutely or long term may have increased vulnerability to local anesthetic toxicity with lidocaine administration.
- Use of ranitidine may be a safer alternative to cimetidine to decrease acid gastric secretion with regard to lowering the likelihood of lidocaine toxicity. Other histamine$_2$-receptor antagonists similar to ranitidine have not been shown to increase the potential toxicities of lidocaine.
- The metabolism, clearance, and subsequent likelihood of toxicity of other local anesthetics, such as bupivacaine, are not altered substantially by treatment with cimetidine.

Summary

Interaction: pharmacokinetic (metabolic)
Substrates: lidocaine
Enzyme: 3A4
Inhibitor: cimetidine
Clinical effect: lidocaine toxicity

References

1. Naguib M, Magboul MM, Samarkandi AH, et al. Adverse effects and drug interactions associated with local and regional anaesthesia. Drug Saf. 1998;18:221–50.
2. Feely J, Wilkinson GR, McAllister CB, et al. Increased toxicity and reduced clearance of lidocaine by cimetidine. Ann Intern Med. 1982;96:592–4.
3. Daneshmend TK, Ene MD, Parker G, et al. Effects of chronic oral cimetidine on apparent liver blood flow and hepatic microsomal enzyme activity in man. Gut. 1984;25:125–8.
4. Bill TJ, Clayman MA, Morgan RF, et al. Lidocaine metabolism pathophysiology, drug interactions, and surgical implications. Aesthet Surg J. 2004;24:307–11.
5. Kim KC, Tasch MD. Effects of cimetidine and ranitidine on local anesthetic central nervous system toxicity in mice. Anesth Analg. 1986;65:840–2.
6. Feely J, Wilkinson GR, Wood AJ. Reduction of liver blood flow and propranolol metabolism by cimetidine. N Engl J Med. 1981;304:692–5.
7. Kuhnert BR, Zuspan KJ, Kuhnert PM, et al. Lack of influence of cimetidine on bupivacaine levels during parturition. Anesth Analg. 1987;66:986–90.

Hello, We Have a Patient With Acute Delirium and We Need an Urgent Psych Consult

45

Lidocaine, metoprolol

Katarina Bojanić MD, Juraj Sprung MD, PhD, and Toby N. Weingarten MD

Abstract
This case discusses a pharmacokinetic drug interaction between lidocaine and metoprolol resulting in changes in drug distribution.

Case

An 80-year-old man with complex regional pain syndrome of his left lower extremity presented to the pain clinic with a severe exacerbation of leg pain leg that developed suddenly that morning while getting out of bed. Fluoroscopic imaging showed that the lead to his spinal cord stimulator had migrated. Because his pain was unmanageable with opiates alone, he was admitted to the telemetry ward of the local hospital for a lidocaine infusion. A loading dose of intravenous lidocaine (100 mg) was administered over 10 minutes, followed by a lidocaine infusion at 4 mg/min. After 6 hours, his lidocaine plasma level was 4 mcg/mL (therapeutic

K. Bojanić MD (✉)
Division of Neonatology, Clinical Hospital Merkur, Zagreb, Croatia
e-mail: sprungkatarina@hotmail.com

J. Sprung MD, PhD
Department of Anesthesiology, Mayo Clinic, Rochester, MN, USA

T.N. Weingarten MD
Department of Anesthesiology, Mayo Clinic, Rochester, MN, USA

Department of Anesthesiology, Mayo Clinic College of Medicine, Rochester, MN, USA

C. Marcucci et al. (eds.), *A Case Approach to Perioperative Drug-Drug Interactions*, DOI 10.1007/978-1-4614-7495-1_45

level, 2–5 mcg/mL) and his pain was controlled. The next day, he underwent successful revision of his spinal cord stimulator lead.

The patient did well over the subsequent 2 years, except that he developed hypertension, which was treated with extended-release metoprolol (100 mg) at night. While moving boxes one morning, he felt pain and a "popping" sensation in his back and felt the stimulation pattern shift from his leg to his flank. At 8:00 PM, the patient went to the emergency department complaining of severe pain which was unresponsive to opioids. He was again admitted to the telemetry ward and a lidocaine infusion was started. At 6:00 AM, the patient had marked improvement of his pain, and his lidocaine plasma level was 4.9 mcg/mL. On morning rounds, it was realized that the patient had missed his evening dose of metoprolol, and he was given extended-release metoprolol (100 mg).

That afternoon, the patient became disoriented and began shouting at the nursing staff and pulling at his intravenous line and monitors. An urgent psychiatry consultation was requested to evaluate the acute delirium, and haloperidol was administered. A toxicology screen was sent, which was positive only for morphine. Fortunately, the psychiatrist also thought to order a serum lidocaine level as well, which was elevated at 6.4 mcg/mL. The lidocaine infusion was discontinued. The patient's mental status cleared after several hours, but unfortunately, his leg pain returned. He underwent a successful revision of the stimulator lead displacement the next day.

Discussion

This is an example of a pharmacokinetic drug–drug interaction resulting in changes in drug distribution.

More specifically, this is an example of lidocaine neurotoxicity caused by reduction in hepatic clearance in the presence of the β-adrenergic blocker metoprolol.

Lidocaine is an amide local anesthetic that blocks fast voltage-gated sodium channels in neurons. Peripheral nerve injury can result in upregulation of tetrodotoxin-resistant sodium channels on nociceptive fibers and dorsal root ganglions.[1] Lidocaine inhibits these channels and has been used to treat pain associated with complex regional pain syndrome.[2] Resorption of lidocaine from block sites is usually rapid, and in some cases, serum lidocaine levels rise at comparable speed to intravenous injection. Systemic toxic reaction from lidocaine may start when serum levels exceed 5 mcg/mL. Steady-state blood lidocaine concentration during an intravenous infusion depends on the infusion rate and hepatic drug clearance. Rapid elimination of lidocaine occurs through hepatic metabolism with cytochrome P450 3A4 (CYP3A4).

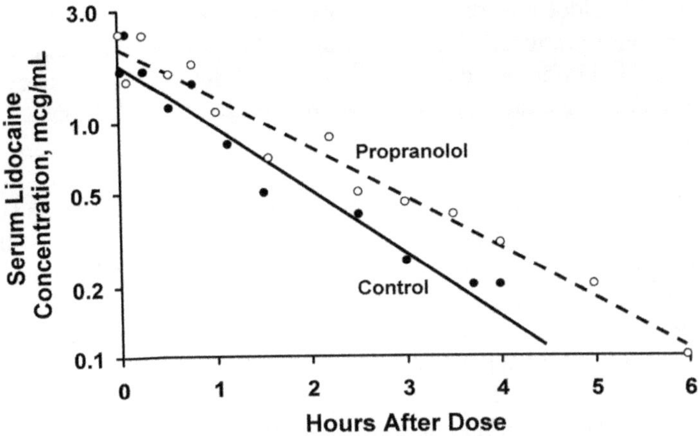

Fig. 45.1 Serum lidocaine concentrations after a single dose of lidocaine in a patient who received propranolol and in a patient who did not receive it. The mean elimination half-life was prolonged from 65 min in the control patient to 101 min in the patient who received propranolol [Adapted from Ochs HR, Carstens G, Greenblatt DJ. Reduction in lidocaine clearance during continuous infusion and by coadministration of propranolol. N Engl J Med. 1980;303:373–377. With permission from Massachusetts Medical Society]

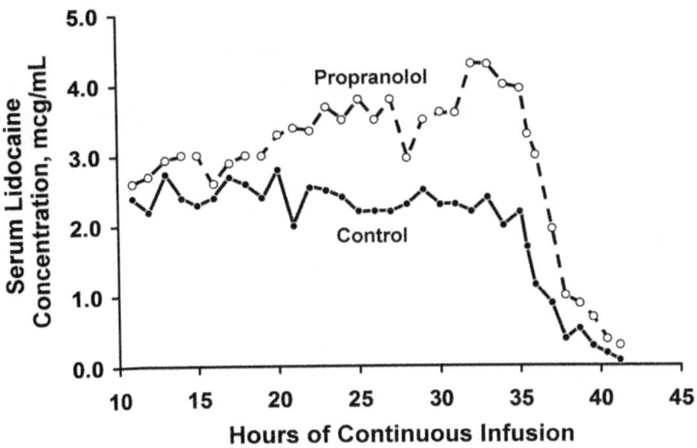

Fig. 45.2 Serum lidocaine concentrations during and after continuous infusion of lidocaine in a patient who received propranolol and in a patient who did not receive it [Adapted from Ochs HR, Carstens G, Greenblatt DJ. Reduction in lidocaine clearance during continuous infusion and by coadministration of propranolol. N Engl J Med. 1980;303:373–377. With permission from Massachusetts Medical Society]

Coadministration of β-adrenoceptor antagonists (eg, propranolol, metoprolol) decreases cardiac output and, consequently, hepatic blood flow, which results in reduction of lidocaine clearance, both after a single bolus of lidocaine (Fig. 45.1) and during continuous lidocaine infusion (Fig. 45.2).[3,4] The coadministration of propranolol with lidocaine results in a 30% increase in mean serum lidocaine steady-state concentrations.[4] Other conditions that decrease hepatic blood flow, such as myocardial infarction and congestive heart failure, as well as advanced age, may result in decreased clearance of lidocaine, resulting in lidocaine accumulation and toxicity.[5,6]

Local anesthetic toxicity manifests with both central nervous system and cardiovascular toxicities. Our octogenarian patient had delirium with a lidocaine plasma concentration of 6.4 mcg/mL. Greater plasma concentrations can be associated with seizures followed by coma. Saravay et al. described patients who had psychiatric presentation of lidocaine toxicity, and the spectrum of signs and symptoms ranged from mood changes, "doom anxiety," confusional states, and hallucinations to delusions.[7] Though lidocaine is less cardiotoxic than other local anesthetics, cardiovascular depression also can occur, although typically at much greater concentrations. Therefore, physicians should anticipate the need to decrease the dosage of lidocaine in situations requiring the coadministration of a β-adrenergic blocker and especially for geriatric patients.

Take-Home Points

- Lidocaine hepatic metabolism is highly dependent on blood flow to the liver, which may be altered in any condition that decreases cardiac index (eg, use of β-adrenergic blockers, myocardial infarction).
- Coadministration of metoprolol and lidocaine significantly influences lidocaine kinetics and reduces its elimination, leading to an increase in lidocaine levels by about 30% on average, which may result in toxic serum concentrations.
- Lidocaine toxicity can present as acute psychiatric disturbance, and high-risk populations include patients with decreased cardiac output and those who are elderly.

Summary

Interaction: pharmacokinetic (distribution)
Substrates: lidocaine and metoprolol
Mechanism/site of action: reduced hepatic metabolism via reduction hepatic blood flow
Clinical effect: local anesthetic toxicity

References

1. Lai J, Hunter JC, Porreca F. The role of voltage-gated sodium channels in neuropathic pain. Curr Opin Neurobiol. 2003;13:291–7.
2. Schwartzman RJ, Patel M, Grothusen JR, et al. Efficacy of 5-day continuous lidocaine infusion for the treatment of refractory complex regional pain syndrome. Pain Med. 2009;10:401–12.
3. Conrad KA, Byers 3rd JM, Finley PR, et al. Lidocaine elimination: effects of metoprolol and of propranolol. Clin Pharmacol Ther. 1983;33:133–8.
4. Ochs HR, Carstens G, Greenblatt DJ. Reduction in lidocaine clearance during continuous infusion and by coadministration of propranolol. N Engl J Med. 1980;303:373–7.
5. Prescott LF, Adjepon-Yamoah KK, Talbot RG. Impaired Lignocaine metabolism in patients with myocardial infarction and cardiac failure. Br Med J. 1976;1:939–41.
6. Bowdle TA, Freund PR, Slattery JT. Age-dependent lidocaine pharmacokinetics during lumbar peridural anesthesia with lidocaine hydrocarbonate or lidocaine hydrochloride. Reg Anesth. 1986;11:123–7.
7. Saravay SM, Marke J, Steinberg MD, et al. "Doom anxiety" and delirium in lidocaine toxicity. Am J Psychiatry. 1987;144:159–63.

Fatal Pain Relief

46

Local anesthetics, intrathecal morphine

Matthew M. Kumar MD
and Richard Levi Boortz-Marx MD, MS

Abstract
This case discusses a synergistic pharmacodynamic interaction between morphine and bupivacaine, resulting in death. This drug pair eliminated both central and peripheral respiratory drive.

Case

A 72-year-old woman was being evaluated for implantation of an intrathecal morphine pump. She had chronic back pain secondary to osteoporosis, numerous old compression fractures of the thoracic and lumbar spines, degenerative disk disease, and spinal stenosis. She was taking oral morphine (60 mg BID) and oxycodone (5 mg every 6 h for breakthrough pain as needed).

On the morning of the intrathecal morphine trial, the patient rated her pain 8 on a 10-point pain scale. She received an intrathecal morphine injection (600 mcg) through an indwelling, lumbar intrathecal catheter. Four hours later, she rated her pain at 6/10. She was given another intrathecal injection (300 mcg). Two hours later, she still rated her pain at 6/10. Her vital signs were normal with a respiratory rate of 20 breaths per minute. A third intrathecal injection of morphine (300 mcg) with bupivacaine (3.25 mg) was administered.

Immediately after the third injection, the patient reported total pain relief and rated her pain at 0/10. Thirty minutes later, the patient was pain-free still and was able to ambulate with adequate motor strength in her lower limbs. Fifteen minutes later,

M.M. Kumar MD (✉)
Department of Anesthesiology & Critical Care Medicine, Mayo Clinic, Rochester, MN, USA
e-mail: mkumar@mayo.edu

R.L. Boortz-Marx MD, MS
Department of Anesthesiology, University of North Carolina, Chapel Hill, NC, USA

C. Marcucci et al. (eds.), *A Case Approach to Perioperative Drug-Drug Interactions*, DOI 10.1007/978-1-4614-7495-1_46

resting comfortably in bed, the patient's pulse oximeter saturation decreased to less than 85%. Oxygen by nasal cannulae (4 L/min) was started. Her vital signs were normal, with a respiratory rate of 10 to 12 breaths per minute.

Thirty minutes later, the patient was found unresponsive and pulseless. Attempts at resuscitation were unsuccessful. She was pronounced dead 75 minutes after her last intrathecal injection. An autopsy showed normal heart, lungs, and brain. The pathologist ascribed the cause of death to opioid-induced respiratory depression.

Discussion

This is an example of a pharmacodynamic drug–drug interaction(DDI).

More specifically, this is an example where abolishing pain with local anesthetic may eliminate the respiratory stimulus and unmask the respiratory depression effects of opiates.

Respiratory depression is a well-recognized complication of intrathecal opioid administration.[1] However, patients taking opioid therapy long term are generally resistant to this adverse effect because tolerance develops against the effects of the opioid medication. In this case, respiratory depression did not appear until the administration of a local anesthetic.

Often, a low dose of bupivacaine is added to intrathecal morphine to improve the quality of pain relief.[2] Devoid of respiratory muscle paralysis, intrathecal bupivacaine administration *per se* does not depress respiration. Pharmacokinetic interaction between morphine and intrathecal bupivacaine is minimal and clinically insignificant. However, an established therapeutic principle states that pain is a physiologic antagonist of opioid analgesia.[3]

Substance P, a strong respiratory stimulant, has effects on respiration opposite to those of morphine and endorphin.[4,5] It enhances the rhythmogenesis of brainstem motorneurons and increases the tidal volume and minute ventilation. On the other hand, substance-P antagonists, applied to the ventral surface of the medulla, blunt the ventilatory response to hypoxia, hypercapnia, and somatosensory-induced stimulation.[6] Laboratory studies show that substance P binding to its receptor (NK1) is inhibited by local anesthetics at concentrations reached in the cerebrospinal fluid after intrathecal injection.[7]

It appears that in this case, the stimulating effect of pain on respiration was abolished by administration of a local anesthetic. Intrathecal morphine administered nearly 7 hours earlier, along with long-term oral opioid ingestion, had predisposed the patient to respiratory depression. Abolishing the pain that was sustaining her respiratory drive probably resulted in respiratory arrest. Similar catastrophic respiratory arrests have been reported after various analgesic techniques that abolish pain in patients who were opioid–dependent long term.[8]

Take-Home Points

- Pain is an important respiratory stimulant for patients who are opioid–dependent long term.
- Abolishing pain may eliminate the respiratory stimulus in these patients and unmask the respiratory depression effects of opiates.
- Respiratory functions should be monitored carefully for patients with long-term opioid dependency who undergo analgesic or anesthetic interventions that abolish pain.

Summary

Interaction: pharmacodynamic
Substrates: morphine and bupivacaine
Mechanism of action: synergy of pain relief (peripheral and central) and opioid-induced respiratory depression
Clinical effect: severe respiratory depression, culminating in death

References

1. Gehling M, Tryba M. Risks and side-effects of intrathecal morphine combined with spinal anaesthesia: a meta-analysis. Anaesthesia. 2009;64:643–51.
2. Akerman B, Arwestrom E, Post C. Local anesthetics potentiate spinal morphine antinociception. Anesth Analg. 1988;67:943–8.
3. Hanks GW, Twycross RG. Pain, the physiological antagonist of opioid analgesics. Lancet. 1984;1:1477–8.
4. Bonham AC. Neurotransmitters in the CNS control of breathing. Respir Physiol. 1995;101: 219–30.
5. Takita K, Herlenius E, Yamamoto Y, et al. Effects of neuroactive substances on the morphine-induced respiratory depression: an in vitro study. Brain Res. 2000;884:201–5.
6. Chen Z, Hedner J, Hedner T. Substance P in the ventrolateral medulla oblongata regulates ventilatory responses. J Appl Physiol. 1990;68:2631–9.
7. Li YM, Wingrove DE, Too HP, et al. Local anesthetics inhibit substance P binding and evoked increases in intracellular Ca2+. Anesthesiology. 1995;82:166–73.
8. Piquet CY, Mallaret MP, Lemoigne AH, et al. Respiratory depression following administration of intrathecal bupivacaine to an opioid-dependent patient. Ann Pharmacother. 1998;32:653–5.

Lipid Lifesaver

47

Local anesthetic, lipid emulsion

Adrian Pichurko MD and Guy Weinberg MD

Abstract
This case discusses the interesting but not fully understood pharmacodynamic interaction between local anesthetics and lipid emulsion.

Case

A 33-year-old, 72 kg man presented for washout of an open humerus fracture under regional anesthesia. The patient complained of dizziness just as the anesthesiologist was completing an infracoracoid block with 30 cc of 0.375% bupivacaine without epinephrine. The injection was stopped and the needle was withdrawn just as the patient had a generalized, tonic-clonic seizure. Oxygen was delivered by mask ventilation and the seizures subsided after the patient was given midazolam (4 mg) intravenously. Vital signs were stable and the patient was breathing spontaneously when, 5 minutes after the seizure, the ECG registered ventricular tachycardia followed rapidly by a slow idioventricular rhythm and then asystole. Chest compressions were begun immediately, the trachea was intubated, and the patient ventilated with 100% oxygen. A few minutes after the cardiac arrest, while chest compressions continued, 150 cc of 20% lipid emulsion were injected intravenously over 2 minutes and followed by a continuous lipid infusion of 20 mL/min. A sinus rhythm with a palpable pulse returned after a few minutes. The blood pressure was 110/70 mm Hg and heart rate was 90 beats per minute(bpm). The lipid infusion was continued for 20 minutes during which the patient awakened, his heart rate slowed to 80 bpm and his blood pressure returned to pre-event levels.

A. Pichurko MD (✉) • G. Weinberg MD
Department of Anesthesiology, University of Illinois, Chicago, IL, USA
e-mail: pichurko@gmail.com

C. Marcucci et al. (eds.), *A Case Approach to Perioperative Drug-Drug Interactions*, DOI 10.1007/978-1-4614-7495-1_47

Discussion

This is an example of a complex and not fully elucidated antagonistic pharmacodynamic interaction.

Local anesthetic systemic toxicity (LAST) results either from the inadvertent intravascular injection, vascular entrainment, or vascular absorption of local anesthetic. It is estimated to occur in as many as 1 in 500 peripheral nerve blocks. Specific at-risk subgroups include patients with ischemic heart disease, conduction defects, or low cardiac output; the very young and old; and patients with specific metabolic defects, such as carnitine deficiency, that affect mitochondrial function. LAST can occur immediately (eg, during injection) or after a substantial delay; however, intervals of 5 to 10 minutes after injection of local anesthetic are very common.[1]

Symptoms of toxicity typically involve the central nervous system (CNS) and cardiovascular system. The brain is more sensitive to local anesthetic overdose and thus symptoms like agitation, seizures, and altered mental status tend to occur earlier and at lower levels of toxicity than cardiovascular compromise. Cardiovascular toxicity often manifests initially with arrhythmias, tachycardia, and hypertension. Signs of worsening toxicity include progressive hypotension, conduction blockade, bradycardia, and even, as in the case described here, asystole. Complete cardiovascular collapse secondary to local anesthetics is classically viewed as refractory to standard resuscitation measures. The lipophilicity of the particular local anesthetic parallels its potential for causing cardiovascular toxicity and among toxic signs of overdose involving the most lipophilic agents, arrhythmias, bradycardia, and hypotension tend to occur earlier in the sequence of toxic effects. The most lipophilic drugs, like bupivacaine, can cause hemodynamic instability without any premonitory CNS symptoms.[1]

Bupivacaine is thought to cause cardiac toxicity by action at several sites including voltage–dependent sodium, potassium, and calcium channels; adrenergic and lipid signaling schemes; and mitochondrial metabolism. This combination of adverse effects may explain why LAST is often refractory to standard resuscitation.

Intravascular infusion of lipid emulsion has been shown over the past several years to effectively reverse both CNS and cardiovascular signs of local anesthetic toxicity. Lipid is thought to exert several effects and the precise mechanism(s) of its benefit have not been irrefutably established. The simplest is a sequestering effect, the so-called "lipid sink" mechanism. It has been demonstrated *in vitro* that local anesthetic partitions into lipid droplets contained in the plasma, thereby decreasing the drug's availability to receptors and reducing free (unbound) local anesthetic concentration at tissue sites of toxicity. This could result from an initial electrostatic interaction between the strong negative surface charge of the lipid membrane and the bupivacaine molecule, which is positively charged at physiological serum pH. This is followed by absorption into the lipid droplet, although the exact interfacial dynamics have not been worked out yet. Such a generic mechanism could account for the ability of lipid emulsion infusion to reverse toxicity involving the CNS, a tissue that does not normally utilize fatty acid substrates for metabolism.

Additional mechanisms including post-ischemic cardioprotection are under investigation. A direct metabolic effect has also been postulated in which increased plasma fatty acids overcome the bupivacaine-induced inhibition of mitochondrial fatty acid transport and metabolism. Fatty acids released by the lipid infusion can also displace and interfere with local anesthetic binding of sodium channels at the plasma membrane.[1] Lipid has also been shown to reduce myocardial stunning and cardiac reperfusion injury by inhibiting mitochondrial glycogen synthase kinase-3β.[2] Its anti-apoptotic effect is also mediated through the well-known Akt cytoprotective pathway.[2] These mechanisms probably do not account for all of the therapeutic benefit of lipid emulsion and research to identify further mechanisms is a focus of several laboratories.[1]

It is noteworthy that several of these mechanisms rely on a bulk-phase effect in which a large initial bolus infusion is required. As demonstrated in the case scenario, lipid rescue guidelines recommend that the initial bolus be followed by a continuing infusion. This was first noted in animal models of LAST where the single bolus alone would result in temporary resuscitation and that a following infusion of lipid for several minutes was needed to prevent recurrence of cardiovascular instability. This could simply indicate a need to counter the metabolic dissipation of lipid droplets to maintain a constant plasma triglyceride or fatty acid concentration. However, the exact pharmacokinetics of lipid-local anesthetic interaction are still under investigation and identifying the optimal dosing regimen for lipid emulsion is a priority of several laboratories.[1]

The American Society of Regional Anesthesia (ASRA) 2010 guidelines emphasize the primacy of airway management, seizure suppression, and Advanced Cardiac Life Support (ACLS).[3] They also recommend a 20% lipid emulsion intravenous bolus of 1.5 mL/kg of lean body mass, followed by a 0.25 mL/kg/min infusion for 10 minutes after hemodynamic stability is attained. Failure to resuscitate should prompt a second bolus; persistent hypotension after resuscitation would indicate the need for an increased infusion rate (eg, 0.5 mL/kg/min). The maximum recommended dose of lipid is approximately 10 mL/kg over 30 minutes. Note that the standard ACLS protocol should be revised in two respects: vasopressin is *not* recommended in LAST and doses of epinephrine should be smaller than usual (eg, ~1 mcg/kg), since doses ≥70 mcg/kg have been shown to impair lipid rescue.[4] ASRA guidelines caution: "*propofol is not a substitute for lipid emulsion therapy* because of its low lipid content (10%), the large volumes required for the benefit of lipid in resuscitation (hundreds of milliliters) and the direct cardiac depressant effects of propofol."[3]

Few adverse effects of lipid emulsion therapy have been reported in the setting of rapid infusion for drug overdose; previous concerns about pulmonary and neurologic damage have not been realized.[1] However, clinical laboratory results will be predictably difficult to interpret for an hour or so following lipid infusion. Most notably, it may falsely elevate hemoglobin and platelet counts on serum analysis and obscure electrolyte analysis. It is advised to draw labs before emulsion, if possible, and to notify the laboratory of the lipemic sample.[5]

Take-Home Points

- Although formal randomized clinical trials are excluded by ethical and practical considerations, there is strong evidence that local anesthetic systemic toxicity can be rapidly reversed by bolus injection and continuous infusion of 20% lipid emulsion.
- There are many proposed mechanisms for this effect and future research will identify the differing contributions of these various effects.
- Current local anesthetic resuscitation guidelines include lipid emulsion along with airway management and ACLS.

Summary

Interaction: pharmacokinetic and possible physicochemical
Substrates: local anesthetics, especially bupivacaine and 20% lipid emulsion
Site of action/mechanism: unknown
Clinical effect: marked decrease in local anesthetic toxicity including recovery from cardiac and central nervous system collapse

References

1. Bern S, Akpa BS, Kuo I, et al. Lipid resuscitation: a life-saving antidote for local anesthetic toxicity. Curr Pharm Biotechnol. 2011;12(2):313–9.
2. Rahman S, Li J, Bopassa JC, et al. Phosphorylation of GSK-3β mediates intralipid-induced cardioprotection against ischemia/reperfusion injury. Anesthesiology. 2011;115(2):242–53.
3. Neal JM, Bernards CM, Butterworth JF, et al. Practice advisory on local anesthetic systemic toxicity. Reg Anesth Pain Med. 2010;35(2):152–61.
4. Hiller DB, Gregorio GD, Ripper R, et al. Epinephrine impairs lipid resuscitation from bupivacaine overdose: a threshold effect. Anesthesiology. 2009;111(3):498–505.
5. Smith NA. Possible side effects of Intralipid rescue therapy. Anaesthesia. 2010;65(2):210–1.

Drug–Drug Interactions Involving Opioids

VII

Introduction

48

Toby N. Weingarten MD

Abstract
This section introduces drug–drug interactions involving opioid pain medications.

New Year's Day, 2001 heralded the decade of pain control and research in the United States, established by an Act of Congress. Even before this Act of Congress, the tide of clinical practice had already shifted towards a more liberal policy of prescribing opioid medication for the treatment of chronic pain. The result has been a dramatic increase in the number of opioid analgesic prescriptions, a practice change not without downsides. Opioids render patients tolerant to their analgesic effects, and in some cases paradoxically make patients hyperalgesic to pain. The therapeutic window between analgesia and respiratory depression narrows, and opioid-tolerant patients are more likely to experience postoperative sedation and respiratory depression. Prescription drug diversion and abuse is rampant. Accidental poisoning from overdose and opioid–drug interactions from prescription opioids has become common in emergency departments across the country. Deaths of celebrities from cardiac dysrhythmias from methadone–drug interactions have captured the national headlines.

With increasing frequency, all anesthesiologists, no matter if we are pain physicians, intensivists, or perioperative physicians, are encountering patients who are on chronic opioid therapy. We are often looked upon as the "experts" of these medications. It is imperative we have a good understanding of the pharmacodynamic and pharmacokinetic properties of opioids. Opioids have numerous drug–drug interactions of important clinical interest. Best known are additive and

T.N. Weingarten MD
Department of Anesthesiology, Mayo Clinic College of Medicine, Rochester, MN, USA

Department of Anesthesiology, Mayo Clinic, Rochester, MN, USA
e-mail: Weingarten.toby@mayo.edu

C. Marcucci et al. (eds.), *A Case Approach to Perioperative Drug-Drug Interactions*, DOI 10.1007/978-1-4614-7495-1_48

synergistic reactions resulting in respiratory depression, typically when opioids are administered with other sedating medications such as benzodiazepines. Less known, but equally important, effects result from interactions that affect the metabolism of opioids. Many opioids are significantly metabolized by the hepatic cytochrome P450 (CYP) system; a metabolic pathway then can be induced or inhibited by numerous medications including antimicrobials, antidepressants, and seizure medications. The resulting interactions may be expected, such as opioid withdrawal or oversedation, but there can be idiosyncratic reactions, such as serotonin syndrome from the interactions of tramadol and paroxetine, or meperidine and phenelzine. The heterogeneity of the P450 system leads to variable metabolism of some opioids. For example, codeine is metabolized by the polymorphic cytochrome 2D6, and patients may be "poor metabolizers" and have limited analgesia from codeine or "ultrafast metabolizers" and experience an exaggerated opioid effect. Thus, a thorough understanding of opioid pharmacokinetics, pharmacodynamics, and idiosyncrasies of the different opioids is needed for safe practice. Understanding opioid–drug interactions is a crucial component of the practicing anesthesiologist's knowledge base.

No 'Subs'titute for Sobriety 49

Buprenorphine, μ-agonist opioids

James Hilliard MSN, CRNA
and Kirk Lalwani MD, FRCA, MCR

Abstract
This case discusses the pharmacodynamic interaction between buprenorphine and opioid μ-receptor agonists resulting in hypoanalgesic effect.

Case

An otherwise healthy 34-year-old man presented to the Emergency Department (ED) after being struck by a motor vehicle in a crosswalk. The patient sustained abrasions to the face, hands, and arms, along with a fracture of the right tibia and fibula. He reported a pain score of 10 out of 10 despite receiving narcotics from the paramedics in transit. The ED team proceeded to administer repeated doses of intravenous short-acting opioids without improvement in the patient's pain score.

After 30 minutes of intractable pain, the patient revealed that he had been abusing Suboxone® (buprenorphine/naloxone) in order to "clear his urine" of detectable cocaine metabolites prior to an employment drug screen. The patient admitted to buying "Subs" or "Subbies" on the street, which he began taking over a week ago.

A toxicology screen demonstrated a buprenorphine serum level of 0.67 ng/mL indicating abuse of Suboxone® within the last 24 hours. The urine toxicology screen was positive for the cocaine metabolite benzoylecgonine. The patient admitted to cocaine use concurrently with Suboxone®.

J. Hilliard MSN, CRNA (✉) • K. Lalwani MD, FRCA, MCR
Department of Anesthesiology and Perioperative Medicine,
Oregon Health and Science University, Portland, OR, USA
e-mail: hillarja@ohsu.edu

C. Marcucci et al. (eds.), *A Case Approach to Perioperative Drug-Drug Interactions*, DOI 10.1007/978-1-4614-7495-1_49

The adult pain service was consulted. After assessing the patient, the team offered a multimodal approach to manage his pain through the perioperative period. The patient was given oral adjuncts, including pregabalin, celecoxib, and acetaminophen, and agreed to femoral and sciatic nerve blocks. Prior to leaving for the operating room, the patient reported a pain score of 4 out of 10, and experienced reasonably good pain control throughout his recovery.

Discussion

This is an example of a pharmacodynamic interaction involving antagonism (competitive binding) at the μ-receptor.

Buprenorphine is a semi-synthetic opioid analgesic derived from thebaine. Thebaine is one of the main alkaloids in the opium poppy *Papaver somniferum*. Buprenorphine is metabolized by cytochrome (CYP) 3A4. Coadministration with 3A4 inhibitors such as diltiazem and erythromycin may result in increased plasma levels. The opposite is true with 3A4 inducers such as phenobarbital and St. John's wort, as concurrent usage of these medications may decrease plasma levels of buprenorphine.

Buprenorphine is a centrally acting partial μ-agonist and a κ and δ antagonist.[1] This agonist-antagonist activity provides utility in the treatment of opiate addiction by avoiding dysphoria associated with naloxone, and euphoria seen with pure μ_1-receptor agonists.[2] While the high lipophilicity of buprenorphine results in rapid onset and a long duration of action, the tight binding and high receptor affinity could result in partial opioid blockage and a reduction in analgesia from full agonist opioids.[3]

Buprenorphine demonstrates a ceiling effect on μ activity, which reduces the risk for respiratory depression in opioid-naïve patients.[4] This characteristic makes buprenorphine a suitable analgesic in many pain management scenarios, especially within the geriatric population.[5] Despite a ceiling effect at high doses, however, there is an increased risk for respiratory depression in pediatric patients.[6] Also, when used with benzodiazepines or in the presence of alcohol, a synergistic effect may result in excessive respiratory depression and sedation.[1] This effect has resulted in fatal overdose.[7,8]

Buprenorphine is available in combination with naloxone as a sublingual tablet, known as Suboxone®, or as a sole agent, Subutex®. Buprenorphine is a schedule III agent with an FDA indication for analgesia and the treatment of opiate addiction. According to the manufacturer, the estimated worldwide use is 400,000 patients.[9] Obviously, this estimate does not include the illicit use of Suboxone for self-detoxification, which has been reported in the literature.[2]

Since the passage of the Drug Addiction Treatment Act in 2000, physicians have been able to prescribe opioid medication for the treatment of opioid addiction and withdrawal. Buprenorphine/naloxone (Suboxone®) is ideal for this treatment, even when compared with methadone.[10,11] The pharmacokinetics and pharmacodynamics of buprenorphine allow for rapid titration with minimal risk for lethal side effects.

This increased margin of safety allows for less monitoring and observation, unlike the requirements of methadone maintenance programs. Additionally, the abuse potential for Suboxone® is low. Any attempt to abuse the drug via illicit preparation releases the antagonist naloxone and precipitates withdrawal symptoms in opioid–dependent patients.[12]

Current literature presents conflicting perioperative pain management strategies for the patient on buprenorphine. Some recommend conversion from buprenorphine to a full opioid agonist like methadone.[13] Others demonstrate the effectiveness of full opioid agonists in patients stabilized on buprenorphine throughout the perioperative period.[14]

A multimodal approach using nonopioid analgesics has proven valuable in managing postoperative pain in the context of Suboxone® use.[1,2,13,14] This approach can employ nonsteroidal anti-inflammatory drugs (NSAIDs), centrally acting analgesic adjuncts such as ketamine, pregabalin, and α_2-agonists, as well as regional anesthesia techniques.

Take-Home Points

- Buprenorphine use and abuse can complicate perioperative pain management.
- In opioid-sensitive individuals, buprenorphine can have a significant μ-receptor effect, including respiratory depression and decreased level of consciousness. Fatal overdose can occur when buprenorphine is taken with other sedatives/hypnotics, or even alcohol.
- Buprenorphine binds to the μ-receptor with high affinity, but its low activity results in partial agonism and reduced efficacy of opioid analgesics. Patients who use or abuse buprenorphine can be refractory to conventional pain management.
- Consider using a multimodal approach to perioperative pain management. A plan that is not dependent on narcotics may be effective in the context of buprenorphine use.

Summary

Interaction: pharmacodynamic
Substrates: Suboxone® and opioid μ-receptor agonists
Mechanism/site of action: central μ-receptor (competitive binding)
Clinical effect: hypoanalgesic effect of opioids

References

1. Vadivelu N, Anwar M. Buprenorphine in postoperative pain management. Anesthesiol Clin. 2010;28:601–9.
2. Marcucci C, Fudin J, Thomas P, et al. A new pattern of buprenorphine misuse may complicate perioperative pain control. Anesth Analg. 2009;108:1996–7.
3. Center for Substance Abuse Treatment. Clinical Guidelines for the Use of Buprenorphine in the Treatment of Opioid Addiction. A Treatment Improvement Protocol (TIP) Series 40, DHHS Publication No. (SMA). Washington, DC: US Department of Health and Human Services, 2004.
4. Dahan A, Yassen A, Romberg R, et al. Buprenorphine induces ceiling in respiratory depression but not analgesia. Br J Anaesth. 2006;96(5):627–32.
5. Pergolizzi J, Böger RH, Budd K, et al. Opioids and the management of chronic severe pain in the elderly: consensus statement of an International Expert Panel with focus on the six clinically most often used World Health Organization Step III opioids (buprenorphine, fentanyl, hydromorphone, methadone, morphine, oxycodone). Pain Pract. 2008;8(4):287–313.
6. Geib AJ, Babu K, Burns M, et al. Adverse effects in children after unintentional buprenorphine exposure. Pediatrics. 2006;118:1746–51.
7. Auriacombe M, Fatseas M, Dubernet J, et al. French field experience with buprenorphine. Am J Addict. 2004;13 Suppl 1:S17–28.
8. Amass L, Ling W, Freese TE, et al. Bringing buprenorphine-naloxone detoxification to community treatment providers: the NIDA Clinical Trials Network field experience. Am J Addict. 2004;(13 Suppl 1):S42–66.
9. Suboxone: facts for patients. Richmond: Reckitt Benckiser Pharmaceuticals, Inc.; 2008.
10. Buprenorphine replacement therapy: a confirmed benefit. Prescrire Int. 2006;15(82):64–70.
11. Gowing L, Ali R, White JM. Buprenorphine for the management of opioid withdrawal. Cochrane Database Syst Rev. 2009;(3):CD002025.
12. Bryson EO, Lipson S, Gervirtz C. Anesthesia for patients on buprenorphine. Anesthesiol Clin. 2010;28:611–7.
13. Alford DP, Compton P, Samet JH. Acute pain management for patients receiving maintenance methadone or buprenorphine therapy. Ann Intern Med. 2006;144:127–34.
14. Kornfield H, Manfredi L. Effectiveness of full agonist opioids in patients stabilized on buprenorphine undergoing major surgery: a case series. Am J Ther. 2010;17:523–8.

A Needle and the Damage Done

50

Fatal Forty DDI: buprenorphine, ritonavir, CYP3A4

James Hilliard MSN, CRNA
and Kirk Lalwani MD, FRCA, MCR

Abstract
This case discusses a pharmacokinetic drug interaction between buprenorphine, ritonavir, and atazanavir. Buprenorphine is a cytochrome P450 3A4 substrate. Ritonavir and atazanavir are both potent 3A4 inhibitors.

Case

A 38-year-old nurse in the preoperative center sustained a needlestick injury while starting an intravenous line and drawing blood from a patient with advanced HIV infection. After washing the puncture, the nurse was directed to Employee Health for further evaluation and management. During the history and physical, out of fear, the nurse failed to disclose his remote recovery from opiate addiction and current substitution therapy with Suboxone® (buprenorphine/naloxone), 12 mg/d.

A regimen for highly active antiretroviral therapy (HAART) with a fixed-dose combination of atazanavir (ATV) and ritonavir (RTV) was prescribed as first-line postexposure prophylaxis (PEP). The nurse filled the prescription and began the treatment. After 5 days, he began to notice worsening daytime somnolence and impaired cognition. He called his addiction counselor, who recalled a significant drug interaction between Suboxone® and protease inhibitors.

The nurse was directed to an emergency room where he was monitored for a few hours and released. His daily Suboxone® dose was reduced to 8 mg/d while on the prophylaxis regimen, which led to resolution of symptoms.

J. Hilliard MSN, CRNA (✉) • K. Lalwani MD, FRCA, MCR
Department of Anesthesiology and Perioperative Medicine,
Oregon Health and Science University, Portland, OR, USA
e-mail: hillarja@ohsu.edu

C. Marcucci et al. (eds.), *A Case Approach to Perioperative Drug-Drug Interactions*, DOI 10.1007/978-1-4614-7495-1_50

Discussion

This is an example of inhibitors added to a substrate.

Buprenorphine, an opioid partial agonist used in the treatment of opioid dependence, is principally metabolized by cytochrome P450 3A4 (CYP3A4).[1] Atazanavir and ritonavir are both potent inhibitors of 3A4. When these drugs are used concomitantly, the inhibition of buprenorphine's metabolic clearance via a clinically significant pharmacokinetic interaction has been described.[2,3]

Interestingly, the pharmacokinetic effects of RTV in combination with other protease inhibitors are not predictable. For example, lopinavir-ritonavir can result in decreased methadone plasma levels and withdrawal symptoms.[4]

The high frequency of HIV infection among intravenous drug abusers requires careful management of both antiretroviral therapy and the treatment of opiate addiction. The known drug interactions between these two regimens can result in clinically significant supratherapeutic or subtherapeutic serum concentrations of opioid agonists and partial agonists.[5]

Take-Home Points

- Protease inhibitors may have an inhibitory effect on the metabolism of buprenorphine and its active metabolite, norbuprenorphine.
- Some protease inhibitor combinations (eg, lopinavir-ritonavir) may reduce plasma levels of methadone, resulting in an opiate withdrawal syndrome.
- Careful dosage adjustments and monitoring are necessary in order to avoid adverse drug interactions, and to maintain compliance with both treatment regimens.

Summary

Interaction: pharmacokinetic
Substrate: buprenorphine
Enzyme: CYP3A4
Inhibitors: ritonavir and atazanavir
Clinical effect: increased opioid effects including somnolence

References

1. Strain EC, Stitzer ML, Liebson IA, et al. Buprenorphine versus methadone in the treatment of opioid dependence: self-reports, urinalysis and addiction severity index. J Clin Psychopharmacol. 1996;16:58–67.
2. McCance-Katz EF, Moody DE, Morse GD, et al. Interaction between buprenorphine and atazanavir or atazanavir-ritonavir. Drug Alcohol Depend. 2007;91:269–78.
3. Bruce RD, Altice FL. Three case reports of a clinical pharmacokinetic interaction with buprenorphine and atazanavir plus ritonavir. AIDS. 2006;20:783–4.
4. McCance-Katz EF, Rainey PM, Friedland G, et al. The protease inhibitor lopinavir-ritonavir may produce opiate withdrawal in methadone-maintained patients. Clin Infect Dis. 2003; 37:476–82.
5. McCance-Katz EF. Treatment of opioid dependence and coinfection with HIV and hepatitis C virus in opioid-dependent patients: the importance of drug interactions between opioids and antiretroviral agents. Clin Infect Dis. 2005;41 Suppl 1:S89–95.

Dad's Not Having Much Pain

51

Fatal Forty DDI: methadone, ciprofloxacin, CYP3A4

Rani Chovatiya MD, Mehmet S. Ozcan MD, FCCP,
and Randal O. Dull MD, PhD

Abstract
This case discusses a pharmacokinetic interaction between methadone and ciprofloxacin resulting in increased sedative and analgesic effects of methadone. Methadone is a cytochrome P450 3A4 substrate and ciprofloxacin is a 3A4 inhibitor.

Case

A 59-year-old housepainter fell off a ladder at a job site and suffered a mild concussion. At the time of the accident, he felt numb from the waist up but recovered an hour later. The patient had a longstanding history of pain due cervical stenosis, which he managed with opioid therapy and the recent addition of amitriptyline to circumvent documented opioid tolerance. His internist felt that a follow-up X-Ray of his cervical spine would be prudent. The film showed advancing degenerative changes (cervical stenosis and multilevel foraminal stenosis) from C3 to C7.

The patient subsequently underwent C5-6 and C6-7 anterior cervical diskectomy and fusion with C3-T2 posterior decompression and fixation/fusion. He was admitted to

R. Chovatiya MD (✉)
Department of Anesthesiology, University of Illinois Medical Center, Chicago, IL, USA
e-mail: Rchova1@uic.edu

M.S. Ozcan MD, FCCP
Department of Anesthesiology, The University of Oklahoma Health Sciences Center, Oklahoma City, OK, USA

R.O. Dull MD, PhD
Department of Anesthesiology, University of Illinois at Chicago, Chicago, IL, USA

C. Marcucci et al. (eds.), *A Case Approach to Perioperative Drug-Drug Interactions*, DOI 10.1007/978-1-4614-7495-1_51

the neurosurgical intensive care unit postoperatively and extubated on postoperative day 1. He complained of excruciating pain. He was started on hydromorphone via patient controlled analgesia, but his pain remained poorly controlled.

On postoperative day 2, the pain service was consulted for recommendations and noted the patient's history of opioid tolerance. He was initiated on oral methadone therapy three times daily along with intravenous (IV) hydromorphone as needed for breakthrough pain. On postoperative day 3, the patient noted that his pain had improved to a tolerable level and was satisfied with his pain management. On postoperative day 4, he was started on PO ciprofloxacin for a urinary tract infection. That evening the patient's daughter spoke to out-of-town family and reported that the patient was comfortable. However, on postoperative day 5, the nurse noted that the patient appeared to be more drowsy and confused. His breathing had also become shallower, and he required supplemental O_2 therapy. He had not requested any IV hydromorphone in the last 24 hours. The methadone therapy was stopped immediately, and IV naloxone was administered. The patient's mental status and respiratory function promptly returned to baseline.

Discussion

This is an example of an inhibitor added to a substrate.

Methadone is metabolized through *N*-demethylation, which is catalyzed by several isoenzymes of the cytochrome P450 (CYP) family including cytochromes 2B6, 2C8, 2C18, 2D6, and 3A4. Among those, 3A4 is suggested as the major enzyme involved in the *N*-demethylation.[1] Ciprofloxacin, a fluoroquinolone antibiotic, is a potent inhibitor of the CYP3A4 isoenzyme in humans.[2] Other fluoroquinolones that inhibit 3A4 are norfloxacin and sparfloxacin. Therefore, in this example, it is highly likely that the administration of ciprofloxacin led to a decrease in the rate of metabolism of methadone, leading to signs and symptoms of opioid overdose. There is also a risk for a pharmacodynamic drug–drug interaction (DDI) in the form of additive QT prolongation and resulting arrhythmias, although that did not occur in this case. In fact, there are several case reports of this drug–drug interaction (DDI) in the literature.[3–5] In these case reports, opioid overdose typically occurred 24 to 48 hours after starting ciprofloxacin in patients receiving methadone. For a patient on a maintenance dose of methadone, it is prudent to choose a different antibiotic than a fluoroquinolone when feasible. When a combination of methadone and fluoroquinolones that inhibit CYP3A4 must be used, signs of opioid overdose should be expected to occur and dosages revised accordingly

Take-Home Points

- Methadone is a substrate of several isoenzymes of the cytochrome P450 family, mainly cytochrome 3A4.
- Ciprofloxacin (ie, a fluoroquinolone antibiotic) is an inhibitor of 3A4. Norfloxacin and sparfloxacin also inhibit 3A4.
- Fluoroquinolones that do not inhibit 3A4 include gatifloxacin, levofloxacin, moxifloxacin, and ofloxacin.
- If feasible, choose a non-fluoroquinolone antibiotic for patients receiving methadone. If it is indicated to use both drugs, closely monitor the patient's level of sedation and consider decreasing the dose of methadone as long as the fluoroquinolone is used.

Summary

Interaction: pharmacokinetic
Substrate: methadone
Inhibitor: ciprofloxacin
Enzyme: CYP3A4
Clinical effects: increased sedative and analgesic effects of methadone

References

1. Iribarne C, Berthou F, Baird S, et al. Involvement of cytochrome P450 3A4 enzyme in the N-demethylation of methadone in human liver microsomes. Chem Res Toxicol. 1996;9(2): 365–73.
2. McLellan RA, Drobitch RK, Monshouwer M, et al. Fluoroquinolone antibiotics inhibit cytochrome P450-mediated microsomal drug metabolism in rat and human. Drug Metab Dispos. 1996;24(10):1134–8.
3. Herrlin K, Segerdahl M, Gustafsson LL, et al. Methadone, ciprofloxacin, and adverse drug reactions. Lancet. 2000;356(9247):2069–70.
4. Nair MK, Patel K, Starer PJ. Ciprofloxacin-induced torsades de pointes in a methadone-dependent patient. Addiction. 2008;103(12):2062–4.
5. Samoy L, Shalansky KF. Interaction between Methadone and Ciprofloxacin. Can J Hosp Pharm. 2010;63(5):382–4.

Royal Flush

52

Fatal Forty DDI: methadone, nortriptyline, CYP2D6, CYP3A4

Kimberly Mauer MD, Catherine Marcucci MD, and Neil B. Sandson MD

Abstract
This case discusses a pharmacokinetic interaction between nortriptyline and methadone, resulting in tricyclic antidepressant toxicity. Nortriptyline is a cytochrome P450 (CYP) 2D6 and 3A4 substrate. Methadone is an inhibitor of those enzymes.

Case

A 45-year-old female black jack dealer on the overnight shift at a Las Vegas casino had hit a run of bad luck. Her years of leaning over the card tables had wrecked her marriage and wrecked her neck. However, knowing how fickle fortune is and having her eye on the resident Elvis impersonator, she finally decided to move on with her life and agreed to start nortriptyline to treat her depression over her divorce. She also finally saw a chronic pain specialist and requested pharmacological management for her cervical facet arthropathy and chronic muscle tension in her neck but requested, "the drug addict drug that lets people work." She was started on methadone 30 mg three times per day.

K. Mauer MD (✉)
Department of Anesthesiology & Perioperative Medicine, Oregon Health and Science University, Portland, OR, USA
e-mail: mauer@ohsu.edu

C. Marcucci MD
Anesthesia Services Department, Philadelphia Veterans Affairs Medical Center, Philadelphia, PA, USA

N.B. Sandson MD
Department of Psychiatry, University of Maryland Medical System, Baltimore, MD, USA

Department of Psychiatry, VA Maryland Health Care System, Baltimore, MD, USA

C. Marcucci et al. (eds.), *A Case Approach to Perioperative Drug-Drug Interactions*, DOI 10.1007/978-1-4614-7495-1_52

Approximately 1 week later, she was out on a date with her new boyfriend when she noticed that her face was red and hot and her mouth was dry. Very worried that she now had to deal with "overactive thyroid," she visited the physician on call at the casino and mentioned that she was also sweating very little during the very crowded and hot evening hours on the Strip.

She reported the nortriptyline and methadone and the physician noticed she was lethargic with a rapid heart rate. An electrocardiogram was ordered which showed sinus tachycardia. He also noticed that she appeared quite red in the face.

Discussion

This is an example of an inhibitor added to a substrate.

Nortriptyline and the other secondary-amine tricyclics are metabolized primarily by cytochrome P450 (CYP) 2D6 but also by CYP3A4.[1] Methadone is a moderately strong 2D6 inhibitor, and also 3A4 substrate.[2] Thus, the introduction of methadone to the patient's medication panel significantly impaired the ability to metabolize the nortriptyline. The introduction of methadone has been shown to increase the level of tricyclic antidepressants (TCAs).[3] This lead to TCA toxicity, including tachycardia, dry mouth, and general anhydrosis.

The blood levels of tertiary amines such as amitriptyline may be elevated by either 2D6 or 3A4 inhibitors. Nortriptyline levels will be increased by 2D6 inhibitors, but not 3A4 inhibitors. This is because the hydroxylation performed by 2D6 is quite important to the metabolism of both secondary and tertiary amine TCAs, whereas the demethylation performed by 3A4 is much less crucial to the metabolism of secondary-amine TCAs.

Take-Home Points

- Nortriptyline is a secondary amine metabolized by 2D6 primarily.
- Methadone is 2D6 inhibitor.
- Coadministration can cause tricyclic antidepressant toxicity.
- Pain physicians should be aware that patients see a variety of practitioners, all of whom prescribe metabolically relevant drugs.

Summary

Interaction: pharmacokinetic
Substrate: nortriptyline
Enzyme: 2D6 and 3A4
Inhibitor: methadone
Clinical effects: antidepressant toxicity

References

1. Dahl ML, Iselius L, Alm C, et al. Polymorphic 2-hydroxylation of desipramine: a population- and family study. Eur J Clin Pharmacol. 1993;44(5):445–50.
2. Maany I, Dhopesh V, Arndt IO, et al. Increase in desipramine serum levels associated with methadone treatment. Am J Psychiatry. 1989;146(2):1611–3.
3. Wu D, Otton SV, Sproule BA, et al. Inhibition of human cytochrome P450 2D6 (CYP2D6) by methadone. Br J Clin Pharmacol. 1993;35(1):30–4.

The Worry That's Always With Us: Afternoon Nap

53

Oxycodone, diazepam

Syed M. Quadri DO and Randal O. Dull MD, PhD

Abstract
This case discusses the pharmacodynamic interaction between oxycodone and diazepam resulting in apnea and decreased level of consciousness in a patient with chronic back pain.

Case

An obese 72-year-old man with a history of hypertension and hyperlipidemia was seen by his regular pain doctor complaining of an exacerbation of chronic low back pain and muscle spasms two days after moving furniture for his daughter. The physician noted the patient's L3-L5 spinal fusion surgery 4 months earlier with a current stable regimen of an extended release oxycodone (40 mg BID) and oxycodone (5 mg q6h prn) for breakthrough pain, which offered him appropriate relief. She felt that the patient's pain exacerbation was mainly related to muscular spasm so instructed him to continue his current regimen, apply heat, rest and given a prescription of diazepam (10 mg q6h prn) for spasm for a duration of 10 days.

The patient's wife called later that afternoon, concerned that she could not arouse her husband long enough to get him to the dinner table. She mentioned that "he wakes up briefly but he's not always breathing." She was told to call the emergency

S.M. Quadri DO (✉)
Department of Anesthesiology, University of Illinois at Chicago
College of Medicine, Chicago, IL, USA
e-mail: Shafquadri@gmail.com

R.O. Dull MD, PhD
Department of Anesthesiology, University of Illinois at Chicago, Chicago, IL, USA

C. Marcucci et al. (eds.), *A Case Approach to Perioperative Drug-Drug Interactions*, DOI 10.1007/978-1-4614-7495-1_53

response team immediately. In the Emergency Department, the patient was found to be unconscious and spontaneously breathing with periods of apnea. He was administered oxygen and intravenous flumazenil. The patient regained consciousness and complained of low back pain. The pain service was consulted. The diazepam was discontinued and he was given a trigger point injection with local anesthetic and methylprednisolone. He was monitored in the Emergency Department and was later discharged home.

Discussion

This is an example of a synergistic pharmacodynamic interaction at the end-organ level.

More specifically, this is an example of central nervous system (CNS) depression resulting from the concomitant use of an opioid and a benzodiazepine.

Opioids are prescribed most commonly for the management of pain. One of the side effects of opioid therapy is respiratory depression. The opioid ligand binding to μ-receptors causes a dose-dependent suppression of respiratory centers in the brainstem and decreased sensitivity to CO_2 levels in the blood thereby increasing apneic thresholds. However, opioids alone rarely cause unconsciousness. The use of a benzodiazepine with an opioid is synergistic in producing unconsciousness and plays a significant role in respiratory depression.[1,2]

The benzodiazepine in this case was prescribed to alleviate muscle spasm. However, one of the side effects of benzodiazepines is sedation. When used alone in healthy adults, benzodiazepines rarely cause unconsciousness or respiratory depression. They work by increasing the affinity for γ-amino-butyric acid (GABA), the principal inhibitory neurotransmitter in the CNS, to its receptor.[3] The respiratory centers in the brain are thought to have a rhythmic balance of excitatory and inhibitory neurotransmitters that modulate breathing. Benzodiazepines may participate in partially disrupting this modulation. However, benzodiazepines do not directly stimulate GABA receptors as does propofol.

Propofol is a potent hypnotic agent used to render patients unconscious or sedated for anesthesia or the intensive care unit. Opioid administration reliably decreases propofol doses needed for anesthesia induction and maintenance.

The concomitant use of long-acting opioids such as extended release morphine, oxycontin, methadone, fentanyl patch, and (to a lesser degree) buprenorphine with benzodiazepines or propofol have a distinct propensity to cause respiratory depression. Indeed, there have been cases reported in which methadone and benzodiazepines were found post mortem in overdose fatalities.[4]

Take-Home Points

- Pure agonist opioids cause respiratory depression in a dose-dependent manner.
- Benzodiazepines cause sedation and tend to have a ceiling effect as they are not direct-acting ligands.
- The concomitant use of benzodiazepines and opioids commonly can lead to increased sedation, and in some case significant respiratory depression.

Summary

Interaction: pharmacodynamic (synergism)
Substrates: oxycontin and diazepam
Mechanisms/sites of action: opioid (oxycodone) binding of μ-receptor in CNS respiratory centers decreases response to CO_2 curve, benzodiazepine (diazepam) increases GABA affinity to GABA receptor in the CNS
Clinical effects: apnea and decreased level of consciousness

References

1. Miller RD, et al., editors. Anesthesia. 7th ed. New York: Churchill Livingstone; 2009. Chapter 27.
2. White JM. Mechanisms of fatal opioid overdose. Addiction. 1999;94(7):961–72.
3. Stoelting RK, Hillier SC. Handbook of pharmacology and physiology in anesthetic practice. Philadelphia: Lippincott Williams & Wilkins; 2006.
4. Shields LB, Hunsaker JC, Corey TS, et al. Methadone toxicity fatalities: a review of medical examiner cases in a large metropolitan area. J Forensic Sci. 2007;52(6):1389–95.

The Bawling Baby

54

Fatal Forty DDI: rifampin, methadone, CYP3A4, CYP2B6

Angela Kendrick MD

Abstract
This case discusses the pharmacokinetic interaction between methadone and rifampin resulting in methadone withdrawal symptoms. Methadone is a cytochrome P450 3A4 and 2B6 substrate and rifampin is a 3A4 and 2B6 inducer. Rifampin induces metabolism of methadone via 3A4 and 2B6 and can cause methadone withdrawal symptoms.

Case

A 5-month-old, 6 kg infant girl underwent a Glenn procedure for a second-stage repair of her hypoplastic left heart syndrome, after a previous Norwood procedure. Following her second cardiac procedure, she had a protracted postoperative course in the pediatric intensive care unit and was placed on vancomycin due to mediastinitis. She received intravenous (IV) midazolam and fentanyl for an extended course of postoperative mechanical ventilation.

The anesthesia pain service recommended a two-stage weaning plan for the opioids and benzodiazepine infusions. During her fourth postoperative week, a conversion of her constant infusions to scheduled IV methadone and lorazepam was accomplished. At the end of her fourth postoperative week, she returned to the operating room for a second debridement of her sternum

The infectious disease team recommended the addition of an additional antibiotic because of the persistent infection.

A. Kendrick MD
Department of Anesthesiology and Perioperative Medicine (APOM),
Doernbecher Children's Hospital, Oregon Health and Science University,
Portland, OR, USA
e-mail: Kendrick@ohsu.edu

C. Marcucci et al. (eds.), *A Case Approach to Perioperative Drug-Drug Interactions*, DOI 10.1007/978-1-4614-7495-1_54

A methadone wean was started after the second postoperative period. Three days after the infant began the new antibiotic, the pain resident was called because the baby had become agitated and was crying inconsolably. He reviewed the infant's recent medications, including vancomycin and the recently added rifampin, and immediately ordered a rescue dose of methadone.

Discussion

This is an example of an inducer added to a substrate.

Methadone is generally thought to be a cytochrome P450 (CYP) substrate that is metabolized by both CYP3A4 (mainly) with a small contribution from 2B6, 2C8, 2C9, 2C19, and 2D6, (although there is at least one published report of a greater role for CYP2B6.[1,2] This complex metabolism of methadone by six different cytochrome P450 enzymes offers significant opportunities for drug interactions.[3] CYP3A4 is found both in the liver and in the intestine and its activity varies greatly among individuals.[4] Rifampin is a potent inducer of virtually all of the P450 enzymes, including 3A4 and 2B6. There are several articles in the literature documenting withdrawal symptoms in patients on methadone maintenance after rifampin was given. Onset of the withdrawal symptoms ranged from one to 33 days after the rifampin was started.[5,6] Decreased serum levels of methadone were also documented in patients receiving rifampin.

Methadone does not produce active metabolites, its active form is the parent compound. Despite the pain team's monitoring of this infant, a withdrawal syndrome did develop, likely as a result of a reduction in serum methadone levels from the increased enzymatic activity or increased production of 3A4.

Take-Home Points

- Methadone undergoes metabolism by more than one CYP enzyme subfamily, but 3A4 is responsible for the main biotransformation (*N*-demethylation) of the parent compound.
- Rifampin is a potent inducer of the cytochrome P450 system.
- Carefully monitoring for changes in sedation level, including the appearance of withdrawal symptoms, is always indicated when adding an enzyme inducer in the presence of methadone.

Summary

Interaction: pharmacokinetic
Substrates: methadone
Enzyme: 3A4 and 2B6
Inducer: rifampin
Clinical effect: opioid withdrawal

References

1. Kapur BM, Hutson JR, Chibber T, et al. Methadone: a review of drug-drug and pathophysiological interactions. Crit Rev Clin Lab Sci. 2011;48(4):171–95.
2. Kharasch ED, Hoffer C, Whittington D, et al. Role of hepatic and intestinal cytochrome P450 3A and 2B6 in the metabolism, disposition, and miotic effects of methadone. Clin Pharmacol Ther. 2004;76(3):250–69.
3. Smith HS. Opioid metabolism. Mayo Clin Proc. 2009;84:613–24.
4. Ferrari A, Coccia CPR, Bertolini A, et al. Methadone–metabolism, pharmacokinetics and interactions. Pharmacol Res. 2004;50:551–9.
5. Bending MR, Skacel PO. Rifampicin and methadone withdrawal (letter). Lancet. 1977;1(8023):1211.
6. Kreek MJ, Garfield JW, Gutjahr CL. Rifampin –induced methadone withdrawal. N Engl J Med. 1976;294:1104–6.

Sleeping Beauty

55

Fatal Forty DDI: fentanyl, ritonavir, CYP3A4

Hans P. Sviggum MD and Juraj Sprung MD, PhD

Abstract
This case discusses the pharmacokinetic interaction between fentanyl and ritonavir, leading to prolonged narcotic action. Fentanyl is a cytochrome P450 3A4 substrate and ritonavir is a 3A4 inhibitor.

Case

A 28-year-old, 49 kg woman who was employed as a runway model was admitted to the surgical intensive care unit after undergoing a 4-hour exploratory laparotomy and repair of multiple liver lacerations after a motor vehicle collision. She had been diagnosed with human immunodeficiency virus (HIV) one week earlier and started on highly active antiretroviral therapy with atazanavir, ritonavir, and tenofovir disoproxil/emtricitabine.

Anesthesia was induced with fentanyl, etomidate, and succinylcholine, and then maintained with desflurane and a continuous infusion of fentanyl (3 mcg/kg/h). Before leaving the operating room, the neuromuscular blockade was fully reversed, the fentanyl infusion was reduced to 2 mcg/kg/h, and a propofol infusion (50 mcg/kg/min) was started.

The patient was hemodynamically stable in the intensive care unit (ICU). Expedient tracheal extubation was planned and the propofol and fentanyl infusions were discontinued. Two hours later, she was making no spontaneous respiratory effort, although she opened her eyes in response to tactile stimulation. The patient received

H.P. Sviggum MD (✉)
Department of Anesthesiology, Mayo Clinic College of Medicine, Rochester, MN, USA
e-mail: sviggum.hans@mayo.edu

J. Sprung MD, PhD
Department of Anesthesiology, Mayo Clinic, Rochester, MN, USA

C. Marcucci et al. (eds.), *A Case Approach to Perioperative Drug-Drug Interactions*, DOI 10.1007/978-1-4614-7495-1_55

naloxone (80 mcg) and became more awake, but only briefly. Her arousal level continued to wax and wane. The ICU fellow shook his head and said, "It's like the fairy tale—she's beautiful, but she won't wake up." A naloxone drip was initiated and she slowly became alert, awake, and aware over the next 16 hours. She was finally extubated the next day.

Discussion

This is an example of a substrate added to an inhibitor.

Fentanyl, a widely used synthetic opioid, is metabolized mainly by the hepatic cytochrome P450 (CYP) 3A4 isozyme to its major oxidative metabolite, norfentanyl.[1] Less than 8% of the drug is excreted unchanged.[2] Ritonavir, a protease inhibitor commonly used in the treatment of HIV infection, is one of the most potent inhibitors of 3A4.[3] It also causes some inhibition of CYP2D6.

A 1999 study by Olkkola et al. showed that 3 days of ritonavir treatment decreased the clearance of fentanyl by 67%.[3] Additionally, the ritonavir treatment more than doubled the elimination half-life of fentanyl after a single bolus dose. However, plasma concentrations of fentanyl at 15 and 30 minutes after injection did not differ significantly between ritonavir and placebo treatments. Likely, initial fentanyl concentrations after a bolus dose are not affected because ritonavir has no marked effect on the volume of fentanyl distribution. Accordingly, Kharasch et al. found that CYP3A alterations did not change peak plasma fentanyl concentrations or the time to peak fentanyl concentration, but substantially affected its elimination.[4]

On the basis of these findings, the interaction between fentanyl and ritonavir appears to have little clinical effect on the onset or peak level of analgesia. However, a high dosing frequency or continuous infusion of fentanyl can drastically increase plasma levels of fentanyl in patients with abnormal 3A4 activity because of impaired elimination. In this instance, dangerous augmentation of fentanyl-induced respiratory depression may occur. It is probable that ritonavir affects the elimination of transdermally administered fentanyl at the same magnitude as that of intravenous fentanyl.[1]

Fentanyl has a high extraction ratio of approximately 0.8, meaning that its elimination by the liver should be more dependent on liver blood flow than on changes in intrinsic clearance.[5] This ratio may be why 3A4 inhibitors less potent than ritonavir do not cause as marked a decrease in the clearance of fentanyl.

Studies by Feierman and Lasker showed that selective inhibitors of other cytochrome P450 enzymes—1A2, 2D6, 2C9, and 2E1—did not inhibit fentanyl metabolism.[6] Liver cytochrome P450 enzymes also participate in the metabolism of other opioids, such as sufentanil and alfentanil. They do not have as large a role in the metabolism of other common opioids, such as morphine and hydromorphone, which are more dependent on glucuronidation in the liver. As with most hepatic enzymes, interindividual variability in the activity of 3A4 can be substantial. However, the impact of variable hepatic 3A4 expression on interpatient variability is difficult to predict in the systemic clearance of fentanyl at this time.[1]

Interestingly, there is some evidence that ritonavir may have varying pharmacokinetic effects when used concomitantly with opioids other than fentanyl. Although ritonavir is a potent inhibitor of the CYP3A family of isozymes, a component of 3A induction may emerge, depending on length of treatment. Specifically, ritonavir has been found to decrease plasma methadone concentrations, which has been attributed to 3A induction.[7] Steady-state compared with acute ritonavir therapy caused mild apparent induction of hepatic CYP3A, but net inhibition still predominated.[7] Additionally, meperidine hydrochloride levels were found to be decreased after 10-day treatment with ritonavir, suggesting induction of hepatic metabolism.[8] At this time, it appears unclear about exactly how the length of ritonavir treatment influences pharmacokinetic effects on various opioid medications. However, if the patient in the above scenario had been taking ritonavir for over 1 month, it is unclear that the above interaction would have proven clinically significant.

Take-Home Points

- Hepatic cytochrome P450 enzymes are crucial to the metabolism of many drugs. The synthetic opioid fentanyl is metabolized largely by the hepatic CYP3A4 isozyme.
- Ritonavir is a protease inhibitor commonly used as part of highly active antiretroviral therapy for HIV infection and is a potent inhibitor of 3A4.
- Ritonavir can substantially decrease the elimination of fentanyl and may dangerously augment and prolong fentanyl-induced effects, including respiratory depression.
- Doses of fentanyl should be reduced when repeated or continuous dosing (including transdermal dosing) of fentanyl is used for patients who are also taking ritonavir, especially at the beginning of ritonavir treatment.
- Ritonavir does not increase the peak concentration of fentanyl after a single bolus dose.
- Ritonavir treatment is unlikely to cause prolonged action of fentanyl when fentanyl is administered in small, intermittent bolus doses.
- After several weeks, ritonavir's inductive profile may mitigate or even overtake its inhibitory affects on 3A4.

Summary

Interaction: pharmacokinetic
Substrate: fentanyl
Enzyme: 3A4
Inhibitor: ritonavir
Clinical effect: prolonged narcotic action

References

1. Labroo RB, Paine MF, Thummel KE, et al. Fentanyl metabolism by human hepatic and intestinal cytochrome P450 3A4: implications for interindividual variability in disposition, efficacy, and drug interactions. Drug Metab Dispos. 1997;25(9):1072–80.
2. McClain DA, Hug Jr CC. Intravenous fentanyl kinetics. Clin Pharmacol Ther. 1980;28(1):106–14.
3. Olkkola KT, Palkama VJ, Neuvonen PJ. Ritonavir's role in reducing fentanyl clearance and prolonging its half-life. Anesthesiology. 1999;91(3):681–5.
4. Kharasch ED, Whittington D, Hoffer C. Minimal influence of hepatic & intestinal CYP3A activity on the acute disposition & effect of oral transmucosal fentanyl (OTFC) [abstract]. Anesthesiology. 2003;99:A515.
5. Rowland M, Tozer TN. Elimination. In: Clinical pharmacokinetics: concepts and applications. 3rd ed. Baltimore: Williams & Wilkins; 1995. p. 156–83.
6. Feierman DE, Lasker JM. Metabolism of fentanyl, a synthetic opioid analgesic, by human liver microsomes: role of CYP3A4. Drug Metab Dispos. 1996;24(9):932–9.
7. Kharasch ED, Bedynek PS, Walker A, et al. Mechanism of ritonavir changes in methadone pharmacokinetics and pharmacodynamics: II. Ritonavir effects of CYP3A and P-glycoprotein activities. Clin Pharmacol Ther. 2008;84(4):506–12.
8. Piscitelli SC, Kress DR, Bertz RJ, et al. The effect of ritonavir on the pharmacokinetics of meperidine and normeperidine. Pharmacotherapy. 2000;20(5):549–53.

Codeine Can't Do It

56

Fatal Forty DDI: codeine, fluoxetine, CYP2D6

Katarina Bojanić MD, Wayne T. Nicholson MD, PharmD, MSc, Erica D. Wittwer MD, PhD, Toby N. Weingarten MD, and Juraj Sprung MD, PhD

Abstract

This case discusses a pharmacokinetic interaction between the prodrug codeine and fluoxetine. Codeine is converted to its active metabolite morphine by cytochrome P450 2D6. Fluoxetine is a 2D6 inhibitor.

Case

A 45-year-old man reported to a surgery center for elective repair of a right inguinal hernia with mesh. The anesthesiologist noted that he had a remote history of dental pain controlled with codeine and a recent history of depression controlled with fluoxetine (40 mg). He underwent an uncomplicated total intravenous general anesthesia with propofol and remifentanil. He also received intravenous hydromorphone (1.0 mg), intravenous ketorolac (15 mg), and had the portal sites infiltrated with 10 mL of 0.50% bupivacaine. On discharge from the surgical center, the patient had only minor discomfort at the surgical site. He received a prescription of 30 acetaminophen/codeine tablets (300 mg/30 mg) and was instructed to take one or two tablets every 4 to 6 hours as needed for pain.

K. Bojanić MD (✉)
Division of Neonatology, Clinical Hospital Merkur, Zagreb, Croatia
e-mail: sprungkatarina@hotmail.com

W.T. Nicholson MD, PharmD, MSc • E.D. Wittwer MD, PhD • J. Sprung MD, PhD
Department of Anesthesiology, Mayo Clinic, Rochester, MN, USA

T.N. Weingarten MD
Department of Anesthesiology, Mayo Clinic, Rochester, MN, USA

Department of Anesthesiology, Mayo Clinic College of Medicine, Rochester, MN, USA

C. Marcucci et al. (eds.), *A Case Approach to Perioperative Drug-Drug Interactions*, DOI 10.1007/978-1-4614-7495-1_56

Eighteen hours later, the patient was in the emergency department, complaining of severe right inguinal pain. He reported the onset of pain 4 hours after discharge with steadily worsening pain, despite taking the codeine as prescribed. Despite taking the codeine tablets, his pain continued to worsen. His physical exam was unremarkable.

The patient received morphine (4 mg) intramuscularly. Within 15 minutes he reported considerable improvement in his pain and was able to go home. His prescription was switched to oxycodone/acetaminophen tablets (5 mg/500 mg). On his follow-up visit to the surgeon the next week, he was comfortable and had used only 18 oxycodone/acetaminophen tablets.

Discussion

This is an example of a prodrug substrate added to an inhibitor.

More specifically, this is a pharmacokinetic interaction due to inhibition of the hepatic *O*-demethylation of codeine to morphine because of suppression of the cytochrome P450 (CYP) 2D6 system (fluoxetine use).

Codeine has weak affinity for the μ-receptor and is considered a prodrug that must be metabolized into morphine to have analgesic properties. Approximately 90% of codeine undergoes either glucuronidation to form codeine-6-glucuronide or *N*-demethylation to form norcodeine (Fig. 56.1). The by-products are then eliminated. Only 10% of codeine undergoes *O*-demethylation and is converted to morphine. The latter pathway is mediated by the cytochrome P450 enzyme 2D6 and is thought to be responsible for the analgesic effects of codeine.[1]

Numerous medications have been shown to inhibit 2D6.[2,3] Pharmacologic inhibition by a strong inhibitor of this enzyme has been shown to completely block the conver-

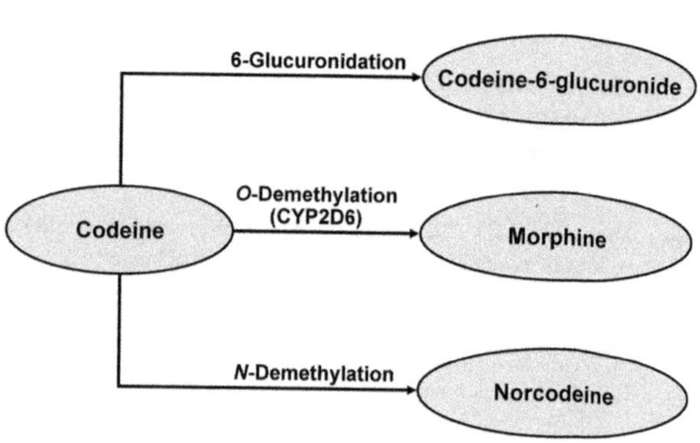

Fig. 56.1 Metabolism of codeine

Table 56.1 *In vitro* dextromethorphan inhibitor constants (K_i) for frequently used drugs with variable CYP2D6 inhibition potential

Inhibitor	*Ki* Value for Substrate Dextromethorphan (*μM*)
Fluoxetine	0.056
Paroxetine	0.23
Propafenone	0.031
Quinidine	0.010
Sertraline	0.47
Amiodarone	11.8
Metoprolol	11.3
Verapamil	38.7

Ki values obtained using pooled human liver microsomes. Dextromethorphan was used as a substrate for CYP2D6 and inhibitors were added to determine the inhibition constants (*Ki*). The inhibition constant describes the potency of an inhibitor and is the concentration required to produce half maximum inhibition. Thus, a lower *Ki* value implies increased inhibitor potency. The *Ki* for fluoxetine is 0.056 μM indicating that a very low concentration is required to inhibit the CYP2D6 enzyme from its metabolism of dextromethorphan. The last three medications in the list of inhibitors have high *Ki* values indicating that they would be less likely than the first five to cause enzyme inhibition and reduce metabolism of CYP2D6 substrates

[Adapted from VandenBrink BM, Foti RS, Rock DA, Wienkers LC, Wahlstrom JL. Prediction of CYP2D6 drug interactions from in vitro data: evidence for substrate-dependent inhibition. *Drug Metab Dispos*. 2012;40(1):47–53. With permission from American Society for Pharmacology and Experimental Therapeutics]

sion of codeine to morphine. For example, plasma morphine levels were undetectable in healthy study participants who received a single dose of quinidine followed by a dose of codeine.[2] Because codeine has almost no affinity for the μ-receptor, this lack of affinity resulted in a loss of its analgesic properties. Fluoxetine is a strong inhibitor of 2D6 and limitation of codeine to morphine conversion by this enzyme is likely if *in vitro* data of dextromethorphan metabolism is considered.[3] Although codeine has not been studied, dextromethorphan undergoes metabolism via *O*-demethylation by 2D6, in a same fashion as codeine, and this process is inhibited by fluoxetine (see Table 56.1).[3] Other 2D6 inhibitors may have varying degrees of inhibition of this enzyme (see Table 56.1),[3] and depending on substrate clinical effects may vary.

Several populations have variability of 2D6 activity due to genetic polymorphisms, which can also affect the *O*-demethylation of codeine and its conversion to morphine. Most individuals are 2D6 extensive metabolizers and convert codeine into morphine normally. However, approximately 7% to 10% of the Caucasian population metabolize drugs poorly through 2D6 and are unable to convert codeine into morphine. In these individuals, codeine has no analgesic properties.[4] Some individuals have ultra-rapid 2D6 metabolism and convert more codeine into morphine and thus are at risk of codeine intoxication.[5] Therefore, the clinical significance of inhibition would depend on the inherent activity of the 2D6 enzyme.

This patient began having postoperative pain as the analgesic effects of the hydromorphone, ketorolac, and local anesthetic began to wane. Previously, he had a normal analgesic response to codeine, indicating he likely has intermediate or extensive 2D6 metabolism. With his long-term use of fluoxetine, 2D6 was inhibited and conversion from codeine into morphine was limited. Thus, the codeine was ineffective as an analgesic, his pain became uncontrollable, and he sought medical help.

When considering other opiates, the P450 enzymes are not involved in the metabolism of morphine, oxymorphone, hydromorphone.[6] For example, oxymorphone is the 2D6 metabolite of oxycodone, which is a potent analgesic itself, so a decreased 2D6 activity should not reduce its analgesic efficacy.[6] Hydrocodone is partially metabolized by 2D6 to hydromorphone although the efficacy is not completely dependent on the metabolite as in the case of codeine. Therefore, because the parent drugs have analgesic efficacy, they still can be used clinically in patients with concomitant use of medication that may inhibit 2D6 activity. In addition, codeine may have varying efficacy due genetic predisposition and possibly drug interactions, therefore all these issues should be considered in pain management strategies.

Take-Home Points

- Codeine is a prodrug of morphine that requires *O*-demethylation by the cytochrome P450 enzyme 2D6.
- Some medications cause strong inhibition of 2D6, which may diminish the analgesic properties of codeine.
- Some populations have genetic polymorphisms of 2D6 that affects the proportion of codeine that undergoes *O*-demethylation. Individuals who have extensive 2D6 metabolism have a normal response to codeine, although individuals with poor 2D6 metabolism have no response and those with ultra-rapid 2D6 metabolism are at risk for codeine intoxication.
- Even after inhibition of 2D6, other opioids—such as morphine, oxycodone, and hydromorphone—continue to be effective.

Summary

Interaction: pharmacokinetic
Substrate: codeine (prodrug)
Enzyme: 2D6
Inhibitor: fluoxetine
Clinical effect: lack of analgesic efficacy due to decreased conversion of codeine to morphine, the pharmacologically active metabolite at the μ-receptor.

References

1. Dayer P, Desmeules J, Leemann T, et al. Bioactivation of the narcotic drug codeine in human liver is mediated by the polymorphic monooxygenase catalyzing debrisoquine 4-hydroxylation (cytochrome P-450 dbl/bufI). Biochem Biophys Res Commun. 1988;152(1):411–6.
2. Sindrup SH, Arendt-Nielsen L, Brosen K, Bjerring P, et al. The effect of quinidine on the analgesic effect of codeine. Eur J Clin Pharmacol. 1992;42(6):587–91.
3. VandenBrink BM, Foti RS, Rock DA, et al. Prediction of CYP2D6 drug interactions from in vitro data: evidence for substrate-dependent inhibition. Drug Metab Dispos. 2012;40(1): 47–53.
4. Desmeules J, Gascon MP, Dayer P, et al. Impact of environmental and genetic factors on codeine analgesia. Eur J Clin Pharmacol. 1991;41(1):23–6.
5. Gasche Y, Daali Y, Fathi M, et al. Codeine intoxication associated with ultrarapid CYP2D6 metabolism. N Engl J Med. 2004;351(27):2827–31. Erratum in: N Engl J Med. 2005 1;352(6): 638.
6. Armstrong SC, Cozza KL. Pharmacokinetic drug interactions of morphine, codeine, and their derivatives: theory and clinical reality, part I. Psychosomatics. 2003;44(2):167–71.

A Shuddering Interaction

57

Meperidine, phenelzine, serotonin toxicity

Christine A. Kenyon Laundre MD, Randall Flick MD, and Juraj Sprung MD, PhD

Abstract
This case discusses a pharmacodynamic interaction between phenelzine and meperidine resulting in serotonin syndrome.

Case

A 35-year-old woman drove into a brick wall in a suicide attempt, even though she had started taking phenelzine sulfate approximately 3 weeks earlier for treatment-resistant depression. She presented for emergency surgery for multiple open fractures.

The patient had an uneventful general anesthetic and intraoperative course and the trachea was extubated in the operating room. She was taken to the postanesthesia care unit, where she remained hemodynamically stable, but had severe postoperative shivering. Per protocol, the recovery room nurse gave meperidine hydrochloride (25 mg) intravenously to the patient.

Ten minutes after receiving meperidine, the patient had agitation, tremor, diaphoresis, and tachycardia. The anesthesiologist was called immediately and noted ankle clonus on physical examination. He quickly reviewed the patient's medical record, noted the treatment with phenelzine, a monoamine oxidase inhibitor (MAOI), and suspected a drug interaction with meperidine. Chlorpromazine (25 mg) and midazolam (2 mg) were administered intravenously, after which the patient's symptoms diminished. Subsequently, she was transferred to the intensive care unit for observation and had no further complications.

C.A.K. Laundre MD (✉)
Anesthesiology Associates of Wisconsin, Milwaukee, WI, USA
e-mail: cakenyon@gmail.com

R. Flick MD • J. Sprung MD, PhD
Department of Anesthesiology, Mayo Clinic, Rochester, MN, USA

C. Marcucci et al. (eds.), *A Case Approach to Perioperative Drug-Drug Interactions*, DOI 10.1007/978-1-4614-7495-1_57

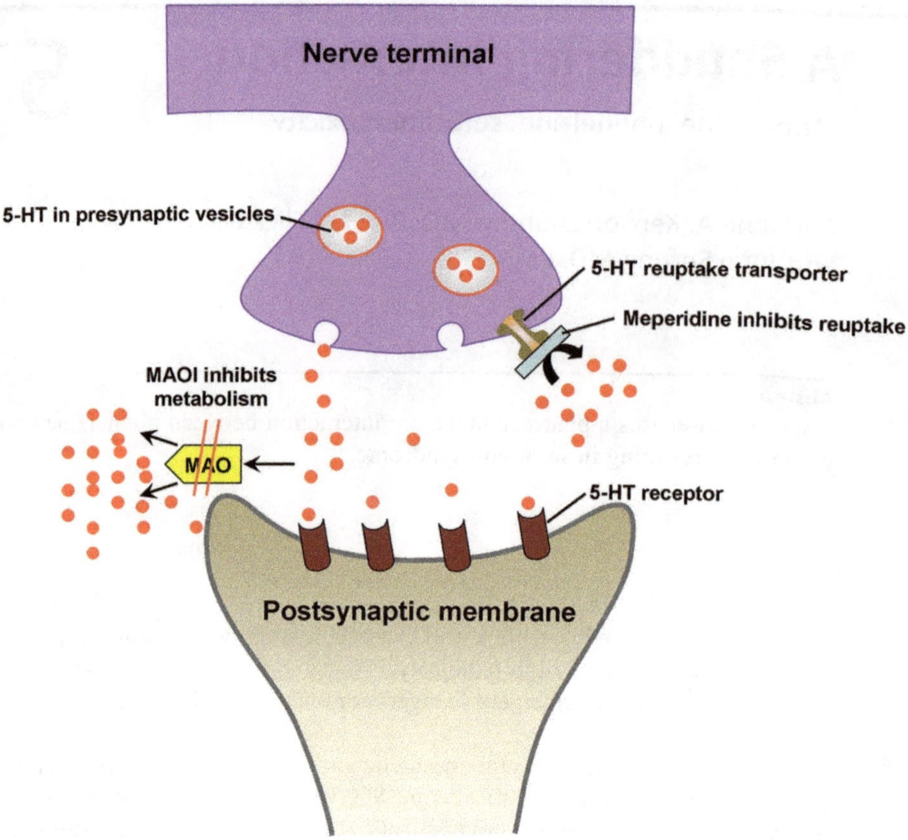

Fig. 57.1 Mechanism of serotonin syndrome. Stimulation of postsynaptic serotonin receptors is excessive because of decreased serotonin metabolism due to an MAOI and decreased uptake into the presynaptic terminal due to meperidine. 5-HT indicates 5-hydroxytryptamine; MAO, monoamine oxidase; MAOI, monoamine oxidase inhibitor; red dot, 5-HT

Discussion

This is an example of a pharmacodynamic interaction at the neurotransmitter level.

More specifically, this is an example of one drug (phenelzine) inhibiting serotonin metabolism combined with another drug (meperidine) inhibiting serotonin reuptake, resulting in serotonin toxicity.

This drug combination results in an increased intrasynaptic serotonin concentration, which then leads to central serotonin syndrome, or serotonin toxicity (Fig. 57.1).[1] MAOIs inhibit monoamine oxidases, the enzymes responsible for inactivation of numerous neurotransmitters, including dopamine, norepinephrine, epinephrine, serotonin, and tyramine.[2] Meperidine is a synthetic opioid analgesic used most commonly for treatment of pain and postoperative shivering.[3] In addition to its action on opioid receptors, meperidine inhibits presynaptic serotonin reuptake.[1] Because of the risk for serotonin toxicity, meperidine is contraindicated in patients who have received an MAOI within the previous 14 days.[3]

Serotonin is produced by the decarboxylation and hydroxylation of L-tryptophan and is found in both the central and peripheral nervous systems. It has numerous actions throughout the body through its interactions with seven families of 5-hydroxytryptamine (5-HT) receptors (5-HT_1 through 5-HT_7).[4] The actions of serotonin include the modulation of thermoregulation, appetite, pain perception, vascular tone, gastrointestinal motility, and sympathetic nervous system function.[2,4] Although serotonin toxicity likely involves multiple types of 5-HT receptors, agonism of 5-HT_{2A} receptors seems to contribute substantially to toxicity development.[4] In addition, serotonin acts as a cotransmitter with γ-aminobutyric acid and norepinephrine, and serotonin receptors exist on some dopaminergic neurons, leading to serotonin-induced dopamine release in the brain.[2] These complex interactions probably contribute to the development of serotonin toxicity, although the exact mechanisms are understood incompletely.[2,4]

The combination of MAOIs with medications that either cause release of serotonin or inhibit serotonin reuptake may precipitate serotonin toxicity by increasing the amount of serotonin available at the synapse. Potent serotonin reuptake inhibitors, such as the selective serotonin reuptake inhibitors, are more likely to cause toxicity than weaker reuptake inhibitors. However, meperidine seems to be an exception to this rule. It is a weak serotonin reuptake inhibitor, yet it has been associated with severe and fatal serotonin toxicity when combined with MAOIs. The reason for this intense response is unknown but may be related to differences in susceptibility and drug metabolism among individual patients.[1]

The first report of interaction between meperidine and an MAOI was published in 1955.[5,6] It involved a physician who was treated for pulmonary tuberculosis with the MAOI iproniazid and received meperidine (100 mg) intramuscularly. Within 20 minutes, he had muscle twitching, nausea, cyanosis, profuse perspiration, hypertension, tachycardia, hyperreflexia, and ankle clonus. He recovered without specific treatment. Since that time, there have been numerous reports of serotonin toxicity—some cases of which have been fatal—due to the combination of an MAOI and meperidine.[1,4,6]

Serotonin toxicity consists of a triad of neuroexcitatory features: neuromuscular hyperactivity (tremor, clonus, myoclonus, hyperreflexia, and pyramidal rigidity), autonomic hyperactivity (diaphoresis, fever, tachycardia, and tachypnea), and altered mental status (agitation, excitement, and, in advanced cases, confusion). Generally, the onset of symptoms is rapid, occurring as the second drug reaches an effective blood level.[1] Toxicity severity ranges from mild, self-limited symptoms to severe neurologic and hemodynamic instability and death. In mild cases, only supportive treatment may be needed, including discontinuing the causative medication and providing intravenous hydration.[2] However, the patient should be monitored closely because rapid deterioration may occur.[1] 5-HT_{2A} antagonists, such as cyproheptadine hydrochloride (oral) and chlorpromazine hydrochloride (intravenous), are effective in reducing the symptoms of toxicity, and benzodiazepines are useful as adjunctive treatment to control agitation and to blunt hyperadrenergic responses.[1,4] In severe cases, intubation, mechanical ventilation, and sedation may be required.[1]

Editor's Note: The specific interaction between phenelzine and meperidine has an important medical historical context in the United States. In 1984, Libby Zion, the daughter of journalist Sidney Zion, died within 24 hours of admission to a New York City hospital. She had been treated with phenelzine prior to admission, and was given meperidine shortly after arriving on the ward. She developed hyperthermia, and suffered unresuscitatable cardiac arrest. Her father believed she died because the medical residents caring for her were careless because of exhaustion, and successfully made this case to the media and New York State legislature. In 1989, New York State instituted work-hour restrictions for postgraduate medical trainees, enshrined in what was named the "Libby Zion Law." These restrictions were then nationally promulgated by the Accreditation Council of Graduate Medical Education in 2003.[7]

Take-Home Points

- MAOIs are effective antidepressants but are typically not used as first-line treatment because of potentially severe interactions with foods and other medications.
- MAOIs inhibit the metabolism of numerous neurotransmitters, including dopamine, norepinephrine, epinephrine, serotonin, and tyramine.
- Meperidine is an opioid analgesic that also inhibits serotonin reuptake at presynaptic nerve terminals.
- Serotonin has numerous effects throughout the body, including the modulation of thermoregulation, appetite, pain perception, vascular tone, gastrointestinal motility, and sympathetic nervous system function.
- The combination of MAOIs and any medication that inhibits serotonin reuptake may lead to serotonin toxicity, which is characterized by neuromuscular hyperactivity, autonomic hyperactivity, and altered mental status.

- Serotonin toxicity may be mild and self-limited or severe and fatal. Treatment consists of careful observation and supportive care, 5-HT_{2A} antagonists (cyproheptadine), and benzodiazepines.

- Meperidine is contraindicated in any patient who has received an MAOI in the previous 14 days.

Summary

Interaction: pharmacodynamic
Substrate: phenelzine and meperidine
Mechanism: serotonin reuptake inhibition
Clinical effects: serotonin syndrome

References

1. Gillman PK. Monoamine oxidase inhibitors, opioid analgesics and serotonin toxicity. Br J Anaesth. 2005;95:434–41.
2. Rapaport MH. Dietary restrictions and drug interactions with monoamine oxidase inhibitors: the state of the art. J Clin Psychiatry. 2007;(68 Suppl 8):42–6.
3. Clark RF, Wei EM, Anderson PO. Meperidine: therapeutic use and toxicity. J Emerg Med. 1995;13:797–802.
4. Boyer EW, Shannon M. The serotonin syndrome. N Engl J Med. 2005;352:1112–20.
5. Mitchell RS. Fatal toxic encephalitis occurring during iproniazid therapy in pulmonary tuberculosis. Ann Intern Med. 1955;42:417–24.
6. Stack CG, Rogers P, Linter SP. Monoamine oxidase inhibitors and anaesthesia: a review. Br J Anaesth. 1988;60:222–7.
7. Lerner B. "A case that shook medicine" Washington Post, November 28, 2006.

Double Indemnity

58

Fatal Forty DDI: morphine, rifampin, P-glycoprotein

Lisa Chan MD, Catherine Marcucci MD,
Neil B. Sandson MD, and Kirk Lalwani MD, FRCA, MCR

Abstract
This case discusses a pharmacokinetic drug interaction involving absorption and the P-glycoprotein (P-gp) transport system. Morphine is a P-gp substrate and rifampin is a P-gp inducer.

Case

A 62-year-old man developed a painful case of shingles complicated by postherpetic neuralgia while serving the last year of an 8-year prison sentence for possession and distribution of narcotics. Treatment options were somewhat limited during his period of incarceration. Fortunately, he experienced reasonable pain relief with an oral dose of morphine, a drug whose side-effect profile he was very willing to tolerate. He was eventually titrated to a dose of MS Contin (120 mg BID). Shortly after his release, he was seen at his local Veterans Affairs (VA) clinic and diagnosed with tuberculosis. He was placed on several medications, including rifampin, and he indicated his willingness to be compliant, as he had seen several prison mates

L. Chan MD (✉)
Department of Pediatric Cardiac Anesthesiology, Memorial Regional Hospital,
Hollywood, FL, USA
e-mail: lisaychan@gmail.com

C. Marcucci MD
Anesthesia Services Department, Philadelphia Veterans Affairs Medical Center,
Philadelphia, PA, USA

N.B. Sandson MD
Department of Psychiatry, University of Maryland Medical System, Baltimore, MD, USA

Department of Psychiatry, VA Maryland Health Care System, Baltimore, MD, USA

K. Lalwani MD, FRCA, MCR
Department of Anesthesiology & Perioperative Medicine, Oregon Health and Science
University, Portland, OR, USA

C. Marcucci et al. (eds.), *A Case Approach to Perioperative Drug-Drug Interactions*, DOI 10.1007/978-1-4614-7495-1_58

succumb to the disease. Sixteen days later, he came to the multidisciplinary pain clinic at the regional VA hospital without an appointment. He described a severe loss of pain relief from the MS Contin, in spite of the fact that he had frequently "doubled up" the dose. Given his history, his primary care provider at the clinic had refused to prescribe a significantly higher dose. He appeared agitated and in extreme pain, shouting "I can't live in this hell, just go ahead and put me back in jail!"

Discussion

This is an example of a (P-glycoprotein) inducer added to a (P-glycoprotein) substrate.

This interesting drug–drug interaction does not occur as a result of alterations in P450-mediated metabolism. Rather, the kinetics of orally administered morphine in this case are mediated by the P-glycoprotein (permeability glycoprotein, or P-gp) transport system; morphine is a substrate molecule that will be continually transported back into the gut lumen by an intact transporter.[1–4] Rifampin, acting as an inducer, increases production of the transport protein, which increased the extrusion of morphine from enterocytes and back into the gut lumen. This serves to decrease systemic absorption. Some morphine is likely to be absorbed into the systemic vasculature despite induction of the P-glycoprotein pump within the plasma membrane of enterocytes. However, distribution from the systemic vasculature to the central nervous system (CNS) is also decreased through induction of the pump within the plasma membrane of blood–brain barrier (BBB) endothelial cells. Induction of the pump at this site leads to more extrusion of morphine from the cytosol of BBB endothelial cells and back into the systemic vasculature.[1–4]

For any given dose of oral morphine, the presence of a P-glycoprotein inducer will cause a decrease in both the plasma level and the concentration of the drug in the central nervous system, rendering the original dose less effective in controlling the patient's pain. Rifampin, in particular, has been demonstrated to cause a loss of analgesic efficacy after coadministration with oral morphine for a period of several weeks.[5]

Take-Home Points

- This is an efflux pump P-glycoprotein mediated drug interaction.
- P-glycoprotein is a transporter, specifically an ATP-binding cassette subfamily B member 1 (ABCB1), between intra- and extracellular membranes most commonly in the gut, liver, kidney, and brain.

- P-glycoprotein has a wide variety of substrates: morphine, methadone, antiretroviral, and chemotherapeutic agents. While there is bidirectional transport, the net efflux of oral morphine by intestinal P-gp reduces morphine's systemic absorption, and the net efflux by blood brain barrier P-gp reduces morphine's distribution into the CNS.

- Rifampin increases the production and thus net activity of P-gp, thereby increasing the amount of morphine extruded and decreasing the systemic levels of morphine.

- Likewise, inhibition of P-gp (by quinidine, for example) will increase the systemic levels and clinical effects of morphine.

- Current research is looking at the manipulation of P-gp to alter the side effect profiles of medications, such as reducing pruritus from morphine.[6]

Summary

Interaction: pharmacokinetic (absorption and distribution)
Substrate: morphine
Transporter: P-glycoprotein
Inducer: rifampin
Clinical effects: decreased bioavailability of morphine leading to loss of analgesia

References

1. Kharasch ED, Hoffer C, Whittington D, et al. Role of P-glycoprotein in the intestinal absorption and clinical effects of morphine. Clin Pharmacol Ther. 2003;74(6):543–54.
2. Wandel C, Kim R, Wood M, et al. Interaction of morphine, fentanyl, sufentanil, alfentanil, and loperamide with the efflux drug transporter P-glycoprotein. Anesthesiology. 2002; 96(4):913–20.
3. Mercer SL, Coop A. Opioid analgesics and P-glycoprotein efflux transporters: a potential systems-level contribution to analgesic tolerance. Curr Top Med Chem. 2011;11(9):1157–64.
4. Padowski JM, Pollack GM. Pharmacokinetic and pharmacodynamic implications of P-glycoprotein modulation. Methods Mol Biol. 2010;596:359–84.
5. Fromm MF, Eckhardt K, Li S, et al. Loss of analgesic effect of morphine due to coadministration of rifampin. Pain. 1997;72(1–2):261–7.
6. Mercadante S, Villari P, Fulfaro F. Rifampicin in opioid-induced itching. Support Care Cancer. 2001;9(6):467–8.

Breaking the Codeine

59

Fatal Forty DDI: codeine, quinidine, CYP2D6

Clint Christensen MD, Nathan G. Orgain MD,
and Randal O. Dull MD, PhD

Abstract
This case discusses the pharmacokinetic interaction between codeine and quinidine. Codeine is a prodrug, metabolized to the active compound morphine by CYP2D6, quinidine is a 2D6 inhibitor.

Case

A 75-year-old man was treated in the pain clinic for chronic back pain due to degenerative joint disease. He was on a stable dose of codeine (60 mg po every 6 hours) for many months with satisfactory pain control. Despite availability of sustained-release analgesics, the patient always elected to remain on codeine, feeling that his evening dose helped him fall asleep, and he didn't want to "use that stronger stuff."

However, one day he presented to the clinic with a 1 week acute exacerbation of pain, despite taking with his usual pain medications. He reported that extra doses of codeine weren't helping, although a dose of acetaminophen seemed to partially alleviate his pain. The anesthesiologist noted that the patient had been seen by his internist 10 days earlier, who placed him on quinidine (300 mg po every 6 hours) for

C. Christensen MD (✉)
Department of Anesthesiology, University of Utah School of Medicine,
Salt Lake City, UT, USA
e-mail: clint.christensen@hsc.utah.edu

N.G. Orgain MD
Department of Anesthesiology, University of Utah, Salt Lake City, UT, USA

R.O. Dull MD, PhD
Department of Anesthesiology, University of Illinois at Chicago, Chicago, IL, USA

C. Marcucci et al. (eds.), *A Case Approach to Perioperative Drug-Drug Interactions*, DOI 10.1007/978-1-4614-7495-1_59

control of his frequent atrial fibrillation episodes. The patient further explained that quinidine was started because sotalol, his previous medication, made him feel dizzy. He denied any other health or medication changes, and was very hesitant to deviate from his analgesic regimen, since he had experienced very good results in pain control until now.

Discussion

This is an example of an inhibitor added to a prodrug substrate.

Codeine is a well-known opioid used most commonly for its analgesic and antitussive effects. Off-label, codeine is also used in the treatment of diarrhea, narcolepsy, and sickle cell crisis. Codeine is a prodrug that undergoes metabolism to three different compounds: norcodeine, codeine-6-glucuronide, and morphine. Morphine is the metabolite responsible for the majority of the analgesic effect of codeine. The conversion of codeine to morphine relies on metabolism via the cytochrome P450 2D6 (CYP2D6) enzyme in the liver.[1–3]

Quinidine is the most potent known inhibitor of CYP2D6. The addition of quinidine to this patient's medications impaired the ability of 2D6 to convert codeine to morphine. The decrease in morphine production resulted in the loss of analgesic efficacy seen in this case. Numerous other drugs, including many antidepressants (eg, fluoxetine, paroxetine, bupropion) and the phenothiazine antipsychotics (perphenazine, fluphenazine, chlorpromazine), also interfere with the 2D6 pathway. In addition, 5% to 10% of Caucasians and 1% to 2% of Asians lack the 2D6 enzyme, and will also obtain an inadequate analgesic response to codeine.[2,4]

Quinidine is a class 1A antiarrhythmic that prolongs the electrocardiac refractory period and reduces automaticity in the heart. It is used primarily to treat atrial fibrillation and flutter, but may also be used in the treatment of malaria. Concerns regarding increased mortality and the pro-arrhythmic potential of quinidine led to a substantial decrease in its use over the past 10 to 15 years, however this reputation has undergone recent reevaluation, and quinidine use may increase.[5]

CYP2D6 metabolizes numerous other analgesics, including oxycodone and the prodrugs hydrocodone and tramadol.[6] Hydromorphone would be a good option for this patient, as it does not undergo 2D6 metabolism. Alternatively, if the quinidine is discontinued, the analgesic efficacy of codeine should return within a few days.

Take-Home Points

- Codeine's analgesic effect depends primarily on its metabolism to morphine via the CYP2D6 pathway.
- Quinidine is one of the most potent inhibitors of CYP2D6. When used in combination with codeine, it will likely result in inadequate analgesia.
- 5% to 10% of Caucasians and 1% to 2% of Asians lack 2D6 and will likely obtain inadequate pain relief from codeine. For them, morphine or hydromorphone might be better alternative analgesics.
- Clinicians may encounter quinidine drug–drug interactions with greater frequency in the future. Although rarely used at present, recent trials suggest that quinidine is a safe and efficacious agent for the treatment of atrial fibrillation. It remains to be seen whether or not the use of this medication will increase based on this data. Quinidine has also been used successfully to treat idiopathic ventricular fibrillation, Brugada syndrome, and short QT syndrome.
- This case demonstrates how the consequences of substrate-inhibitor pairings differ depending on whether the substrate is a prodrug or a "standard" drug. All substrate–inhibitor pairings raise substrate levels. In the case of a "standard" analgesic, such as oxycodone or methadone, the result is a possible increase in efficacy or even toxicity. In the case of prodrug analgesics, such as codeine, hydrocodone, and tramadol, this interaction can produce a loss of efficacy.

Summary

Interaction: pharmacokinetic
Substrate: codeine (prodrug)
Enzyme: 2D6
Inhibitor: quinidine
Clinical effect: decreased conversion to active metabolite (morphine)

References

1. Poulsen L, Brosen K, Arendt-Nielsen L, et al. Codeine and morphine in extensive and poor metabolizers of sparteine: pharmacokinetics, analgesic effect and side effects. Eur J Clin Pharmacol. 1996;51(3–4):289–95.

2. Desmeules J, Gascon MP, Dayer P, et al. Impact of environmental and genetic factors on codeine analgesia. Eur J Clin Pharmacol. 1991;41(1):23–6.
3. Sindrup SH, Arendt-Nielsen L, Brosen K, et al. The effect of quinidine on the analgesic effect of codeine. Eur J Clin Pharmacol. 1992;42(6):587–91.
4. Caraco Y, Sheller J, Wood A. Impact of ethnic origin and quinidine co-administration on codeine's disposition and pharmacodynamic effects. J Pharmacol Exp Ther. 1999;290(1):413–22.
5. Yang F, Hanon S, Lam P, Schweitzer P. Quinidine revisited. Am J Med. 2009;122(4):317–21.
6. Neil B, Sandson M. Drug-drug interaction primer: a compendium of case vignettes for the practicing clinician. Washington, DC: American Psychiatric Press, Inc.; 2007. p. 345.

The Ultimate Ultram Primer I: My Mood Is Better, but Boy Do I Hurt!

60

Fatal Forty DDI: tramadol, paroxetine, CYP2D6

Toby N. Weingarten MD and Juraj Sprung MD, PhD

Abstract
This case discusses a pharmacokinetic interaction between tramadol and paroxetine. Tramadol is a prodrug cytochrome P450 2D6 substrate and paroxetine is a 2D6 inhibitor.

Case

A 45-year-old woman with a long history of depression and fibromyalgia presented for a scheduled visit to her pain clinic. At her last appointment 3 months ago, she reported good control of symptoms and an average pain of 3/10 on an analog pain scale by taking only tramadol (50 mg) several times per day.

However, she now reported an average pain score of 8/10 that was interfering with her sleep, job, and other daily activities. Curiously, she reported not feeling as anxious and upset as she expected when her troubled marriage finally ended and credited her psychiatrist with "staving off a mental collapse" by changing her standing citalopram dose (20 mg daily) to paroxetine (40 mg daily). The psychiatrist was contacted by phone and it was agreed that the patient should change back to

T.N. Weingarten MD (✉)
Department of Anesthesiology, Mayo Clinic College of Medicine, Rochester, MN, USA

Department of Anesthesiology, Mayo Clinic, Rochester, MN, USA
e-mail: Weingarten.toby@mayo.edu

J. Sprung MD, PhD
Department of Anesthesiology, Mayo Clinic, Rochester, MN, USA

C. Marcucci et al. (eds.), *A Case Approach to Perioperative Drug-Drug Interactions*, DOI 10.1007/978-1-4614-7495-1_60

citalopram, but increase the dose to 40 mg daily. A return appointment to the pain clinic 2 weeks later revealed that her pain intensity had returned to a manageable level and that both her mood and anxiety had improved with the increased dose of citalopram.

Discussion

This is an example of an inhibitor added to a prodrug substrate.

Tramadol is a commonly prescribed opioid analgesic for the management of both acute and chronic pain conditions. Tramadol produces analgesia through varied mechanisms. The preparation of tramadol consist of two isomers (+)-tramadol and (−)-tramadol and these produce analgesia through monoaminergic activity via the inhibition of serotonin and norepinephrine reuptake, respectively.[1] Tramadol hydrochloride is also a prodrug that undergoes hepatic *O*-demethylation by the cytochrome P450 (CYP) isoenzyme 2D6 into (+) and (−) O-desmethyltramadol, which is also known as M1.[2] The (+)-M1 metabolite is the primary contributor to the opioid activity of tramadol. There is substantial genetic variability of the CYP2D6 system among Caucasians, and it has been shown that less tramadol is metabolized to M1 and therefore has less analgesic activity among subjects who are poor metabolizers compared to those who are extensive metabolizers.[2]

Multiple medications are known to inhibit the CYP2D6 system including the selective serotonin reuptake inhibitor (SSRI) class of antidepressants.[3] However, the degree of 2D6 inhibition varies among different SSRIs: paroxetine and fluoxetine are the most potent inhibitors, sertraline is a moderate inhibitor, and citalopram only weakly inhibits this system.[3] It has been demonstrated that clinically used doses of paroxetine can inhibit the metabolism of tramadol to (+)-M1 by 67% and result in diminish the analgesic activity (see Fig. 60.1).[4]

In this patient, the use of the potent 2D6 inhibitor, paroxetine, resulted in decreased metabolism of tramadol to M1. This inhibition resulted in lower levels of M1 and less opioid activity of tramadol, as evidenced by the abrupt increase in her pain intensity. Tramadol regained its opioid-mediated analgesic properties when her antidepressant was changed back again to citalopram. Even though citalopram is an inhibitor of 2D6, its action on this system is much less pronounced than paroxetine, and in this patient was insufficient to reduce the analgesia produced by tramadol. It should be noted that the adverse interactions between SSRIs and tramadol hydrochloride are not limited to decreased analgesic efficacy of tramadol, but can also produce a life-threatening serotonergic syndrome, and patients should be monitored for this interaction when combining these medications.[5]

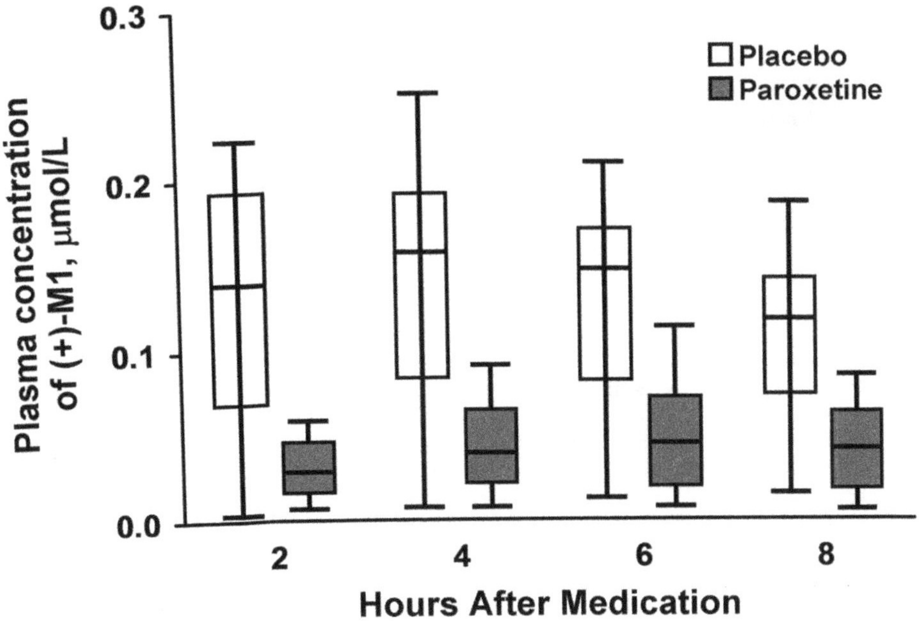

Fig. 60.1 Median, 25th and 75th percentiles, and range of the metabolite (+)-M1 in 16 extensive metabolizers of sparteine after single oral dose of 150 mg tramadol after 3 days of pretreatment with either 20 mg/d paroxetine (shaded box) or placebo (white box). All measurements were made at 2, 4, 6, and 8 hours after medication [Modified from Laugesen S, Enggaard TP, Pedersen RS et al. Paroxetine, a cytochrome P450 2D6 inhibitor, diminishes the stereoselective O-demethylation and reduces the hypoalgesic effect of tramadol. *Clin Pharmacol Ther*. 2005;77:312–23. With permission from Nature Publishing Group]

Take-Home Points

- Tramadol produces analgesia via multiple mechanisms including inhibition of the uptake of monoamines in the central nervous system and opioid activity by its metabolite (+)-*O*-desmethyltramadol (M1).
- Metabolism of tramadol into the M1 metabolite is mediated by the cytochrome P450 enzyme 2D6.
- Multiple medications, including serotonin reuptake inhibitors (SSRIs), inhibit the 2D6 and can reduce the analgesic effect of tramadol by limiting its conversion to the M1 metabolite. However, the degree of 2D6 varies among the different SSRIs.
- The combination of SSRIs and tramadol can also result in the development of the serotonin syndrome and patients should be monitored for the development of this syndrome.

Summary

Interaction: pharmacokinetic
Substrate: tramadol (prodrug)
Enzyme: 2D6
Inhibitor: paroxetine
Clinical effects: decreased conversion of the prodrug tramadol to the more potent opioid metabolite led to decreased analgesic effect

References

1. Raffa RB, Friderichs E, Reimann W, et al. Complementary and synergistic antinociceptive interaction between the enantiomers of tramadol. J Pharmacol Exp Ther. 1993;267:331–40.
2. Poulsen L, Arendt-Nielsen L, Brosen K, et al. The hypoalgesic effect of tramadol in relation to CYP2D6. Clin Pharmacol Ther. 1996;60:636–44.
3. Crewe HK, Lennard MS, Tucker GT, et al. The effect of selective serotonin re-uptake inhibitors on cytochrome P4502D6 (CYP2D6) activity in human liver microsomes. Br J Clin Pharmacol. 1992;34:262–5.
4. Laugesen S, Enggaard TP, Pedersen RS, et al. Paroxetine, a cytochrome P450 2D6 inhibitor, diminishes the stereoselective O-demethylation and reduces the hypoalgesic effect of tramadol. Clin Pharmacol Ther. 2005;77:312–23.
5. Mahlberg R, Kunz D, Sasse J, et al. Serotonin syndrome with tramadol and citalopram. Am J Psychiatry. 2004;161:1129.

The Ultimate Ultram Primer II: I "Haight" Narcotics, but I Hate Seizures More

61

Fatal Forty DDI: tramadol, bupropion, CYP2D6, seizures

Bruce T. Dumser MD and Neil B. Sandson MD

Abstract
This case discusses the synergistic pharmacodynamic interaction between tramadol and bupropion resulting in new-onset seizures. A possible pharmacokinetic interaction is also discussed.

Case

Late on a Sunday morning, the anesthesiologist on call at a small regional hospital received a message from the operating room desk that Dr. Ashbury was posting an urgent case. The patient was a 32-year-old woman who was admitted to the orthopedics service for a tibial fracture sustained during a fall while mountain biking. Dr. Ashbury had initially planned open reduction for the following day, but there were moderate concerns for the patient's distal perfusion and she was bumped up to a Level II weekend case. She was very fit and in good health. Her only standing outpatient medication were bupropion (Wellbutrin XL® 300 mg/d) and nortriptyline (50 mg qhs) which she had been prescribed with good result for postpartum depression 9 months earlier. She asked to have this continued, as her depression had been

B.T. Dumser MD (✉)
Anesthesiology Consultants of Walla Walla, Walla Walla, WA, USA
e-mail: bruce.medicine@gmail.com

N.B. Sandson MD
Department of Psychiatry, University of Maryland Medical System, Baltimore, MD, USA

Department of Psychiatry, VA Maryland Health Care System, Baltimore, MD, USA

C. Marcucci et al. (eds.), *A Case Approach to Perioperative Drug-Drug Interactions*, DOI 10.1007/978-1-4614-7495-1_61

very distressing to both her and her husband. On admission to the hospital the previous Friday, she had adamantly refused narcotics including morphine, hydromorphone, and fentanyl, stating, "Like the song says, I've seen the needle and the damage done." The empathic orthopedics resident (yes, that could happen) finally elicited the history that her parents met in 1967 while living in a certain section in San Francisco during the Summer of Love and that both parents had struggled with lifelong addiction issues involving heroin and other opioids. She finally consented only to tramadol (Ultram®, 75 mg po) every 4 hours as needed, not to exceed 300 mg per day.

The patient spent a weary 6 hours waiting to go into the operating room as the anesthesiologist was very busy with other trauma cases and the labor and delivery deck. Fortunately, she was not in significant pain as she had continued to receive tramadol as needed. Just as the nurses were pulling the trays for her case, there was a STAT overhead call from the nurse covering the preoperative area as the patient had just had a seizure. After stabilization and successful completion of the surgical repair, she was admitted to the intensive care unit, where pain medicine and psychiatric consults were obtained. Both the tramadol and bupropion were discontinued and the patient ultimately agreed to a fentanyl patch with adjuvant patient-controlled analgesia. The psychiatric consultation-liaison service recommended that her nortriptyline be continued. She was ultimately discharged with a planned consultation with the outpatient psychiatry service to discuss if it would be necessary to restart bupropion.

Discussion

This is an example of a synergistic pharmacodynamic interaction leading to a new-onset seizure. It is also an example of a possible pharmacokinetic interaction involving a substrate (tramadol) added to an inhibitor (bupropion), impairing the metabolism to a pharmacologically more active compound at the μ-receptor.

Seizures are a known concern with both bupropion and tramadol, and to a greater extent than most other antidepressants and analgesics, respectively.[1–3] When these two agents are coadministered, the likelihood of new-onset seizures increases synergistically.[4–6]

In addition to this pharmacodynamic drug–drug interaction (DDI), this combination also presents the possibility of an additional pharmacokinetic DDI. Tramadol is a synthetic analog of codeine with an analgesic efficacy and potency less than that of morphine but greater than nonopioids. Metabolism includes a Phase I reaction to *O*-desmethyltramadol (M1) mediated by cytochrome P450 (CYP) 2D6.[7,8] There are other metabolites from other CYP reactions, but the M1 metabolite is notable since it has affinity 300 times greater than that of the parent compound for μ-opioid receptors. Tramadol also inhibits neuronal reuptake of norepinephrine and serotonin, while also increasing presynaptic release of serotonin. Since bupropion is a meaningful CYP2D6 inhibitor, it would be expected that bupropion could interfere with this conversion and accordingly impair tramadol's analgesic efficacy.[9] However, while this DDI is theoretically sound, it has not yet been empirically demonstrated.

Take-Home Points

- Bupropion and tramadol are both known seizure-genic medications. Coadministering these medications synergistically increases this already elevated risk of new-onset seizures.
- Inhibitors of CYP2D6 can decrease the analgesic efficacy of tramadol by impairing tramadol's conversion to its more potent μ-receptor agonist metabolite, *O*-desmethyltramadol (M1). Although this has not yet been empirically demonstrated, it is reasonable to suspect that this could also occur when tramadol is coadministered with bupropion.

Summary

Interaction 1: pharmacodynamic
Substrates: tramadol and bupropion
Mechanism of action: synergistic lowering of the seizure threshold
Clinical effect: new-onset seizure

Interaction 2 (theoretical): pharmacokinetic
Substrate: tramadol
Enzyme: 2D6
Inhibitor: bupropion
Clinical effect: loss of analgesic effect

References

1. Sansone RA, Sansone LA. Tramadol: seizures, serotonin syndrome, and coadministered antidepressants. Psychiatry (Edgmont). 2009;6(4):17–21.
2. Bupropion package insert. Mylan Pharmaceuticals, Morgantown. http://dailymed.nlm.nih.gov/dailymed/lookup.cfm?setid=59a7cda8-34b4-4c02-b100-91f274918eef. Last accessed 11 July 2012.
3. Ultram® (tramadol) package insert. Ortho-McNeil Pharmaceutical Inc., Raritan. 2001 Aug. http://rx-s.net/weblog/more/tramadol_interactions/#ixzz20MIYFNnI. Last accessed 11 July 2012.

4. Labate A, Newton MR, Vernon GM, et al. Tramadol and new-onset seizures. Med J Aust. 2005;182(1):42–3.
5. Boyd IW. Tramadol and seizures. Med J Aust. 2005;182(11):595–6.
6. Stellpflug SJ, Roberts DJ. Which xenobiotic(s) could be responsible for the radiologic findings below? Answer: any proconvulsant xenobiotic, in this case tramadol, bupropion, and nortriptyline. J Med Toxicol. 2010;6(1):72–3.
7. Grond S, Sablotzki A. Clinical pharmacology of tramadol. Clin Pharmacokinet. 2004;43:879–923.
8. Poulsen L, Arendt-Nielsen L, Brosen K, et al. The hypoalgesic effect of tramadol in relation to CYP2D6. Clin Pharmacol Ther. 1996;60:636–44.
9. Kotlyar M, Brauer LH, Tracy TS, et al. Inhibition of CYP2D6 activity by bupropion. J Clin Psychopharmacol. 2005;25(3):226–9.

The Ultimate Ultram Primer III: Tremor-dol Trigger in Serotonin Syndrome

62

Fatal Forty DDI: tramadol, paroxetine, CYP2D6, serotonin syndrome

Bryan C. Hoelzer MD and Stephanie Neuman MD

Abstract
This case discusses pharmacokinetic and pharmacodynamic drug–drug interactions between tramadol and paroxetine resulting in serotonin syndrome.

Case

A 67-year-old woman underwent a right total knee arthroplasty for chronic osteoarthritis. Her medical history was also notable for chronic back pain, fibromyalgia, and a 30-year history of recurrent depression, which was well controlled with paroxetine (20 mg daily). Her other medical problems included urinary incontinence and a history of painful herpes zoster. Other medications included diclofenac and acetaminophen.

Before surgery, the patient underwent a single-injection sciatic nerve block and placement of a femoral nerve catheter for postoperative pain control. She had an uncomplicated intraoperative course and was ordered for supplemental oral acetaminophen and tramadol (50 mg, 6 h) as needed. She had good pain control postoperatively with the femoral nerve catheter and required only one dose of

B.C. Hoelzer MD (✉)
Department of Anesthesiology, Mayo Clinic, Rochester, MN, USA
e-mail: hoelzer.bryan@mayo.edu

S. Neuman MD
Department of Anesthesiology, Gundersen Lutheran, La Crosse, WI, USA

C. Marcucci et al. (eds.), *A Case Approach to Perioperative Drug-Drug Interactions*, DOI 10.1007/978-1-4614-7495-1_62

tramadol during her hospital stay. The femoral nerve catheter was removed in the afternoon on postoperative day 2, and she was discharged to home early on postoperative day 3. She was instructed to continue the scheduled acetaminophen and was given a prescription to continue tramadol therapy as needed.

The patient's knee pain had become intolerable shortly after arriving home, so she began taking twice the prescribed dose of tramadol. The next day, the paramedics were called when the patient had a sudden onset of confusion, myotonic jerks, labored breathing, and increased salivation. She was noted to have a temperature of 38.7°C; blood pressure, 176/102 mm Hg; heart rate, 100 beats per minute; respiratory rate, 16 breaths per minute. Her oxyhemoglobin saturation on room air was 98%. She had dilated pupils, a mild, bilateral 10-Hz hand tremor, and was diaphoretic with flushed skin. Her neurologic exam and head computed tomography were normal and serum laboratory studies were also normal. The patient was admitted to the hospital and her home medications were withheld. The embarrassed resident apologized, saying, "I missed it. Her medication list looked routine to me for a lady her age." The patient improved to baseline condition on hospital day 2.

Discussion

This is an example of a pharmacokinetic interaction involving a substrate added to an inhibitor. It is also an example of a pharmacodynamic interaction leading to serotonin syndrome.

Serotonin (5-hydroxytryptamine [5-HT]) syndrome is characterized by the triad of altered mental status, autonomic dysfunction, and neuromuscular abnormalities.[1] The revised diagnostic criteria for serotonin syndrome described by Radomski et al. require either the addition or an increased dose of a serotonergic medication, along with four major symptoms or three major symptoms plus two minor symptoms.[2] The major symptoms include mental status changes of confusion, euphoria, obtundation, or coma; autonomic dysfunction demonstrated by hyperthermia or diaphoresis; and neuromuscular dysfunction demonstrated by myoclonus, tremors, chills, rigidity, or hyperreflexia. Minor symptoms include mental status agitation and nervousness or insomnia; autonomic dysfunction demonstrated by tachycardia, tachypnea and dyspnea, diarrhea, and low or high blood pressure; and neuromuscular dysfunction resulting in ataxia, mydriasis, or akathisia. These symptoms cannot be due to a preexisting psychiatric disorder, infection, a toxic-metabolic or endocrine cause, or recent treatment with a neuroleptic agent. A diagnosis of the syndrome can be made clinically after both recognition of the signs and symptoms and a careful review of the patient's medications.

The pathophysiologic characteristics of serotonin syndrome are not completely clear.[3] Although no single receptor appears to be responsible for its development, several lines of evidence converge to suggest that agonism of 5-HT_{2A} receptors contributes substantially to the condition.[1] The population at risk for serotonin syndrome includes patients taking one or more medications that increase serotonin levels, such as monoamine oxidase inhibitors (MAOIs), tertiary amine tricyclic antidepressants, selective serotonin receptor inhibitor (SSRIs), meperidine, over-the-counter cough medicines containing dextromethorphan, linezolid (a synthetic antibiotic with MAOI activity), ritonavir (an antiviral), weight-reduction agents (sibutramine), antiemetics (ondansetron, granisetron, metoclopramide), antimigraine agents (triptans), drugs of abuse (methylenedioxymethamphetamine or "ecstasy," lysergic acid diethylamide or "LSD," Syrian rue), and herbal supplements (tryptophan, St. John's wort, ginseng).[1]

Several published case reports describe serotonin syndrome attributed to the concomitant use of an SSRI and tramadol.[3–7] Tramadol is a unique analgesic medication with both opioid and nonopioid properties. Studies *in vitro* and *in vivo* have shown that tramadol-induced pain relief is mediated through binding of μ-opioid receptors, as well as inhibiting reuptake of norepinephrine and serotonin.[4] Tramadol is metabolized through the cytochrome P450 (CYP) isozyme 2D6, and many SSRIs (fluoxetine, paroxetine, high-dose sertraline) are known to have a moderate to potent inhibitory effect on this isozyme,[4,5] Therefore, in addition to aggregate serotonin agonism, another contributing mechanism in serotonin syndrome development with concurrent use of tramadol and certain SSRIs is the inhibition of CYP2D6 by the SSRI, leading to increased tramadol levels with subsequent increased serotonin levels.

Additionally, seizures have been reported in patients taking tramadol in excessive doses, persons predisposed to seizures (those who abuse drugs or alcohol or those with stroke, head injury, or epilepsy), and patients taking antidepressants or other medications that lower the seizure threshold.[7] In the absence of these factors, tramadol alone has not been linked to an increased rate of seizures.[7] Goldsmith et al. described the case of a patient with obsessive-compulsive disorder who achieved complete remission after the addition of tramadol to his fluoxetine therapy, suggesting relevant serotoninergic properties of tramadol.[8]

Most cases of serotonin syndrome are managed adequately with supportive care that includes intravenous fluid therapy, cardiovascular monitoring, and removal of the offending drug or drugs. No standard pharmacologic therapies exist for serotonin syndrome; however, benzodiazepines, cyproheptadine, and chlorpromazine have been reported to be helpful.[1,7] Most cases have acute onset (<24 h) and resolve within 24 hours after therapy initiation and the discontinuation of the offending agent or agents.[1] Admission to an intensive care unit may be required with severe serotonin syndrome.[7]

Little is known about 5-HT concentrations in cerebrospinal fluid. However, several cases of serotonin syndrome with increased 5-HT concentrations have been reported, suggesting that cerebrospinal 5-HT may be a useful test in correctly identifying serotonin syndrome.[3]

Take-Home Points

- Tramadol is a unique analgesic that has opioid and nonopioid properties. Its proposed mechanisms of action include binding to μ-opioid receptors and inhibiting the reuptake of norepinephrine and serotonin.

- The concomitant administration of an SSRI and tramadol increases the risk for serotonin syndrome.

- Serotonin syndrome is characterized by the triad of altered mental status, autonomic dysfunction, and neuromuscular abnormalities.

- Seizures have been reported in patients taking tramadol excessively or taking it concomitantly with drugs that lower the seizure threshold.

- Most cases of serotonin syndrome are self-limited and resolve within 24 hours of initiating supportive care and discontinuing the offending agent or agents.

- Tramadol and SSRIs are commonly used medications. Education of physicians, modification in prescribing practices, and patient education are important steps to take for the detection and avoidance of adverse drug–drug interactions.

Summary

Interaction 1: pharmacokinetic
Substrate: tramadol
Enzyme: 2D6
Inhibitor: paroxetine
Clinical effect: serotonin syndrome

Interaction 2: pharmacodynamic
Substrates: tramadol and fluoxetine
Mechanism/site of action: inhibition of reuptake of serotonin in peripheral and central neurons, agonism of 5-HT_{2A} receptors
Clinical effect: serotonin syndrome

References

1. Boyer EW, Shannon M. The serotonin syndrome. N Engl J Med. 2005;352:1112–20.
2. Radomski JW, Dursun SM, Reveley MA, et al. An exploratory approach to the serotonin syndrome: an update of clinical phenomenology and revised diagnostic criteria. Med Hypotheses. 2000;55:218–24.
3. Mittino D, Mula M, Monaco F. Serotonin syndrome associated with tramadol-sertraline coadministration. Clin Neuropharmacol. 2004;27:150–1.
4. Egberts AC, ter Borgh J, Brodie-Meijer CC. Serotonin syndrome attributed to tramadol addition to paroxetine therapy. Int Clin Psychopharmacol. 1997;12:181–2.
5. Mahlberg R, Kunz D, Sasse J, et al. Serotonin syndrome with tramadol and citalopram. Am J Psychiatry. 2004;161:1129.
6. Kesavan S, Sobala GM. Serotonin syndrome with fluoxetine plus tramadol. J R Soc Med. 1999;92:474–5.
7. Freeman WD, Chabolla DR. 36-year-old woman with loss of consciousness, fever, and tachycardia. Mayo Clin Proc. 2005;80:667–70.
8. Goldsmith TB, Shapira NA, Keck Jr PE. Rapid remission of OCD with tramadol hydrochloride. Am J Psychiatry. 1999;156:660–1.

Too Much of a Good Thing

63

Fatal Forty DDI: codeine, drug–gene interaction, CYP2D6

Erica D. Wittwer MD, PhD, Juraj Sprung MD, PhD, and Wayne T. Nicholson MD, PharmD, MSc

Abstract
This case discusses the drug–gene interaction between cytochrome P450 2D6 and the prodrug codeine resulting in enhanced narcotic effects.

Case

At 2:30 AM, the on-call anesthesia resident was called to a floor "code" and discovered an unresponsive 60-year-old male patient with a pulse of 60 beats per minute. After establishing successful bag-mask ventilation, the resident asked to speak to the patient's spouse who had been dozing in the day lounge, but discovered that the patient and spouse were from Saudi Arabia and did not speak English.

The nurse reported that 3 days earlier, the patient underwent a left total hip arthroplasty. He had hypertension treated with lisinopril and diabetes, which he was trying to manage with diet. He had renal insufficiency after surgery, and his postoperative creatinine value was 1.8 mg/dL. His other laboratory results earlier that day were normal, including values of both hemoglobin and an electrolyte panel. He had been using patient-controlled analgesia with fentanyl, which was changed the previous morning to a combination of acetaminophen and codeine (300 mg/60 mg) for pain. The nurse noted that the patient seemed sleepier throughout the day, but he had continued to report pain and was given his codeine as scheduled. The nurse came in

E.D. Wittwer MD, PhD (✉) • J. Sprung MD, PhD • W.T. Nicholson MD, PharmD, MSc
Department of Anesthesiology, Mayo Clinic, Rochester, MN, USA
e-mail: Wittwer.erica@mayo.edu

C. Marcucci et al. (eds.), *A Case Approach to Perioperative Drug-Drug Interactions*, DOI 10.1007/978-1-4614-7495-1_63

about 1 hour after his last dose of codeine to obtain vital signs and assess his pain level and discovered that the patient was unresponsive.

An arterial blood gas showed respiratory acidosis with an arterial partial pressure of carbon dioxide of 105 mm Hg. Naloxone was given intravenously, and a few minutes later the patient became fully responsive and, fortunately, stated that his pain was tolerable. The patient was transferred to a monitored care unit and a low-dose naloxone infusion was initiated.

Discussion

This is an example of a pharmacogenomic-related problem caused by ultra-rapid metabolism of codeine, leading to toxicity.

Codeine is a prodrug that is metabolized by the hepatic enzyme cytochrome P450 (CYP) 2D6 to its active metabolite, morphine.[1] Morphine is subsequently glucuronidated to its primary metabolites, morphine-3-glucuronide and morphine-6-glucuronide, through the enzyme UDP-glucuronosyltransferase 2B7 (UGT2B7). Morphine and morphine-6-glucuronide both contain active analgesic and sedative properties.

Genetic variants related to codeine metabolism have been identified. Patients who have poor CYP2D6 metabolism metabolize codeine to the active metabolites to a lesser degree than patients with extensive 2D6 metabolism, who metabolize codeine in a normal manner. Persons with a poor metabolizer genotype receive less analgesia from codeine than those with an extensive metabolizer genotype.[2] In contrast, some individuals have ultra-rapid metabolism of codeine, and they produce greater concentrations of morphine than individuals with the extensive metabolizer genotype.[2]

The patient in this example presented as someone with an ultrarapid metabolism of codeine due to a duplication of the *CYP2D6* gene, which led to greater-than-average conversion of codeine to morphine. These increased concentrations of morphine subsequently rely on normal morphine metabolism and clearance. Up to 55% of morphine may be renally excreted as morphine-3-glucuronide, 10% as the parent compound (morphine), 4% as normorphine, and approximately 10% as morphine-6-glucuronide, which has twice the potency of morphine.[3] In this case, clearance of morphine and morphine-6-glucuronide was impaired because of the patient's renal insufficiency, resulting in severe respiratory depression and, ultimately, respiratory arrest.[4] Naloxone was given, successfully antagonizing the respiratory depression of morphine and morphine-6-glucuronide. However, the patient was transferred to a monitored care unit for close observation and the administration of a naloxone infusion because the half-life of naloxone is shorter than the half-life of morphine.

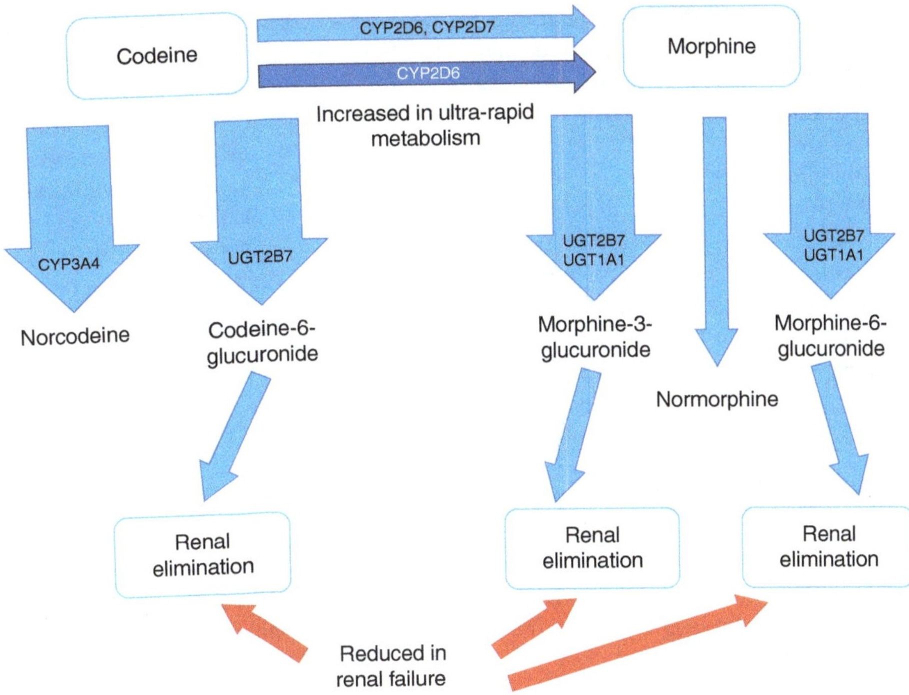

Fig. 63.1 Codeine metabolism pathways. Codeine is primarily metabolized by the enzyme CYP3A4 to norcodeine and by the UGT2B7 enzyme to codeine-6-glucuronide. Codeine is also metabolized, usually to a lesser extent, by the CYP2D6 and CYP2D7 enzymes to morphine. In individuals with ultra-rapid metabolism, the activity of the CYP2D6 enzyme is increased, which increases the conversion of codeine to morphine. After codeine is converted to morphine, morphine is metabolized to morphine-3-glucuronide and morphine-6-glucuronide by the enzyme UGT2B7 and, to a lesser extent, the enzyme UGT1A1. Morphine is also transformed to normorphine. The metabolites that have been glucuronidated are renally excreted, including codeine-6-glucuronide, morphine-3-glucuronide, and morphine-6-glucuronide. In renal failure or renal insufficiency, the elimination of these metabolites is reduced. Therefore, in patients with ultra-rapid metabolism and reduced renal function, levels of morphine and morphine-6-glucuronide, which may cause sedation and respiratory depression, are increased [Based on data from Ref. [5]]

Likely, this pharmacogenomic metabolic problem may be further compounded by other pharmacokinetic issues. Drugs that inhibit CYP34A may cause inhibition of a metabolic pathway of codeine also. In one case report, the use of the macrolide antibiotic clarithromycin in combination with the azole antifungal voriconazole resulted in 3A4 inhibition and prevented the conversion of codeine to norcodeine (Fig. 63.1).[5] This "perfect storm" caused by ultra-rapid 2D6 metabolism (preferential conversion to morphine), renal failure (inhibition of glucuronide metabolite excretion), and 3A4 inhibition resulted in a life-threatening codeine intoxication.

The frequency of the 2D6 ultrarapid metabolizer genotype is variable. In white persons, the frequency is low—from 1% to 5%—and depends on the geographic location of their ancestry. In Asian individuals, the frequency is even lower. By comparison, persons of Mediterranean, Saudi Arabian, and Ethiopian descent have greater frequencies of ultra-rapid metabolism, with almost one-third of individuals in Ethiopia having the ultra-rapid metabolizer genotype.[6] Of note, the opioid tramadol hydrochloride is also a prodrug metabolized through the CYP2D6 enzyme to an active metabolite, (+)-*O*-desmethyltramadol. Thus, individuals with the ultra-rapid metabolizer genotype are also at risk for toxicity with tramadol administration.[6] Patients from these geographic regions may require a heightened level of suspicion for the ultra-rapid metabolizer genotype, and it may be prudent to avoid the use of codeine or tramadol in these individuals.

Take-Home Points

- When administering a prodrug, health care providers should be aware that patients may experience less drug effect than expected (poor metabolism) versus greater effect or more adverse effects than expected (ultra-rapid metabolism).
- Toxicity, including respiratory depression, is possible for patients who are taking codeine or tramadol and possess the ultra-rapid metabolizer genotype.
- The frequency of the ultra-rapid metabolizer genotype varies on the basis of geographic location. When caring for patients from geographic locations with increased frequencies of this genotype, providers should give consideration to the use of alternatives to codeine or tramadol.
- Renal insufficiency or renal failure can lead to the accumulation of many drugs and, when combined with altered metabolism due to genetic variation, can become especially dangerous.

Summary

Interaction: pharmacogenomic (drug–gene)
Substrate: codeine
Enzyme: CYP2D6
Mechanism: ultra-rapid metabolism
Clinical effects: enhanced narcotic effects including somnolence and respiratory depression

References

1. Eichelbaum M, Evert B. Influence of pharmacogenetics on drug disposition and response. Clin Exp Pharmacol Physiol. 1996;23(10–11):983–5.
2. Kirchheiner J, Schmidt H, Tzvetkov M, et al. Pharmacokinetics of codeine and its metabolite morphine in ultra-rapid metabolizers due to CYP2D6 duplication. Pharmacogenomics J. 2007; 7(4):257–65.
3. Razaq M, Balicas M, Mankan N. Use of hydromorphone (Dilaudid) and morphine for patients with hepatic and renal impairment. Am J Ther. 2007;14(4):414–6.
4. Osborne R, Joel S, Grebenik K, et al. The pharmacokinetics of morphine and morphine glucuronides in kidney failure. Clin Pharmacol Ther. 1993;54(2):158–67.
5. Gasche Y, Daali Y, Fathi M, et al. Codeine intoxication associated with ultrarapid CYP2D6 metabolism. N Engl J Med. 2004;351(27):2827–31. Erratum in: N Engl J Med. 2005;352(6):638.
6. Stamer UM, Stuber F, Muders T, et al. Respiratory depression with tramadol in a patient with renal impairment and CYP2D6 gene duplication. Anesth Analg. 2008;107(3):926–9.

Drug–Drug Interactions Involving Nonopioid Pain Medications

VIII

Introduction

64

Toby N. Weingarten MD

Abstract
This section introduces drug–drug interactions involving nonopioid pain medications.

The armamentarium of analgesic medications is not limited to opioids, but consists of a wide variety of drugs including nonsteroidal antiinflammatory drugs (NSAIDs), acetaminophen, muscle relaxants, ergot alkaloids, antidepressants, and anticonvulsants. Complicating the situation for the pain practitioner is the reality that pharmacotherapy for many patients with chronic debilitating pain very often consists of multiple drugs, which increases the risk for drug–drug interactions (DDIs). The presence of significant psychiatric comorbidities in this most deserving, yet often clinically challenging, cohort of patients mandates a constant vigilance against DDIs.

Unfortunately for both the patient and the practitioner, DDIs involving the nonopioid pain medications have a high degree of clinical acuity and can be fatal. This is reflected by the number of non-opioid pain medications that appear on the **Fatal Forty**[1]—namely, NSAIDs, cyclobenzaprine, carbamazepine, and tricyclic antidepressants.

The best way to start the process of weeding through the thicket of possible non-opioid DDIs is to acquire a working knowledge of the cytochrome P450 (CYP) 2D6 enzyme. Next, the tricyclic antidepressants—amitriptyline, nortriptyline, desipramine, imipramine and others—are a good jumping-off point into this material. They all act as CYP2D6 substrates, some preferentially. Although intentional overdoses with tricyclic antidepressants have become less common in clinical practice, these antidepressants are still an important source of serious or fatal arrhythmias, especially when used in conjunction with other medications.

[1] The Forty Drugs You Must Know To Keep Your Patients and Yourself Safe from Harm

T.N. Weingarten MD
Department of Anesthesiology, Mayo Clinic College of Medicine, Rochester, MN, USA

Department of Anesthesiology, Mayo Clinic, Rochester, MN, USA
e-mail: Weingarten.toby@mayo.edu

C. Marcucci et al. (eds.), *A Case Approach to Perioperative Drug-Drug Interactions*, DOI 10.1007/978-1-4614-7495-1_64

Next, we would recommend giving attention to the NSAIDs. These are ubiquitous medications in the acute and chronic pain populations and, really, in the general population as well. Since NSAIDS are available over the counter, patients may not disclose their regular use. However, they are often not benign. NSAID–induced gastropathies result in tens of thousands of hospitalizations and countless deaths per year. The cardiovascular and renal toxicities secondary to NSAIDs harm thousands more annually. What is less appreciated is the potential for serious drug–NSAID interactions.

For example, NSAIDs when administered with phenytoin can result in significant phenytoin toxicity. Similarly, acetaminophen, also ubiquitous in clinical practice, is often overlooked as it is formulated with opioid analgesics as well as over the counter cough, cold, fever, and headache remedies. However, its potential to induce life-threatening hepatotoxicity cannot be ignored.

A representative array of clinical cases is presented in this section to remind the reader, that although nonopioid analgesics may have higher therapeutic indices than narcotics, one must always be mindful that they can produce DDIs that range from unpleasant to lethal.

Pining for Pete in the Pain Clinic

65

Fatal Forty DDI: nortriptyline, paroxetine, CYP2D6

Steven S. Liu MD, Toby N. Weingarten MD, and Catherine Marcucci MD

Abstract
This case discusses the interaction of nortriptyline and paroxetine. Nortriptyline is a tricyclic antidepressant (TCA) that is a cytochrome P450 2D6 substrate and paroxetine is a 2D6 inhibitor. The interaction resulted in TCA toxicity. The metabolism of other TCAs is discussed.

Case

A 59-year-old woman with chronic neuropathic pain associated with postherpetic neuralgia reported to the pain clinic for a regular visit. She had been on a 4-year stable regimen of oral nortriptyline, (100 mg taken at night). Her neuropathic pain was well controlled, but over the past month she noticed frequent palpitations, dizziness, and dry mouth. Her physical exam was remarkable for mydriasis and decreased bowel sounds. On further questioning, she began to weep and stated that she had been struggling with several months of severe grief because her beloved companion dog Pete was struck and killed by a car. She was worried she was becoming depressed and 6 weeks ago sought treatment from a psychiatrist. The

S.S. Liu MD (✉)
Department of Anesthesiology and Critical Care, University of Pennsylvania, Philadelphia, PA, USA

T.N. Weingarten MD
Department of Anesthesiology, Mayo Clinic, Rochester, MN, USA

Department of Anesthesiology, Mayo Clinic College of Medicine, Rochester, MN, USA

C. Marcucci MD
Department of Anesthesiology, Mayo Clinic College of Medicine, Rochester, MN, USA
e-mail: sandson.marcucci@comcast.net

C. Marcucci et al. (eds.), *A Case Approach to Perioperative Drug-Drug Interactions*, DOI 10.1007/978-1-4614-7495-1_65

psychiatrist diagnosed an adjustment disorder and initiated had recently started her on oral paroxetine (20 mg). An electrocardiogram was obtained in the office and was notable for sinus tachycardia with a heart rate of 135 beats per minute. A phone call was immediately placed to the psychiatrist's office.

Discussion

This is an example of an inhibitor added to a substrate.

The interaction between nortriptyline and paroxetine is a recognized and clinically significant drug–drug interaction (DDI).[1]

Nortriptyline is a tricyclic antidepressant (TCA) approved for use of the treatment of symptoms of depression. However, in contemporary practice it is often used to treat neuropathic pain, postherpetic neuralgia, fibromyalgia, anxiety, and enuresis. Nortriptyline is a secondary amine TCA (along with desipramine and protriptyline). Nortriptyline undergoes hepatic metabolism primarily by hydroxylation by the cytochrome P450 (CYP) 2D6 isoenzyme and to a lesser extent by demethylation by the CYP3A4, 2C19, and 1A2 isoenzymes.[2] CYP2D6 is believed to be responsible for 90% of nortriptyline metabolism.[3] Typical side effects of TCA relate to their anticholinergic actions including dryness of the mouth and drowsiness.[4] Toxicity from nortriptyline and other TCA drugs can manifest as more severe anticholinergic effects including tachycardia, hyperpyrexia, tremors, convulsions and death.[4]

Paroxetine is a selective serotonin reuptake inhibitor (SSRI) used in the treatment of depression, social anxiety, and post-traumatic stress disorder. It is one of the most potent competitive 2D6 inhibitors of clinically used SSRIs.[5,6] The pharmacokinetic DDI between nortriptyline and paroxetine is recognized. Briefly, the addition of paroxetine represented a disruption of the metabolic equilibrium of nortriptyline. Although the case does not specify an increase in nortriptyline blood levels, up to a four-fold increase would be possible in such a scenario. Hence, this patient presented with a state of mild TCA toxicity.

This case also demonstrates the multiple problems faced by pain practitioners prescribing tricyclic antidepressants. All TCAs are at least partial substrates of 2D6[7] (Table 65.1). The tertiary amine TCAs (imipramine, clomipramine, and amitriptyline) also undergo differential metabolism by the enzymes CYP3A4, 2C19, and 1A2, depending on the individual TCA in question. This mandates an awareness of the inhibitors of each of the enzymes. Many patients with chronic pain also suffer from major depression and other psychiatric illnesses. Much like intensive care physicians, chronic pain physicians must carefully choose and prescribe in a complicated pharmacologic milieu. Even so, as in this case, the most careful prescriber can get tripped up by the other practitioner. Robust and continuous education by the pain practitioner of himself and the patient, and ongoing communication with the

Table 65.1 Cytochrome P450s of primary importance for the metabolism of antidepressant and neurologic drugs: a schematic presentation

Cytochrome P450	Antidepressants	Neuroleptics
CYP1A2	Fluvoxamine	Clozapine
		Olanzapine
CYP2C19	Amitriptyline	
	Citalopram	
	Clomipramine	
	Moclobemide	
CYP2D6	Amitriptyline	Haloperidol
	Clomipramine	Perphenazine
	Desipramine	Risperidone
	Fluoxetine	Thioridazine
	Imipramine	
	Mianserin	
	Mirtazapine	
	Nortriptyline	
	Paroxetine	
	Venlafaxine	
CYP3A4/5	Mirtazapine	Haloperidol[a]
	Reboxetine	Minor enzyme(s) for most neuroleptics
	Minor enzyme(s) for most antidepressants	

[a]CYP3A4/5 is only important at high haloperidol doses
[Reprinted from Bertilsson L. Metabolism of antidepressant and neuroleptic drugs by cytochrome p450s: clinical and interethnic aspects. *Clin Pharmacol Ther.* 2007;82:606-9. With permission from Nature Publishing Group]

other prescribing physicians is imperative. A better choice by the psychiatrist, given the preexisting stable efficacy of the nortriptyline and the patient's symptoms was an antidepressant with less inhibition of CYP2D6, such as citalopram or venlafaxine (neither of which is a potent CYP2D6 inhibitor).

Take-Home Points

- All tricyclic antidepressants are at least partially metabolized by CYP2D6.
- Nortriptyline, as a secondary amine TCA, is preferentially a 2D6 substrate.
- Paroxetine is a strong competitive 2D6 inhibitor.
- This recognized DDI will produce up to fourfold increases in nortriptyline levels and clinical TCA toxicity.

Summary

Interaction: pharmacokinetic
Substrate: nortriptyline
Inhibitor: paroxetine
Enzyme: CYP2D6
Clinical effect: quinidine-like effects on cardiac conduction from nortriptyline toxicity

References

1. Leucht S, Hackl HJ, Steimer W, et al. Effect of adjunctive paroxetine on serum levels and side-effects of tricyclic antidepressants in depressive inpatients. Psychopharmacology (Berl). 2000;147(4):378–83.
2. Venkatakrishnan K, von Moltke LL, Greenblatt DJ. Nortriptyline E-10-hydroxylation in vitro is mediated by human CYP2D6 (high affinity) and CYP3A4 (low affinity): implications for interactions with enzyme-inducing drugs. J Clin Pharmacol. 1999;39(6):567–77.
3. Olesen OV, Linnet K. Hydroxylation and demethylation of the tricyclic antidepressant nortriptyline by cDNA-expressed human cytochrome P-450 isozymes. Drug Metab Dispos. 1997;25:740–4.
4. A new antidepressant of the tricyclic group: nortriptyline hydrochloride (aventyl hydrochloride). JAMA. 1965;194:727–8.
5. Crewe HK, Lennard MS, Tucker GT, et al. The effect of selective serotonin re-uptake inhibitors on cytochrome P4502D6 (CYP2D6) activity in human liver microsomes. Br J Clin Pharmacol. 1992;34:262–5.
6. von Moltke LL, Greenblatt DJ, Court MH, et al. Inhibition of alprazolam and desipramine hydroxylation in vitro by paroxetine and fluvoxamine: comparison with other selective serotonin reuptake inhibitor antidepressants. J Clin Psychopharmacol. 1995;15(2):125–31.
7. Bertilsson L. Metabolism of antidepressant and neuroleptic drugs by cytochrome p450s: clinical and interethnic aspects. Clin Pharmacol Ther. 2007;82:606–9.

You Do Not Look Well Today, Mon Ami

66

Fatal Forty DDI: amitriptyline, amiodarone, QRS widening

Kimberly Mauer MD, Catherine Marcucci MD, and Neil B. Sandson MD

Abstract
This case discusses pharmacokinetic and pharmacodynamic interactions between amitriptyline and amiodarone, resulting in QRS widening.

Case

A 62-year-old man presented to the operating room for a microvascular trigeminal nerve decompression. He suffered greatly from right-sided V2 distribution trigeminal neuralgia and had failed conservative management with a 6-month course of amitriptyline (100 mg per night) and numerous peripheral nerve blocks. He had also failed previous trials of carbamazepine, oxcarbazepine, topiramate, phenytoin, and gabapentin.

K. Mauer MD (✉)
Department of Anesthesiology & Perioperative Medicine, Oregon Health and Science University, Portland, OR, USA
e-mail: mauer@ohsu.edu

C. Marcucci MD
Anesthesia Services Department, Philadelphia Veterans Affairs Medical Center, Philadelphia, PA, USA

N.B. Sandson MD
Department of Psychiatry, University of Maryland Medical System, Baltimore, MD, USA

Department of Psychiatry, VA Maryland Health Care System, Baltimore, MD, USA

C. Marcucci et al. (eds.), *A Case Approach to Perioperative Drug-Drug Interactions*, DOI 10.1007/978-1-4614-7495-1_66

A brief, nonsustained burst of ventricular fibrillation was noted right after induction of anesthesia and the surgery was cancelled. Amiodarone(150 mg) was given intravenously (IV) in the operating room and the patient was admitted to the intensive care unit postoperatively. He received amiodarone(360 mg) over the next 6 hours and 540 mg in the remaining 18 hours to complete his dosing schedule. However, the patient continued to have infrequent but persistent runs of ventricular fibrillation. Each episode was appropriately controlled with further IV dosing of amiodarone. The Cardiology service was consulted and he was discharged home after two "arrhythmia-free" days with an oral loading dose of amiodarone (800 mg daily for 1-3 weeks). He was then to reduce his dose to 400 mg daily for the next month.

The patient's trigeminal neuralgia pain continued unabated and the patient continued taking his usual dose of amitriptyline. One week after returning home, his partner noticed that his pupils appeared dilated and he seemed unusually listless and restless. The patient admitted to his partner that he had had difficulty urinating for the last 24 hours, who took him immediately to the emergency department. His electrocardiogram was notable for widened QRS complexes and he was admitted to the Coronary Care Unit.

Discussion

This is a mixed example of both a pharmacodynamic interaction and also a pharmacokinetic interaction in which an inhibitor is added to a substrate.

Tricyclic antidepressants (TCAs) are particularly important drugs with regard to drug–drug interactions (DDIs). They have a low therapeutic index by virtue of their quinidine-like effects on cardiac conduction. Additionally, they are quite susceptible to being "victims" in DDIs. These traits explain why TCAs are included in the **Fatal Forty**.

The pharmacodynamic dimension of this interaction is straightforward. Both amitriptyline and amiodarone exert effects in cardiac conduction. When coadministered, these agents can produce synergistic QT prolongation which can progress to potentially fatal arrhythmias such as torsades de pointes or even ventricular fibrillation.[1,2]

In terms of the pharmacokinetic interaction, amitriptyline, as a tertiary amine TCA, undergoes both hydroxylation by cytochrome P450 (CYP) enzyme 2D6 and also demethylation by CYP2C19, 3A4, and 1A2.[3,4] The latter process actually catalyzes the hepatic conversion of amitriptyline into nortriptyline. Amiodarone is basically a paninhibitor, and accordingly inhibits the activity of these enzymes.[2,5] As a result, the addition of amiodarone to the patient's regimen elevated amitriptyline levels, further increasing the arrhythmogenic potential of this drug combination. The patient's difficulty in micturition is due to the enhanced anticholinergic effects from elevated amitriptyline levels.

Take-Home Points

- Tricyclic antidepressants are used in a variety of neuropsychiatric conditions including chronic pain and are worthy of attention whenever they appear in a medication list.
- Tricyclic antidepressants have a low therapeutic index and have quinidine-like effects on cardiac conduction.
- Amitriptyline is a substrate of 2C19, 3A4, and 1A2.
- Amiodarone is a paninhibitor.

Summary

Interaction 1: pharmacodynamic
Substrates: amitriptyline and amiodarone
Site of action/mechanism: synergistic arrhythmogenic effects on cardiac conduction
Clinical effect: cardiac arrhythmias

Interaction 2: pharmacokinetic (so obviously dumb that not enough folks have done it to produce an extensive literature of reported cases)
Substrate: amitriptyline
Inhibitor: amiodarone
Enzymes: CYP2D6, 1A2, 3A4
Clinical effect: elevated amitriptyline levels and thus greater arrhythmia risk

References
1. Amitriptyline Package Insert: Sandoz Inc., Princeton, NJ 08540. Revised Apr 2010.
2. Amiodarone Package Insert: Taro Pharmaceuticals U.S.A., Inc. Hawthorne, NY 10532.
3. Leucht S, Hackl HJ, Steimer W, et al. Effect of adjunctive paroxetine on serum levels and side-effects of tricyclic antidepressants in depressive inpatients. Psychopharmacology (Berl). 2000;147(4):378–83.
4. Venkatakrishnan K, Greenblatt DJ, von Moltke LL, et al. Five distinct human cytochromes mediate amitriptyline N-demethylation in vitro: dominance of CYP 2C19 and 3A4. J Clin Pharmacol. 1998;38(2):112–21.
5. Yamreudeewong W, DeBisschop M, Martin LG, et al. Potentially significant drug interactions of class III antiarrhythmic drugs. Drug Saf. 2003;26(6):421–38.

My Headache Is Gone, But My Leg Now Hurts

67

Fatal Forty DDI: methysergide, erythromycin, CYP3A4

Jessica D. Lorenz MD, Juraj Sprung MD, PhD, and Wayne T. Nicholson MD, PharmD, MSc

Abstract
This case discusses the pharmacokinetic interaction between methysergide and erythromycin resulting in vasospasm. Methysergide is a cytochrome P450 3A4 substrate and erythromycin is a 3A4 inhibitor.

Case

A 60-year-old woman presented to a hospital multidisciplinary pain clinic for evaluation of migraine headaches and cluster headaches. She complained also of sinus pain precipitated by multiple episodes of acute and chronic sinusitis. She resided both in Europe and the United States and stated that she obtained medical care and medications "on both sides of the Atlantic, but not penicillin, I'm deathly allergic," as she travelled back and forth frequently and was a dual citizen. She requested a refill of methysergide as she felt that ameliorated her migraine symptoms most effectively. She was frustrated to learn it was not available in the United States but stated that she had a large stockpile in Europe and she would continue to get it there.

J.D. Lorenz MD (✉) • J. Sprung MD, PhD • W.T. Nicholson MD, PharmD, MSc
Department of Anesthesiology, Mayo Clinic, Rochester, MN, USA
e-mail: Lorenz.jessica@mayo.edu

C. Marcucci et al. (eds.), *A Case Approach to Perioperative Drug-Drug Interactions*, DOI 10.1007/978-1-4614-7495-1_67

On a return visit, the patient reported continued use of methysergide for frequent migraines and a recent prolonged bout of sinusitis that caused great pain and required a 10-day course of erythromycin. She stated that her migraine and sinus pain were quiet that day, but "now I seem to be a leg pain patient." Examination showed a cold, pale foot with no appreciable capillary refill. Posterior tibial and dorsalis pedis pulses were neither palpable nor detectable with a Doppler examination. She received an angiogram, which showed vasospasm of the right popliteal artery. She was treated with intra-arterial vasodilator therapy, and blood flow was restored to the foot.

Discussion

This is an example of an inhibitor added to a substrate.

More specifically, it is an example an inhibitor of the cytochrome P450 (CYP) isozyme 3A (erythromycin) added to a substrate (methysergide), leading to methysergide toxicity.

The serotonin 5-hydroxytryptamine (5-HT) receptors are present in the central and peripheral nervous system and mediate both excitatory and inhibitory neurotransmission. The contemporary migraine-specific drugs all act as agonists at certain subclasses of serotonin 5-HT receptors. The pharmacology of ergot alkaloids is complex and effects differ depending on the drug. Methysergide is used prophylactically in the treatment of migraine headaches.[1] Methysergide is an antagonist of several receptors including 5-HT_{2A}, 5-HT_{2B}, 5-HT_{2C}, and an agonist of the 5-HT_{1B} receptor and, possibly, the 5-HT_{1D} receptor.[2]

In vitro studies suggest that methysergide contracts arteries, possibly through 5-HT_{1B} receptors. In addition, antagonism of the 5-HT_{2B} and 5-HT_{2C} receptors leads to increased levels of neuropeptide Y with acute drug administration and increased levels of neuropeptide Y mRNA with long-term drug administration. Neuropeptide Y, a vasoconstrictor found in some sympathetic nerves, blocks neurogenic inflammation.[2] In addition to these serotonergic effects, peripheral vasoconstriction may be due in part to partial agonist or antagonist effects at adrenergic and dopaminergic receptors.[3] In a more complete review, Silberstein discusses the pharmacology of methysergide and its metabolite for migraine therapy.[2]

Methysergide is only one of the ergot alkaloids employed in the therapy of migraine headaches. Other agents used for migraine include ergotamine and dihydroergotamine. Methysergide is metabolized into its active metabolite methylergometrine (also known as methylergonovine) and this ergot derivative is also a potent vasoconstrictor.[2] Although methylergometrine (methylergonovine) is also available for therapeutic use, it is used more commonly for the management of postpartum hemorrhage rather than for migraine.

Methysergide extensively undergoes hepatic first-pass metabolism.[2] Animal studies indicate that CYP3A is involved with the biotransformation of ergotamine and other ergot alkaloids.[4] By comparison, erythromycin, a macrolide antibiotic, is a potent inhibitor of CYP3A. It inhibits both the intestinal and hepatic CYP systems.[5] However, when concomitantly administered with methysergide, erythromycin reduces the metabolism of both methysergide and methylergometrine, leading to an increase in their plasma concentrations. In addition, erythromycin is a potent inhibitor of P-glycoprotein. Therefore, caution should be exercised when it is used simultaneously with drugs that depend on the P-glycoprotein transport system.

Accumulation of methysergide, methylergometrine, and other ergot alkaloids can result in symptoms similar to those seen in ergotism. In the Middle Ages, ergotism causing painful burning sensations and blackened limbs was referred to as *Holy fire* or *St. Anthony's fire.*[3,6] Ergot alkaloids responsible are produced by the fungus *Claviceps purpurea* and historically epidemics of ergotism occurred when rye grain became infected with this fungus. Ergot toxicity can present with central nervous system effects (eg, hallucinations, psychosis), in addition to vasospastic ischemia that may lead to gangrene.

Due to the high first-pass metabolism of ergot compounds, vasoconstriction may also present when one of these compounds metabolism is inhibited. Ergotism has been demonstrated with ergotamine and other potent CYP 3A inhibitors.[6–8] Before the advent of vasodilating medications, serious morbidity was reported with vasospastic ischemia, including myocardial infarction, abdominal angina with bowel infarction, and gangrene that necessitated limb amputation.[8–10] This interaction concern is clearly demonstrated by product *black box warnings* about ergot derivatives and concomitant CYP3A inhibitor use.[11]

Methysergide therapy is also associated with other adverse effects, such as retroperitoneal and pleuropulmonary fibrosis and fibrosis of the cardiac valves and mesenteric arteries. Because of these adverse effects, the use of methysergide was discontinued in the United States in 2002, but it is used therapeutically outside the United States. Although residents in the United States are unlikely to be using methysergide, visitors from other countries may present for evaluation in a US hospital or clinic while taking it. However since ergotamine and dihydroergotamine are prescribed for migraine therapy, there is a potential for US physicians to encounter vasospastic ischemia when patients use ergot derivatives with CYP3A inhibitors such as erythromycin.

Take-Home Points

- Methysergide and its active metabolite, methylergometrine, and other ergot alkaloids are metabolized by the 3A class of cytochrome P450 enzymes.
- Erythromycin and other potent CYP3A inhibitors reduce metabolism. This inhibition may decrease the metabolism of ergot alkaloids leading to toxicity.
- Vasospastic ischemia may result from inhibition of metabolism, potentially resulting in coronary ischemia, small bowel infarction, or peripheral limb ischemia.
- Although the use of methysergide was discontinued in the United States in 2002, people visiting the United States from other countries may be taking this medication. Additionally, other ergot alkaloids (eg, ergotamine and dihydroergotamine) are available in the United States.
- Due to the potential of vasospastic ischemia, potent CYP3A inhibitors are contraindicated with ergot alkaloid therapy.

Summary

Interaction: pharmacokinetic
Substrate: methysergide
Enzyme: CYP3A4
Inhibitor: erythromycin
Clinical effect: methysergide toxicity manifesting as vasospasm

References

1. Koehler PJ, Tfelt-Hansen PC. History of methysergide in migraine. Cephalalgia. 2008;28:1126–35.
2. Silberstein SD. Methysergide. Cephalalgia. 1998;18:421–35.
3. Dam AK, Mishra JC. Managing ergot-induced gangrene: the anesthesiologist as a key player. Anesth Analg. 2002;95(2):409–10.
4. Moubarak AS, Rosenkrans Jr CF. Hepatic metabolism of ergot alkaloids in beef cattle by cytochrome P450. Biochem Biophys Res Commun. 2000;274(3):746–9.
5. Eadie MJ. Clinically significant drug interactions with agents specific for migraine attacks. CNS Drugs. 2001;15:105–18.
6. Fröhlich G, Kaplan V, Amann-Vesti B. Holy fire in an HIV-positive man: a case of 21st-century ergotism. CMAJ. 2010;182(4):378–80.
7. Mortier E, Pouchot J, Vinceneux P, et al. Ergotism related to interaction between nelfinavir and ergotamine. Am J Med. 2001;110(7):594.
8. Horowitz RS, Dart RC, Gomez HF. Clinical ergotism with lingual ischemia induced by clarithromycin-ergotamine interaction. Arch Intern Med. 1996;156:456–8.

9. Vaughan-Lane T. Gangrene induced by methysergide and ergotamine: a case report. J Bone Joint Surg Br. 1979;61-B:213–4.
10. Menzies KE, Isbister WH. Gangrene of the small bowel: a complication of methysergide therapy. Aust N Z J Surg. 1982;52:510–1.
11. D.H.E. 45® *(dihydroergotamine mesylate)* Injection, USP: Product information, Novartis Pharmaceuticals Corporation, East Hanover, New Jersey, 31 July 2002.

Special 'K'ase

Oral S-ketamine, ticlopidine

68

Lisa Chan MD and Kirk Lalwani MD, FRCA, MCR

Abstract
This case discusses the pharmacokinetic interaction between oral S-ketamine and ticlopidine resulting in enhanced ketamine effects. Ketamine is a cytochrome P450 2B6 substrate and ticlopidine is a 2B6 inhibitor.

Case

The first case of the day was an arthroscopic meniscectomy for a patient listed only as "Dr. K." He was a 58-year-old anesthesia attending at that institution who had been in a motor vehicle accident resulting in a series of orthopedic reconstructions to his lower limb, complicated by a perioperative myocardial infarction for which he had subsequently received a drug-eluting stent.

The anesthesiologist, who of course was also Dr. K.'s colleague and friend, saw Dr. K. in the preoperative area to make sure he had stopped his ticlopidine a week in advance and would restart it postoperatively. Dr. K. then quietly confided that he had been taking oral ketamine for his knee pain, prescribed by a pain specialist he had seen while on a trip outside the United States, and that he had doubled the dose in the last several days due to severe pain. He was anxiously hoping that this procedure "would be the end of the issues" and he would suffer less pain. He asked his friend for "confidentiality" in the matter and judicious use of a "balanced" anesthetic during the procedure.

L. Chan MD (✉)
Department of Pediatric Cardiac Anesthesiology, Memorial Regional Hospital, Hollywood, FL, USA
e-mail: lisaychan@gmail.com

K. Lalwani MD, FRCA, MCR
Department of Anesthesiology & Perioperative Medicine, Oregon Health and Science University, Portland, OR, USA

C. Marcucci et al. (eds.), *A Case Approach to Perioperative Drug-Drug Interactions*, DOI 10.1007/978-1-4614-7495-1_68

The anesthesiologist was on call a few days nights later when he got a call from the Emergency Department (ED) physician. The ED doctor reported that Dr. K. had been brought in for somnolence and "crazy talk." Mrs. K was in tears and reported that her husband had been in pain and acting strangely at dinner after picking apples with the grandchildren and had taken a dose of hydrocodone after dinner. Worried about accusations of narcotic overuse, she brought along the bottle of hydrocodone. It was nearly full.

The anesthesiologist then realized that his friend had experienced increased pain the week prior to surgery because the preoperative cessation of ticlopidine was no longer potentiating the effects of his oral ketamine, leading him to increase the dose. After returning home from surgery, he had restarted this higher dose of ketamine, supplemented by hydrocodone for postoperative pain relief. When he then resumed his ticlopidine, he experienced ketamine's adverse effects of somnolence and hallucinations.

Discussion

This is an example of an inhibitor added to a substrate.

Ketamine is a phencyclidine derivative, and is used as a general (dissociative) anesthetic agent, or as a sedative–analgesic at subanesthetic doses.[1] Ketamine is thought to exert its analgesic effect by antagonizing *N*-methyl-D-aspartate (NMDA) receptors.[2] These receptors are thought to be instrumental in the pathogenesis of chronic pain, particularly neuropathic pain for which ketamine has been beneficial.[3] Ketamine is commercially available in the United States as a 1:1 racemic mixture, and in addition as a S-ketamine isomer in Europe. The purer S-ketamine form is believed to be two to four times more potent than the racemic mixture and possibly has a safer side-effect profile by reducing adverse central nervous system (CNS) effects such as somnolence, hallucinations, dissociative feelings, and blurred vision.[4,5]

Ketamine is demethylated into the metabolite norketamine by the cytochrome P450 system (CYP) 3A4 and 2B6 enzymes.[5] Norketamine is pharmacologically active, it is one-third as potent as ketamine and norketamine may contribute to the overall analgesic effect.[6] Oral administration provides the highest level of norketamine.[7] Synergistic and additive effects have been described when ketamine is used with other forms of pain medications that act via different receptors such as opioids and local anesthetics, providing "balanced" analgesia.[8]

Most clinical data about ketamine is descriptive (ie, case reports, case series) rather than controlled studies. One of the few randomized, blinded studies in humans has shown that ticlopidine, which is a CYP2B6 inhibitor, greatly decreases the metabolism of ketamine.[9] In light of this finding, it is prudent to prescribe a decreased dose of ticlopidine when coprescribing ketamine. Unexpectedly, this same study on ticlopidine also found that itraconazole, a CYP3A4 inhibitor, did not change the metabolism of ketamine, while clarithromycin, another 3A4 inhibitor, did decrease its metabolism.[10] The reason is unknown. There are other drugs metabolized by the same enzymes such as bupropion and methadone. The prudent approach to a drug with similar metabolism as ketamine is to start at a low dose and titrate to effect, keeping in mind that addition of other drugs may change its pharmacodynamic profile.

Take-Home Points

- Ketamine is a phencyclidine derivative used for anesthesia and sedation-analgesia. It is a NMDA receptor antagonist, and is available in two forms: racemic, and S-isomer (available in Europe), with the S-isomer more potent and exhibiting a safer side-effect profile. The cytochrome P450 (CYP) enzymes 3A4 and 2B6 metabolize ketamine into a pharmacologically active metabolite, norketamine. Ketamine works synergistically with narcotics and local anesthetics to accentuate analgesia. Of all routes of administration, oral ketamine has the most analgesia and longest duration due to its highest level of norketamine.

- Ticlopidine is a potent inhibitor of 3A4 and 2B6 enzymes. Therefore, when prescribing ticlopidine for its antiplatelet effect, it may be prudent to start with a lower dose of ketamine.

- Enzyme inducers such as rifampicin and St. John's wort (CYP3A4) have been shown to accelerate the elimination of S-ketamine and S-norketamine from the central compartment, leading to reduced plasma concentrations and therapeutic effect.[9,10]

- Not all inhibitors of the 3A4 and 2B6 enzymes follow the predicted pharmacodynamic profile; some seem to have no effect. Therefore, the cautious approach to a drug with metabolism similar to ketamine is to start at a low dose and titrate to effect, keeping in mind that the addition of other drugs may change its pharmacodynamic profile.

Summary

Interaction: pharmacokinetic
Substrate: oral S-ketamine
Enzyme: CYP2B6
Inhibitor: ticlopidine
Clinical effects: enhanced dissociative and somnolent effects of ketamine

References

1. Visser E, Schug SA. The role of ketamine in pain management. Biomed Pharmacother. 2006;60:341–8.
2. Fisher K, Coderre TJ, Hagen NA. Targeting the N-methyl-D-aspartate receptor for chronic pain management. Preclinical animal studies, recent clinical experience and future research directions. J Pain Symptom Manage. 2000;20:358–73.
3. Eide PK. Wind-up and the NMDA receptor complex from a clinical perspective. Eur J Pain. 2000;4:5–15.
4. Arendt-Nielsen L, Nielsen J, Petersen-Felix S, et al. Effect of racemic mixture and the (S+)-isomer of ketamine on temporal and spatial summation of pain. Br J Anaesth. 1996;77:625–31.
5. White PF, Way WL, Trevor AJ. Ketamine – its pharmacology and therapeutic uses. Anesthesiology. 1982;56:119–36.
6. Noppers I, Olofsen E, Niesters M, et al. Effect of rifampicin on S-ketamine and S-norketamine plasma concentrations in healthy volunteers after intravenous S-ketamine administration. Anesthesiology. 2011;114(6):1435–45.
7. Grant IS, Nimmo WS, Clements JA. Pharmacokinetics and analgesic effects of IM and oral ketamine. Br J Anaesth. 1981;53:805–10.
8. Schmid RL, Sandler AN, Katz J. Use and efficacy of low-dose ketamine in the management of acute postoperative pain: a review of current techniques and outcomes. Pain. 1999;82:111–25. Peltoniemi MA, Saari TI, Hagelberg NM, et al. Exposure to oral S-ketamine is unaffected by itraconazole but greatly increased by ticlopidine. Clin Pharmacol Ther. 2011;90(2):296–302. doi: 10.1038/clpt.2011.140. Epub 2011 Jun 29.
9. Peltoniemi MA, Saari TI, Hagelberg NM, et al. St John's wort greatly decreases the plasma concentrations of oral S-ketamine. Fundam Clin Pharmacol. 2012;26(6):743–50. Epub 2011 Jun 2.
10. Hagelberg NM, Peltoniemi MA, Saari TI, et al. Clarithromycin, a potent inhibitor of CYP3A, greatly increases exposure to oral S-ketamine. Eur J Pain. 2010;14:625–9.

Not Manic About NSAIDS

69

Fatal Forty DDI: ketorolac, lithium, toxicity

Allen N. Gustin MD, FCCP and Michael J. Bishop MD

Abstract
This case discusses a pharmacokinetic interaction between lithium and ketorolac. Lithium is excreted by the kidneys and ketorolac is an inhibitor of renal excretion.

Case

A 62-year-old woman with chronic right knee and lower lumbar osteoarthritis presented to the operating room for a right total knee arthroplasty. Her past medical history included hypertension treated with a calcium channel antagonist, and bipolar disease treated with lithium. The patient was very concerned about postoperative pain, but refused an epidural, given her lumbar osteoarthritis. The anesthesiology team planned a femoral nerve catheter, intravenous (IV) nonsteroidal anti-inflammatory drugs (NSAIDs), and an opioid patient-controlled anesthesia (PCA).

A femoral nerve catheter was placed preoperatively. Intravenous ketorolac was given on induction of general anesthesia. After a prolonged operative procedure, the patient was slow to emerge from anesthesia. In the postanesthesia care unit (PACU), her pain was treated with a constant infusion of her femoral nerve catheter and an

A.N. Gustin MD, FCCP (✉)
Department of Anesthesia and Critical Care, University of Chicago Pritzker School of Medicine, Chicago, IL, USA
e-mail: agustin@dacc.uchicago.edu

M.J. Bishop MD
Department of Anesthesiology, University of Washington School of Medicine, Seattle, WA, USA

C. Marcucci et al. (eds.), *A Case Approach to Perioperative Drug-Drug Interactions*, DOI 10.1007/978-1-4614-7495-1_69

opioid PCA with hydromorphone. Despite this, her pain score was 10+ on a 10-point scale. The anesthesiologist in the PACU gave a bolus via the femoral nerve catheter, decreased the interval dosing of the PCA, and gave a second dose of IV ketorolac in the PACU (with a plan to continue the ketorolac for 48 hours). Her pain score decreased to a 5 and the patient appeared much more comfortable. Over the next 30 minutes, the patient became progressively more somnolent and then had a brief seizure. The patient received IV phenytoin and was transferred to the intensive care unit. Her workup revealed only a serum lithium level was found to be three times the normal therapeutic level (2.6 mEq/L). An osmotic diuretic was administered, and IV bicarbonate was started. The patient's lithium levels normalized 36 hours after discontinuation of the ketorolac with continuing supportive care, and the patient's mental status returned to baseline.

Discussion

This is an example of an inhibitor of renal excretion added to a substrate.

Patients on chronic lithium therapy have large stores of lithium in their body. Small changes in renal function, or changes in intravascular volume, can lead to dramatic changes in serum lithium concentrations. Thus, patients on chronic lithium therapy can be at risk for lithium toxicity in the perioperative period.

The therapeutic dosage of lithium ranges between 150 and 2700 mg/day, with therapeutic serum levels ranging between 0.6 and 1.2 mEq/L.[1] Lithium clearance is predominantly renal. Because of minimal protein binding, lithium is freely filtered at a rate dependent on glomerular filtration rate (GFR). Consequently, lithium dosing must be adjusted based on renal function. Individuals with chronic renal insufficiency must be closely monitored for lithium toxicity.[2] Reabsorption of lithium is increased, and toxicity is more likely, in patients who are hyponatremic or volume depleted. Also, medications that decrease GFR can cause increases of serum lithium levels quite quickly. The plasma elimination half-life of a single dose of lithium is from 12 to 27 hours, which varies with age. Lithium half-life increases to approximately 36 hours in the elderly and is believed to be secondary to decreased GFR.[1]

Three drug classes have been identified as potential precipitants of lithium toxicity in the perioperative period. There is a high variability of individual risks associated with these medications in patients:[2]

- Thiazide diuretics will increase excretion of sodium but will enhance reuptake of lithium ions in the kidney.[2]

- Angiotensin-converting enzyme (ACE) inhibitors and angiotensin II receptor blockers (ARBs) that reduce GFR and enhance the tubular reabsorption of lithium.[1]
- NSAIDs that reduce GFR and interrupt renal prostaglandin synthesis. All NSAIDs appear to raise lithium levels except for aspirin and sulindac (Clinoril).[1–6]

The clinical symptoms of lithium toxicity range from mild to severe:

- **Mild lithium toxicity:** Serum lithium concentrations will usually range between 1.2 and 1.5 mEq/L. Mild toxicity is reflected by sedation, nausea, skeletal muscle weakness, and changes on the ECG characterized by widening of the QRS complex. All of these factors can confuse anesthesiology providers in the perioperative period. Also, it is common for elderly patients (who excrete lithium slowly) to become confused, even in the presence of normal therapeutic plasma concentrations of this lithium.[1]
- **Moderate lithium toxicity:** Serum lithium concentrations will range between 1.6 and 2.5 mEq/L. Moderate lithium toxicity can include confusion, drowsiness, restlessness, unsteady gait, coarse tremor, dysarthria, skeletal muscle fasciculation, and vomiting. Atrioventricular heart block, hypotension, cardiac dysrhythmias, and seizures may occur when plasma concentrations of lithium are > 2 mEq per liter.[1]
- **Severe lithium toxicity:** Serum lithium concentrations will be > 2.5 mEq/liter. Symptoms include seizures, coma, and cardiovascular collapse. Patients with severe lithium toxicity can even develop a syndrome of irreversible lithium-effectuated neurotoxicity (SILENT) such as cognitive impairment, sensorimotor peripheral neuropathy, and cerebellar dysfunction.[1] Severe lithium toxicity is a medical emergency that may require aggressive treatment, including hemodialysis.[2] If renal function is adequate, increasing renal excretion of lithium can be accelerated by osmotic diuresis and IV administration of sodium bicarbonate.[1]

Treatment for lithium toxicity is based on clinical severity:

- The care for the patient with lithium toxicity is mainly supportive.
- Cases of mild to severe lithium toxicity may be managed with correction of hypovolemia (if present) and with removal of any medications that reduce GFR.
- Cases of severe toxicity may require hemodialysis.

Take-Home Points

- Lithium toxicity can mimic many of the postoperative symptoms that are associated with exposure to general anesthesia. These symptoms can be either gastrointestinal symptoms (nausea and vomiting) or neurological symptoms (tremors, lethargy, confusion). Thus, anesthesiologists should always keep a high level of suspicion for lithium toxicity during the perioperative period.
- Avoid introducing NSAIDS or ACE inhibitors to patients on chronic lithium therapy in the perioperative period. Anesthesiologists should avoid NSAIDs as adjuncts for postoperative pain in patients on chronic lithium therapy.
- Procedures involving the kidneys (nephrectomy, vascular procedures of the abdominal aorta) may cause changes in GFR, which puts patients on chronic lithium therapy at risk for lithium toxicity.
- Avoid prolonged periods of NPO status in patients on chronic lithium therapy as this alone could precipitate toxicity.
- Avoid hypovolemia in patients on chronic lithium therapy in the operating room.

Summary

Interaction: pharmacokinetic
Substrate (renal): lithium
Inhibitor (of renal excretion): ketorolac
Clinical effect: lithium toxicity

References

1. Stoelting RH. Pharmacology and physiology of anesthesia practice. 6th ed. Philadelphia: Lippincott Williams and Wilkins; 2006.
2. Finley PR, Peabody CA. Clinical relevance of drug interactions with lithium. Clin Pharmacokinet. 1995;29:172–91.
3. Phelan K, Mosholder AD, Lu S. Lithium interaction with the cyclooxygenase 2 inhibitors rofecoxib and celecoxib and other nonsteroidal anti-inflammatory drugs. J Clin Psychiatry. 2003;64:1328–34.
4. Johnson AG, Day RO. NSAID related adverse drug interactions with clinical relevance. An update. Int J Clin Pharmacol Ther. 1994;32(10):509–32.
5. Cold JA, Simpson MA, Augustin BG, et al. Increased lithium serum and red blood cell concentrations during ketorolac coadministration. J Clin Psychopharmacol. 1998;18(1):33–7.
6. Juurlink DN, Kopp A, Rochon PA, et al. Drug-induced lithium toxicity in the elderly: a population based study. J Am Geriatr Soc. 2004;52:794–8.

Keep It Capped!

Acetaminophen, ethanol

70

Christine M. Formea PharmD, BCPS
and Wayne T. Nicholson MD, PharmD, MSc

Abstract
This case discusses the pharmacokinetic interaction between acetaminophen and ethanol.

Case

A 58-year-old woman was seen in the preoperative clinic for 2 weeks before a scheduled total knee replacement. The nurse practitioner was alarmed by the patient's obvious jaundice and contacted the anesthesiologist. The patient reported that she had consumed a large quantity of extra-strength acetaminophen in the previous 2 days (15 g in 48 hours) for severe, intermittent, shooting pain that radiated down her left leg and had made standing and sitting difficult and painful. She complained of nausea as well and vomited in the clinic. She reluctantly admitted to a long history of heavy social drinking and admonished herself for not leaving the whiskey in the liquor cabinet. Preoperative laboratory values were consistent with acetaminophen-induced hepatotoxicity and the patient was admitted to the hospital.

Acetaminophen was immediately discontinued, the patient received *N*-acetylcysteine to treat acetaminophen overdose, and she was referred to the acute pain service to treat a newly diagnosed L1-L3 nerve root compression. The pain service anesthesiologist prescribed oxycodone to control her acute, severe pain and discussed the paramount importance of maintaining a daily acetaminophen dose of less than 4 g. She was referred to an alcohol addiction program. When the patient returned to the

C.M. Formea PharmD, BCPS (✉)
Pharmacy Research, Mayo Clinic, College of Medicine, Rochester, MN, USA
e-mail: Formea.Christine@mayo.edu

W.T. Nicholson MD, PharmD, MSc
Department of Anesthesiology, Mayo Clinic, Rochester, MN, USA

C. Marcucci et al. (eds.), *A Case Approach to Perioperative Drug-Drug Interactions*, DOI 10.1007/978-1-4614-7495-1_70

preoperative clinic a few months later for her elective total knee replacement surgery, she had been alcohol free for 10 weeks, her laboratory values had returned to baseline, and she had no further complications.

Discussion

This is an example of a substrate added to an inducer.

Acetaminophen is an over-the-counter drug commonly used for its antipyretic and analgesic properties. The maximum recommended therapeutic acetaminophen dose for adults is 4 g per day, which generally is well tolerated.[1] The cytochrome P450 (CYP) isozyme 2E1 is responsible for generating toxic *N*-acetyl-*p*-benzoquinone imine (NAPQI).[1] At recommended doses and in the presence of adequate physiologic glutathione, acetaminophen is 95% detoxified by glucuronidation and sulfation; 5% becomes a toxic NAPQI intermediate, which subsequently is inactivated by glutathione conjugation and finally is excreted in the urine as a thiol metabolite.[2]

In an acetaminophen overdose, glucuronidation and sulfation hepatic detoxification pathways become saturated, resulting in increased cytochrome P450 metabolism and enhanced production of NAPQI. Glutathione stores become depleted, causing reduced capacity to inactivate toxic NAPQI. Increased NAPQI generation, coupled with reduced NAPQI inactivation, results in characteristic hepatic centrilobular necrosis.[1,2]

The pattern of ethanol consumption (binge or long term), genetics, and total intake of ethanol can contribute to variability in alcoholic liver disease occurrence.[3] Ethanol is metabolized by oxidative pathways in the liver through ethanol dehydrogenase, cytochrome P450 enzymes, and catalase enzymes that form acetaldehyde, which negatively affects the oxidative metabolic ability of hepatocytes.[1,3] Long-term ethanol use induces CYP2E1, the isozyme also responsible for metabolizing drugs, including acetaminophen.

When acutely combined with acetaminophen, ethanol inhibits the oxidative metabolism of acetaminophen, thus preventing toxic NAPQI formation, and appears to decrease hepatotoxicity because of competitive inhibition.[3] Long-term ethanol use induces 2E1; however, increased toxicity of acetaminophen and increased production of toxic NAPQI are not usually seen with therapeutic doses.[4] This effect may be due to the inhibition of 2E1 by the ethanol. Therefore, long-term ethanol users who take an overdose of acetaminophen in the absence of acute use of ethanol may have increased vulnerability to hepatotoxicity because induced 2E1 increases production of NAPQI but no acute ethanol level is present to inhibit CYP2E1.[3,4]

The controversy continues on whether long-term ethanol users have an increased sensitivity to acetaminophen toxicity because of depleted hepatic stores of glutathione.[4] Health care providers should critically evaluate the timing of ethanol and acetaminophen consumption and their relationship to provide acetaminophen toxicity treatment if needed.[4]

Case reports and studies link acetaminophen hepatotoxicity potentiation to ethanol consumption.[5–7] In one case report, a 48-year-old patient with a 33-year history of ethanol use ingested 10 g of acetaminophen 2 days before hospital admission. After receiving treatment, the patient was discharged without further complications.[5] A 43-year-old patient with a history of ethanol use ingested 50 g of acetaminophen in 3 days before hospital admission. After resolution of renal and hepatic failure, the patient was discharged.[5]

In 10 healthy study volunteers, NAPQI formation was increased by 22% when a single oral treatment of acetaminophen (500 mg) was administered 8 hours after a 6-hour continuous intravenous infusion of ethanol.[6] When a group of long-term ethanol users received 2 g of acetaminophen, the group showed significantly lower plasma levels of glutathione compared with healthy volunteers, suggesting that long-term use of ethanol may result in low levels of glutathione and may be a risk factor for acetaminophen toxicity.[7]

Caution with this interaction was reaffirmed in a recent release by the US Food and Drug Administration.[8] Advisory committees recommended that the maximum safe dose may not be the same for all individuals. Some persons who take acetaminophen may have toxic effects at lower acetaminophen doses than others. Current information suggests that some individuals, such as those who use ethanol or have liver disease, may have increased sensitivity to the effects of the toxic metabolite because of increased production or a decreased ability of the liver to clear it from the body.

Take-Home Points

- Health care providers must be alert to patients with a history of ethanol use and be familiar with the potential complications and interactions of ethanol with prescription drugs, over-the-counter drugs, and dietary and herbal supplements.

- Health care providers must carefully collect a patient's history of use of over-the-counter drugs, because many patients do not believe that these agents can be harmful.

- All patients should be counseled that acetaminophen use should not exceed 4 g per day and that larger doses may cause severe hepatotoxicity.
- Long-term ethanol use may result in a reduction of protective hepatic glutathione, and thus even 4 g of acetaminophen per day may be excessive for some users.

Summary

Interaction: pharmacokinetic
Substrate: acetaminophen
Enzyme: CYP2E1
Inducer: ethanol
Clinical effect: increased production of hepatotoxic NAPQI metabolite

References

1. Graham GG, Scott KF, Day RO. Tolerability of paracetamol. Drug Saf. 2005;28:227–40.
2. Riordan SM, Williams R. Alcohol exposure and paracetamol-induced hepatotoxicity. Addict Biol. 2002;7:191–206.
3. Zakhari S, Li TK. Determinants of alcohol use and abuse: impact of quantity and frequency patterns on liver disease. Hepatology. 2007;46:2032–9.
4. Prescott LF. Paracetamol, alcohol and the liver. Br J Clin Pharmacol. 2000;49:291–301.
5. McClain CJ, Kromhout JP, Peterson FJ, et al. Potentiation of acetaminophen hepatotoxicity by alcohol. JAMA. 1980;244:251–3.
6. Thummel KE, Slattery JT, Ro H, et al. Ethanol and production of the hepatotoxic metabolite of acetaminophen in healthy adults. Clin Pharmacol Ther. 2000;67:591–9.
7. Lauterburg BH, Velez ME. Glutathione deficiency in alcoholics: risk factor for paracetamol hepatotoxicity. Gut. 1988;29:1153–7.
8. U. S. Food and Drug Administration [Internet]. Joint meeting of the Drug Safety and Risk Management Advisory Committee with the Anesthetic and Life Support Drugs Advisory Committee and the Nonprescription Drugs Advisory Committee: meeting announcement. Rockville: Department of Health and Human Services; June 29–30, 2009. Available from: http://www.fda.gov/AdvisoryCommittees/Calendar/ucm143083.htm. Last Accessed on 4 June 2012.

The ACE Is Not Always High

Fatal Forty DDI: ketorolac, lisinopril

71

Wayne T. Nicholson MD, PharmD, MSc

Abstract
This case discusses a pharmacodynamic interaction between ketorolac and lisinopril that resulted in acute renal failure.

Case

A 64-year-old woman weighing 51 kg underwent an uncomplicated general anesthetic for an abdominal hysterectomy. On her preoperative evaluation, she reported hypertension, well controlled with daily lisinopril (10 mg) and hydrochlorothiazide (25 mg) and her creatinine was noted to be 1.3 mg/dL. She had an uneventful intraoperative course under general anesthesia with propofol, fentanyl, and isoflurane.

Postoperatively, the patient was normotensive. She had mild nausea and one episode of vomiting that resolved with intravenous (IV) ondansetron hydrochloride (4 mg). She received a total of 10 mg of IV morphine sulfate and 30 mg of IV ketorolac tromethamine. The Acute Pain Service initiated morphine patient-controlled analgesia (PCA) and IV ketorolac (30 mg q6h) as needed. On the floor, the patient was mildly hypertensive and the surgical resident restarted her outpatient medications. Her pain was under good control overnight well with only one additional dose of ketorolac. Urine output decreased throughout the night, and, despite receiving maintenance hydration, the patient had minimal urine output (<30 mL/h) the following morning.

Routine follow-up labs showed an increase in creatinine to 2.9 mg/dL. The ketorolac, lisinopril, hydrochlorothiazide, and morphine were discontinued immediately and the patient's PCA was changed to fentanyl. The patient's serum creatinine value peaked at 4.6 mg/dL early the following day. Over the next 3 days, the patient was

W.T. Nicholson MD, PharmD, MSc
Department of Anesthesiology, Mayo Clinic, Rochester, MN, USA
e-mail: Nicholson.wayne@mayo.edu

C. Marcucci et al. (eds.), *A Case Approach to Perioperative Drug-Drug Interactions*, DOI 10.1007/978-1-4614-7495-1_71

adequately hydrated, her urine output gradually increased, and her serum creatinine value decreased to 1.4 mg/dL. Treatment with lisinopril and hydrochlorothiazide was restarted, and she was discharged from the hospital later that day. Subsequent follow-up showed no further renal issues.

Discussion

This is an example of a pharmacodynamic interaction between ketorolac and an ACE inhibitor.

More specifically, this is an example of a pharmacodynamic interaction between a nonsteroidal antiinflammatory drug (NSAID) (ketorolac) and an angiotensin-converting enzyme (ACE) inhibitor (lisinopril) on glomerular filtration rate.

Ketorolac use may induce acute renal failure.[1] In most cases, NSAID use does not pose a significant risk to kidney function.[2] However, situations that reduce volume (eg, diuretic use, vomiting, postoperative blood loss) increase the risk involved with NSAID use. This risk is further increased by the concomitant use of ACE inhibitors. Known in the medical literature as the *triple whammy*, the combination of diuretics, NSAIDs, ACE inhibitors, or angiotensin receptor II blockers, may cause renal dysfunction.[3]

The mechanism of injury involves the different actions of these agents on renal hemodynamics. Adequate glomerular blood flow is dependent on prostaglandin-mediated afferent arteriolar vasodilation; angiotensin II–mediated efferent arteriolar vasoconstriction, and cardiac output.[4] NSAIDs inhibit cyclooxygenase, causing the reduction of prostaglandin production and resulting in reduced afferent vasodilation. ACE inhibition decreases the production of angiotensin II, resulting in reduced efferent vasoconstriction. A volume state lowered by pathologic factors or hypovolemia reduces cardiac output. This combination causes a drop in glomerular blood flow and a subsequent reduction in glomerular filtration rate.

This drug combination is frequently prescribed for older patients, and severe renal adverse effects may present in this high-risk population.[5] Many physiologic changes are associated with aging. Renal aging is associated with alterations in renal morphologic characteristics and a decline in renal function, which is accelerated or accentuated, or both, by such diseases as diabetes mellitus and hypertension.[6] Alterations in cardiac function have been described in this population and also may be a consequence of aging. Additionally, there may be an altered production of or response to endogenous vasodilating substances on aging vasculature.[7] Likely, one or more of these physiologic changes elevate the risk for renal adverse effects in the aging individual.

Since it is possible for selective (ie, cyclooxygenase-2 inhibitors) or nonselective NSAIDs to cause adverse renal effects, dosage should continue to be a consideration for the older population. In practice, an "adult dose" of these agents is often used without the consideration of treatment individualization.

NSAIDs have a ceiling effect on the treatment of pain. However, the adverse effects of these agents continue to be dose related. There are likely instances in clinical practice where NSAID dosage exceeds the ceiling effect, shifting the risk–benefit ratio. Also, in practice, the serum creatinine level alone is often used to assess the renal function of an older patient. Since many older individuals may present with normal serum creatinine levels, renal function in this population cannot adequately be predicted with serum creatinine values.[8] Instead, an estimate of clearance calculated with the Cockroft-Gault equation or the Modification of Diet in Renal Disease formula should be performed. Aside from the interactions discussed herein, proper assessment of renal function in this case should have resulted in a reduction of the ketorolac use to a safer, more individualized dose.

Take-Home Points

- Nonselective NSAIDs and cyclooxygenase-2 selective inhibitors may cause dose-related toxicities. The lowest dose for the shortest period of use should be a primary consideration, especially in the older individual.
- The risks for adverse effects with NSAID use are likely increased in the older population because of the physiologic changes (renal and cardiovascular) associated with aging.
- Risk for renal adverse effects associated with NSAIDs is increased by hypovolemic states (postoperative fluid loss or vomiting), diuretic use, or conditions of poor cardiac output.
- Risk of renal adverse effects associated with NSAID use increases with the concomitant use of angiotensin-converting enzyme inhibitors or angiotensin receptor II blockers, or both, and these adverse effects further compromise renal hemodynamics.
- Renal function should be assessed before NSAID use. However, in older individuals, adequacy of renal function cannot be judged simply by serum creatinine value. An estimate of clearance should be calculated for dosage considerations.
- Recognition of this interaction and the prompt discontinuation of the offending agents usually results in recovery of renal function.

Summary

Interaction: pharmacodynamic
Substrates: ketorolac and lisinopril
Mechanism/site of action: decreased renal function through synergistic reduction of glomerular filtration rate
Clinical effect: renal failure

References

1. Quan DJ, Kayser SR. Ketorolac induced acute renal failure following a single dose. J Toxicol Clin Toxicol. 1994;32(3):305–9.
2. Pannu N, Nadim MK. An overview of drug-induced acute kidney injury. Crit Care Med. 2008;36(4 Suppl):S216–23.
3. Loboz KK, Shenfield GM. Drug combinations and impaired renal function: the 'triple whammy'. Br J Clin Pharmacol. 2005;59(2):239–43.
4. Adhiyaman V, Asghar M, Oke A, et al. Nephrotoxicity in the elderly due to co-prescription of angiotensin converting enzyme inhibitors and nonsteroidal anti-inflammatory drugs. J R Soc Med. 2001;94(10):512–4.
5. Smets HL, De Haes JF, De Swaef A, et al. Exposure of the elderly to potential nephrotoxic drug combinations in Belgium. Pharmacoepidemiol Drug Saf. 2008;17(10):1014–9.
6. Zhou XJ, Rakheja D, Yu X, et al. The aging kidney. Kidney Int. 2008;74(6):710–20. Epub 2008 Jul 9.
7. Nicholson WT, Vaa B, Hesse C, et al. Aging is associated with reduced prostacyclin-mediated dilation in the human forearm. Hypertension. 2009;53(6):973–8. Epub 2009 May 4.
8. Lash JP, Gardner C. Effects of aging and drugs on normal renal function. Coron Artery Dis. 1997;8(8–9):489–94.

When the Smoke Clears, Relaxation Disappears

72

Fatal Forty DDI: cyclobenzaprine, smoked tobacco, CYP1A2

Avinash Ramchandani MD
and Julio A. Gonzalez-Sotomayor MD

Abstract
This case discusses the pharmacokinetic interaction between cyclobenzaprine and smoked tobacco resulting in cyclobenzaprine toxicity due to reversal of enzyme induction. Cyclobenzaprine is a cytochrome P450 1A2 substrate. Smoked tobacco is a 1A2 inducer.

Case

A 32-year-old woman with a history of anxiety disorder and a one-pack-per-day smoking habit fell and injured her back at work, causing significant muscle spasms and general and localized back pain. An orthopedic surgeon advised her that surgery was possible if her symptoms did not improve and urged her to stop smoking. She was started on oral ibuprofen (400 mg orally q6h), cyclobenzaprine (5 mg orally three times a day), physical therapy due to suspected radiculopathy, and scheduled for a follow-up scan in 3 weeks.

The patient struggled through the next week as best she could, gradually the cyclobenzaprine dose to 15 mg orally three times a day, but counting her disinclination for cigarettes as a hidden blessing. Unfortunately, she developed cauda equina

A. Ramchandani MD (✉)
Pain Care Physicians, Austin, TX, USA
e-mail: avinashr@paincaretx.com

J.A. Gonzalez-Sotomayor MD
Pain Division, Department of Anesthesiology and Perioperative Medicine,
Oregon Health and Science University, Portland, OR, USA

C. Marcucci et al. (eds.), *A Case Approach to Perioperative Drug-Drug Interactions*, DOI 10.1007/978-1-4614-7495-1_72

syndrome and underwent emergent and successful laminectomy and diskectomy with significant improvement in her pain. Right before her scheduled discharge, she began experiencing lethargy and mild blurred vision, but did not discuss these with the surgeons as she was desperate to get home to her young children. She insisted to her husband that she could "sleep it off" when she got home and was duly discharged with oral opioids, cyclobenzaprine, gabapentin, nicotine replacement therapy to maintain her tobacco-free status, and instructions to continue physical therapy.

Four days later, the patient was seen in the emergency department for new-onset hypertension and palpitations. Sinus tachycardia and frequent premature ventricular complexes (PVCs) were noted with no clear etiology for these signs and symptoms. She was admitted to the cardiology step down unit, where the consulting pharmacist recommended immediate discontinuation of the cyclobenzaprine. Her symptoms and electrocardiogram changes resolved over the next 36 to 48 hours.

Discussion

This is an example of reversal of induction.

This clinical scenario illustrates the impact that smoking has on cyclobenzaprine metabolism and the risk for developing cyclobenzaprine toxicity after smoking cessation.

Cyclobenzaprine is a skeletal muscle relaxant acting at the central nervous system, where it influences α and γ motor systems. Cyclobenzaprine undergoes extensive metabolism at the level of the hepatic cytochrome P450 (CYP) system. CYP1A2 and CYP3A4 are the major enzymes responsible for its metabolism. CYP2D6 seems to play only a minor role.[1]

Polycyclic aromatic hydrocarbons found in tobacco smoke induce CYP1A2, resulting in faster metabolism of many drugs, including cyclobenzaprine. Smoking cessation reverses smoking-induced 1A2 levels to normal, increasing plasma concentrations of drugs whose dose was established while smoking. Increased plasma concentrations after smoking cessation may cause serious clinical consequences, particularly in drugs with narrow therapeutic ratio.[2] Nicotine replacement treatment to assist smoking cessation will not prevent this effect because cytochrome enzyme induction is not related to the nicotine component of tobacco, but to polycyclic aromatic hydrocarbons in tobacco smoke.

Caffeine is also metabolized by CYP1A2 and its clearance has been used to study 1A2 activity in smokers subjected to sudden smoking cessation. By the second day after smoking cessation, caffeine clearance decreases 20% and by the seventh day the clearance decrease is about 36%.[3] These results have led to recommendations for immediate reduction in dose of CYP1A2- metabolized drugs whenever patients stop smoking. These recommendations are particularly relevant for hospitalized patients who are abruptly subjected to involuntary smoking cessation due to the speed at which the induction of 1A2 dissipates.

Cyclobenzaprine is structurally related to the tricyclic antidepressant amitriptyline. Cyclobenzaprine toxicity may produce similar life-threatening neurologic and cardiovascular effects seen with tricyclic antidepressant overdose.[4] A 5-year multicenter retrospective review of cyclobenzaprine toxicity confirmed the clinical picture characterized by prominent central nervous system depression and anticholinergic effects.[5] In that review, symptomatic patients had a mean dose ingested of 184 mg. Some cases were serious enough to require intensive care unit admission and mechanical ventilation but there was no report of life-threatening events. Previous reports of deaths involving cyclobenzaprine were in situation of multiple drug intoxication, including drugs with documented cardiovascular toxicity. The limited toxicity from cyclobenzaprine, when compared with amitriptyline, may be the relatively smaller doses ingested by cyclobenzaprine overdose patients vs the tricyclic-overdose patients.

Take-Home Points

- Tobacco smoking increases cyclobenzaprine metabolism by inducing cytochrome P450 1A2 activity.
- Smoking cessation will rapidly reverse this induction and result in increased plasma concentration of cyclobenzaprine, possibly attaining toxic levels.
- Nicotine replacement therapy will not prevent reversal of CYP1A2 induction.
- Smoking cessation may require immediate dose reduction of cyclobenzaprine and other drugs metabolized at CYP1A2 level.

Summary

Interaction: pharmacokinetic (enzyme induction)
Substrate: cyclobenzaprine
Enzyme: cytochrome CYP1A2
Inducer: polycyclic aromatic hydrocarbons found in tobacco smoke
Clinical effect: smoking cessation may result in cyclobenzaprine toxicity by reversal of CYP1A2 induction

References

1. Wang RW, Liu L, Cheng H. Identification of human liver cytochrome P450 isoforms involved in the in vitro metabolism of cyclobenzaprine. Drug Metab Dispos. 1996;24(7):786–91.
2. Schaffer SD, Yoon S, Zadezensky I. A review of smoking cessation: potentially risky effects on prescribed medications. J Clin Nurs. 2009;18(11):1533–40.
3. Faber MS, Fuhr U. Time response of cytochrome P450 1A2 activity on cessation of heavy smoking. Clin Pharmacol Ther. 2004;76:178–84.
4. Chabria SB. Rhabdomyolysis: a manifestation of cyclobenzaprine toxicity. J Occup Med Toxicol. 2006;1:16.
5. Spiller HA, Winter ML, Mann KV, et al. Five-year multicenter retrospective review of cyclobenzaprine toxicity. J Emerg Med. 1995;13(6):781–5.

Befuddled by Aspirin

73

Fatal Forty DDI: aspirin, valproic acid, protein binding

Melisa N. Weingarten RN, MS, Juraj Sprung MD, PhD, and Toby N. Weingarten MD

Abstract
This case discusses dual pharmacokinetic drug–drug interactions that occur with coadministration of valproic acid and aspirin. There is mutual plasma-protein–binding displacement that will increase free valproic acid. Also, valproic acid is a substrate of mitochondrial β-oxygenase and aspirin is an inhibitor of mitochondrial ß-oxygenase.

Case

An 80-year-old woman (45 kg) presented to the Emergency Department with a complex head laceration that she sustained after rising too quickly during a commercial break from her favorite television show and striking her head against the coffee table. She was confused and appeared tentative and frail but she was able to report that she had been feeling lightheaded or dizzy upon standing over the past several weeks. She had a history of generalized seizures well controlled with a stable dose of divalproex sodium (500 mg BID), and mild hypertension treated with hydrochlorothiazide (25 mg daily). Two months ago, her granddaughter, who was a fourth-year medical student, recommended that she take a daily morning aspirin for mild to moderate osteoarthritis in her knees and hips and also for its cardioprotective properties. Dutifully, she had been taking aspirin 325 mg daily.

After surgical repair of the laceration, the patient was admitted to the intensive care unit. The patient was confused and uncertain about what was going on and why she was there, but the anesthesia team was neither of these things and strongly

M.N. Weingarten RN, MS (✉)
Patient Education, Mayo Clinic, Rochester, MN, USA
e-mail: Weingarten.melisa@mayo.edu

J. Sprung MD, PhD • T.N. Weingarten MD
Department of Anesthesiology, Mayo Clinic, Rochester, MN, USA

C. Marcucci et al. (eds.), *A Case Approach to Perioperative Drug-Drug Interactions*, DOI 10.1007/978-1-4614-7495-1_73

suspected two related drug–drug interactions (DDIs) involving the coadministration of aspirin and valproic acid. Sure enough, her valproic acid level was measured and the total valproic acid level was found to be 90 ng/mL, within the therapeutic range (therapeutic level, 40 [trough]–100 [peak] ng/mL), but the free valproic acid level was found to be above therapeutic range, 20 ng/mL, (therapeutic levels, 4–15 ng/mL). She was also found to have mild hypoalbuminemia. Her aspirin was discontinued and her divalproex sodium was decreased to 250 mg twice a day for a few days, and then retitrated back to 500 mg twice a day. After several weeks, she no longer experienced lightheadedness when standing and her total and free serum valproic acid concentrations had returned within therapeutic levels.

Discussion

This is an example of a pharmacokinetic drug–drug interaction involving distribution. It is also an example of an inhibitor added to a substrate.

Valproic acid is a commonly used anticonvulsant and mood stabilizer. Valproic acid is tightly bound to plasma proteins, such as albumin, and in this form it is pharmacologically inactive.[1] Approximately 5% is not bound to proteins, or "free," and this "free fraction" is able to cross into the central nervous system, and is thus pharmacologically active.[2] The therapeutic index of valproic acid is sufficiently narrow that higher levels can result in central nervous system toxicity, manifesting initially as lightheadedness and dizziness, that can progress to confusion and increasing somnolence.

Aspirin also binds to plasma proteins.[3] When it is administered with valproic acid there is mutual displacement of both drugs with resultant increase in the free fraction of both.[4,5] In situations where there is at the same time a decrease in plasma proteins this affect maybe more pronounced.[6,7] In our case, the patient was malnourished as evidenced by her low weight and mild hypoalbuminemia, which also may have contributed to the increased free fraction of valproic acid.

Additionally, valproic acid is metabolized via several pathways, of which 40% is by the mitochondrial β-oxidation pathway.[8] Aspirin inhibits ß-oxidation.[9] When there is both an increase in the free fraction of valproate as well as meaningful metabolic inhibition, then free concentrations of valproate can rise up to fourfold.[7] There are numerous reports of valproic toxicity in the context of aspirin therapy.[5–7] The standard clinical practice of a patient taking valproic acid is to measure total serum valproic acid concentrations.[7] However, the therapeutic range of valproic acid based on total levels is dependent on a predictable relationship between total and free valproate serum concentrations, based on the assumption of normal albumin levels, absence of displacement of valproic acid from plasma proteins, and absence of co-occurring metabolic inhibition. Thus, in clinical situations where these assumptions cannot be met, as they were not in this case, monitoring free valproic acid concentration is more appropriate for the titration of valproic acid.[6,7]

In conclusion, drugs such as aspirin, which can both displace valproic acid from plasma proteins, (thus increasing the free fraction) and inhibit the metabolism of valproic acid, can increase the free valproic acid concentration and lead to toxicity. Hypoalbuminemia can contribute to this affect. In these situations, free valproic acid concentration measurements are a better guide to titrate this antiepileptic medication.

Take-Home Points

- Valproic acid is tightly bound to plasma proteins. Only the free form is pharmacologically active.
- Aspirin displaces valproic acid from plasma proteins, resulting in an increased fraction of the unbound, or free form.
- Aspirin also inhibits the metabolism of valproic acid and can increase both total and free levels.
- Hypoalbuminemia increases the fraction of free valproic acid.
- Though usually total valproic acid levels are used manage valproic therapy, free valproic acid levels may be more appropriate in the setting of coadministration of aspirin.

Summary

Interaction 1: pharmacokinetic (distribution)
Substrates: valproic acid and aspirin
Mechanism: mutual protein binding displacement with rise in free fraction of valproic acid
Clinical effects: valproic acid toxicity including lightheadedness and dizziness

Interaction 2: pharmacokinetic (metabolism)
Substrate: valproic acid
Enzyme: mitochondrial ß-oxidation
Inhibitor: aspirin
Clinical effects: decreased elimination of valproic acid leading to toxicity

References

1. Klotz U, Antonin KH. Pharmacokinetics and bioavailability of sodium valproate. Clin Pharmacol Ther. 1977;21:736–43.
2. DeVane CL. Pharmacokinetics, drug interactions, and tolerability of valproate. Psychopharmacol Bull. 2003;37 Suppl 2:25–42.
3. Ali MA, Routh JI. The protein binding of acetylsalicylic acid and salicylic acid. Clin Chem. 1969;15:1027–38.
4. Farrell K, Orr JM, Abbott FS, et al. The effect of acetylsalicylic acid on serum free valproate concentrations and valproate clearance in children. J Pediatr. 1982;101:142–4.
5. Orr JM, Abbott FS, Farrell K, et al. Interaction between valproic acid and aspirin in epileptic children: serum protein binding and metabolic effects. Clin Pharmacol Ther. 1982;31:642–9.
6. Goulden KJ, Dooley JM, Camfield PR, et al. Clinical valproate toxicity induced by acetylsalicylic acid. Neurology. 1987;37:1392–4.
7. Sandson NB, Marcucci C, Bourke DL, et al. An interaction between aspirin and valproate: the relevance of plasma protein displacement drug-drug interactions. Am J Psychiatry. 2006;163:1891–6.
8. Van den Branden C, Roels F. Peroxisomal beta-oxidation and sodium valproate. Biochem Pharmacol. 1985;34:2147–9.
9. Abbott FS, Kassam J, Orr JM, et al. The effect of aspirin on valproic acid metabolism. Clin Pharmacol Ther. 1986;40:94–100.

You Can't Trick Us! 74

Fatal Forty DDI: ibuprofen, phenytoin, CYP2C9, protein binding

Catherine Marcucci MD and Neil B. Sandson MD

Abstract
This case discusses two pharmacokinetic interactions between ibuprofen and phenytoin, resulting in phenytoin toxicity.

Case

The anesthesia department and the various surgical subspecialty departments at an academic medical center were in the habit of having a "stump the service" contest four times per year, with the losing service buying pizza. It was the orthopedic residents' turn to present. Their favorite internal medicine consultant had found them a good case and they were very confident they had a case that no one on the anesthesia service would be able to untangle, as it would look, for all the world, like an infectious disease (ID) case.

The patient was an otherwise healthy 72-year-old woman except for trigeminal neuralgia that was managed stably and effectively with phenytoin (300 mg/day). She had presented to the orthopedics clinic fearful that she had "torn a ligament" after a fall from her bicycle. She had a swollen painful right knee and intermittent fevers and flu-like symptoms three weeks after vacationing on the Eastern Shore of Maryland. She was given the presumptive diagnosis of Lyme disease and

C. Marcucci MD (✉)
Anesthesia Services Department, Philadelphia Veterans Affairs Medical Center, Philadelphia, PA, USA
e-mail: sandson.marcucci@comcast.net

N.B. Sandson MD
Department of Psychiatry, University of Maryland Medical System, Baltimore, MD, USA

Department of Psychiatry, VA Maryland Health Care System, Baltimore, MD, USA

C. Marcucci et al. (eds.), *A Case Approach to Perioperative Drug-Drug Interactions*, DOI 10.1007/978-1-4614-7495-1_74

started on doxycycline, with a plan to refer her to the ID clinic for additional testing and therapy for babesiosis if her Lyme symptoms did not improve. She requested oxycodone for the knee pain, but was advised to initiate management of her knee pain ibuprofen, maximum daily of 2400 mg, in divided doses. Two days later, the patient's husband called the clinic, stating, "it's gone to her nerves, she's wobbly and her eyes are googly." The "stumper" question for the anesthesiologists was whether ID had diagnosed tertiary Lyme disease or babesiosis. The anesthesia residents took a moment to huddle and then announced that Ortho would be buying the food for next conference as the correct answer was actually to ask for the baseline and follow-up phenytoin levels before and after starting ibuprofen therapy

More than a little impressed, the surgeons admitted that the patient's baseline phenytoin trough level had been 18 mcg/mL. Repeat trough level three days later was 25 mcg/mL. Her "disseminated Lyme" symptoms were actually the unsteadiness and nystagmus of moderate phenytoin toxicity.

Discussion

This is a combined pharmacokinetic drug–drug interaction (DDI) in which an inhibitor was added to a substrate, in addition to the occurrence of mutual plasma-protein–binding displacement.

The paninducer (and **Fatal Forty** member) phenytoin is itself metabolized primarily by the cytochrome 450 (CYP) enzymes 2C9 and 2C19, with greater reliance on 2C9.[1,2] Ibuprofen, a ubiquitous nonsteroidal anti-inflammatory drug (NSAID) and also a **Fatal Forty** drug, is a moderate inhibitor of CYP2C9, as is the case for many other NSAIDs as well.[3] By itself, this inhibitor–substrate interaction would probably not be sufficient to generate significant phenytoin toxicity. However, a synergistic contribution from another dimension of pharmacokinetic drug handling, namely plasma–protein–binding displacement, magnifies this effect. Both phenytoin and ibuprofen (and again, most other NSAIDs as well) are highly bound and have blood concentrations in the mcg/mL range, rather than the ng/mL range, as is the case with most other medications.[4,5] This leads to significant mutual displacement from plasma proteins. In a manner analogous to the interaction of aspirin and valproate (see "**Befuddled by Aspirin**"), the addition of ibuprofen increases the free fraction of phenytoin, and then the inhibition of 2C9 disproportionately increases free phenytoin concentrations, even though there may not be much evident change in total phenytoin concentrations. As in this case, this can lead to phenytoin toxicity.[6]

Take-Home Points

- Phenytoin is a preferential CYP2C9 and CYP2C19 substrate.
- Ibuprofen is a moderate 2C9 inhibitor.
- The effect of the DDI is magnified by a protein-binding displacement interaction.
- DDIs are all around us, occur in the setting of acute on chronic medical conditions, and can present with symptoms that are easily mistaken for other conditions.

Summary

Interaction 1: pharmacokinetic (metabolic)
Substrate: phenytoin
Inhibitor: ibuprofen
Enzyme: CYP2C9
Clinical effect: phenytoin toxicity

Interaction 2: pharmacokinetic (distribution)
Substrates: ibuprofen and phenytoin
Site of action: plasma proteins
Clinical effect: phenytoin toxicity

References

1. Cadle RM, Zenon 3rd GJ, Rodriguez-Barradas MC, et al. Fluconazole-induced symptomatic phenytoin toxicity. Ann Pharmacother. 1994;28(2):191–5.
2. Mamiya K, Ieiri I, Shimamoto J, et al. The effects of genetic polymorphisms of CYP2C9 and CYP2C19 on phenytoin metabolism in Japanese adult patients with epilepsy: studies in stereoselective hydroxylation and population pharmacokinetics. Epilepsia. 1998;39(12):1317–23.
3. Kumar V, Wahlstrom JL, Rock DA, et al. CYP2C9 inhibition: impact of probe selection and pharmacogenetics on in vitro inhibition profiles. Drug Metab Dispos. 2006;34(12):1966–75. Epub 2006 Sep 8.
4. Phenytoin Package Insert. PARKE-DAVIS (Division of Pfizer Inc) NY, NY 10017. Revised 10/2009.
5. Hydrocodone Bitartrate and Ibuprofen Tablets Package Insert -- Bryant Ranch Prepack, North Hollywood, CA. Revised 9/2009.
6. Sandyk R. Phenytoin toxicity induced by interaction with ibuprofen. S Afr Med J. 1982;62(17):592.

IX

Drug–Drug Interactions Involving Benzodiazepines and Other Sedatives

Introduction

75

Catherine Marcucci MD

Abstract
This introduces drug–drug interactions involving benzodiazepines and other sedatives.

Drug–drug interactions (DDIs) involving benzodiazepines and other sedatives are worthy of our study because these drugs, as well drugs that are not nominally sedatives but have as their side effect central nervous system (CNS) depression, are used ubiquitously in the perioperative period.

The interactions themselves, both pharmacokinetic DDIs and pharmacologic DDIs, are relatively straightforward. The benzodiazepines, including midazolam, are cytochrome P450 (CYP) 3A4 substrates. The list of CYP3A4 inhibitors is fairly well-identified (eg, protease inhibitors, some macrolide antibiotics, ketoconazole, itraconazole, verapamil). One would hope that prescribing practitioners in all medical subspecialties would already be in a state of vigilance regarding benzodiazepine DDIs and had taken steps to ensure that their patients are in a state of vigilance regarding DDIs. But, unfortunately these DDIs still happen with distressing frequency.

This is even more true when pharmacodynamic DDIs are considered. Central nervous system depression resulting from sedative DDIs ranges from somnolent-but-arousable to true changes in mental status. Associated clinical sequelae range from increased incidence of hypoxia, hypercarbia, aspiration, falls, and prolonged hospital stays. Interventions range from flumazenil to oxygen to intubation.

Of course, it is not always possible to avoid administering DDI drug pairs to patients. Patients on protease inhibitors come to the operating room or the procedure room and need benzodiazepines. Nobody would suggest that these patients forego

C. Marcucci MD
Anesthesia Services Department, Philadelphia Veterans Affairs Medical Center, Philadelphia, PA, USA
e-mail: sandson.marcucci@comcast.net

C. Marcucci et al. (eds.), *A Case Approach to Perioperative Drug-Drug Interactions*, DOI 10.1007/978-1-4614-7495-1_75

sedation and amnestic agents or that their providers make that choice for them. But this is where the time invested in reading and studying these cases is time well spent. It should serve to make the perioperative practitioner able to mitigate the potential the distressing and deleterious clinical sequelae, even if the coadministration of specific drug pairs cannot be avoided. This will make the perioperative period safer for our patients. And, of course, as the title of several cases alludes to, this should also help to alleviate "the worry that's always with us."

The Worry That's Always With Us: Now I'm Depressed

76

Benzodiazepines, opioids, propofol

Kelly T. Peretich MD and Raymond M. Planinsic MD

Abstract
This case discusses the pharmacodynamic interactions seen with the coadministration of propofol, opioids, and benzodiazepines.

Case

The anesthesia chief resident went to the preoperative area to talk to her first patient of the day, a 70-year-old man scheduled for foot surgery. He was accompanied by his wife and daughter and stated he was very nervous and did not like hospitals. He confirmed that he took no regular medications except for lisinopril and simvastatin. The plan was for ankle block and sedation as needed under monitored anesthesia care (MAC).

The patient remained anxious in the operating room (OR) and was given midazolam (2 mg) and fentanyl (50 mcg) before the block was performed. The patient startled with the incision and received fentanyl (50 mcg) and propofol (20 mg). He was also started on a propofol infusion. He began to breathe more slowly and became apneic despite chin lift and jaw thrust maneuvers. He was intubated after bag-mask ventilation proved difficult. The rest of the case proceeded without incident and the patient was extubated in the OR before being transported to the post-anesthesia care unit.

K.T. Peretich MD (✉) • R.M. Planinsic MD
Department of Anesthesiology, University of Pittsburgh Medical Center, Pittsburgh, PA, USA
e-mail: peretichkt@upmc.edu

C. Marcucci et al. (eds.), *A Case Approach to Perioperative Drug-Drug Interactions*, DOI 10.1007/978-1-4614-7495-1_76

Later, the anesthesia resident visited the patient in the recovery room to update him and his family about what happened during the case. The resident explained that the reason he required intubation was likely due to medication effects and, as she had explained while obtaining consent, this was a known risk of such procedures. The wife was very understanding but the daughter appeared uneasy. She approached the resident later and admitted that she gave her father one of her "alprazolams" that morning because he seemed so nervous about his surgery. The resident accompanied the daughter back to her father's bedside and explained to both the patient and family how important it is to be up front about any and all medications taken because of the effects they have on the body, especially in combination with other mediations. The resident went home that evening and discharged her frustration by recounting the whole story in minute detail to her spouse.

Discussion

This is an example of multiple synergistic pharmacodynamic interactions.

The combination of propofol, benzodiazepines, and opioids is one that is used commonly with general anesthesia and is being used increasingly more often in routine sedation. Procedures such as colonoscopy or those involving extremities lend themselves well to the combination of regional anesthesia with MAC.[1,2] The likely reason for the popularity of this combination is that when propofol, opioids, and benzodiazepines are administered together they act synergistically to produce a hypnotic effect as well as to induce immobility.[3] This means that, in addition to the decreased anxiety obtained with benzodiazepines and the pain control achieved with opioids, these drugs also work to accomplish the level of decreased awareness and decreased response to stimuli desired for surgical procedures. Several studies have demonstrated this point.

Most of the research has investigated combinations of two of these agents rather than all three at once. However, interactions between the two-drug combinations of propofol and benzodiazepines, propofol and opioids, and benzodiazepines and opioids have shown that each of these pairs exhibits synergistic activity in terms of producing hypnosis.[3] Also, although opioids and benzodiazepines cannot produce immobility on their own, when each agent is combined with propofol it causes left-shifts in the propofol immobility dose response curves.[3] Furthermore, giving opioids has been shown to yield higher concentrations of propofol in the blood than when the same dose of propofol is administered alone.[4] Interestingly, although opioids enhance the hypnotic effects of propofol, this is not reflected by a change in the bispectral index.[5,6] The synergistic effects of propofol, benzodiazepines, and opioids on awareness as well as immobility allow for the desired level of sedation to be achieved using reduced dosages of each individual drug. Using lower doses of multiple drugs may decrease the incidence of side effects caused by any individual drug. This is suggested by studies in the intensive care setting that show increased hemodynamic stability in patients receiving a combination of these drugs for sedation versus one drug alone.[7,8]

Even though combining these drugs has clear benefits that can be used to the anesthetist's advantage, it is not without risks. Propofol, benzodiazepines, and opioids all have the potential to cause respiratory depression independently and, when given together, these effects are additive and respiratory depression can occur at lower doses.[6] Propofol alone has the potential to decrease hypoxic respiratory drive up to 80%.[9] Under general anesthesia this is not as much of a concern until assessing for readiness to extubate. It is not surprising that depressive effects on ventilation become more significant in situations where it is desirable to have the patient breathe spontaneously. One retrospective study on sedation for gastrointestinal endoscopy cites the need for intubation during these procedures as occurring in 0.07%-0.1% of cases.[1] The effects on respiratory depression are dose-dependent for each agent as well as being additive when combining agents.

The cumulative nature of respiratory depression in response to these drugs may be more apparent in certain patient populations that are more sensitive to the effects of these drugs. This is the case in older patients who generally have reduced metabolism and/or clearance of the drug itself and may benefit from dose decreases.[8] Another patient population that would be expected to have more profound respiratory depression at standard doses and would benefit from decreased doses is the group of patients with liver disease. Although even cirrhotic liver changes do not affect the clinically relevant actions of propofol, the normal metabolism of both benzodiazepines and opioids occur in the liver and are highly impacted by decreased liver function.[8,9] The potential for the combination of these drugs to cause increased respiratory depression may be the reason why some studies show an increase in weaning time from the ventilator with a combination regimen as compared with a single drug regimen.[7,8]

Take-Home Points

- In combination, propofol, opioids, and benzodiazepines work synergistically to produce hypnotic and immobilizing effects and therefore allow decreased doses of each drug when they are used together. The decreased doses may lead to more hemodynamic stability and decreased incidence of side effects from each individual drug.

- Propofol, opioids, and benzodiazepines all have the potential to cause respiratory depression, and when these drugs are used in combination, their effects on respiratory depression are additive. These effects are especially pronounced in older patients and patients with liver disease.

- The importance of an accurate and complete history and physical cannot be overemphasized.

Summary

Interaction: pharmacodynamic
Substrates: propofol, opioids, benzodiazepines
Mechanism/sites of action: multiple central nervous system sites
Clinical effect: increased hypnosis and sedation, decreased respiratory drive

References

1. Agostoni M, Fanti L, Gemma M, et al. Adverse events during monitored anesthesia care for GI endoscopy: an 8-year experience. Gastrointest Endosc. 2011;74(2):266–71.
2. McQuaid KR, Laine L. A systematic review and meta-analysis of randomized, controlled trials of moderate sedation for routine endoscopic procedures. Gastrointest Endosc. 2008;67:910–23.
3. Hendrickx JFA, Eger EI, Sonner JM, et al. Is synergy the rule? A review of anesthetic interactions producing hypnosis and immobility. Anesth Anal. 2008;107(2):494–506.
4. Yufune S, Takamatsu I, Masui K. Effect of remifentanil on plasma propofol concentration and bispectral index during propofol anaesthesia. Br J Anaesth. 2011;106(2):208–14.
5. Lysakowski C, Dumont L, Pellegrini M, et al. Effect of fentanyl, alfentanil, remifentanil and sufentanil on loss of consciousness and bispectral index during propofol induction of anaesthesia. Br J Anaesth. 2001;86(4):523–7.
6. Nieuwenhuijs DJ, Olofsen E, Romberg RR, et al. Response surface modeling of remifentanil-propofol interaction on cardiorespiratory control and bispectral index. Anesthesiology. 2003;98(2):312–22.
7. Devlin JW, Roberts RJ. Pharmacology of commonly used analgesics and sedatives in the ICU: benzodiazepines, propofol, and opioids. Anesthesiol Clin N Am. 2011;29(4):567–85.
8. Eilers H, Niermann CU. Clinically important drug interactions with intravenous anaesthetics in older patients. Drugs Aging. 2003;20(13):969–80.
9. Fassoulaki A, Theodoraki K, Melemeni A. Pharmacology of sedation agents and reversal agents. Digestion. 2010;82(2):80–3.

The Worry That's Always With Us: Tragic but Not Rare

77

Alprazolam, clonazepam, and buprenorphine

Phillip Adams DO and Ibtesam A. Hilmi MB, CHB, FRCA

Abstract
This case discusses the additive respiratory effects of benzodiazepines and opioid narcotics. The case was complicated by obstructive sleep apnea.

Case

A 37-year-old man with past medical history of generalized anxiety disorder, intravenous heroin abuse, morbid obesity, and obstructive sleep apnea (OSA) who was followed in the sleep clinic was in recovery for his heroin abuse for over a year. He was prescribed buprenorphine/naloxone (Suboxone®) 24 mg sublingual daily to help with his recovery, as well as clonazepam (1 mg orally), which he took twice daily for his anxiety.

He was increasingly anxious for the past couple of days and acquired several tablets of alprazolam from a friend. One day his girlfriend found him unconscious in his recliner. She immediately called paramedics, who found him apneic and unresponsive. The first responders administered advanced cardiac life support as well as several doses of naloxone but the patient unfortunately expired.

There was no drug paraphernalia anywhere in the residence, nor did the patient have any signs of recent intravenous drug use. His girlfriend adamantly insisted that he

P. Adams DO (✉)
Department of Anesthesiology, University of Pittsburgh Medical Center, Pittsburgh, PA, USA
e-mail: adamsp@upmc.edu

I.A. Hilmi MB, CHB, FRCA
Department of Anesthesiology, University of Pittsburgh Medical Center, UPMC-Presbyterian Hospital, Pittsburgh, PA, USA

C. Marcucci et al. (eds.), *A Case Approach to Perioperative Drug-Drug Interactions*, DOI 10.1007/978-1-4614-7495-1_77

had not used illegal drugs in over a year and had been "clean" during that time. Ultimately, the cause of death was determined to be cardiac arrest due to severe hypoxia, which was likely a result of respiratory arrest following respiratory depression worsened by airway obstruction.

Discussion

This is an example of a pharmacodynamic drug–drug interaction.

More specifically, ventilatory responsiveness to rises in $PaCO_2$ is depressed in patients who have received opioids or benzodiazepines and the effect is augmented when the two drug classes are administered concurrently.

Benzodiazepines (BZs) and opioids are commonly used as preoperative sedatives, general anesthetic adjuncts, and as sole agents for intravenous (IV) sedation cases. Their use as anxiolytics and analgesics, respectively, is also quite common in the outpatient population.

BZs have several clinical uses including sedation, amnesia, anxiolysis, and as anticonvulsants. BZs mimic the inhibitory neurotransmitter γ-aminobutyric acid (GABA) and exert their action by binding allosterically to the $GABA_A$ receptor subtype.[1] The BZ effect on $GABA_A$ receptors allows for chloride channel opening and an influx of chloride ion, leading to hyperpolarization of the neuron.[2] Opioid medications are used mostly for their analgesic effects. There are several opioid receptor subtypes including mu (μ), delta (δ), kappa (κ), and nociceptin orphanin FQ.[3] All of the receptor subtypes are associated with some degree of analgesia; however different subtypes are responsible for the various adverse effects observed (Table 77.1).

Both classes of medications are associated with respiratory depression. Opioids are known for their effects on respiratory depression and are sometimes implicated in cases of severe respiratory depression with respiratory acidosis, hypoxia, and even death. Opioid agonists have the ability to push the CO_2 responsiveness curve to right and also decrease the slope of the curve, which means a higher $PaCO_2$ is required to drive respirations.[4] This occurs in a dose dependent fashion such that a large dose of opioid can shift the CO_2 response curve so far that apnea and hypoxia ensue. BZs can independently decrease the slope of the CO_2 response curve in a dose-dependent fashion, however, this effect is much less pronounced than that of opioid-induced respiratory depression (Fig. 77.1).[5–8]

When BZs and opioid medications are combined, their respiratory depressant effects are additive.[9] When using a small dose of a BZ, such as midazolam, as a premedication, significant respiratory depression is unlikely. However, when combined with an opioid, such as fentanyl, patients can experience severe respiratory

Table 77.1 Opioid Receptor Subtypes

Receptor	Distribution	Effect
μ_1	Brain, spinal cord, periphery	Analgesia
μ_2	Brain, spinal cord, periphery	Analgesia, GI transit, respiratory depression, pruritus
μ_3	Immune cells, amygdale, peripheral neural, CV endothelial cells	Various including nitric oxide release
δ_1	Brain, periphery	Analgesia, cardioprotection
δ_2	Brain, spinal	Analgesia, cardioprotection, thermoregulation
κ_{1a}	Brain (nucleus accumbens, neocortex, cerebellum)	Analgesia, feeding
κ_{1b}		
κ_{2a}	Brain (hippocampus, thalamus, brainstem)	Analgesia, diuresis, neuroendocrine
κ_{2b}		
κ_3	Brain	Spinal analgesia, peripheral effects

Table illustrating receptor subtypes, distribution, and effects. Nociceptin orphanin FQ is not included due to lack of definitive data.
[Adapted from Dietis N, Rowbotham DJ, Lambert DG. Opioid receptor subtypes: Fact or artifact? Br J Anaesth 2011; 107 (1): 8-18. With permission from Oxford University Press.]

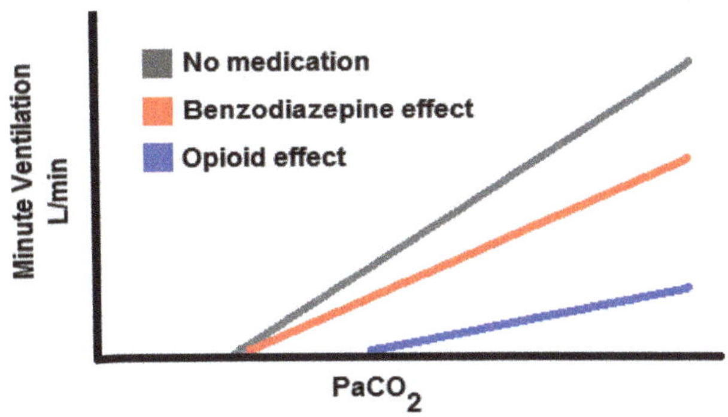

Fig. 77.1 Figure illustrating the carbon dioxide-ventilatory response curve and the effects of different medications. Benzodiazepines can reduce the slope of the curve, whereas opioids can both reduce the slope of the curve and move the curve to the right. These effects necessitate a higher $PaCO_2$ to drive minute ventilation [Based on data from refs.[4–8]]

depressant effects to the point of needing assisted mask ventilation. Similar events can occur in the endoscopy suite where the combination of fentanyl and midazolam is commonly utilized.

In what is probably the most uncontrolled setting, patients are often prescribed a BZ and an opioid analgesic in the outpatient setting and it is not uncommon that these prescriptions may come from different practitioners.[10] These medications can be taken in large dosages and in a discrete manner, in such a way that overconsumption with sedation and respiratory depression can go unnoticed to the point of apnea, hypoxia, and eventual brain death. Death rates from unintentional prescription drug overdose rose 142% from 1999-2004.[11] Naloxone and flumazenil can be given as opioid and BZ antagonists, respectively; however, they may not be administered in sufficient time to prevent irreversible injury. Buprenorphine, a long-acting opioid used for the treatment of chronic pain and recovery from opioid addiction, has respiratory depressant effects and has led to several deaths when combined with a BZ.[12,13] If taken parenterally, the naloxone component of the buprenorphine/naloxone combination (Suboxone®) becomes active and antagonizes the effects of buprenorphine.[14] However, the respiratory depressant effects of buprenorphine are more resistant to antagonism by naloxone and an additional intravenous infusion of naloxone may be required.[15]

Furthermore, the use of sedative medications in patients with obstructive sleep apnea further increases the risk for developing respiratory complications, even with light sedation. OSA is present in 3% to 7% of middle-age adults and patients with OSA carry a higher risk for postoperative respiratory depression and airway obstruction.[16,17] This same risk carries over to the outpatient setting where medications, such as BZs and opioids, can lead to sedation, respiratory depression, and obstruction that can further augment hypercarbia and hypoxia. Opioid therapy alone can lead to both obstructive and central sleep apnea.[18] Extreme caution should be used when choosing to treat patients with known OSA with combinations of opioids and BZs in the outpatient setting due to the increased risk sedation, obstruction and possible profound hypercarbia.

In addition to patients with OSA, any disease state that puts a patient at risk for hypoventilation should have their BZ and opioid therapy managed cautiously. Patients with chronic obstructive pulmonary disease (COPD) and neuromuscular diseases, such as myasthenia gravis, muscular dystrophy, and amyotrophic lateral sclerosis to name a few, can also be negatively impacted by concurrent BZ and opioid therapy.

BZs and opioids have great clinical efficacy in the perioperative, inpatient, and outpatient settings. These benefits do not come without risks, and one that must not be overlooked is the potential for respiratory depression. Knowledge of the additive effects of these medications, and vigilance in the management of their use, can help to limit these adverse effects.

Take-Home Points

- Benzodiazepines and opioids alone can cause a dose-dependent shift in the CO_2 responsiveness curve, necessitating higher $PaCO_2$ to drive spontaneous ventilation.
- When drugs from these classes are used concurrently, their effects on ventilation are additive and ventilation can be significantly depressed.

- Certain patient populations are at an increased risk for respiratory depression and the development of profound hypercarbia.
- Patients who suffer from obstructive sleep apnea can develop obstruction and respiratory depression due to sedation and a decrease in CO_2 responsiveness that is inherent to benzodiazepines and opioids.

Summary

Interaction: pharmacodynamic
Substrates: buprenorphine/naloxone, clonazepam, and alprazolam
Mechanism/site of action: additive respiratory depression
Clinical effects: hypoventilation leading to hypercarbia, hypoxia, and death

References

1. Campo-Soria C, Change Y, Weiss DS. Mechanism of action of benzodiazepines on $GABA_A$ receptors. Br J Pharmacol. 2006;148:984–90.
2. Akaike N, Inoue M, Krishtal OA. 'Concentration-clamp' study of gamma-aminobutyric-acid-induced chloride current kinetics in frog sensory neurones. J Physiol. 1986;379:171–85.
3. Dietis N, Rowbotham DJ, Lambert DG. Opioid receptor subtypes: fact or artifact? Br J Anaesth. 2011;107(1):8–18.
4. Bourke DL, Warley A. The steady-state and rebreathing methods compared during morphine administration in humans. J Physiol. 1989;419:509–17.
5. Gross JB, Blouin RT, Zandsberg S. Effect of flumazenil on ventilatory drive during sedation with midazolam and alfentanil. Anesthesiology. 1996;85(4):713–20.
6. Forster A, Gardaz JP, Suter PM. Respiratory depression by midazolam and diazepam. Anesthesiology. 1980;53:494–7.
7. Forster A, Morel D, Bachmann M. Respiratory depressant effects of different doses of midazolam and lack of reversal with naloxone: a double-blind randomized study. Anesth Analg. 1983;62:920–4.
8. Gross JB, Smith L, Smith TC. Time course of ventilatory response to carbon dioxide after intravenous diazepam. Anesthesiology. 1982;57:18–21.
9. Van den Hoogen RHV, Bervoets KJW, Colpaert FR. Respiratory effects of epidural morphine and sufentanil in the absence and presence of chlordiazepoxide. Pain. 1989;37:103–10.
10. Wilsey BL, Fishman SM, Gilson AM, et al. Profiling multiple provider prescribing of opioids, benzodiazepines, stimulants, and anorectics. Drug Alcohol Depend. 2010;112(1–2):99–106.
11. Paulozzi LJ, Kilbourne EM, Desai HA. Prescription drug monitoring programs and death rates from drug overdose. Pain. 2011;12(5):747–54.
12. Pirnay SO, Mégarbane B, Borron SW, et al. Effects of various combinations of benzodiazepines with buprenorphine on arterial blood gases in rats. Basic Clin Pharmacol Toxicol. 2008;103:228–39.
13. Mégarbane B, Hreiche R, Pirnay S, et al. Does high-dose buprenorphine cause respiratory depression: possible mechanisms and therapeutic consequences. Toxicol Rev. 2006;25(2):79–85.

14. Orman JS, Keating GM. Spotlight on buprenorphine/naloxone in the treatment of opioid dependence. CNS Drugs. 2009;23(10):899–902.
15. van Dorp E, Yassen A, Sarton E, et al. Naloxone reversal of buprenorphine-induced respiratory depression. Anesthesiology. 2006;105(1):51–7.
16. den Herder C, Schmeck J, Appelboom DJK, et al. Risks of general anaesthesia in people with obstructive sleep apnoea. BMJ. 2004;329:955–9.
17. Punjabi NM. The epidemiology of adult obstructive sleep apnea. Proc Am Thorac Soc. 2008;5(2):136–43.
18. Mogri M, Desai H, Webster L. Hypoxemia in patients on chronic opiate therapy with and without sleep apnea. Sleep Breath. 2009;13:49–57.

Lack of Sedation

78

Fatal Forty DDI: midazolam, carbamazepine, CYP3A4

Erica D. Wittwer MD, PhD, Juraj Sprung MD, PhD, and Wayne T. Nicholson MD, PharmD, MSc

Abstract
This case discusses a pharmacokinetic interaction between midazolam and carbamazepine. Midazolam is a cytochrome P450 3A4 substrate and carbamazepine is a 3A4 inducer. Coadministration significantly decreases the sedative effects of oral midazolam.

Case

A 15-year-old, 40 kg girl was scheduled to undergo tonsillectomy with general anesthesia. She had frequent migraine headaches that disrupted her life considerably. She had tried numerous medication regimens and was currently taking sumatriptan and caffeine to treat her headaches and carbamazepine for migraine prophylaxis.

The patient was extremely nervous about having an intravenous (IV) line placed and began to cry. The anesthesia team decided to do an inhalation induction, and discussed the technique with the patient and her parents. The patient's mother asked whether the patient could take something to help her relax before going to the operating room. The resident ordered oral midazolam (20 mg) for the patient.

On arrival at the operating room 45 minutes later, the patient was still tearful and asked when the "relaxing medicine" would begin to work. She reported that she felt no relief from her anxiety and still was very nervous. She was reassured by the resident and the nurse and began to relax after breathing a nitrous oxide–oxygen

E.D. Wittwer MD, PhD (✉) • J. Sprung MD, PhD • W.T. Nicholson MD, PharmD, MSc
Department of Anesthesiology, Mayo Clinic, Rochester, MN, USA
e-mail: Wittwer.erica@mayo.edu

C. Marcucci et al. (eds.), *A Case Approach to Perioperative Drug-Drug Interactions*, DOI 10.1007/978-1-4614-7495-1_78

mixture for several minutes. The remainder of the inhalation induction was uneventful. When the attending anesthesiologist visited the patient before discharge to home, the patient's mother questioned why the sedation medication did not help her.

Discussion

This is an example of a substrate added to an inducer.

More specifically, this is an example of a pharmacokinetic interaction of an inducer (carbamazepine) and a substrate (midazolam).

Midazolam is a benzodiazepine metabolized by the cytochrome P450 3A4 (CYP3A4) isozyme and commonly used for its anxiolytic and sedative properties. It may be used as a premedicant for patients going to the operating room for surgery and also is used in the intensive care unit as a sedative for patients receiving mechanical ventilation. Commonly, oral midazolam is used as a premedicant for children and IV midazolam is used for adults. In the case described, the teenager was so anxious about the IV line placement that oral midazolam was administered.

The patient had been taking carbamazepine, a commonly used antiepileptic drug that is also used as a prophylactic agent in the treatment of migraine headaches. It is metabolized by CYP3A4 and also has the ability to induce this enzyme to increase metabolism. Induction of CYP3A4 results in increased metabolism of other 3A4 substrates, such as midazolam. Another frequently used antiepileptic, phenytoin, has the same effects on 3A4. In one study of patients taking carbamazepine or phenytoin, the area under the plasma concentration–time curve (AUC), maximum concentration, and half-life of a single dose of oral midazolam were shown to be significantly reduced, and the patients taking these antiepileptics did not have sedation.[1] In contrast, the comparative participants not taking the antiepileptics had significant sedation (Fig. 78.1).

Several other medications can affect midazolam serum levels. For example, rifampin is an antibiotic used to treat certain infections, including tuberculosis, and also has the ability to induce CYP3A4. Its use has been shown to decrease both the AUC and the half-life of oral midazolam when midazolam was administered after 5 days of rifampin treatment.[2] The reduction in the pharmacokinetic parameters was also paralleled with a reduction in the pharmacodynamics of midazolam to such a degree that midazolam completely lost its effectiveness. Armodafinil, used to promote wakefulness, such as in the treatment of narcolepsy, is also a moderate 3A4 inducer and has been shown to reduce the AUC and maximum concentration of oral midazolam.[3] Armodafinil is a less commonly used medication; however, rifampin,

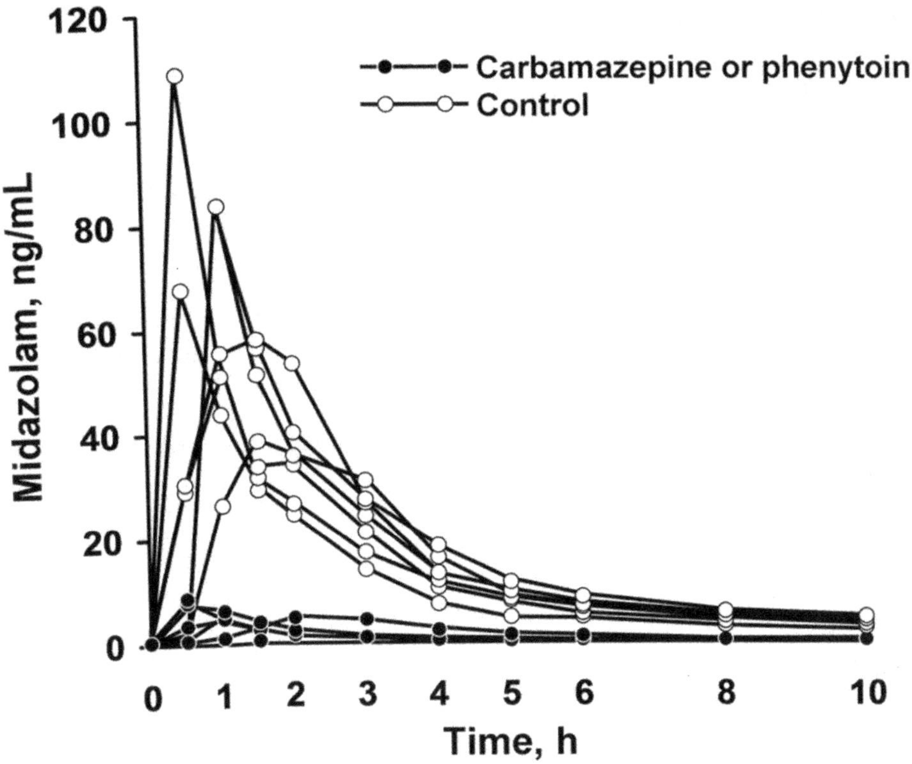

Fig. 78.1 Plasma midazolam concentrations over the 10 hours after a 15-mg oral dose of midazolam in six patients with epilepsy taking carbamazepine or phenytoin and in seven healthy control subjects [Adapted from Backman JT, Olkkola KT, Ojala M et al. Concentrations and effects of oral midazolam are greatly reduced in patients treated with carbamazepine or phenytoin. *Epilepsia.* 1996;37(3):253-7. with permission from John Wiley & Sons, Inc.]

phenytoin, and carbamazepine are frequently encountered medications, and the interaction with midazolam should be considered when a sedative or anxiolytic is needed for patients taking these medications. Midazolam may be administered in the clinical setting of a seizure in patients taking these antiepileptics, and increased doses may be required to achieve effect.

Of note, these studies investigated the effect of 3A4 inducers on orally dosed midazolam.[1-3] Although the effect on IV midazolam has not been elucidated, it is likely that the oral interaction is more substantial because of first-pass metabolism. CYP3A4 inducers will reduce the pharmacokinetic and pharmacodynamic parameters of IV midazolam, but IV administration likely gains greater importance when metabolism through 3A4 has an increased role (ie, multiple boluses or infusion).

Take-Home Points

- Carbamazepine, phenytoin, rifampin, and armodafinil are inducers of the CYP3A4 enzyme.
- Midazolam is metabolized through CYP3A4, and induction of this enzyme increases midazolam metabolism.
- In the presence of 3A4 inducers, the effect of oral midazolam can be completely obliterated. This response is especially relevant when midazolam is prescribed as a premedicant for children who are taking these medications, because midazolam is frequently administered in oral form to children.
- The impact of 3A4 induction on the pharmacokinetics and pharmacodynamics of IV midazolam has not been elucidated but may be reduced to some degree.

Summary

Interaction: pharmacokinetic
Substrate: oral midazolam
Enzyme: CYP3A4
Inducer: carbamazepine
Clinical effects: obliteration of sedative effects

References

1. Backman JT, Olkkola KT, Ojala M, et al. Concentrations and effects of oral midazolam are greatly reduced in patients treated with carbamazepine or phenytoin. Epilepsia. 1996;37(3):253–7.
2. Backman JT, Olkkola KT, Neuvonen PJ. Rifampin drastically reduces plasma concentrations and effects of oral midazolam. Clin Pharmacol Ther. 1996;59(1):7–13.
3. Darwish M, Kirby M, Robertson Jr P, Hellriegel ET. Interaction profile of armodafinil with medications metabolized by cytochrome P450 enzymes 1A2, 3A4 and 2C19 in healthy subjects. Clin Pharmacokinet. 2008;47(1):61–74.

A Cold Isn't Going to Slow Me Down

79

Midazolam, goldenseal, CYP3A4, CYP3A5, CYP2D6

Leelee Thames MD and Jessica Miller MD

Abstract

This case discusses a pharmacokinetic interaction between midazolam and goldenseal. Midazolam is a cytochrome P450 3A4, 3A5, and 2D6 substrate and goldenseal is an inhibitor of these enzymes. Coadministration leads to prolonged sedative effects of midazolam.

Case

The outpatient surgical center had eighteen cataract surgeries scheduled. The resident recognized it was going to be another fast-paced Friday with no time for slow case starts or delayed recoveries. Her last patient of the day was a 68-year-old man (90 kg) who drank two beers daily. He had a history of type 2 diabetes mellitus that was controlled with metformin and two episodes of pneumonia in the past year, one of which caused had caused the cancellation of a previously scheduled cataract surgery. His preoperative serum glucose and creatinine values were normal. Two previous episodes of upper respiratory tract infection in the past year had caused his cataract surgery to be cancelled several times. To circumvent this, the patient had taken herbal supplements in the prior month to "build up my immune system and help speed my recovery."

The anesthesia team planned sedation with midazolam and alfentanil. They anticipated his tolerance for benzodiazepines might be elevated due to his alcohol

L. Thames MD (✉)
Oregon Anesthesiology Group, Portland, OR, USA
e-mail: leeleethames.md@gmail.com

J. Miller MD
Oregon Anesthesiology Group, Providence St. Vincent's Hospital, Portland, OR, USA

C. Marcucci et al. (eds.), *A Case Approach to Perioperative Drug-Drug Interactions*, DOI 10.1007/978-1-4614-7495-1_79

intake, so the resident gave midazolam (2 mg IV) right after monitors were placed. When the attending arrived, the patient was very drowsy and the resident decreased the dose of alfentanil prior to surgical manipulation, The case went smoothly; however, the patient continued to be somnolent and required placement of a nasal trumpet.

At the end of the case, the surgeon thanked the resident for a smooth and fast day. However, the patient remained somnolent in the postanesthesia care unit, despite loud verbal and strong tactile stimulation. The patient's wife was interviewed and she restated how hard they had worked to make sure he was ready for this surgery.

Discussion

This is an example of an inhibitor added to a substrate.

An appropriate history and physical is essential to good anesthesia practice. However, even the most careful practitioner may fail to elicit information regarding herbal medications. Patients may not consider herbal supplements as medications or deem them as harmless. Specific questioning regarding herbal medications should be included in the preoperative evaluation. This can help reduce potentially harmful drug–drug interactions that may affect anesthetic or surgical outcome.

Goldenseal is readily available and commonly used for the prevention of upper respiratory infections, aid digestion, topical antimicrobial effects, and commonly combined with other herbals to enhance medicinal effects. It is also known for hiding toxins on urine drug screens, specifically marijuana.[1]

Goldenseal is composed of two principal isoquinoline alkaloid compounds; hydrastine and berberine. It is also sold under the alternative names Indian pain, eye balm, and ground raspberry.[1] It is a known cytochrome P450 (CYP) 3A4 and CYP2D6 inhibitor.[2,3]

Midazolam, a triazolobenzodiazepine, is a CYP3A4 substrate.

The mechanism of this drug interaction, therefore is due to inhibition of various CYP isoforms, specifically CYP3A4/5 and CYP2D6. Approximately 50% of all prescription drugs undergo metabolism by 3A4.[1] Drugs with a narrow therapeutic index that are metabolized by 3A4 (such as tacrolimus and cyclosporine) and 2D6 (nortriptyline) have the potential for toxicity when administered concurrently with goldenseal.[2,3] Goldenseal has moderate to major interactions with many medications commonly used for anesthesia including triazolobenzodiazepines, opioids such as methadone and alfentanil, volatile agents, antiemetics such as ondanestron and dexamethasone, and local anesthetics like lidocaine.[4,5]

Goldenseal is contraindicated in patients who are pregnant or have glucose-6-phosphate deficiency.[1]

To determine the cause of this patient's prolonged recovery time, the differential diagnosis of prolonged emergence should be considered. Advanced age slows drug metabolism. Chronic alcohol intake can cause liver disease, thus reducing the liver's detoxification/metabolism ability. Chronic alcohol intake may cause poor nutrition and reduce albumin synthesis. Low albumin increases the amount of ionized or "active" drug, thus increasing the medications clinical effect. Renal failure is a common complication with poorly controlled DM. The clearance of midazolam could be reduced by decreased renal function. Blood glucose levels should be determined to eliminate hypoglycemia. Errors in drug administration may have resulted in excess drug administration. The patient may be taking other drugs not mentioned on the medication list, or have other medical problems not revealed in the patient interview.

In this case, the patient was normoglycemic and had normal preoperative kidney and renal function. On discussion with his wife, further details were obtained about the herbal supplement which was likely a combination of echinacea with goldenseal. Midazolam is a known substrate for CYP3A4 metabolism.[2–4] The concurrent use of goldenseal with midazolam resulted in decreased metabolism, thus increasing the clinical effect of the midazolam.

Take-Home Points

- Herbal supplements can have significant drug–drug interactions.
- Goldenseal is a CYP3A4 and CYP2D6 inhibitor.
- Midazolam is a CYP3A4 substrate.
- Know all medications (including herbals) and doses taken by patients prior to drug administration.
- If the patient is taking goldenseal, check the medication list for 3A4 and 2D6 substrates such as benzodiazepines, tacrolimus, cyclosporine, nortriptyline, methadone, alfentanil, ondansetron, dexamethasone, and lidocaine.
- Watch especially for the presence of tacrolimus, cyclosporine, and nortriptyline on the drug list as these drugs have a narrow therapeutic index and impaired metabolism can easily cause clinical toxicity.
- With chronic alcohol intake, poor nutrition should also be considered in drug interactions. Preoperative labs may include albumin to assess nutritional status. Lower levels of albumin increase the ionized (active) form of drugs.

Summary

Interaction: pharmacokinetic
Substrate: midazolam
Enzyme: CYP3A4, CYP3A5, and CYP2D6
Inhibitor: goldenseal
Clinical effects: prolonged sedation

References

1. Complementary Medicine, Goldenseal. University of Maryland Medical Center. http://www.umm.edu/altmed/articles/goldenseal-000252.htm. Accessed 20 Sept 2009.
2. Gurley BJ, Swain A, Hubbard MA, et al. Supplementation with goldenseal (*Hydrastis Canadensis*), but not kava kava (*Piper methysticum*), inhibits human CYP3A activity *in vivo*. Clin Pharmacol Ther. 2008;83(1):61–9.
3. Gurley BJ, Gardner SF, Hubbard MA, et al. In vivo effects of goldenseal, kava kava, black cohosh, and valerian on human cytochrome P450 1A2, 2D6, 2E1, and 3A4/5 phenotypes. Clin Pharmacol Ther. 2005;77(5):415–26.
4. Goldenseal. In: AltMedDex System [Internet database]. Greenwood Village: Thomas Reuters (Healthcare) Inc. Updated periodically.
5. Flockhart DA. Drug Interactions: Cytochrome P450 Drug Interaction Table. Indiana University School of Medicine. 2007. http://medicine.iupui.edu/clinpharm/ddis/table.aspx. Accessed 26 Mar 2012.

Her Patients Never Wake Up on Time

80

Fatal Forty DDI: midazolam, diltiazem, alfentanil, CYP3A4, CYP3A5, CYP3A7

Toby N. Weingarten MD, Erica D. Wittwer MD, PhD, and Wayne T. Nicholson MD, PharmD, MSc

Abstract
This is an example of one drug (diltiazem hydrochloride) suppressing hepatic metabolism of two other drugs (midazolam hydrochloride and alfentanil hydrochloride) through inhibition of several isoenzymes in the cytochrome P450 3A family

Case

A cardiac anesthesia group at a large academic center was examining its anesthetic practice of patients undergoing coronary artery bypass graft surgery (CABG) in an effort to streamline postoperative patient care and reduce demands on the intensive care unit. The new cardiac anesthesia fellow was given the task of analyzing the time from surgery completion to extubation to determine the variation of extubation times. When he reviewed the charts of several hundred recent cases, he noticed that the extubation times of patients of one anesthesiologist in particular were consistently several hours longer than the times of other anesthesiologist. Intrigued, the fellow started looking at individual practice patterns. He noticed that the "slow" anesthesiologist regularly administered a loading dose of diltiazem prior to induction and then a diltiazem infusion during the case. Her intraoperative use of intravenous infusions of midazolam and alfentanil was also unique. When queried, she explained that she used diltiazem as prophylaxis against postoperative atrial fibrillation. Also she felt the use of midazolam and alfentanil infusions provided a

T.N. Weingarten MD (✉) • E.D. Wittwer MD, PhD • W.T. Nicholson MD, PharmD, MSc
Department of Anesthesiology, Mayo Clinic, Rochester, MN, USA
e-mail: Weingarten.toby@mayo.edu

C. Marcucci et al. (eds.), *A Case Approach to Perioperative Drug-Drug Interactions*, DOI 10.1007/978-1-4614-7495-1_80

consistent level of anesthesia and allowed for the use of a lower concentration of isoflurane resulting in more stable patient hemodynamics during the case.

Discussion

This is an example of coadministration of an inhibitor and two substrates.

More completely, this is an example of one drug (diltiazem) suppressing hepatic metabolism of two other drugs (midazolam and alfentanil) through inhibition of cytochrome P450 3A (CYP3A).

Diltiazem is a calcium ion influx inhibitor during membrane depolarization of cardiac and vascular smooth muscle. Diltiazem has been shown to reduce the incidence of postoperative atrial fibrillation in patients undergoing open heart surgery.[1] Diltiazem undergoes extensive hepatic biotransformation by *N*-demethylation by CYP3A and is also a competitive inhibitor of that enzyme.[2]

The subfamily of CYP3A includes CYP3A4, CYP3A5, and CYP 3A7. In adults, 3A4 and 3A5 are the most frequently considered in biotransformation, since 3A7 is found primarily in fetal tissue. Midazolam is metabolized by CYP3A into 1′-hydroxymidazolam and 4–hydroxymidazolam.[3] Alfentanil undergoes dealkylation metabolism by CYP3A into noralfentanil and *N*-phenylpropionamide.[4] *In vitro* midazolam has been shown to act as a competitive inhibitor in relation to the metabolism of alfentanil and thus reduce the formation rates of alfentanil metabolites via inhibition of CYP3A4.[5] In addition, elevations in plasma concentrations of both midazolam and alfentanil have been clearly demonstrated following CYP3A inhibition in human studies.[6]

The use of diltiazem in conjunction with alfentanil and midazolam has been shown to result in a delay in extubation by several hours.[7] Although no "perfect" cardiac anesthetic exists, many clinicians employ combinations of different anesthetic agents to provide a balanced anesthetic that minimizes hemodynamic instability. Many cardiac anesthetic groups are focusing on "fast-track" postoperative recovery including reducing the time to extubation. A thorough appreciation of drug–drug interactions can help minimize postoperative oversedation.

Take-Home Points

- Diltiazem, midazolam, and alfentanil are metabolized by CYP3A.
- Several drugs, including diltiazem, are potent inhibitors of CYP3A.

- Inhibition of CYP3A can slow the metabolism of midazolam and alfentanil. This can result in clinically relevant prolongation of sedation from these medications especially when these are administered via continuous infusion.

Summary

Interaction: pharmacokinetic
Substrates: midazolam and alfentanil
Enzyme: CYP3A subfamily
Inhibitor: diltiazem
Clinical effects: prolonged anesthetic effect and delayed extubation

References

1. Dobrilovic N, Vadlamani L, Buchert B, et al. Diltiazem prophylaxis reduces incidence of atrial fibrillation after coronary artery bypass grafting. J Cardiovasc Surg (Torino). 2005;46:457–61.
2. Jones DR, Gorski JC, Hamman MA, et al. Diltiazem inhibition of cytochrome P-450 3A activity is due to metabolite intermediate complex formation. J Pharmacol Exp Ther. 1999;290(3):1116–25.
3. Gorski JC, Hall SD, VandenBranden M, et al. Regioselective biotransformation of midazolam by members of the human cytochrome *P*450 3A (CYP3A) subfamily. Biochem Pharmacol. 1994;47:1643–53.
4. Klees TM, Sheffels P, Dale O, et al. Metabolism of alfentanil by cytochrome p4503a (cyp3a) enzymes. Drug Metab Dispos. 2005;33(3):303–11.
5. Labroo RB, Thummel KE, Kunze KL, et al. Catalytic role of cytochrome P4503A4 in multiple pathways of alfentanil metabolism. Drug Metab Dispos. 1995;23:490–6.
6. Chaobal HN, Kharasch ED. Single-point sampling for assessment of constitutive, induced, and inhibited cytochrome P450 3A activity with alfentanil or midazolam. Clin Pharmacol Ther. 2005;78(5):529–39.
7. Ahonen J, Olkkola KT, Salmenpera M, et al. Effect of diltiazem on midazolam and alfentanil disposition in patients undergoing coronary artery bypass grafting. Anesthesiology. 1996;85:1246–52.

When Enough Is Now Too Much

81

Fatal Forty DDI: midazolam, itraconazole, CYP3A4

Erica D. Wittwer MD, PhD, Juraj Sprung MD, PhD, and Wayne T. Nicholson MD, PharmD, MSc

Abstract
This case discusses the pharmacokinetic interaction between midazolam and itraconazole, resulting in increased sedation. Midazolam is a cytochrome P450 3A4 substrate and itraconazole is a 3A4 inhibitor.

Case

On a Friday night, the junior anesthesiology resident on call was assigned to do the preoperative evaluation for a 10-year-old girl who would be coming to the operating room the following morning for a repeat irrigation and debridement of an infected right lower extremity wound right, sustained along with open fractures in a car crash 2.5 weeks previously. She was receiving antibiotics, including vancomycin. A recent culture was concerning for fungal infection, and she had started receiving itraconazole 4 days ago. Previous anesthesia notes indicated an uneventful endotracheal intubation and anesthesia course.

The nurse told the resident that the patient had been doing well except that she was very anxious about waking up from the procedure in severe pain, as she had previously. The resident ordered oral midazolam (18 mg) for the patient. Forty minutes later, the resident and the was summoned by her parents to come to her room because they were not able to arouse her. The patient was breathing at a rate of 5 breaths per minute; with some stimulation, her respirations increased to 10 per minute. It was apparent that the patient was oversedated from the midazolam.

E.D. Wittwer MD, PhD (✉) • J. Sprung MD, PhD • W.T. Nicholson MD, PharmD, MSc
Department of Anesthesiology, Mayo Clinic, Rochester, MN, USA
e-mail: Wittwer.erica@mayo.edu

C. Marcucci et al. (eds.), *A Case Approach to Perioperative Drug-Drug Interactions*, DOI 10.1007/978-1-4614-7495-1_81

However, the parents did not understand why because the child had tolerated midazolam with minimal sedation a few days ago.

The patient was transferred to the monitored care unit, where she continued to be sedated and somnolent overnight. Gradually, she became more responsive and was appropriately answering questions in the morning. It was decided that she should come to the operating area for surgery as scheduled, but she was not given a benzodiazepine. The procedure was uneventful, and the patient woke up without difficulty.

Discussion

This is an example of an inhibitor added to a substrate.

Itraconazole is an antifungal that is metabolized by the cytochrome P450 (CYP) isozyme 3A4 to metabolites, including hydroxyitraconazole. Both itraconazole and hydroxyitraconazole are potent inhibitors of CYP3A4.[1,2] Administration of medications that are also substrates for CYP3A4 may lead to decreased metabolism of those drugs and, subsequently, to increased plasma levels and increased effect or toxicity (Fig. 81.1).

Midazolam is a commonly used anxiolytic and sedative that is metabolized by 3A4. Studies have shown significantly altered pharmacokinetics, including an increased area-under-the-concentration curve versus the time curve, peak concentration levels, and half-life when midazolam was administered to study participants taking itraconazole orally[3,4] (Fig. 81.1).

When midazolam is administered in the oral form, the pharmacokinetics and pharmacodynamics are significantly altered because of an inhibition of metabolism due to itraconazole. However, when midazolam is administered in the intravenous form, the impact of itraconazole on the pharmacokinetics and pharmacodynamics of midazolam is reduced.[5] This difference in interaction is likely because oral midazolam goes through substantial first-pass metabolism in the liver. When the pharmacodynamics of orally administered midazolam are altered because of CYP3A4 inhibition, the clinical picture is increased sedation and an extended period before the sedation resolves. Caution should still be used when administering midazolam in intravenous form for patients receiving itraconazole because the interaction potentially could cause clinically significant pharmacodynamic alterations, especially when large doses are administered or midazolam is used in multiple doses or infusions (ie, the intensive care unit setting) for an extended period.

Itraconazole is not the only azole antifungal that interacts with drug metabolism. Posaconazole and ketoconazole also inhibit CYP3A4 and have been found to impair

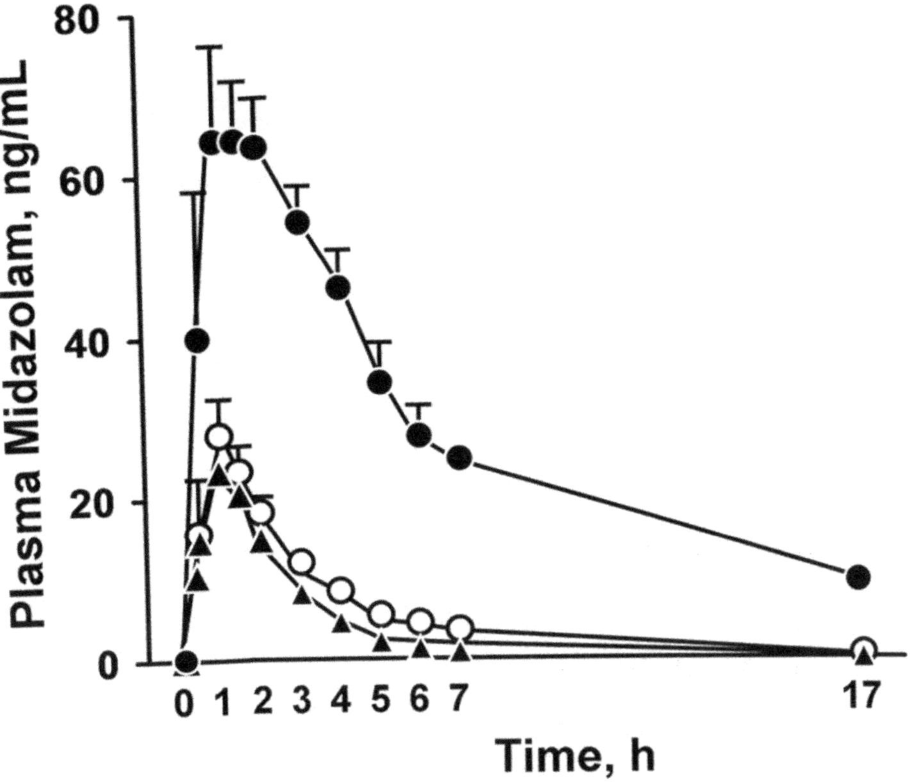

Fig. 81.1 Concentrations of midazolam in plasma after oral midazolam (7.5 mg) administration following pretreatment with placebo (open circle), itraconazole (100 mg; closed circle), and terbinafine (250 mg; closed triangle). (The allylamine antifungal terbinafine does not inhibit cytochrome P450 in vitro.) [Adapted from Ahonen J, Olkkola KT, Neuvonen PJ. Effect of itraconazole and terbinafine on the pharmacokinetics and pharmacodynamics of midazolam in healthy volunteers. *Br J Clin Pharmacol.* 1995;40:270-272. With permission from Wiley-Blackwell.]

the metabolism of midazolam.[6] The clinical interactions of CYP3A substrates with fluconazole are of lesser magnitude and generally are observed only with daily doses of 200 mg or more.[7] In addition to midazolam interactions, the coadministration of ketoconazole or itraconazole with other CYP3A substrates—such as cyclosporine, tacrolimus, alprazolam, triazolam, nifedipine, felodipine, simvastatin, lovastatin, vincristine sulfate, terfenadine, and astemizole—may also result in clinically significant drug interactions, some of which can be life threatening.[7] Therefore, it is prudent to avoid the use of oral midazolam for patients receiving these antifungals. Intravenous midazolam should be used with caution and with close observation for increased or extended effects.

Take-Home Points

- Itraconazole, posaconazole, and ketoconazole inhibit CYP3A4, the isozyme responsible for the metabolism of midazolam.
- Prolonged and increased sedation is observed when itraconazole is used with oral midazolam.
- These effects are not as pronounced after intravenous midazolam administration; however, this route should also be used with caution for patients receiving itraconazole, posaconazole, or ketoconazole.
- Oral midazolam should be avoided for patients receiving itraconazole, posaconazole, or ketoconazole.

Summary

Interaction: pharmacokinetic
Substrate: midazolam
Enzyme: CYP3A4
Inhibitor: itraconazole
Clinical effects: increased sedative effects

References

1. Quinney SK, Galinsky RE, Jiyamapa-Serna VA, et al. Hydroxyitraconazole, formed during intestinal first-pass metabolism of itraconazole, controls the time course of hepatic CYP3A inhibition and the bioavailability of itraconazole in rats. Drug Metab Dispos. 2008;36:1097–101.
2. Isoherranen N, Kunze KL, Allen KE, et al. Role of itraconazole metabolites in CYP3A4 inhibition. Drug Metab Dispos. 2004;32:1121–31.
3. Olkkola KT, Backman JT, Neuvonen PJ. Midazolam should be avoided in patients receiving the systemic antimycotics ketoconazole or itraconazole. Clin Pharmacol Ther. 1994;55:481–5.
4. Ahonen J, Olkkola KT, Neuvonen PJ. Effect of itraconazole and terbinafine on the pharmacokinetics and pharmacodynamics of midazolam in healthy volunteers. Br J Clin Pharmacol. 1995;40:270–2.
5. Olkkola KT, Ahonen J, Neuvonen PJ. The effects of the systemic antimycotics, itraconazole and fluconazole, on the pharmacokinetics and pharmacodynamics of intravenous and oral midazolam. Anesth Analg. 1996;82:511–6.
6. Krishna G, Moton A, Ma L, et al. Effects of oral posaconazole on the pharmacokinetic properties of oral and intravenous midazolam: a phase I, randomized, open-label, crossover study in healthy volunteers. Clin Ther. 2009;31:286–98.
7. Venkatakrishnan K, von Moltke LL, Greenblatt DJ. Effects of the antifungal agents on oxidative drug metabolism: clinical relevance. Clin Pharmacokinet. 2000;38:111–80.

The Distressed Daughter

82

Fatal Forty DDI: alprazolam, carbamazepine, CYP3A4

Jennifer Egan MD, Kirk Lalwani MD,
and Catherine Marcucci MD

Abstract
This case discusses a pharmacokinetic interaction between carbamazepine and alprazolam leading to sedation. Alprazolam is a cytochrome P450 3A4 substrate. Carbamazepine is a 3A4 inducer. Discontinuation of carbamazepine leads to less metabolism of alprazolam and greater sedation.

Case

The anesthesiologist taking care of a 72-year-old man scheduled for rhizotomy was paged by the nurse checking him in. She asked to have someone from the anesthesia service come over to the preoperative area, saying "He still needs anesthesia consent, but he's really sleepy. I can't even get him undressed." When the anesthesiologist arrived, she found a somewhat disheveled elderly man, who appeared quite sedated but conscious, and a very distressed daughter. By the daughter's report, the patient had always been in generally good health, except for trigeminal neuralgia, for which he had been taking carbamazepine (Tegretol®) 400 mg twice daily for the past 3 years. He had also suffered from persistent generalized anxiety since the death of his wife 2 months earlier, although his distress and agitation had remitted

J. Egan MD (✉)
Department of Anesthesia, Indiana University School of Medicine, Indianapolis, IN, USA
e-mail: Jennifer.egan22@gmail.com; eganj@ohsu.edu

K. Lalwani MD, FRCA, MCR
Department of Anesthesiology and Perioperative Medicine, Oregon Health and Science University, Portland, OR, USA

C. Marcucci MD
Anesthesia Services Department, Philadelphia Veterans Affairs Medical Center, Philadelphia, PA, USA

C. Marcucci et al. (eds.), *A Case Approach to Perioperative Drug-Drug Interactions*, DOI 10.1007/978-1-4614-7495-1_82

somewhat after titration of a standing alprazolam dosage of 1 mg twice daily. He had been seen by his internist 2 weeks earlier for a preoperative history and physical. His internist had noted a mild leukopenia on his preoperative labs and quite correctly surmised that the carbamazepine might be the culprit. Due to the patient's age and since he was "getting the nerve zapped anyway," the internist advised the patient to discontinue the carbamazepine. The patient's daughter confirmed the recent history, stating that after the surgery she was planning on looking at nursing homes as her father seemed to be getting senile rapidly. She confided that she had cried that morning when he been unable to dress himself.

Discussion

This is an example of reversal of induction.

By discontinuing the carbamazepine without decreasing the alprazolam dose, the internist inadvertently exposed the patient to the increased sedating effects of elevated serum benzodiazepine levels.

The triazolobenzodiazepines (alprazolam, midazolam, triazolam, and estazolam), as well as other drugs such as haloperidol are all 3A4 substrates.[1,3] Carbamazepine is an inducer of cytochrome P450 (CYP) 3A4, in addition to multiple other P450 enzymes.[1,4,5] The original presence of the carbamazepine (inducer) in the standing medication panel resulted in titration to a higher dose of alprazolam (substrate) than otherwise would have been required to achieve the desired clinical effect. Abrupt discontinuation of the carbamazepine led to a reversal of 3A4 induction. In such cases, the resulting decrease in available 3A4 will lead to less active metabolism of the alprazolam, yielding higher alprazolam blood levels at the same alprazolam dosage and subsequent oversedation.

Take-Home Points

- This is an example of a classic DDI than can occur because drugs are *stopped* in the perioperative period. Carbamazepine was *removed* from the patient's medication list, and therefore, is not an obvious contributor to the patient's sedated state when reviewing only the current medications.
- Anesthesiologists may be the first to detect DDIs set in motion by providers from other specialties.
- Remember that induction of a P450 enzyme means "more enzyme, not more powerful" enzyme. It is a quantitative rather than qualitative issue. "De-induction" will mean that less total enzyme is available.

- Because enzymes are complex proteins, it takes time for the liver to synthesize them—induction generally becomes clinically significant over the course of weeks, not hours or days.

- Carbamazepine is an inducer of multiple P450 enzymes.[2]

Summary

Interaction: pharmacokinetic
Substrate: alprazolam
Enzyme: CYP3A4
Inducer: carbamazepine
Clinical effect: removal of the inducer leads to less metabolism of the benzodiazepine and greater sedation

References

1. Arana GW, Epstein S, Molloy M, et al. Carbamazepine-induced reduction of plasma alprazolam concentrations: a clinical case report. J Clin Psychiatry. 1988;49(11):448–9.
2. Arana GW, Goff DC, Friedman H, et al. Does carbamazepine-induced reduction of plasma haloperidol levels worsen psychotic symptoms? Am J Psychiatry. 1986;143(5):650–1.
3. Dresser GK, Spence JD, Bailey DG. Pharmacokinetic-pharmacodynamic consequences and clinical relevance of cytochrome P450 3A4 inhibition. Clin Pharmacokinet. 2000;38(1):41–57.
4. Spina E, Pisani F, Perucca E. Clinically significant pharmacokinetic drug interactions with carbamazepine. An update. Clin Pharmacokinet. 1996;31(3):198–214.
5. Ucar M, Neuvonen M, Luurila H, Dahlqvist R, Neuvonen PJ, Mjorndal T. Carbamazepine markedly reduces serum concentrations of simvastatin and simvastatin acid. Eur J Clin Pharmacol. 2004;59(12):879–82.

Check Check and Double Check

83

Fatal Forty DDI: diazepam, fluvoxamine, CYP3A4, CYP2C19

Catherine Marcucci MD and Neil B. Sandson MD

Abstract
This case discusses the pharmacokinetic interaction between diazepam and fluvoxamine resulting in excessive sedation. Diazepam is a cytochrome P450 3A4 and 2C19 substrate and fluvoxamine is a cytochrome P450 3A4 and 2C19 inhibitor.

Case

A 29-year-old female triathlete was admitted to the step-down unit for intravenous administration of vancomycin, fluid and wound management, and intravenous hydromorphone patient-controlled analgesia (PCA). She had just undergone extensive soft tissue debridement and fasciotomy of her right perineum, groin, and lower extremity due to a virulent community-acquired methicillin-resistant *Staphylococcus aureus* infection. She had a remote history of Tourette's syndrome as an adolescent and an anxiety disorder due to the tragic murder of her parents in a robbery 2 years ago. Her only standing medication was diazepam (Valium®, 5 mg three times a day), which was continued in the perioperative period as she had failed an attempt to taper the diazepam dosage some months earlier. On the second postoperative day, the

C. Marcucci MD (✉)
Anesthesia Services Department, Philadelphia Veterans Affairs Medical Center, Philadelphia, PA, USA
e-mail: sandson.marcucci@comcast.net

N.B. Sandson MD
Department of Psychiatry, University of Maryland Medical System, Baltimore, MD, USA

Department of Psychiatry, VA Maryland Health Care System, Baltimore, MD, USA

C. Marcucci et al. (eds.), *A Case Approach to Perioperative Drug-Drug Interactions*, DOI 10.1007/978-1-4614-7495-1_83

surgical service increased the diazepam to 10 mg three times daily as the patient was very anxious about the application of the vacuum wound dressing. On the fourth postoperative day, the step-down nurses urgently paged the anesthesia fellow covering the unit. The patient now had extreme anxiety and distress with an overwhelming urge to repeatedly take off the vacuum dressing and check the incision sites, even after the nurses had carefully shown her the wounds twice in an attempt to reassure her that the infection was gone and she was not bleeding.

The anesthesiologist, fearful of "mixing benzodiazepines," ordered a stat extra dose of Valium with additional dosing as needed and consulted the psychiatric service. The consulting team saw the patient and entered a provisional diagnosis of obsessive-compulsive disorder (OCD) precipitated by acute stressors. They prescribed fluvoxamine (Luvox®, 25 mg twice a day), as the patient had responded well to it during a brief Tourette's-associated OCD flare as a child. Over the next 2 days, there was no appreciable diminution of OCD symptoms while the patient was awake, but her periods of wakefulness decreased to just a few hours per day, during which time she also began to complain bitterly of pain. Ultimately she became so sleepy, she choked while nodding off with a bite of dinner in her mouth.

Discussion

This is an example of an inhibitor added to a substrate.

Diazepam is a substrate of two cytochrome P450 enzymes, 2C19 and 3A4, with primary metabolism via 2C19.[1] Fluvoxamine is a strong 2C19 inhibitor and a moderate 3A4 inhibitor.[2–4] Thus, the addition of fluvoxamine impaired the metabolism of diazepam via both 2C19 and 3A4 and led to a significant increase in the blood level of diazepam.[5] Fluvoxamine, while superficially a reasonable choice (the patient had previously responded well to it for OCD), was not advantageous in terms of its pharmacokinetic profile. This is because onset of clinical efficacy of fluvoxamine for remission of OCD symptoms is on the order of 6 weeks. Unfortunately, the kinetics of P450 inhibition typically are much shorter (on the order of days), so the deleterious effects of increased sedation (such as a near-aspiration event) appeared long before the OCD symptoms could have been expected to remit.

Unwittingly, the clinicians caring for this patient committed several other blunders. For instance, it was not necessarily inappropriate for the patient to remain on diazepam after the fluvoxamine was started, so long as the diazepam dose was appropriately adjusted downward to account for the drug–drug interaction (DDI). The standing order of diazepam (10 mg three times daily) should have been rewritten, perhaps as low as 2 mg three times daily, and orders for as needed diazepam doses should have been similarly decreased. Alternatively, the prescribing doctors could have instead started the patient on a different benzodiazepine altogether. Because lorazepam and oxazepam are metabolized by phase II conjugation and do not rely on Phase I (P450) metabolism, they would have been better choices. Lastly, the increase in overall sedation decreased the awake cycles of the patient both in frequency and duration to the point that there was a decrease in her demand-dosing via PCA, which caused her to "get behind the pain curve."

Take-Home Points

- Inhibition of Phase I oxidative metabolism (P450 metabolism) takes place over a relatively short time frame, often days, not weeks or months.
- Consultants will sometimes recommend a medication that is suitable for the very specific problem they have been asked to address, without considering the whole medication regimen.
- What has worked for the patient in the past must still be looked at critically– patients' medication regimens are in a constant state of flux.
- Remember that drugs within a drug class are not necessarily metabolized via the same pathways! In North America, diazepam is the benzodiazepine that is "outside the family group," it is the only widely used benzodiazepine to undergo significant metabolism via CYP2C19. Etizolam, a benzodiazepine whose metabolism has been studied in Japan, is also a 2C19 substrate. It is not available in the United States or Canada. A number of widely used benzodiazepines are metabolized by CYP3A4 or by phase II conjugation (glucuronidation).
- When evaluating a medication panel for potential DDIs, it is as important to know what *isn't* the culprit as it is to know what "the suspects" are. In this case, neither the administration of vancomycin nor hydromorphone are relevant to the DDI in question, as neither one undergoes appreciable Phase I oxidative metabolism. Vancomycin is largely (80% to 90%) excreted unchanged by the kidney and hydromorphone undergoes extensive metabolism via glucuronidation (Phase II metabolism) in the liver.

Summary

Interaction: pharmacokinetic
Substrate: diazepam
Enzyme: CYP3A4 and CYP2C19
Inhibitor: fluvoxamine
Clinical effects: excessive sedation

References

1. Ono S, Hatanaka T, Miyazawa S, et al. Human liver microsomal diazepam metabolism using cDNA-expressed cytochrome P450s: role of CYP2B6, 2C19 and the 3A subfamily. Xenobiotica. 1996;26:1155–66.
2. Christensen M, Tybring G, Mihara K, et al. Low daily 10-mg and 20-mg doses of fluvoxamine inhibit the metabolism of both caffeine (cytochrome P4501A2) and omeprazole (cytochrome P4502C19). Clin Pharmacol Ther. 2002;71:141–52.
3. Niemi M, Backman JT, Neuvonen M, et al. Effects of fluconazole and fluvoxamine on the pharmacokinetics and pharmacodynamics of glimepiride. Clin Pharmacol Ther. 2001;69:194–200.
4. von Moltke LL, Greenblatt DJ, Court MH, et al. Inhibition of alprazolam and desipramine hydroxylation in vitro by paroxetine and fluvoxamine: comparison with other selective serotonin reuptake inhibitor antidepressants. J Clin Psychopharmacol. 1995;15:125–31.
5. Perucca E, Gatti G, Cipolla G, et al. Inhibition of diazepam metabolism by fluvoxamine: a pharmacokinetic study in normal volunteers. Clin Pharmacol Ther. 1994;56:471–6.

Doggone It—The Case Is Cancelled

84

Fatal Forty DDI: midazolam, lopinavir/ritonavir, CYP3A4

Erica D. Wittwer MD, PhD,
Wayne T. Nicholson MD, PharmD, Msc, Corinne Wisdo DPM,
and Catherine Marcucci MD

Abstract
This case discusses a pharmacokinetic drug interaction between midazolam and ritonavir/lopinavir. Midazolam is a cytochrome P450 3A4 substrate and ritonavir/lopinavir is a 3A4 inhibitor.

Case

A 68-year-old HIV-positive man presented to the OR for repair of closed metatarsal fracture he incurred after tripping over his dog. As instructed, he had taken his morning medications with a sip of water at 6 AM, including his morning dose of lopinavir/ritonavir 400/100 mg.

The patient had a life-long fear of paralysis and was terribly afraid of general anesthesia, stating "I don't do well being put under." He refused both general and spinal anesthesia and could not be reassured, eventually consenting to general anesthesia only in the case of a life-threatening emergency. He did agree to an ankle block and sedation. While waiting in the preoperative area the patient was extremely nervous

E.D. Wittwer MD, PhD (✉) • W.T. Nicholson MD, PharmD, MSc
Department of Anesthesiology, Mayo Clinic, Rochester, MN, USA
e-mail: Wittwer.erica@mayo.edu

C. Wisdo DPM
Dunes Podiatry, Murrells Inlet, SC, USA

C. Marcucci MD
Anesthesia Services Department, Philadelphia Veterans Affairs Medical Center, Philadelphia, PA, USA

C. Marcucci et al. (eds.), *A Case Approach to Perioperative Drug-Drug Interactions*, DOI 10.1007/978-1-4614-7495-1_84

and agitated. He requested something to help him relax and midazolam (2 mg) was administered intravenously (IV). One hour later, he was next to go to the operating room and his block was accomplished in the block area with monitoring, supplemental oxygen, and an additional dose of midazolam (4 mg IV).

As the nurses were pulling the instruments, the podiatry attending paged the anesthesiologist. Review of the films had indicated fracture also of the distal tibia, necessitating a longer, more involved repair including use of a thigh tourniquet and placement of an external fixation device. A "bigger anesthetic" was requested. When the anesthesiologist approached the patient to revisit the question of a general or spinal anesthesia, she found that he lacked capacity to consent to an elective spinal anesthetic as he was sedated to the point of being nonverbal, even while conscious. The case was cancelled since repair of a closed ankle fracture did not meet the "emergency" criterion. The patient was transferred to the PACU where he had an extended stay and eventually required admission to a monitored bed. He underwent surgery under general anesthesia the following afternoon when he was alert and able to provide consent.

Discussion

This is an example of a substrate added to an inhibitor.

Lopinavir is a protease inhibitor that is used in the treatment of HIV to reduce virus proliferation in the body. It is completely metabolized by the cytochrome P450 3A family of enzymes (CYP 3A). Although ritonavir is also a protease inhibitor, the lower dose present within this combination is used to inhibit CYP3A metabolism of the lopinavir to increase efficacy. In addition, this ritonavir enzyme inhibition also leads to increased levels of other drugs that are metabolized by CYP3A enzymes.

Midazolam is a benzodiazepine commonly used in the operating room, procedure suites, and the intensive care unit for sedation and anxiolysis. Administration is usually by either IV or oral routes. Several protease inhibitors (eg, indinavir, nelfinavir, saquinavir) are known to inhibit CYP3A enzymes and their manufacturers' product information sheets contraindicate or caution the concomitant use of midazolam.

Significant decreases in midazolam clearance are observed by both the IV and oral administration demonstrating the inhibitory effects of lopinavir/ritonavir on both absorption and metabolism. Hepatic inhibition of CYP3A4 by lopinavir/ritonavir results in a 77% reduction in midazolam clearance following IV administration.[1] With oral midazolam administration, inhibition of both intestinal and hepatic CYP3A enzymes should be considered. Lopinavir/ritonavir results in an increase in intestinal midazolam availability from 78% to 87%, along with a decrease in hepatic clearance.[2] Overall, inhibition of CYP3A by the lopinavir/ritonavir combination demonstrates a 92% decrease in clearance of oral midazolam.[1] Decreased clearance results in an increased plasma concentration of the midazolam which can prolong sedation. Since increases in the concentration of midazolam are expected to be higher with oral vs IV administration, lopinavir/ritonavir and oral midazolam is contraindicated.[3] However in a recent retrospective study, a sixfold risk for severe prolonged sedation was associated with the coadministration of intravenous midazolam with either lopinavir/ritonavir or atazanavir/ritonavir in a population HIV-positive patients receiving sedation during bronchoscopy.[4] Therefore, selection of a sedative that does not undergo significant CYP3A metabolism (eg, lorazepam) should be a consideration.[5]

It should be noted that administration of protease inhibitors can result in very complicated drug–drug interactions. The CYP3A inhibition can be variable with among different protease inhibitors although, ritonavir is the most potent.[4] Following multiple dose therapy the CYP3A activity is reduced by 90%.[6] However, it is important that inhibition should be considered with other ritonavir metabolic effects. Although many drugs undergo metabolism by CYP3A there are often other metabolic pathways involved in biotransformation of a given drug. In addition to 3A inhibition, ritonavir may also cause induction of several CYP450 enzymes including 1A2, 2B6, 2C9 and 2C19.[1,6] Possibly these or other inductive effects may result in drug–drug interactions that appear paradoxical when only CYP3A inhibition is considered. Here, other minor metabolic pathways might now have a greater importance once induced.

In a properly monitored setting, a single bolus of IV midazolam is generally considered to be safe in patients taking protease inhibitors, however, the combination of two IV boluses and the patient's age contributed to his oversedation.[7] Oral administration of midazolam in a patient taking protease inhibitors would not be recommended. Additionally, a continuous midazolam infusion should be avoided with patients receiving protease inhibitor therapy.[7]

Take-Home Points

- Protease inhibitors such as lopinavir/ritonavir may have complex drug interactions because enzyme induction or inhibition may occur depending on metabolic pathway.
- Midazolam is a substrate of CYP3A and coadministration with lopinavir/ritonavir may lead to increased levels resulting in prolonged sedation.
- Although a single dose of IV midazolam may be used in a properly monitored setting, benzodiazepines that do not undergo significant CYP3A metabolism (eg, lorazepam) should be considered.

Summary

Interaction: pharmacokinetic
Substrate: midazolam
Enzyme: CYP3A4
Inhibitor: lopinavir/ritonavir
Clinical effects: extended and exaggerated effect of midazolam

References

1. Yeh RF, Gaver VE, Patterson KB, et al. Lopinavir/ritonavir induces the hepatic activity of cytochrome P450 enzymes CYP2C9, CYP2C19, and CYP1A2 but inhibits the hepatic and intestinal activity of CYP3A as measured by a phenotyping drug cocktail in healthy volunteers. J Acquir Immune Defic Syndr. 2006;42(1):52–60.
2. Wyen C, Fuhr U, Frank D, et al. Effect of an antiretroviral regimen containing ritonavir boosted lopinavir on intestinal and hepatic CYP3A, CYP2D6 and P-glycoprotein in HIV-infected patients. Clin Pharmacol Ther. 2008;84(1):75–82.
3. Product information: Kaletra tablets (lopinavir/ritonavir). North Chicago: Abbott Laboratories; 2011.
4. Hsu AJ, Carson KA, Yung R, Pham PA. Severe prolonged sedation associated with coadministration of protease inhibitors and intravenous midazolam during bronchoscopy. Pharmacotherapy. 2012;32(6):538–45.
5. Dresser GK, Spence JD, Bailey DG. Pharmacokinetic-pharmacodynamic consequences and clinical relevance of cytochrome P450 3A4 inhibition. Clin Pharmacokinet. 2000;38:41–57.
6. Kirby BJ, Collier AC, Kharasch ED, Dixit V, Desai P, Whittington D, Thummel KE, Unadkat JD. Complex drug interactions of HIV protease inhibitors 2: in vivo induction and in vitro to in vivo correlation of induction of cytochrome P450 1A2, 2B6, and 2C9 by ritonavir or nelfinavir. Drug Metab Dispos. 2011;39(12):2329–37. Epub 2011 Sep 19.
7. HIV InSite, Database of antiretroviral drug Interactions, interactions with Midazolam (Versed) and antiretrovirals, University of California, San Francisco. http://hivinsite.ucsf.edu/insite?page=ar-00-02&post=8&param=73#60. Accessed 1/10/2012.

Noct' Out

Fatal Forty DDI: chloral hydrate, phenobarbital, furosemide

85

Michael Wollenberg MD and Kirk Lalwani MD, FRCA, MCR

Abstract

This case discusses a complex interaction involving chloral hydrate. A synergistic pharmacodynamics interaction occurred between chloral hydrate and other sedatives. A protein-binding displacement reaction between chloral hydrate and furosemide also occurred.

Case

Jimmy, a 3-year-old, 14 kg boy, was admitted to the intensive care unit (ICU) after he had required resuscitation during magnetic resonance imaging (MRI) under routine sedation. He had a history of low-grade astrocytoma, which had been debulked 6 months ago, and he was on an antiepileptic medication, which he took regularly. He was in his usual state of health when he presented for the surveillance imaging. Prior to starting the scan, he received a sedating dose of chloral hydrate (Noctec®, 100 mg/kg orally). He was positioned in the MRI scanner 30 minutes later with adequate sedation. Twenty minutes later, Jimmy's SpO_2 was noted to be 55% and his heart rate 40 beats per minute (bpm). He was quickly removed from the MRI suite, evaluated, and noted to be pulseless. CPR was initiated. He was intubated, ventilated with 100% O_2, given one dose of epinephrine and 450 mL. of normal saline. Approximately 6 minutes passed between removal from the MRI suite and return of spontaneous circulation.

Jimmy was taken to the ICU where he remained sedated and ventilated, now 4 hours after the aborted scan. His medical history was reviewed with his mother

M. Wollenberg MD (✉) • K. Lalwani MD, FRCA, MCR
Department of Anesthesiology and Perioperative Medicine, Oregon Health and Science University, Portland, OR, USA
e-mail: wollenbm@ohsu.edu

C. Marcucci et al. (eds.), *A Case Approach to Perioperative Drug-Drug Interactions*, DOI 10.1007/978-1-4614-7495-1_85

and it was ascertained that he had been receiving phenobarbital (50 mg po every 12 hours) since being diagnosed with seizures secondary to his astrocytoma. His ICU nurse also noted that he had made almost no urine in the first 4 hours of his ICU stay despite receiving 30 mL/kg of crystalloid during resuscitation. A decision was made to administer one dose of IV furosemide. A few minutes after the dose, Jimmy became flushed, diaphoretic, tachycardic, and appeared restless in the ICU bed. The symptoms lasted approximately 20 minutes and resolved spontaneously. His urine output picked up and he awoke 1 hour later. He was extubated that night and discharged the next morning with no residual sequelae.

Discussion

This is an example of a mixed pharmacodynamic and pharmacokinetic drug–drug interaction.

More specifically, this case demonstrates several concerns when using chloral hydrate. First, there is a significant risk for synergy between chloral hydrate and sedative medications such as benzodiazepines, opioids, or in this case, barbiturates. Second, chloral hydrate and its metabolites will displace or be displaced by other protein-bound medications and give rise to transient symptoms of toxicity.

Chloral hydrate is a commonly used synthetic sedative/hypnotic agent used primarily for sedation and analgesia in children. Both chloral hydrate and its primary active metabolite cause nonspecific sedation of the central nervous system (CNS) through an unknown mechanism. Therapeutic doses range from 25 to 125 mg/kg and result in sedation in approximately 30 minutes.[1] Sedation is long lasting, 80 minutes ±15 minutes in one study, and deeper than the sedation achieved with comparable doses of midazolam.[2] Chloral hydrate is rapidly metabolized by alcohol dehydrogenase in the liver and erythrocytes resulting in trichloroethanol (TCE). TCE is the primary active metabolite of chloral hydrate. A portion of the TCE produced is conjugated with glucuronic acid to form TCE-glucuronide, which is excreted in the urine (primarily) and bile. The remainder is oxidized to trichloroacetic acid (TCA), which is less active than the primary active metabolite TCE. Direct oxidation of chloral hydrate to TCA also occurs, primarily in the liver and kidney.[3] The half-life of TCE is in the range of 7 to 10 hours while the half-life of TCA is much longer, 60+ hours.[4] The unlucky patient in this case suffered from two separate drug–drug interactions associated with chloral hydrate.

Chloral hydrate is capable of causing vomiting, stupor, coma, respiratory depression, hypotension, and even arrhythmias in high doses. Excessive sedation and respiratory depression is a serious concern when combining chloral hydrate with benzodiazepines, opioids, barbiturates, or other CNS depressant drugs.[5] In our case, Jimmy had been receiving barbiturates, which should have led to reconsideration of the dose of chloral hydrate administered, or selection of a short-acting drug such as propofol.

The dose of furosemide Jimmy received in the ICU triggered the second of the described interactions, that of displacement of the drug from protein-binding sites resulting in symptoms of overdose. Furosemide displaces TCA from its binding site within albumin. It is unclear whether the now displaced TCA directly causes the symptoms described above, or if TCA displaces thyroxine from its thyroid-binding proteins resulting in tachycardia, flushing, diaphoresis, and agitation.[6] Either way, elevated TCA due to displacement by furosemide is associated with this short-lived toxicity. A similar effect is seen when chloral hydrate is administered with warfarin. Chloral hydrate displaces warfarin from its protein-binding site resulting in a transient increase in the anticoagulant effect, the clinical significance of which is unclear.[7]

Take-Home Points

- CNS depressants may act synergistically when combined, resulting in excessive sedation or respiratory depression. When multiple CNS depressant medications are given in combination, it is imperative that adequate monitoring be provided and that staff trained in airway management and resuscitation are available.

- When furosemide and chloral hydrate are combined, symptoms of agitation, tachycardia, flushing, and diaphoresis may result from displacement of chloral hydrate metabolites from their binding sites on albumin.

- When chloral hydrate is combined with warfarin, a transient increase in warfarin activity may be observed due to displacement of warfarin from its protein-binding sites.

Summary

Interaction 1: pharmacodynamic
Substrates: chloral hydrate and phenobarbital
Site of action: CNS
Clinical effects: synergistic sedation and cardiopulmonary depression

Interaction 2: pharmacokinetic (distribution)
Substrates: chloral hydrate and furosemide
Mechanism: plasma protein displacement
Sites of action: multiple systemic end-organs
Clinical effects: sympathetic discharge symptoms including tachycardia and diaphoresis

References

1. Napoli KL, Ingall CG, Martin GR. Safety and efficacy of chloral hydrate sedation in children undergoing echocardiography. J Pediatr. 1996;129:287–91.
2. D'Agostino J, Terndrup TE. Chloral hydrate versus midazolam for sedation of children for neuroimaging: a randomized clinical trial. Pediatr Emerg Care. 2000;16:1–4.
3. Buck ML. The use of chloral hydrate in infants and children. Pediatr Pharm. 2005;11(9):1–4.
4. Breimer DD. Clinical pharmacokinetics of hypnotics. Clin Pharmacokinet. 1977;2:93–109.
5. Pershad J, Palmisano P, Nichols M. Chloral hydrate: the good and the bad. Pediatr Emerg Care. 1999;15:432–5.
6. Dean RP, Rudinsky BF, Kelleher MD. Interaction of chloral hydrate and intravenous furosemide in a child. Clin Pharm. 1991;10:385–7.
7. Griner PF, Raisz LG, Rickles FR, et al. Chloral hydrate and warfarin interaction: clinical significance? Ann Intern Med. 1971;74:540–3.

Predisposed to Doze

Promethazine, CYP2D6 poor metabolizer

86

Erica D. Wittwer MD, PhD, Juraj Sprung MD, PhD, and Wayne T. Nicholson MD, PharmD, MSc

Abstract
This case discusses a drug–gene interaction. Promethazine is a cytochrome P450 (CYP) 2D6 substrate. Patients who are CYP2D6 poor metabolizers exhibit greater sedation for a given promethazine dose.

Case

A 63-year-old woman experienced persistent nausea and vomiting in the postanesthesia care unit (PACU) after an uncomplicated general anesthesia for right total knee arthroplasty, despite treatment with ondansetron, granisetron, and droperidol. In addition, she had moderately severe postoperative pain and required supplemental hydromorphone. She was otherwise healthy and took only nonsteroidal anti-inflammatory drugs for knee pain. She had no known adverse drug reactions, but did report that codeine had been ineffective in treating her pain after a dental procedure several years earlier. The anesthesiologist administered one dose of ketorolac (15 mg) intravenously to improve her pain control to minimize sedation or potential for respiratory depression, as well as promethazine (12.5 mg) for persistent nausea. Her pain decreased significantly and she continued receiving hydromorphone as needed while in the PACU.

On the Orthopedics floor, the patient had orders for a hydromorphone patient-controlled administration pump and ketorolac every 6 hours for pain, granisetron once daily as needed for nausea, and promethazine every 4 to 6 hours as needed for nausea. She continued to require promethazine and hydromorphone for treatment of nausea and pain. On the night of surgery the surgical resident was urgently called

E.D. Wittwer MD, PhD (✉) • J. Sprung MD, PhD • W.T. Nicholson MD, PharmD, MSc
Department of Anesthesiology, Mayo Clinic, Rochester, MN, USA
e-mail: Wittwer.erica@mayo.edu

C. Marcucci et al. (eds.), *A Case Approach to Perioperative Drug-Drug Interactions*, DOI 10.1007/978-1-4614-7495-1_86

because the patient was very sleepy and apneic when not stimulated. She had received a total of three doses of promethazine and 2.2 mg of hydromorphone, including the doses in the PACU. Naloxone was administered and although the respirations improved, she remained quite somnolent. The patient gradually became more alert in the intensive care unit and hydromorphone was resumed the following day without noticeable sedation. After discussion with the pharmacist it was postulated that poor metabolism of the promethazine may have resulted in this case of excessive sedation. She was later tested and found to have a genotype consistent with poor cytochrome P450 2D6 metabolism.

Discussion

This is an example of a pharmacogenomic or drug–gene interaction characterized by poor metabolism.

Promethazine is a histamine-1 antagonist used, among other indications, to treat nausea and vomiting and may cause increased sedation. Promethazine is metabolized by P450 (CYP) 2D6.[1] The 2D6 isozyme is responsible for approximately 25% of all drug metabolism by cytochrome P450 enzymes. Genetic polymorphisms can alter the activity or concentration of CYP2D6, significantly changing plasma levels of drugs dependent on 2D6 for clearance. Poor metabolism of promethazine can potentially lead to increased adverse effects and toxicity.

Different phenotypical presentations in metabolism can present depending on genotype. Metabolism can be described as poor, intermediate, extensive (normal) or ultra-rapid and depending on allelic activity. Individuals who metabolize drugs poorly have no active copy of the CYP2D6 allele; those with intermediate metabolism phenotypes have one active copy. Extensive metabolizers have two active copies, and those with ultra-rapid metabolism have duplicate or multiple active copies. Phenotypes for extensive metabolizers of 2D6 clear these substrates normally. An intermediate metabolism phenotype is less predictable since it can result in drug clearance that might resemble normal to less than normal. Those who metabolize drugs poorly and who metabolize drugs ultra-rapidly have decreased and increased drug clearance, respectively.

Several categories of drugs such as antidepressants (including amitriptyline, fluoxetine, duloxetine, venlafaxine, etc.), antipsychotics (including haloperidol, chlorpromazine, risperidone, aripiprazole, etc.), antiemetics (including metoclopramide, ondansetron, etc), codeine, dextromethorphan, and some cardiac drugs (including metoprolol, carvedilol, propranolol, timolol, etc.) are biotransformed by CYP2D6. As codeine is a prodrug, individuals who are 2D6 poor metabolizers do not metabolize codeine to its active metabolite morphine, and thus do not receive the analgesic effect as those who metabolize codeine normally.[2] Our patient reported that codeine was ineffective in treating her pain which was a clue for the pharmacist that she might be a CYP2D6 poor metabolizer when taken together with this outcome.

Foster et al. described an interesting case that emphasized the interaction between promethazine and opioids that caused intolerable adverse effects.[3] Administration of promethazine with other medications that can cause sedation or respiratory depression, may worsen the adverse effects for a patient with poor CYP2D6 metabolism, and this was a most plausible explanation for the excessive sedation with promethazine encountered in our patient.

Take-Home Points

- Promethazine is metabolized through the isozyme CYP2D6. Individuals can have poor drug metabolism with no active copy of the CYP2D6 allele, leading to increased adverse effects or toxicity, or both, from promethazine use.
- The 2D6 isozyme is responsible for approximately 25% of all drug metabolism and different phonotypical presentations may be seen in metabolism by CYP2D6.
- Reduced clearance resulting in promethazine toxicity can manifest as somnolence, blurred vision, confusion, extrapyramidal symptoms, uncoordination, and seizures.

Summary

Interaction: pharmacogenomic (drug–gene)
Substrates: promethazine
Enzyme: CYP2D6
Clinical effect: sedation

References

1. Nakamura K, Yokoi T, Inoue K, et al. CYP2D6 is the principal cytochrome P450 responsible for metabolism of the histamine H1 antagonist promethazine in human liver microsomes. Pharmacogenetics. 1996;6:449–57.
2. Kirchheiner J, Schmidt H, Tzvetkov M, et al. Pharmacokinetics of codeine and its metabolite morphine in ultra-rapid metabolizers due to CYP2D6 duplication. Pharmacogenomics J. 2007;7(4):257–65.
3. Foster A, Mobley E, Wang Z. Complicated pain management in a CYP450 2D6 poor metabolizer. Pain Pract. 2007;7:352–6.

Synergistic Sedation

87

Fatal Forty DDI: midazolam, clozapine, synergism and clozapine, sertraline, CYP2D6

Michael P. Hutchens MD, Paul Schipper MD, FACS, FACCP, and Catherine Marcucci MD

Abstract
This case discusses a pharmacodynamic interaction between clozapine, midazolam, fentanyl, hydromorphone, and oxycodone resulting in central nervous system depression. It also discusses a pharmacokinetic interaction between clozapine and sertraline resulting in increased bioavailability of clozapine.

Case

A 50-year-old man with a history of schizophrenia was stably maintained on clozapine (Clozaril®, 300 mg TID) and sertraline (Zoloft®, 100 mg qd). He developed hemoptysis and underwent lung resection for squamous carcinoma of his left lung. He was anxious in the holding area and received midazolam (2 mg) intravenously. An epidural was placed and anesthesia was induced. Intraoperatively, the patient was persistently and severely hypotensive and required repeated boluses of phenylephrine and a phenylephrine infusion despite minimal blood loss. Over the last 2.5 hours of the procedure, fentanyl (250 mcg) was given via the epidural catheter to augment postoperative analgesia. An epidural infusion of 0.1% bupivacaine with hydromorphone 10 mcg/mL was started in the postanesthesia care unit.

M.P. Hutchens MD (✉)
Department of Anesthesiology and Perioperative Medicine,
Oregon Health and Science University, Portland, OR, USA
e-mail: hutchenm@ohsu.edu

P. Schipper MD, FACS, FACCP
Section of General Thoracic Surgery, Division of Cardiothoracic Surgery,
Department of Surgery, Oregon Health and Sciences University, Portland, OR, USA

C. Marcucci MD
Anesthesia Services Department, Philadelphia Veterans Affairs Medical Center,
Philadelphia, PA, USA

C. Marcucci et al. (eds.), *A Case Approach to Perioperative Drug-Drug Interactions*, DOI 10.1007/978-1-4614-7495-1_87

Because he could not be weaned from the phenylephrine infusion in the postoperative period, the intensive care team decided to decrease the epidural infusion postoperative period. Interestingly, although the patient aroused to stimulus, he was also noted to be sleeping on all nursing assessments. When the patient finally awoke and drowsily complained of pain, he was given a total two doses of oxycodone (5 mg orally) over a 10-hour period. He subsequently exhibited mental status changes and respiratory depression. He suffered an early aspiration pneumonia that was likely due to excessive sedation. Reintubation was considered, however, he was ultimately managed on bi-level positive airway pressure (BiPAP) therapy for several hours. The psychiatric consultation service was called, and they recommended a decrease of his clozaril dose to a total of 500 mg/day and discontinuation of the sertraline. By the third postoperative day, the patient had striking improvement in his mental status, was off phenylephrine, and was awake and appropriate. *(Personal communication 2014, Michael Hutchens MD)*

Discussion

This is an example of a pharmacodynamic drug–drug interaction (DDI) between several central nervous system depressants. This is also an example of a pharmacokinetic DDI involving reversal of inhibition.

Clozapine is an atypical antipsychotic with especially potent central nervous system (CNS) depressant capabilities. The package insert for clozapine specifically lists a "black box" warning of "…collapse, respiratory arrest, and cardiac arrest" when clozapine is coadministered with benzodiazepines during the early titration phase.[1] While this patient had been on clozapine chronically before the lung resection, the black box warning indicates clozapine's ability to synergize with other CNS depressants, such as benzodiazepines and narcotic analgesics, to produce mental status changes and impairments in cardiopulmonary function.

The addition not only of midazolam, but also oxycodone, high-dose epidural fentanyl, and epidural hydromorphone, to clozapine likely produced synergistic CNS depression that led to the patient's hemodynamic and respiratory depression. Additionally, clozapine is a P450 substrate and is specifically metabolized by several CYP450 enzymes, including 2D6.[2]

Sertraline is a mildly sedating CNS depressant as well as a dose-dependent CYP2D6 inhibitor.[3] Discontinuation of the sertraline served to remove one of several sedating medication and eliminate a potential, although probably mild, impediment to enzymatic elimination of clozapine.[4]

Take-Home Points

- Clozapine is an antipsychotic medication with strong CNS depressant effects.
- Clozapine carries a black box warning with respect to CNS sedation when it is coadministered with benzodiazepines.
- Clozapine is a CYP2D6 substrate.
- Coadministration of sertraline, a dose-dependent CYP2D6 inhibitor, was a potential contributor to the clinical situation by impeding clozapine metabolism.

Summary

Interaction 1: pharmacodynamic
Substrates: clozapine, midazolam, fentanyl, hydromorphone, and oxycodone
Mechanism/site of action: synergistic CNS depression
Clinical effect: sedation

Interaction 2: pharmacokinetic (mild)
Substrate: clozapine
Enzyme: CYP2D6
Inhibitor: sertraline
Clinical effect: increased bioavailability of clozapine

References

1. Clozaril Package Insert, Novartis, Basel, Switzerland, 2002. Viewed 16 July 2012.
2. Olesen OV, Linnet K. Contributions of five human cytochrome P450 isoforms to the N-demethylation of clozapine in vitro at low and high concentrations. J Clin Pharmacol. 2001;41(8):823–32.
3. Solai LK, Mulsant BH, Pollock BG, et al. Effect of sertraline on plasma nortriptyline levels in depressed elderly. J Clin Psychiatry. 1997;58(10):440–3.
4. Pinninti NR, de Leon J. Interaction of sertraline with clozapine. J Clin Psychopharmacol. 1997;17(2):119–20.

Drug–Drug Interactions Involving Neuromuscular Blockade Agents

X

Introduction

88

David G. Metro MD

Abstract
This section introduces drug–drug and drug–gene interactions involving neuromuscular blocking agents.

"You must not be in much of a rush to get home," my attending said to me as he walked out of the operating room. This was said on a Friday evening around 7:00 PM and I, as a CA-1, had just simultaneously given a dose of pancuronium along with starting a vancomycin infusion right before the surgeon decided he was done for the night. Ultimately, I ended up staying a couple of hours later but had learned a valuable lesson about drug interactions.

Since curare was introduced as a muscle relaxant for use in surgery in the 1940s, neuromuscular blocking (NMB) agents have become an important tool in the armamentarium of the anesthesia provider. We believe that mastery of neuromuscular blockade is a *sine qua non* of mastering the practice of anesthesiology. Part and parcel of the requisite intimate knowledge of the effects of neuromuscular blockers is knowledge of the associated interactions.

These drugs are particularly interesting because they are involved in both drug–gene and drug–drug interactions with effects mediated at the neuromuscular junction, plasma cholinesterases, and the hepatic enzymes. Also, the effects of NMBs can either be prolonged or shortened by the addition of other agents and these effects can have results from minor annoyances to a significant impact in patient safety. We have included more than one succinylcholine case scenario, because, although the debate rages on about succinylcholine and its role in rapid sequence and/or emergent intubation, it is a drug that has been in constant and enormous clinical use for 60 years. Additionally, it's been our experience that *nobody* can ever remember the basics of pseudocholinesterase and how it relates to the dibucaine number without sneaking away and reviewing the information on the sly. We felt, therefore, that a

D.G. Metro MD
Department of Anesthesiology,
University of Pittsburgh School of Medicine, Pittsburgh, PA, USA
e-mail: metrodg@upmc.edu

C. Marcucci et al. (eds.), *A Case Approach to Perioperative Drug-Drug Interactions*, DOI 10.1007/978-1-4614-7495-1_88

second (or third) opportunity to review this material might be of benefit to the reader.

We hope you enjoy this section and that we've achieved our goal of explaining these drug–drug and drug–gene interactions in clear and memorable detail. Of course, we hope also to maybe save you some day from ruining the start of your weekend……….

Blocked Again: Effects of Repeated Doses of Succinylcholine

89

Succinylcholine, repeated doses

Matthew Patrick Feuer MD and Thomas M. Chalifoux MD

Abstract
This case discusses the effects of repeated doses of succinylcholine.

Case

A 51-year-old woman with an elevated body mass index presented for a bronchoscopy and lung biopsy. Her past surgical history included a colonoscopy, knee arthroscopy, and childhood tonsillectomy without anesthesia or airway difficulties. Her airway exam revealed a Mallampati 2 airway, thyromental distance of two finger-widths, normal mouth opening, and normal cervical range of motion. Her preoperative laboratory values were normal.

After preoxygenation, the patient received a 4 mg defasciculating dose of rocuronium, propofol (200 mg) and succinylcholine (120 mg). Endotracheal tube placement, using both MacIntosh 3 and Miller 2 blades, was unsuccessful. She was ventilated by mask and a #4 LMA was placed. The difficult airway cart was requested. The patient's vital signs remained stable with a heart rate of 77 beats per minute but she began to cough a little. With about 5 minutes elapsed since induction, she received additional propofol (200 mg) and succinylcholine (80 mg) in order to intubate with a 8.0 endotracheal tube via video laryngoscope. The patient's heart rate dropped

M.P. Feuer MD (✉)
Department of Anesthesiology, Frederick Memorial Hospital, Frederick, MD, USA
e-mail: matthewpatrickfeuer@yahoo.com

T.M. Chalifoux MD
Department of Anesthesiology, University of Pittsburgh School of Medicine, Magee-Womens Hospital Anesthesiology, Pittsburgh, PA, USA

C. Marcucci et al. (eds.), *A Case Approach to Perioperative Drug-Drug Interactions*, DOI 10.1007/978-1-4614-7495-1_89

into the range of 30 to 40 beats per minute (bpm) from a baseline rate of 65 bpm. Following administration of 0.5 mg atropine, the heart rate increased to 80 bpm.

Since the thoracic surgeon was extremely fast, muscle relaxation was maintained with a succinylcholine infusion at 85 mcg/kg/min. Nerve stimulation monitoring ensured that twitches were palpable for the duration of the 30 minute case. After cessation of the infusion, the anesthesiologist was surprised to find that patient's response to train-of-four (TOF) stimulation exhibited fade and post-tetanic facilitation. Recovery of the TOF ratio to greater than 75% took about 6 minutes and the patient was safely extubated and taken to the recovery room.

Discussion

Technically speaking, this is not an example of a classic drug–drug interaction. But you still need to know it and you had *better* know it.

Drug–drug interactions are most correctly defined as occurring between two drugs of the same class or drugs interacting across drug class or type. However, the preceding case scenario highlights a different issue for the anesthesia provider, one that is important enough to conceptualize it, if you will, as a "temporal" drug interaction., ie, the interaction of "new" succinylcholine with "old" succinylcholine.

Succinylcholine consists of two acetylcholine molecules joined end to end and, therefore, can stimulate all cholinergic receptors. Succinylcholine's primary action is at the nicotinic receptors of the neuromuscular junction but it can also act at the sympathetic and parasympathetic ganglia, the adrenal medulla, and the muscarinic receptors of the sinus node. Hence, succinylcholine can lead to increased or decreased heart rate and blood pressure. Most commonly, succinylcholine can cause sinus bradycardia or nodal bradycardia in children (who have high parasympathetic tone) or in adults, following administration of a second dose.

A second dose of succinylcholine given five minutes after the first will frequently cause bradydysrhythmias.[1] The "self-taming" technique (pretreatment with a small dose of succinylcholine in an effort to decrease the incidence of muscle fasciculations and myalgia following succinylcholine administration) has been shown to significantly increase the likelihood of bradycardia after both a single and a second dose of succinylcholine.[2] The higher incidence of bradycardia after a second dose suggests that products of succinylcholine hydrolysis (choline and succinylmonocholine) may sensitize the heart to subsequent doses. The bradycardic effect is usually transient and is attenuated by prior intravenous administration of atropine,[3] glycopyrrolate,[4] d-tubocurarine,[5] thiopentone,[6] ganglionic blockers, or ketamine.[7] The efficacy of these treatments suggests that muscarinic stimulation, direct myocardial effects, and ganglionic stimulation may all play a role in the bradycardia produced by succinylcholine. In our clinical scenario, the anesthesiologist might have chosen to pretreat with atropine (0.01 mg/kg) prior to the second dose of succinylcholine.

Phase II block is a neuromuscular block, with characteristics similar to blocks by nondepolarizing neuromuscular agents, that can be caused by prolonged succinylcholine infusion. Succinylcholine infusion can cause three distinct phases of neuromuscular blockade. Initially, the patient exhibits a profound block with diminished twitch height, no fade on TOF stimulation or tetanic stimulation, no potentiation of twitch height after tetanus, and no reversibility with anticholinesterase administration. This can be followed by a period of tachyphylaxis with increased infusion requirements and subsequent Phase II block. Phase II block results in a profound block which shows fade on TOF and tetanic stimulation, post-tetanic potentiation, and variable reversibility with anticholinesterase drugs. Some of these Phase II characteristics have more recently been shown to occur after single intubating doses of succinylcholine.[8] When Phase II block occurs, allowing for spontaneous recovery is recommended.

Classically, Phase II block was thought to show prolonged recovery times in comparison to Phase I block, however, a study of succinylcholine infusions by Chen and colleagues showed no significant difference in recovery time between patients who developed Phase I and those who developed Phase II blocks.[9] This study used lower average total doses (4.3 mg/kg) and shorter average infusion durations (52 min) compared to earlier studies. The authors also found no simple correlation between dose, duration, and the occurrence of Phase II. The incidence of Phase II block was about 30%. It would appear that infusions of 2 to 6 mg/kg total dose and up to 80 minutes total duration can be used with no abnormal prolongation of recovery time.

Take-Home Points

- Succinylcholine can cause significant bradycardia, particularly in children, and with a second dose, in adults.
- Atropine (0.01 mg/kg), given prior to a second dose of succinylcholine, may prevent bradycardia.
- Phase II block can occur with succinylcholine infusion; but prolonged recovery is less likely if infusions of 2 to 6 mg/kg total dose for less than 80 minutes are used.
- The preferred treatment for Phase II block is allowing for spontaneous recovery.

Summary

Interaction: "pharmacodynamic"
Substrates: repeated succinylcholine doses
Mechanism/sites of action: cholinergic receptors
Clinical effect: Phase II block, bradycardia, other cholinergic responses

References

1. Luprian KG, Churchill-Davidson HC. Effect of suxamethonium on cardiac rhythm. BMJ. 1960;4:1774–7.
2. Magee DA, Sweet PT. Cardiac effects of self-taming of succinylcholine and repeated succinylcholine administration. Can Anaesth Soc J. 1982;29(6):577–9.
3. Viby-Mogensen J, Wisborg K. Thiopentone-nitrous oxide-halothane anaesthesia and suxamethonium: the significance of preoperative atropine and gallamine administration. Br J Anaesth. 1980;52(11):1137–42.
4. Sørensen O, Eriksen S, Hommelgaard P, et al. Thiopental-nitrous oxide-halothane anesthesia and repeated succinylcholine: comparison of preoperative glycopyrrolate and atropine administration. Anesth Analg. 1980;59(9):686–9.
5. Magee DA, Sweet PT, Holland AJ. Effect of atropine on bradydysrhythmias induced by succinylcholine following pretreatment with D-tubocurarine. Can Anaesth Soc J. 1982;29(6):573–6.
6. Williams CH, Deutsch S, Linde HW, et al. Effects of intravenously administered succinyldicholine on cardiac rate, rhythm, and arterial blood pressure in anesthetized man. Anesthesiology. 1961;22:947–54.
7. Sears DH, Abdul-Rasool IH, Katz RL. The effect of a second dose of succinylcholine on cardiac rate and rhythm following induction of anesthesia with ketamine. Anesthesiology. 1988;68(4):644.
8. Naguib M, Lien CA, Aker J, et al. Posttetanic potentiation and fade in the response to tetanic and train-of-four stimulation during succinylcholine-induced block. Anesth Analg. 2004;98(6):1686–91.
9. Chen YA, Fan SZ, Lee PC, et al. Continuous succinylcholine infusion and phase II block in short surgical procedures. Acta Anaesthesiol Sin. 1993;31(4):253–6.

Irreversibility Sux

90

Succinylcholine, neostigmine

Joseph C. Shy MD and David G. Metro MD

Abstract
This case discusses the pharmacodynamic interaction between neostigmine and succinylcholine, resulting in increased neuromuscular weakness.

Case

A 60 kg 74-year-old woman with past medical history significant for coronary artery disease, hypertension, hyperlipidemia, diabetes mellitus type 2, peripheral vascular disease, and chronic kidney disease on dialysis three times weekly presented for left femoral-popliteal bypass. After, induction of general anesthesia, succinylcholine (120 mg) was then given to facilitate intubation. A nerve stimulator was placed and after return-of-four twitches, the patient was given rocuronium to maintain paralysis. Surgery was uneventful and, upon completion, testing with nerve stimulator revealed 2/4 twitches. The patient was given glycopyrrolate (0.6) along with neostigmine (5 mg) for reversal of paralysis. She was extubated without complication and transported to the postanesthesia care unit (PACU).

In the PACU, the patient was tachycardic and hypotensive. Ten minutes into the PACU stay, significant swelling of her left lower extremity edema was noted and she was taken back to the operating room emergently for suspected arterial bleed. Etomidate and succinylcholine were again given to facilitate replacement of the endotracheal tube. Upon completion of the repair, nerve stimulator failed to demonstrate any twitches. Return of spontaneous ventilation was not observed. The patient required intubation and mechanical ventilation for 2 hours postoperatively.

J.C. Shy MD (✉)
Department of Anesthesiology, University of Pittsburgh Medical Center, Pittsburgh, PA, USA
e-mail: shyjc@upmc.edu

D.G. Metro MD
Department of Anesthesiology, University of Pittsburgh School of Medicine, Pittsburgh, PA, USA

C. Marcucci et al. (eds.), *A Case Approach to Perioperative Drug-Drug Interactions*, DOI 10.1007/978-1-4614-7495-1_90

Discussion

This is an example of an antagonistic pharmacodynamic interaction.

Succinylcholine (suxamethonium chloride) is a quaternary ammonium compound consisting of two acetylcholine molecules linked together. Clinically, it is a depolarizing neuromuscular blocking agent that binds to nicotinic M receptors for acetylcholine. It initially causes depolarization of the neuromuscular junction leading to "desensitization" and paralysis. The onset of action of succinylcholine is quite rapid, on the order of 30 to 60 seconds, and it ordinarily has a short duration of action, about 3 to 5 minutes. Succinylcholine is broken down by butyrylcholinesterase, or pseudocholinesterase, found in the plasma. Succinylcholine is capable of producing two types of neuromuscular blockade, a Phase I or a Phase II block. Phase I blockade is the depolarizing block mentioned above. Phase II blockade is characteristic of a nondepolarizing block which becomes apparent after large doses of succinylcholine are given.[7]

Acetylcholinesterase inhibitors (such as neostigmine, pyridostigmine, and edrophonium) are used to reverse neuromuscular blockade due to nondepolarizing agents. They block the enzyme acetylcholinesterase from breaking down acetylcholine, allowing for a build up of this molecule and the ability to overcome the competitive blockade from nondepolarizing agents. However, in addition to acetylcholinesterase, these medications inhibit the enzyme pseudocholinesterase.[4] Neostigmine, pyridostigmine, and edrophonium are all eliminated by renal excretion.[5,8,10]

If given concomitantly, succinylcholine and acetylcholinesterase inhibitors are capable of prolonging the neuromuscular blockade.[3] In a Phase I or depolarizing block, neostigmine will directly potentiate the block by inhibiting the metabolism of succinylcholine. This leads to a prolonged requirement for intubation and mechanical ventilation.

In Phase II blockade the effects of acetylcholinesterase inhibitors can be difficult to determine. In a pure Phase II blockade, paralysis would be reversed by these agents.[1] However, if there were an aspect of Phase I blockade intermixed with Phase II, acetylcholinesterase inhibitors would potentiate the blockade. Even with a nerve stimulator and train-of-four monitoring it can be difficult to ascertain whether a pure Phase II block or mixed block is present. The recommended course of action for a Phase II block is to allow for spontaneous recovery.

Certain disease processes can amplify the interaction between succinylcholine and acetylcholinesterase inhibitors. This includes patients that have reduced or atypical pseudocholinesterase, or the presence of renal failure leading to reduced plasma clearance of the acetylcholinesterase inhibitor.[6,11] The timing between administrations of these drugs also requires close monitoring. In the absence of renal disease, the half-life of neostigmine is from 51 to 90 minutes, the half-life of edrophonium is 33 to 110 minutes, and the half-life of pyridostigmine is 63 to112 minutes. In regards to pseudocholinesterase activity, it will have returned to roughly half of its baseline value ninety minutes after the administration of neostigmine.

It should be mentioned that acetylcholinesterase inhibitors have other clinical uses and their presence needs to be elicited by a thorough history. Specifically, they have been used in eye drop medications for the treatment of glaucoma and strabismus. Of these, echothiophate has been shown to be absorbed systemically in an amount sufficient to inhibit pseudocholinesterase leading to prolonged blockade with succinylcholine.[2,9] It is debated whether the other acetylcholinesterase inhibitors have systemic absorption in amounts high enough to inhibit pseudocholinesterase to a clinically relevant level, however the theoretical interaction remains. Most of these agents, including echothiophate have fallen into disuse in clinical medicine.

Take-Home Points

- Succinylcholine is a depolarizing neuromuscular blocking agent that is broken down by pseudocholinesterase found in plasma.
- Acetylcholinesterase inhibitors such as neostigmine, pyridostigmine, and edrophonium will inhibit pseudocholinesterase in addition to acetylcholinesterase.
- If given concomitantly with succinylcholine, acetylcholinesterase inhibitors will prolong a phase I blockade.
- Abnormal or decreased pseudocholinesterase, and renal failure can exacerbate the interaction between succinylcholine and acetylcholinesterase inhibitors.

Summary

Interaction: pharmacodynamic (competitive antagonism)
Substrates: neostigmine, succinylcholine
Enzyme/site of action: pseudocholinesterase
Inhibitor: neostigmine
Clinical effect: decreased metabolism of succinylcholine leading to increased neuromuscular weakness

References

1. Donati F, Bevan DR. Antagonism of phase II succinycholine block by neostigmine. Anesth Analg. 1985;64:773–6.
2. Pantuck EJ. Echothiphate iodide eye drops and prolonged response to suxamethonium. Br J Anaesth. 1966;38:406–7.
3. Valdrighi JB, Fleming NW, Smith BK, et al. Effects of cholinesterase inhibitors on the neuromuscular blocking action of suxamethonium. Br J Anaesth. 1994;72(2):237–9.
4. Sunew KY, Hicks RG. Effects of neostigmine and pyridostigmine on duration of succinylcholine action and pseudocholinesterase activity. Anesthesiology. 1978;49:188–91.
5. Williams AR, Bailey M, Joye T, Burt N. Marked prolongation of the succinycholine effect two hours after neostigmine reversal of neuromuscular blockade in a patient with chronic renal insufficiency. South Med J. 1999;92:77–9.
6. Ramirez JG, Sprung J, Keegan MT, Hall BA, Bourke DL. Neostigmine-induced prolonged neuromuscular blockade in a patient with atypical pseudocholinesterase. J Clin Anesth. 2005;17:221–4.
7. Naguib M, Lien CA. Pharmacology of muscle relaxants and their antagonists. In: Miller RD, Eriksson LI, Fleisher LA, Wiener-Kronish JP, Young WL, editors. Miller's anesthesia. 7th ed. Philadelphia: Churchill Livingstone; 2010. p. 859–911.
8. Bishop MJ, Hornbein TF. Prolonged effect of succinylcholine after neostigmine and pyridostigmine administration in patients with renal failure. Anesthesiology. 1983;58(4):384–6.
9. Elderton TE, Formati O, Zsigmund EK. Reduction in plasma cholinesterase levels after prolonged administration of echothiophate iodide eyedrops. Can Anaesth Soc J. 1968;15(3):291–6.
10. Cronnelly R, Stanski DR, Miller RD, Sheiner LB, Sohn YJ. Renal function and the pharmacokinetics of neostigmine in anesthetized man. Anesthesiology. 1979;51:222–6.
11. Baraka A. Suxamethonium-neostigmine interaction in patients with normal or atypical cholinesterase. Br J Anaesth. 1977;49(5):479–84.

Keep an "Ion" the Twitches

91

Magnesium, neuromuscular blockade

Brian Gierl MD and Ferenc E. Gyulai MD

Abstract
This case discusses the antagonistic pharmacodynamics interaction between magnesium and calcium at the neuromuscular junction, causing neuromuscular weakness.

Case

A 35-year-old parturient at 36 weeks gestation presented to the obstetric ward in active labor with a blood pressure of 178/87 mm Hg. She was morbidly obese (body mass index 49 kg/m^2) and had undergone one prior Caesarean section (C-section). She was diagnosed with preeclampsia and started on a magnesium sulfate infusion. Despite her risk factors, the obstetrician agreed to the patient's desire for a trial of vaginal birth after Caesarean section.

After 12 hours of active labor, the patient complained of 10/10 pain radiating to her left shoulder. The obstetrician diagnosed uterine rupture and an emergent Caesarean section was performed under general anesthesia. The patient received fentanyl, propofol, and succinylcholine (180 mg) for intubation. The nurse anesthetist also gave vecuronium (5 mg) to provide relaxation during the vertical incision C-section. The obstetrical team estimates the blood loss to be 1500 cc, so a basic metabolic panel and complete blood count were obtained that showed hematocrit 26% and electrolytes within normal limits. At the end of the case, the patient received neostigmine (5 mg) and glycopyrrolate (0.6 mg) to reverse neuromuscular blockade. Her respiratory rate was 30 breaths per minute with tidal volumes of ~100 cc. Train-of-four showed two weak twitches with fade. She was transferred to the intensive care use with sedation where her strength improved and she was extubated 5 hours later.

B. Gierl MD (✉)
Department of Anesthesiology, University of California San Diego, San Diego, CA, USA
e-mail: gierl.brian@gmail.com

F.E. Gyulai MD
Department of Anesthesiology, University of Pittsburgh Medical Center, Pittsburgh, PA, USA

C. Marcucci et al. (eds.), *A Case Approach to Perioperative Drug-Drug Interactions*, DOI 10.1007/978-1-4614-7495-1_91

Discussion

This is an example of a pharmacodynamic interaction (antagonism).

Calcium is a divalent cation that is essential to neuron and muscle function. The neuron transmits an electrical impulse to the neuromuscular junction where it causes presynaptic voltage-gated calcium channels to open. Calcium then enters the cell and mobilizes acetylcholine (ACh) vesicles for ACh release. Once released, it traverses the neuromuscular junction, binds acetylcholine receptors (AChRs), and depolarizes the postsynaptic myocyte. Extracellular calcium concentration strongly influences intracellular calcium levels and ACh release—such that doubling extracellular calcium concentration increases ACh release 16-fold. By subjecting a nerve to a tetanic stimulus, calcium accumulates in the neurons faster than it can be removed. This intracellular calcium overload increases ACh release with subsequent train-of-four stimulation and may be sufficient to overcome existing muscle blockade. Conversely, conditions that reduce intracellular calcium will decrease ACh release with the potential to block neuromuscular transmission.

Magnesium is another divalent cation that is a cofactor for many essential enzymes in the body. Its ability to block calcium entry at calcium channels has several neuromuscular effects that are relevant in the perioperative period. The administration of 2 to 4 g of $MgSO_4$ with a muscle relaxant shortened the time to relaxation by 33%, and extended the duration of blockade by 25%.[1] In a case report, $MgSO_4$ dosed in the PACU setting for atrial fibrillation was shown to cause recurarization and respiratory failure that required intubation.[2] The preeclamptic parturient classically exhibits magnesium toxicity and may also require general anesthesia for an obstetric procedure. Case reports detail patients with magnesium levels of 5 to 6 mg/dL that have required 3 to 4 hours to recover after a standard (0.05-0.1 mg/kg) dose of vecuronium.[3] Magnesium sulfate has minimal impact on the function of depolarizing muscle relaxants, but may reduce succinylcholine-induced fasciculations and hyperkalemia.[4] In sum, magnesium decreases calcium entry pre- and postsynaptically, leading to decreased ACh release and muscle contraction, respectively.

Lithium is a monovalent cation whose size approximates that of magnesium. In the 1980s, case reports of lithium extending neuromuscular blockade after electroconvulsive therapy (ECT) led scientists to investigate the effect of lithium on the neuromuscular junction. *In vitro* studies showed that neuromuscular function was only impacted with toxic lithium levels.[5] Lithium appears to activate adenosine triphosphate-sensitive potassium (K_{ATP}) channels pre- and postsynaptically. These effects decrease calcium entry leading to decreased presynaptic ACh release and postsynaptic muscle contraction.

Take-Home Points

- Magnesium can antagonize the effect of calcium at the neuromuscular junction with the potential to unmask an underlying neuromuscular junction disease, extend the duration of neuromuscular blockade, or lead to recurarization in the susceptible individual.
- Lithium only causes clinically significant muscle weakness at toxic concentrations.

Summary

Interaction: pharmacodynamic (antagonistic)
Substrates: magnesium and calcium
Mechanism/sites of action: neuromuscular junction
Clinical effect: neuromuscular weakness

References

1. Czarnetzki C, Lysakowski C, Elia N, et al. Time course of rocuronium-induced neuromuscular block after pre-treatment with magnesium sulphate: a randomised study. Acta Anaesthesiol Scand. 2010;54:299–306.
2. Fawcett WJ, Stone JP. Recurarization in the recovery room following the use of magnesium sulphate. Br J Anaesth. 2003;91(3):435–8.
3. Yoshida A, Itoh Y, Nagaya K, et al. Prolonged relaxant effects of vecuronium in patients with deliberate hypermagnesemia: time for caution in cesarean section. J Anesth. 2006;20:33–5.
4. James MF, Cork RC, Dennett JE, et al. Succinylcholine pretreatment with magnesium sulfate. Anesth Analg. 1986;65:373–6.
5. Waud BE, Farrell L, Waud DR. Lithium and neuromuscular transmission. Anesth Analg. 1982;61(5):399–402.

A Reversal of Misfortune

92

Neostigmine, glycopryrolate

Thomas N. Talamo MD and Richard J. Kuwik MD

Abstract

This case discusses a pharmacodynamic interaction between glycopyrrolate and acetylcholine. Neostigmine, when given before or out of proportion to glycopyrrolate can cause bradyarrhythmia and sinus arrest.

Case

An 18-year-old, 80 kg, otherwise healthy man presented for knee reconstruction following an athletic injury. He underwent unremarkable placement of femoral and sciatic nerve blockade catheters and induction of general anesthesia. Rocuronium was administered for muscle relaxation at the surgeon's request and there were 0/4 twitches on train-of-four (TOF) testing 5 minutes later. Bispectral index (BIS) monitoring was employed to assess and monitor anesthetic depth.

Following exsanguination of the lower extremity, a thigh tourniquet was inflated to 300 mm Hg. Surgical incision was made and the procedure proceeded without incident for the next 2 hours. At this time, with the tourniquet still inflated, the skin closure was completed. As the surgical dressings were applied, the patient's heart rate gradually increased to 120 beats per minute. The BIS monitor read 39. There were 4/4 twitches with presence of fade on tetanic stimulation.

In order to reverse residual muscle relaxation without exacerbating the patient's tachycardia, he received neostigmine (4 mg) followed immediately by glycopyrrolate (0.2 mg). Within several minutes, the patient's heart rate dropped to 25 beats per minute followed by sinus arrest and asystole. Chest compressions were immediately started, and atropine administered with epinephrine. Within a minute, the

T.N. Talamo MD (✉) • R.J. Kuwik MD
Department of Anesthesiology, University of Pittsburgh Medical Center, Pittsburgh, PA, USA
e-mail: talamotn@upmc.edu

C. Marcucci et al. (eds.), *A Case Approach to Perioperative Drug-Drug Interactions*, DOI 10.1007/978-1-4614-7495-1_92

patient recovered sinus rhythm with tachycardia and hypertension. Thereafter, the patient's emergence from anesthesia proceeded without incident and the patient was taken to the recovery room.

Discussion

This is an example of a pharmacodynamic interaction (antagonism)

Neostigmine (along with edrophonium and pyridostigmine) belongs to the class of pharmacologic agents called anticholinesterases. Also known as acetylcholinesterase inhibitors, drugs from this class reversibly inhibit the enzyme acetylcholinesterase, thereby preventing the rapid hydrolysis of acetylcholine and ultimately increasing the concentration of this neurotransmitter at its sites of action.[1,3] Among these sites of action is the neuromuscular junction (NMJ) where nondepolarizing muscle relaxants act competitively to inhibit the interaction of acetylcholine with its receptor. Neostigmine is therefore commonly used for the reversal of neuromuscular blockade as the increased concentration of acetylcholine it produces overcomes the competitive inhibition of muscle relaxants.

In addition to its action at the NMJ, acetylcholine is also released at all preganglionic autonomic nerve endings and at all postganglionic parasympathetic nerve endings.[1,3] At the NMJ and autonomic ganglia, acetylcholine acts on nicotinic receptors whereas it acts on muscarinic receptors at postganglionic parasympathetic nerve endings. Among these postganglionic parasympathetic nerve endings is the vagus innervation of the heart. Increased availability of acetylcholine at the muscarinic receptor sites on the heart can produce bradycardia, bradyarrhythmias (including nodal and ventricular escape beats), heart block, and even asystole.[1,3–5,7–9]

Glycopyrrolate (along with atropine and scopolamine) belongs to the class of pharmacologic agents called anticholinergics. It acts as a competitive antagonist at muscarinic receptors, thereby antagonizing the effect of acetylcholine (and anticholinesterases by extension) at these sites.[2] It is commonly used in combination with neostigmine to antagonize the cardiac side-effects associated with anticholinesterase use.

Both the dose and timing of neostigmine administration relative to glycopyrrolate can modify cardiac effect. The onset of action for neostigmine is 7 to 11 minutes as determined by studies using reversal of muscle relaxant, rather than heart rate, as the endpoint.[1,3,10] It is known that the muscarinic effects of anticholinesterases are apparent at lower concentrations than the nicotinic effects, however, and it follows that the cardiac effects present earlier.[1] Glycopyrrolate has an onset of action of 2 to 3 minutes.[2,3] A study by Mirakhur et al. demonstrated that combined administration of neostigmine and glycopyrrolate in a 5:1 ratio was optimal for cardiac stability, while lower relative doses of glycopyrrolate led to a high incidence of conduction disturbances and bradyarrhythmias.[4]

In addition to dosage and timing, several patient-specific factors may contribute or predispose to the adverse cardiac effects of anticholinesterases. Among these factors are β-adrenergic blockade,[5,6] co-existing heart disease,[7] diabetic neuropathy,[8] and previous heart transplantation.[9] In theory, ongoing ß-adrenergic blockade preoperatively may predispose to exaggerated and unopposed parasympathetic stimulation upon administration of anticholinesterases. While there are case reports of prolonged bradycardia in patients under β-blockade, this has not been demonstrated in animal studies.[5,6] An increased incidence of dysrhythmia has been observed with reversal of neuromuscular blockade in patients with pre-existing coronary artery disease, conduction defects, or hypertension.[7] Heart transplant patients with denervated hearts and diabetic patients with autonomic neuropathy (functionally denervated hearts) may also be at increased risk for bradyarrhythmia and arrest following reversal of muscle relaxation as has been seen in several case studies.[8,9] Perhaps this is explained by receptor upregulation and hypersensitivity in the denervated heart, which would lead concurrently to an exaggerated response to increased acetylcholine concentration and possibly a blunted response to anticholinergic agents.[1,8,9]

Take-Home Points

- Administration of neostigmine before, or at high doses relative to glycopyrrolate can result in bradycardia, bradyarrhythmias, heart block, and even asystole.
- Patient-specific factors and co-existing disease may predispose to adverse cardiac events following reversal with neostigmine and glycopyrrolate.

Summary

Interaction: pharmacodynamic
Substrate: acetylcholine and glycopyrrolate
Mechanism/site of action: muscarinic receptor, neuromuscular junction
Clinical effect: mitigation of effects of increased acetylcholine

References

1. Stoelting RK, Hillier SC. Anticholinesterase drugs and cholinergic agonists. In: Pharmacology and physiology in anesthetic practice. 4th ed. Philadelphia: Lippincott Williams & Wilkins; 2006. p. 251–65.

2. Stoelting RK, Hillier SC. Anticholinesterase drugs and cholinergic agonists. In: Pharmacology and physiology in anesthetic practice. 4th ed. Philadelphia: Lippincott Williams & Wilkins; 2006. p. 266–75.
3. Bevan DR, Donati F, Kopman AF. Reversal of neuromuscular blockade. Anesthesiology. 1992;77:785–805.
4. Mirakhur RK, Dundee JW, Jones CJ, et al. Reversal of neuromuscular blockade: dose determination studies with atropine and glycopyrolate given before or in a mixture with neostigmine. Anesth Analg. 1981;60:557–62.
5. Seidl DC, Martin DE. Prolonged bradycardia after neostigmine administration in a patient taking nadolol. Anesth Analg. 1984;63:365–7.
6. Wagner DL, Moorthy SS. Stoelting RK Administration of anticholinesterase drugs in the presence of beta-adrenergic blockade. Anesth Analg. 1982;61:153–4.
7. Owens WD, Waldbaum LS, Stephen CR. Cardiac dysrhythmia following reversal of neuromuscular blocking agents in geriatric patients. Anesth Analg. 1978;57:186–90.
8. Triantafillou AN, Tsueda K, Berg J, et al. Refractory bradycardia after reversal of muscle relaxant in a diabetic with vagal neuropathy. Anesth Analg. 1986;65:1237–41.
9. Beebe DS, Shumway SJ, Maddock R. Sinus arrest after intravenous neostigmine in two heart transplant recipients. Anesth Analg. 1994;78:779–82.
10. Miller RD, Van Nyhuis LS, Eger EI, et al. Comparative times to peak effect and durations of action of neostigmine and pyridostigmine. Anesthesiology. 1974;41:27–33.

Stop Moving

93

Fatal Forty DDI: vecuronium, phenytoin

Michael D. Olson PA-C and Randall Flick MD

Abstract
This case discusses a pharmacokinetic interaction between phenytoin and vecuronium. Vecuronium is a substrate of the cytochrome P450 system and is metabolized in the liver. Phenytoin is an inducer of many subenzymes of the cytochrome P450 system.

Case

A 52-year-old, 90 kg man presented to the operating room for elective repair of his large, painful ventral hernia. The patient had a history of posttraumatic epilepsy managed with phenytoin sodium and essential hypertension controlled with hydrochlorothiazide. General anesthesia was induced with propofol and succinylcholine. After recovery from succinylcholine, as confirmed by train-of-four (TOF) monitoring, vecuronium (9 mg) was given to ensure abdominal muscle relaxation. Anesthesia was maintained with isoflurane and fentanyl. Approximately 20 minutes after the incision, the surgeon reported that the abdominal musculature was not relaxed, and immediately thereafter the patient began to move spontaneously. The anesthesiology resident quickly assessed the patient and elected to give an additional 5 mg of vecuronium. Twenty-five minutes after the second dose of vecuronium, the surgeon again noted a lack of abdominal muscle relaxation. The anesthesiology resident decided to deepen the anesthetic by increasing the end-tidal isoflurane concentration, which resulted in improved surgical conditions. The operation was successfully completed, and the patient received reversal medication for neuromuscular blockade, despite the presence of four twitches on the TOF monitor. His emergence from general anesthesia was uneventful.

M.D. Olson PA-C (✉)
Department of Otolaryngology, Mayo Clinic, Rochester, MN, USA
e-mail: olson.michael@mayo.edu

R. Flick MD
Department of Anesthesiology, Mayo Clinic, Rochester, MN, USA

C. Marcucci et al. (eds.), *A Case Approach to Perioperative Drug-Drug Interactions*, DOI 10.1007/978-1-4614-7495-1_93

Discussion

This is an example of a substrate added to an inducer.

Phenytoin is an antiepileptic drug that is thought to enhance sodium efflux from neurons in the motor cortex. This cellular event tends to stabilize the threshold against hyperexcitability, which is thought to contribute to disorders of cortical hyperexcitability, the most common of which is seizures. Phenytoin metabolism occurs primarily through the cytochrome P450 (CYP) system and, more specifically, its isozymes 2C9 and 2C19. Phenytoin is extensively protein bound in plasma, such that nearly 90% of the drug is bound and less than 5% of any dose is excreted unchanged in the urine.

Vecuronium, an intermediate-acting, nondepolarizing neuromuscular blocking agent, acts as a competitive antagonist at the acetylcholine receptors of the end plate of the neuromuscular junction. Metabolism of vecuronium primarily occurs in the liver through deacetylation by liver microsomes, but up to 25% of its metabolism can occur in the kidney.[1] Most of vecuronium metabolism is either by conversion to the principal metabolite, 3-desacetylvecuronium, or by direct excretion of the parent compound into the bile.[1,2]

The induction of the CYP system by phenytoin, as well as other antiepileptics, has been well described.[3,4] Drugs that induce hepatic microsomal enzymes, such as phenytoin, allow the rapid metabolism of certain drugs, including vecuronium, thereby reducing the drug's duration of action. Alloul and colleagues demonstrated that a single dose of vecuronium can be metabolized rapidly in patients receiving long-term anticonvulsant therapy.[5] They concluded that the mechanism of action was increased hepatic clearance, although it remains unclear which of the numerous enzymes induced by phenytoin (CYP3A4, 2C9, 2C19, or phase II/UGT) is involved in this interaction. Clearly this is a repeatedly observed phenomenon most prevalent in those who have taken anticonvulsants long term but the exact mechanism is as yet unknown.

In contrast, Gray and colleagues showed that in anticonvulsant-naïve patients, acute administration of an anticonvulsant drug can actually enhance the effects of nondepolarizing neuromuscular agents.[6] This enhancement was thought to occur through a suppression of the posttetanic potentiation of the muscle and end plate or because of a decrease in acetylcholine release at the nerve terminal. Finally, in addition to these mechanisms, most anticonvulsants have been shown to increase α_1-acid glycoprotein concentrations.[7] An increase in α_1-acid glycoprotein can increase the protein binding of drugs and alter their distribution.[8] This increased binding is thought to be an additional mechanism of resistance that is mediated by the lack of the active circulating free fraction.

In conclusion, careful analysis of a patient's medication list is essential. If the patient is taking anticonvulsant therapy, the anesthesiologist should pick a neuromuscular blocking agent that is not affected by these mechanisms (eg, atracurium metabolism and elimination are not affected by anticonvulsant therapy).

Take-Home Points

- Phenytoin is metabolized widely by the CYP system—specifically, the isozymes CYP2C9 and CYP2C19.
- Vecuronium is an aminosteroidal nondepolarizing neuromuscular blocking agent metabolized primarily in the liver and secondarily in the kidney.
- Patients who have been taking phenytoin or carbamazepine long term have reduced clearance of nondepolarizing neuromuscular blocking agents. This is thought to occur through either an induction of the liver enzymes that metabolize these agents or increased protein binding of these drugs, thereby reducing their active free fractions.
- Patients who have not been taking anticonvulsant therapy and have received acute doses of these drugs may show prolonged effects of nondepolarizing neuromuscular agents.

Summary

Interaction: pharmacokinetic
Substrate: vecuronium
Enzyme/transporter: unclear
Inducer: phenytoin
Clinical effect: decreased neuromuscular blockade

References

1. Caldwell JE, Szenohradszky J, Segredo V, et al. The pharmacodynamics and pharmacokinetics of the metabolite 3-desacetylvecuronium (ORG 7268) and its parent compound, vecuronium, in human volunteers. J Pharmacol Exp Ther. 1994;270:1216–22.
2. Lebrault C, Berger JL, D'Hollander AA, et al. Pharmacokinetics and pharmacodynamics of vecuronium (ORG NC 45) in patients with cirrhosis. Anesthesiology. 1985;62:601–5.
3. Pirttiaho HI, Sotaniemi EA, Pelkonen RO, et al. Hepatic blood flow and drug metabolism in patients on enzyme-inducing anticonvulsants. Eur J Clin Pharmacol. 1982;22:441–5.
4. Brodie MJ, Dichter MA. Antiepileptic drugs. N Engl J Med. 1996;334:168–75.

5. Alloul K, Whalley DG, Shutway F, et al. Pharmacokinetic origin of carbamazepine-induced resistance to vecuronium neuromuscular blockade in anesthetized patients. Anesthesiology. 1996;84:330–9.
6. Gray HS, Slater RM, Pollard BJ. The effect of acutely administered phenytoin on vecuronium-induced neuromuscular blockade. Anaesthesia. 1989;44:379–81.
7. Kremer JM, Wilting J, Janssen LH. Drug binding to human alpha-1-acid glycoprotein in health and disease. Pharmacol Rev. 1988;40:1–47.
8. Wood M. Plasma binding and limitation of drug access to site of action. Anesthesiology. 1991;75:721–3.

There's Just Not Enough Roc in the World

94

Fatal Forty DDI: rocuronium, carbamazepine

Tammara S. Goldschmidt MD and Randal O. Dull MD, PhD

Abstract
This case discusses the pharmacokinetic interaction between rocuronium and carbamazepine, resulting in shortened duration of neuromuscular blockade.

Case

On a busy Friday afternoon, a 3-year-old, 20 kg boy was added to the operating room (OR) schedule for an urgent revision a ventriculoperitoneal (VP) shunt revision procedure due to mental status changes. The patient had a history of congenital hydrocephalus and birth trauma and suffered from tonic-clonic seizures. His seizures had been difficult to control and he had been on several different seizure medications in the past. The conscientious CA-1 posted to do the case with a pediatric anesthesiology attending "had heard" about the increased neuromuscular requirements of patients on chronic phenytoin therapy. When she called her attending to review the case, she specifically mentioned that the patient was not on phenytoin therapy.

The previous VP shunt removal and replacement in this patient had been difficult secondary to adhesions. The surgeon requested "really good" muscle relaxation to provide optimal conditions for placing the new shunt. The patient was brought to the OR and received an intravenous induction with propofol (3 mg/kg) followed byrocuronium(0.6 mg/kg). The patient was intubated without difficulty and prepared for surgery. About 15 minutes later, on incision, it was noted that the patient was attempting spontaneous ventilation over the mechanical ventilator. The surprised resident elicited train-of-four twitch response of 4/4.

T.S. Goldschmidt MD (✉)
Department of Anesthesiology, University of Illinois, Chicago, IL, USA
e-mail: dtgoldschmidt@yahoo.com

R.O. Dull MD, PhD
Department of Anesthesiology, University of Illinois at Chicago, Chicago, IL, USA

C. Marcucci et al. (eds.), *A Case Approach to Perioperative Drug-Drug Interactions*, DOI 10.1007/978-1-4614-7495-1_94

The patient was redosed with rocuronium (0.1 mg/kg) immediately and twitches were rechecked ten minutes later. The patient already had return of two to three twitches and was redosed with rocuronium (0.1 mg/kg). The puzzled resident called her attending to discuss the situation. When the chart was rechecked for concurrent administration of phenytoin, she discovered that the patient was on Neurotol® for seizure prophylaxis. The chagrined resident realized that she had missed the presence of a slow-release carbamazepine preparation on the patient's medication panel, mistaking it for a neurontin preparation.

She then checked twitches and redosed rocuronium approximately every 10 minutes in order to provide adequate muscle relaxation during the case. Her attending came to the room presently to bring some extra rocuronium vials and give her a break, joking as he came into the room, "I guess the rocuronium factory will be working the midnight shift tonight!" After the surgeons had closed the wound and applied the dressings, twitches were again checked and the patient already had nearly full return to baseline of twitch response. The patient was taking adequate tidal volumes and demonstrated adequate strength return by lifting his legs prior to extubation. The resident was asked to present her case at the upcoming weekly resident case conference, which was scheduled to be on drug–drug interactions mediated by the P450 system.

Discussion

This is an example of a substrate added to an inducer.

Rocuronium is an aminosteroid nondepolarizing neuromuscular blocker (NMB) that is metabolized in the liver by deacetylation.

Phenytoin, an antiepilepsy medication approved for use in children, is a potent inducer of the cytochrome P450 (CYP) enzyme system, particularly CYP3A4, but also CYP2B6, 2C9, and 2C19.[2,3]

Carbamazepine is used also used widely for prophylaxis of seizures in children. It comes in both standard and slow-release formulations. The standard formulation is trademarked as Tegretol® and the slow-release formulation is trademarked as Neurotol®. Neurotol® helps to stabilize carbamazepine blood levels and reduce dosing frequency.[6] Carbamazepine is a paninducer, including CYP3A4, 2B6, 2C9, and 1A2.[1,4]

The chronic nature of this child's carbamazepine use ensured steady-state blood levels. It is not yet fully known which of the P450 enzymes play a role in the enhanced metabolism of rocuronium. However, the shortened neuromuscular blockade seen with coadministration of carbamazepine (or phenytoin) with the aminosteroid NMBs has been extensively reported.[1–5]

As a final note, it is imperative for anesthesiologists to acquaint themselves with the "true identity" of every drug on a patient's medication list.

Take-Home Points

- Phenytoin and carbamazepine are pan-inducers of the cytochrome P450 enzyme system.
- Rocuronium, vecuronium, and other aminosteroid nondepolarizing muscle relaxants undergo metabolism by deacetylation in the liver. The primary enzyme mechanism is not known.
- Rocuronium's neuromuscular blocking action will be attenuated by both phenytoin and carbamazepine.
- Careful twitch monitoring is required during a case when aminosteroid nondepolarizing muscle relaxants are used in the presence of chronic anti-seizure medications.
- Extra dosing of—and quick recovery time from—nondepolarizing muscle relaxants may need to be planned for patients on chronic anti-seizure medication regimens.

Summary

Interaction: pharmacokinetic
Substrate: rocuronium
Enzyme: unclear
Inducer: carbamazepine
Clinical effect: shortened neuromuscular blockade

References

1. Hernandez-Palazon J, Tortosa J, Martinez-Lage J, et al. Rocuronium-induced neuromuscular blockade is affected by chronic phenytoin therapy. J Neurosurg Anesthesiol. 2001;13(2): 79–82.
2. Soriano SG, Kaus SJ, Sullivan LJ, et al. Onset and duration of action of rocuronium in children receiving chronic anticonvulsant therapy. Paediatr Anaesth. 2000;10:133–6.
3. Lee CR, Goldstein JA, Pieper JA. Cytochrome P450 2C9 polymorphisms: a comprehensive review of the in-vitro and human data. Pharmacogenetics. 2002;12(3):251–63.
4. Spacek A, Neiger FX, Krenn CG, et al. Rocuronium-induced neuromuscular block is affected by chronic carbamazepine therapy. Anesthesiology. 1999;90:109–12.
5. Soriano SG, Sullivan LJ, Venkatakrishnan K, et al. Pharmacokinetics and pharmacodynamics of vecuronium in children receiving phenytoin or carbamazepine for chronic anticonvulsant therapy. Br J Anaesth. 2001;86(2):223–9.
6. Sivenius J, Heinonen E, Lehto H, et al. Reduction of dosing frequency of carbamazepine with a slow-release preparation. Epilepsy Res. 1988;2(1):32–6.

Slow Sux I: A Lengthy Wake-up Period After Electroconvulsive Therapy

95

Succinylcholine, atypical plasma cholinesterase

Jennifer A. Rabbitts MB, ChB and Juraj Sprung MD, PhD

Abstract
This case discusses a drug–gene interaction between succinylcholine and a pseudocholinesterase variant, resulting in prolonged action of succinylcholine.

Case

A 23-year-old woman presented for her first electroconvulsive therapy (ECT) for depression after being admitted for a major depressive episode. ECT was being used urgently as first-line treatment because of a suicide attempt. She had no prior medical history and was taking no medications. The anesthesia induction for this ECT was her first experience with anesthetics, and she had no known medication allergies.

Anesthesia for ECT was induced with thiopental (3 mg/kg) and succinylcholine (1 mg/kg), and the airway was managed by bag-mask ventilation. Thirty minutes after ECT, she still was not breathing on her own and showed no muscle function. Given the absence of both a confounding medical condition and a medication cause for the prolonged wake-up period, a diagnosis of pseudocholinesterase deficiency was considered. A nerve stimulator showed no twitches on train-of-four stimulation.

J.A. Rabbitts MB, ChB (✉)
Department of Anesthesiology, Seattle Children's Hospital and University of Washington, Seattle, WA, USA
e-mail: jennifer.rabbitts@seattlechildrens.org

J. Sprung MD, PhD
Department of Anesthesiology, Mayo Clinic, Rochester, MN, USA

C. Marcucci et al. (eds.), *A Case Approach to Perioperative Drug-Drug Interactions*, DOI 10.1007/978-1-4614-7495-1_95

A propofol infusion was started, and the patient was transferred to the postanesthesia recovery unit. After 210 minutes, the patient had four twitches on TOF with no fade. Sedation was stopped, she had normal muscle function, and her trachea was extubated. The patient continued to receive ECT three times weekly with good clinical results, using atracurium besylate or rocuronium bromide for the subsequent anesthetics.

The patient was determined to have low plasma pseudocholinesterase levels and a dibucaine number (DN) of 21%. She and her family were counseled about hereditary pseudocholinesterase deficiency and scheduled for an anesthesia consultation. Testing of family members showed that two of her three siblings had pseudocholinesterase deficiency; genetic testing showed that one was heterozygous for atypical enzyme, and the other was homozygous for atypical enzyme, as was the patient. They were issued medic alert bracelets and received education about pseudocholinesterase deficiency.

Discussion

This is an example of a drug–gene interaction.

More specifically, this is an example of a pharmacogenetic abnormality in a patient homozygous for atypical pseudocholinesterase, resulting in pseudocholinesterase deficiency and prolonged apnea after succinylcholine administration.

Pseudocholinesterase (also known as *plasma cholinesterase* and *butyrylcholinesterase*) is an enzyme synthesized in the liver. It circulates in plasma and hydrolyzes exogenous choline esters, such as succinylcholine, mivacurium chloride, and ester local anesthetics (eg, chloroprocaine, procaine). Pseudocholinesterase is differentiated from true cholinesterase, which is present in red blood cells and nerve tissue and breaks down acetylcholine. Whether it has a biologic function is unclear.

Various medical conditions (eg, liver disease, uremia, hyperpyrexia, malignancy, collagen vascular disease, pregnancy, burns, malnutrition secondary to Crohn's disease or anorexia) and medications (eg, oral contraceptives, cytotoxic drugs, metoclopramide hydrochloride, anticholinesterase insecticides) can cause decreased pseudocholinesterase levels. However, these decreased levels are seldom of clinical consequence because a 75% decrease in pseudocholinesterase is required before succinylcholine effect is prolonged. Furthermore, decreased pseudocholinesterase levels in an individual with the normal chromosomes results in less than 25 minutes of paralysis after succinylcholine administration.[1]

A single gene at the E_1 locus on the long arm of chromosome 3 encodes for pseudocholinesterase. A single amino acid substitution error or a sequencing error at or

Table 95.1 Relationship between dibucaine number and duration of succinylcholine effects

Type of Pseudocholinesterase	Genotype	Prevalence	Dibucaine Number[a]	Response to Succinylcholine or Mivacurium
Homozygous typical	$E_1^uE_1^u$	Normal	70-80	Normal
Heterozygous atypical	$E_1^uE_1^a$	1/480	50-60	Lengthened by 50%-100%
Homozygous atypical	$E_1^aE_1^a$	1/3,200	20-30	Prolonged to 4-8 h

[Adapted from Savarese JJ, Caldwell JE, Lien CA et al: Pharmacology of muscle relaxants and their antagonists. In: Miller RD, ed. Anesthesia. 5th ed. Vol. 1. Philadelphia, PA: Churchill Livingstone; 2000: 412-490. With permission from Elsevier.]
Abbreviations: E_1, long arm of chromosome 3, E_1 locus; E_1^u, usual/normal gene; E_1^a, abnormal gene
[a] Dibucaine number shows percentage of enzyme inhibited

near the enzyme active site can result in production of an abnormally functioning enzyme. Variants of the enzyme include usual variant, atypical variant (dibucaine resistant), silent variant, F variant (fluoride resistant), Newfoundland variant, and K, H, and J variants.

A person may be homozygous for the usual gene (wild type), homozygous for the atypical gene (most severe form; prevalence, 1 in 3,200 persons), heterozygous for one abnormal gene (usually clinically significant only when heterozygous for atypical or silent type; prevalence, 1 in 480 persons for atypical type), or heterozygous for two abnormal genes (intermediate forms) (Table 95.1).[2] Thus, numerous different genotypes with various combinations of these genes are possible.[2] In addition, new genotype variants continue to be discovered.

Usually, heterozygosity for atypical pseudocholinesterase delays by up to 35 minutes a patient's recovery from succinylcholine.[2] In homozygous abnormality, maximal recovery time after succinylcholine is much longer.[2] More specifically, sufficient recovery of neuromuscular function after succinylcholine (1.0-1.5 mg/kg^{-1}) was 15 to 30 minutes for patients heterozygous for one abnormal gene, 35 to 45 minutes for those heterozygous for two abnormal genes, and 90 to 180 minutes, or even longer, for those homozygous for the abnormal gene.[2] Therefore, the anesthesiologist always should use a peripheral nerve stimulator, which can help determine whether the patient is homozygous or heterozygous for abnormal gene.

The dibucaine-resistant variant is the most important clinically. Diagnosis is confirmed with the test that uses amide-type local anesthetic dibucaine (dibucaine test).[3] DN is the percent inhibition or hydrolysis of benzyl choline with dibucaine added to the plasma sample. Dibucaine inhibits normal pseudocholinesterase by 80% and the atypical enzyme by 20%. DN can be used to determine the genetic makeup: homozygous typical individuals have a DN of 70 to 80; homozygous atypical individuals, 20 to 30; and heterozygous atypical individuals, 50 to 60.[4]

DN is a qualitative test and cannot determine the actual enzyme levels or activity. Plasma pseudocholinesterase activity (IU/volume unit) and level may be determined by a quantitative test that detects micromoles of substrate hydrolyzed by pseudocholinesterase per unit of time.

Use of blood products and anticholinesterase drugs can interfere with DN testing, and in order to avoid confusing results, it is best to perform this testing at least 24 hours after their last administrations. Additionally, genotyping for known genes can be done. However, none of these tests predicts the response to succinylcholine precisely.

Management is as described in the present case, with sedation and ventilation until muscle function is normal and the patient can be extubated. Fresh frozen plasma contains pseudocholinesterase but is seldom given. Electromyography or intermittent use of a nerve stimulator should be used to monitor the nerve block.[5] Patients with prolonged blockade after succinylcholine should be tested and anesthesia counseling of the patient and the patient's family members should be conducted.

Take-Home Points

- A quantitative pseudocholinesterase deficiency may occur with several medical conditions and medications; however, it is seldom clinically relevant.
- Qualitatively atypical pseudocholinesterase or decreased pseudocholinesterase production, or both, are caused by several rare genetic variants of the gene encoding for pseudocholinesterase, the most important being dibucaine-resistant variants.
- Pseudocholinesterase deficiency is suspected with prolonged relaxation after succinylcholine administration and is confirmed with a nerve stimulator after other causes have been ruled out.
- The diagnosis is made through measurement of pseudocholinesterase activity, DN, and genetic tests.
- Treatment consists of immediate sedation and ventilatory support and subsequent testing and counseling of the patient and the family members.

Summary

Interaction: pharmacogenomic (drug–gene)
Substrates: succinylcholine and gene located at E1 locus of long arm of chromosome 3
Mechanism: gene deletions produce pseudocholinesterase variant
Clinical effect: prolonged action of succinylcholine

References

1. Viby-Mogensen J. Correlation of succinylcholine duration of action with plasma cholinesterase activity in subjects with the genotypically normal enzyme. Anesthesiology. 1980;53:517–20.
2. Jensen FS, Viby-Mogensen J. Plasma cholinesterase and abnormal reaction to succinylcholine: twenty years' experience with the Danish Cholinesterase Research Unit. Acta Anaesthesiol Scand. 1995;39:150–6.
3. Kalow W, Genest K. A method for the detection of atypical forms of human serum cholinesterase: determination of dibucaine numbers. Can J Biochem Physiol. 1957;35:339–46.
4. Kalow W, Staron N. On distribution and inheritance of atypical forms of human serum cholinesterase, as indicated by dibucaine numbers. Can J Biochem Physiol. 1957;35:1305–20.
5. Cherington M, Lasater G. Prolonged paralysis in pseudocholinesterase deficiency. Arch Neurol. 1973;28:274–5.

Slow Sux II: I Remember Reviewing This for the Boards

96

Succinylcholine, atypical plasma cholinesterase

Andrew Oken MD and Scott Richins MD

Abstract
This case discusses a drug–gene interaction involving the inborn genetic variability of plasma cholinesterase causing prolonged neuromuscular weakness after succinylcholine.

Case

Early one morning at the end of a long night on call, Dr. Green was paged for an emergent laparoscopic appendectomy. The patient was an otherwise healthy 28-year-old woman with no significant past medical history other than a vaginal delivery notable for a "really good epidural." She had a BMI of 27 kg/m^2, was able to do >10 METS of activity and had never had a general anesthetic. She denied allergies to any medications, and took only birth control pills. She denied any family history of problems with anesthesia. She was NPO for more than 6 hours. A brief physical exam was done and was unremarkable.

After speaking with his attending, Dr. Green planned to do a rapid-sequence induction with propofol, succinylcholine, and fentanyl using desflurane for maintenance. No additional muscle relaxant was used. The case proceeded smoothly without incident. She received a total of 200 mcg of fentanyl through the case. After skin closure, the patient was continued on mechanical ventilation to facilitate

A. Oken MD (✉)
Operative Care Division, Portland VAMC, Portland, OR, USA
e-mail: andrew.oken@va.gov

S. Richins MD
Pikes Peak Anesthesia Associates, Colorado Springs, CO, USA

C. Marcucci et al. (eds.), *A Case Approach to Perioperative Drug-Drug Interactions*, DOI 10.1007/978-1-4614-7495-1_96

elimination of desflurane. The patient opened her eyes spontaneously at an end-tidal percent of 0.2 of desflurane. The attending was called in for extubation and a trial of spontaneous breathing was attempted. The patient however subsequently appeared anxious and weak and was noted to be taking inadequate tidal volumes. Dr. Green checked his syringe to verify that 100 mg of succinylcholine was given 60 minutes previously. The patient continued to struggle. She became tachycardic, hypertensive, and then began to desaturate. Train-of-four (TOF) monitoring showed four significantly diminished twitches. A propofol bolus was given and mechanical ventilation was resumed. She was transferred to the postanesthesia care unit (PACU) still intubated and sedated for presumed prolonged neuromuscular weakness secondary to residual succinylcholine. She was mechanically ventilated, monitored, and observed until her neuromuscular function returned to baseline. She was subsequently safely extubated 2 hours later.

Discussion

This is an example of a drug–gene interaction.

This clinical scenario in part represents an example of the interface between genetics and the practice of anesthesiology and, specifically, interpatient variability regularly observed in drug metabolism. These differences can lead to unpredictable responses, toxicities and sensitivities, as well as variations in duration of action. In this circumstance, succinylcholine metabolism is presumed to be effected. Plasma cholinesterase, otherwise known as pseudocholinesterase or butyrylcholinesterase (and not to be confused with RBC cholinesterase) is the plasma protein responsible for metabolism of acetylcholine, succinylcholine, and other esters including mivacurium and ester type local anesthetics. If this enzyme is not present in normal form or quantity, the duration of action these drugs can be prolonged. This might in part explain the patient's prior history of a "really good epidural."[1] The many causes of decreased enzymatic activity of plasma cholinesterase can be categorized as genetic, physiologic, pathologic, or pharmacologic in nature. A few of the most relevant causes in each category are listed below in Table 96.1.

Table 96.1 Causes of decreased plasma cholinesterase activity

Genetic	**Pathologic**	**Pharmacologic**
Atypical, silent, and fluoride resistant genes	Liver disease	Echothiophate iodine
	Renal disease	Neostigmine
Physiologic	Alcoholism	Pyridostigmine
Newborn	Malnutrition	Bambuterol
Advanced age	Myxedema	Monoamine oxidase inhibitors
Pregnancy	Neoplastic disease	Organophosphates
	Plasmapheresis	Cytotoxic drugs
	Thyrotoxicosis	

While there are many causes for decreased enzyme quantity, clinically relevant effects are usually only seen after levels are reduced to ~20% to 30% of normal. Therefore, succinylcholine-associated apnea is most often seen in patients who have some sort of pseudocholinesterase gene mutation.[2] Homozygotes for the atypical, silent, and fluoride resistant mutations can have significantly prolonged effects from succinylcholine.[3] Heterozygote combinations of the three can also have prolonged effects, although individuals who carry one wild enzyme do not typically manifest significantly prolonged succinylcholine blocks unless they have an associated abnormality leading to diminished levels of enzyme.

Plasma cholinesterase is synthesized in the liver and the coding sequence is located on chromosome 3q26. Mutations associated with prolonged apnea have been well described and are mostly point mutations causing deletions or substitutions of nucleotides. New enzyme polymorphisms continue to be described in the literature. The incidence of the most common polymorphisms has been studied in Europe with the following percentages: homozygous wild type 96%, heterozygous wild/atypical 2.5%, wild/fluoride or wild/silent 0.3%, atypical/fluoride 0.005%, fluoride/silent or fluoride/fluoride 0.006%, and atypical/atypical 0.05%.[4]

When prolonged succinylcholine block is suspected, a dibucaine number and enzyme activity measurement can aid in the diagnosis.[5] Dibucaine is a local anesthetic that inhibits the normal enzyme by 80% and the homozygous atypical enzyme by 20% (heterozygous ~40% to 60%). The dibucaine number is simply a number indicating the percentage by which plasma cholinesterase is inhibited. Each polymorphism is associated with a different amount of enzyme inhibition by dibucaine, but this test alone is not sensitive for the silent, fluoride, and other type mutations that require further testing not discussed here. It should also be noted that the dibucaine number reflects only the qualitative activity of the enzyme not the quantity, hence the value in assaying total enzyme activity as well.

Treatment of prolonged neuromuscular blockade is supportive in nature. Generally, patients can be transferred to the PACU or intensive care unit intubated and ventilated where mechanical ventilation and close supervision can continue until the patient's neuromuscular function returns and they can be safely extubated. Attempted reversal of depolarizing neuromuscular block with neostigmine is controversial. If given without any evidence of fade on TOF monitoring neostigmine will only prolong the block, since neostigmine is itself a potent inhibitor of pseudocholinesterase. There is some thought that if a phase II type block is present a dose of <0.3 mg/kg of reversal can be helpful.

After identification of the cause, patients with prolonged weakness should receive counseling and possibly identification bands warning of prolonged effects of these medications. Routine screening of relatives isn't suggested, but relatives should notify physicians of a family history of atypical pseudocholinesterase.

Take-Home Points

- Clinically significant prolongation of succinylcholine may be secondary to decreased levels of enzyme, drug related changes in enzyme activity, or genetically atypical enzyme.
- When genetically normal pseudocholinesterase is present, levels may be reduced to ~20% of normal before clinically relevant prolongation of succinylcholine is recognized.
- Homozygous atypical, silent, and fluoride types, as well as heterozygote atypical/silent and atypical/fluoride are associated with significant prolonged succinylcholine effects.
- Close clinical monitoring return of neuromuscular blockade when administering any neuromuscular blocking agent, including succinylcholine, is strongly recommended.
- The dibucaine number is a laboratory test that assists in characterizing the abnormality. When added to plasma *in vitro*, dibucaine inhibits normal enzyme by 80%. Normal cholinesterase therefore has a dibucaine number of 80 while homozygous atypical enzyme has dibucaine number of 20. Heterozygotes typically show a ~40% to 60% inhibition. Fluoride resistant or silent types exist as well but are far less common.
- Treatment of prolonged succinylcholine neuromuscular blockade is supportive in nature with continued mechanical ventilation until neuromuscular function returns
- Patient counseling and name band identification is suggested following diagnosis.

Summary

Interaction: pharmacogenomic
Substrates: succinylcholine and plasma cholinesterase
Gene: point mutations causing deletion or substitutions of nucleotides located at chromosome 3q26
Mechanism: decreased metabolism of succinylcholine
Clinical effect: prolonged neuromuscular weakness

References

1. Kuhnert BR, Philipson EH, Pimetal R, et al. A prolonged chloroprocaine epidural block in a postpartum patient with abnormal pseudocholinesterase. Anesthesiology. 1982;56(6):477–8.
2. Naguib M, Lien CA. Pharmacology of muscle relaxants and their antagonists. In: Miller RD, Fleisher LA, Eriksson LI, Wiener-Kronish JP, Young WL, editors. Miller's anesthesia. 7th ed. Philadelphia: Churchill Livingston; 2009. p. 1043–5.
3. Rosenberg H, Brandom BW, Sambuughin N. Malignant hyperthermia and other inherited disorders. In: Barasch PG, Cullen BF, Stoelting RK, Cahalan MK, Stock MC, editors. Clinical anesthesia. 6th ed. Philadelphia: Lippincott Williams & Wilkins; 2009. p. 613–6.
4. Hanel HK, Viby-Mogensen J, Schaffalitzky de Muckadell OB. Serum cholinesterase variants in the Danish population. Acta Anaesthesiol Scand. 1978;22:505.
5. Viby-Mogensen J. Correlation of succinylcholine duration of action with plasma cholinesterase activity in subjects with normal enzyme. Anesthesiology. 1980;53:517.

Slow Sux III: Where Did the Twitches Go?

97

Succinylcholine, donepezil, atypical pseudocholinesterase

Katarina Bojanić MD, Juraj Sprung MD, PhD, and Toby N. Weingarten MD

Abstract
This case discusses prolonged paralysis after succinylcholine administration in a patient with atypical pseudocholinesterase and potentiation of the paralytic effects by inhibition of donezepil metabolism by verapamil (cytochrome P450 3A4) and paroxetine (cytochrome P450 2D6).

Case

A 70-year-old, 80 kg woman with a history of mild Alzheimer's disease, depression, and hypertension presented to the operating room for a repair of a small ventral hernia. She had a history of one unremarkable general endotracheal anesthesia 8 years ago. She reported that she had taken her outpatient daily medications that morning, which were donepezil (10 mg), paroxetine (20 mg), and sustained-release verapamil hydrochloride (240 mg).

At induction, she received fentanyl (100 mcg), propofol (130 mg), and succinylcholine (140 mg). She received vecuronium (5 mg) before skin incision and a peripheral nerve monitor was then placed in the preauricular area over the facial nerve. Forty minutes later, the hernia was repaired and skin closure began. The peripheral nerve train-of-four (TOF) stimuli produced three of four twitches. To reverse the neuromuscular block, the patient received neostigmine (5 mg) and glycopyrrolate

K. Bojanić MD (✉)
Division of Neonatology, Clinical Hospital Merkur, Zagreb, Croatia
e-mail: sprungkatarina@hotmail.com

J. Sprung MD, PhD • T.N. Weingarten MD
Department of Anesthesiology, Mayo Clinic, Rochester, MN, USA

C. Marcucci et al. (eds.), *A Case Approach to Perioperative Drug-Drug Interactions*, DOI 10.1007/978-1-4614-7495-1_97

(1 mg). Desflurane was discontinued, and the ventilator respiratory rate was reduced to 6 breaths per minute to facilitate the initiation of spontaneous respirations.

Ten minutes after skin closure, the patient had made no respiratory efforts and triggering of the peripheral nerve stimulator produced no twitches. The anesthesia gas monitoring system detected zero end-tidal desflurane and the patient had become tachycardic and hypertensive. A propofol infusion was initiated and the patient was transferred to the intensive care unit for continued mechanical ventilation. Subsequently, the test for atypical pseudocholinesterase (dibucaine number) was 45% (reference range, 70%-80%).

Eight hours later, the TOF stimuli spontaneously produced four strong twitches, and the patient initiated respiratory effort and was able to follow commands. Her trachea was extubated without further incident.

Discussion

This is an example of multiple inhibitors added to multiple substrates.

Donepezil is a reversible inhibitor of central acetylcholinesterase and is used to treat mild to moderate dementia associated with Alzheimer's disease. It has been shown to inhibit pseudocholinesterase peripherally only at increased plasma concentrations; at typical clinical doses, it usually does not interfere with succinylcholine metabolism.[1] This inhibition is dose dependent (Fig. 97.1). Donepezil is metabolized by the cytochrome P450 (CYP) isozymes 2D6 and 3A4.[2] The present patient was taking both verapamil, which inhibits CYP3A4, and paroxetine, which inhibits CYP2D6.[3,4] The combination of these two medications may have resulted in considerable inhibition of donepezil metabolism and thus increased its plasma levels, potentiating anticholinesterase activity.

The patient also received neostigmine to reverse the nondepolarizing neuromuscular blockade of vecuronium. The peripheral TOF obtained at the end of the operation produced a fade pattern, but it is not clear from this scenario whether the fade represented a partial reversal of the vecuronium block or a Phase II block from succinylcholine (secondary to prolonged effects of succinylcholine). The TOF should have been measured before administration of vecuronium, to ensure that the patient had normally functioning pseudocholinesterase (ie, to confirm that the patient recovered four strong twitches without fade) and that the neuromuscular effects of succinylcholine had dissipated. However, given that the patient had an uneventful anesthesia previously, there was no reason to suspect that she may have atypical pseudocholinesterase.

Neostigmine can potentiate the neuromuscular blockade produced by succinylcholine and also inhibits plasma pseudocholinesterase (the only reversal agent that does

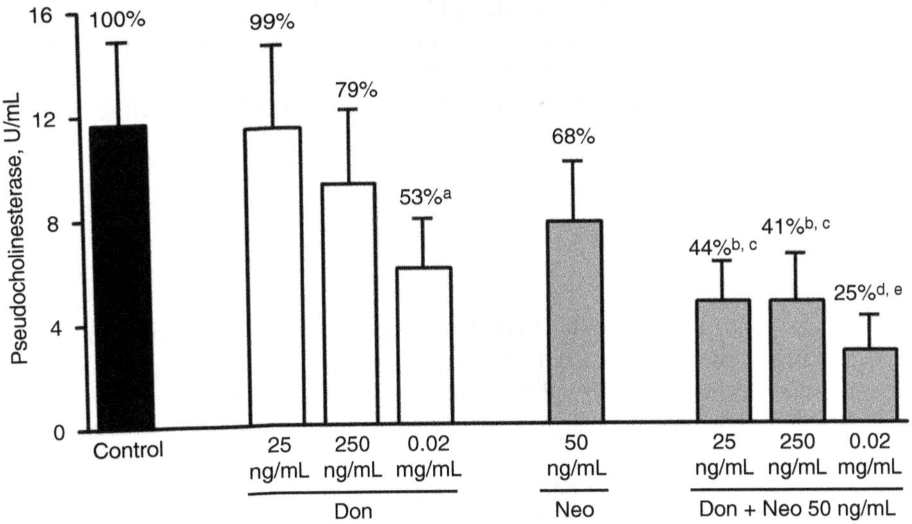

Fig. 97.1 Mean serum pseudocholinesterase activity of five patients taking donepezil (don), neostigmine (neo), and three doses of neostigmine plus donepezil. Error bars indicate SD. Percents cited above the respective histograms indicate remaining pseudocholinesterase activity based on the control activity equaling 100%. [a] $P<.01$ vs control; [b] $P<.007$ vs control; [c] $P<.05$ vs neostigmine; [d] $P<.0001$ vs control; [e] $P<.003$ vs neostigmine [Adapted from Sprung J, Castellani WJ, Srinivasan V et al: The effects of donepezil and neostigmine in a patient with unusual pseudocholinesterase activity. Anesth Analg 1998; 87: 1203-1205. With permission from Wolter Kluwers Health.]

not have an effect on plasma cholinesterase activity is edrophonium chloride).[5] Although reversal of Phase II block after excessive use of succinylcholine can be accelerated with neostigmine, reversal of Phase II block that is present in patients with atypical plasma cholinesterase may not be reliable.[6] The combination of neostigmine and donepezil has an additive effect on pseudocholinesterase inhibition.[1]

In a patient with normal pseudocholinesterase levels (ie, the patient is homozygous for normal pseudocholinesterase), it is doubtful that a moderately depressed pseudocholinesterase level induced by donepezil would cause prolonged neuromuscular block in response to succinylcholine. However, the present patient was heterozygous for atypical pseudocholinesterase, as indicated by the dibucaine number of 45%, and had decreased levels of normal pseudocholinesterase at baseline. The increased plasma donepezil concentrations secondary to its suppressed metabolism and in conjunction with the administration of neostigmine could inhibit plasma pseudocholinesterase sufficiently to cause prolonged paralysis due to nonhydrolyzed acetylcholine.

Donepezil has a good safety record, but still there are reports of some patients who have muscle weakness and muscle fasciculations with its use (signs and symptoms related to acetylcholine-induced depolarization). This observation suggests that in some rare instances and in some susceptible individuals, donepezil may induce clinically significant cholinesterase inhibition. It also is plausible that this response may occur when pathways for donepezil metabolism are inhibited, as was the case in our patient who received verapamil (inhibits CYP3A4) and paroxetine (inhibits CYP2D6).[3,4]

Take-Home Points

- Donepezil is a reversible inhibitor of central acetylcholinesterase and modestly inhibits plasma cholinesterase. In patients with normal pseudocholinesterase activity, this inhibition has no clinical effect on neuromuscular transmission.

- Drugs that inhibit CYP3A4 and CYP2D6 may slow elimination of donepezil and therefore may enhance its otherwise small physiologic effects on plasma cholinesterase.

- It is always important to assess whether paralysis from succinylcholine has resolved before the administration of nondepolarizing neuromuscular blocking drugs or anticholinesterases. This practice avoids the potential for substantial drug–drug interaction that may complicate spontaneous recovery from neuromuscular blockade.

Summary

Interaction: pharmacokinetic (complex)
Substrate: donezepil
Enzyme: CYP3A4 and CYP2D6, pseudocholinesterase
Inhibitor: verapamil (3A4), paroxetine (2D6), and neostigmine (pseudocholinesterase)
Clinical effects: prolonged paralysis after succinylcholine administration in a patient with atypical pseudocholinesterase; potentiation of the paralytic effects by inhibition of donezepil metabolism

References

1. Sprung J, Castellani WJ, Srinivasan V, et al. The effects of donepezil and neostigmine in a patient with unusual pseudocholinesterase activity. Anesth Analg. 1998;87:1203–5.
2. Tiseo PJ, Perdomo CA, Friedhoff LT. Metabolism and elimination of 14C-donepezil in healthy volunteers: a single-dose study. Br J Clin Pharmacol. 1998;46 Suppl 1:19–24.

3. Ma B, Prueksaritanont T, Lin JH. Drug interactions with calcium channel blockers: possible involvement of metabolite-intermediate complexation with CYP3A. Drug Metab Dispos. 2000;28:125–30.
4. Crewe HK, Lennard MS, Tucker GT, et al. The effect of selective serotonin re-uptake inhibitors on cytochrome P4502D6 (CYP2D6) activity in human liver microsomes. Br J Clin Pharmacol. 1992;34:262–5.
5. Clutton RE, Glasby MA. A comparison of edrophonium and neostigmine for the reversal of mivacurium-induced neuromuscular blockade in sheep. Res Vet Sci. 1998;64:265–6.
6. Bevan DR, Donati F. Succinylcholine apnoea: attempted reversal with anticholinesterases. Can Anaesth Soc J. 1983;30:536–9.

Weakened All Weekend

98

Vecuronium, amikacin

Daniel W. Johnson MD

Abstract
This case discusses the complex pharmacodynamic interaction between vecuronium and amikacin resulting in increased neuromuscular blockade.

Case

When Mr. Johnson's retirement funding ran dry, he reluctantly moved to a less-expensive facility. Three days after the transfer, he developed severe abdominal pain. The staff thought this was "his way of adjusting." Two days later, Mr. Johnson was in the operating room (OR) for repair of a perforated bowel and washout of abdominal sepsis.

In the intensive care unit (ICU), the patient suffered from multiorgan system failure with acute kidney and liver function derangements. He was diagnosed with pneumonia with cultures that were positive for *Pseudomonas aeruginosa* and therapy with piperacillin/tazobactam and amikacin was initiated. Mr. Johnson's family was heartbroken and scared as they visited him every day, especially when he returned to the OR for exploratory laparotomy to rule out an anastomotic leak.

The case started smoothly with low doses of fentanyl, sevoflurane, and vecuronium. As the patient's hemodynamics worsened and multiple vasoactive drugs became necessary, the attending anesthesiologist set up an infusion of vecuronium so that they could be sure of neuromuscular blockade while they focused on other issues. With an open abdomen the patient's core temperature dropped to 32°C.

After returning to the ICU, the patient was surprisingly stable, although on a low dose of sedation to help facilitate mechanical ventilation. On his postoperative

D.W. Johnson MD
Department of Anesthesia, Critical Care and Pain Medicine, Massachusetts General Hospital, Boston, MA, USA
e-mail: DWJOHNSON@PARTNERS.ORG

C. Marcucci et al. (eds.), *A Case Approach to Perioperative Drug-Drug Interactions*, DOI 10.1007/978-1-4614-7495-1_98

check, the surgical resident was pleasantly surprised to see that Mr. Johnson had been weaned from all pressors. In fact, he was slightly hypertensive and tachycardic. A neurologic exam revealed no response to commands. “He needs to wake up from the anesthetic, so turn off all the sedation and pain meds,” he instructed the nurses. After the sedative had worn off, the tachycardia and hypertension worsened, but Mr. Johnson would still not open his eyes or follow commands. Prior to departing after a long night of call, the patient’s anesthesiologist went to the ICU to do a postanesthesia check. A review of the situation prompted the anesthesiologist to consider the possibility of prolonged neuromuscular blockade. Eight hours after surgery, a train-of-four (TOF) monitor revealed just one faint twitch out of four stimuli. The anesthesiologist recommended re-sedating the patient until the neuromuscular function recovered to the point that the TOF would result in four strong, equal twitches.

Discussion

This is an example of a complex pharmacodynamic interaction.

Vecuronium is an intermediate-acting neuromuscular blocking agent in the steroidal class. Like the other nondepolarizing neuromuscular blockers, it acts by competing with acetylcholine at the postsynaptic receptor of the neuromuscular junction. The normal duration of action of vecuronium after a dose for tracheal intubation is approximately 30 to 50 minutes.[1] Normally, 30% to 40% of a dose of vecuronium is metabolized by the liver, and elimination is accomplished both by renal (40% to 50%) and hepatic (50% to 60%) pathways. One of the metabolites, 3-desacetylvecuronium, exhibits slower plasma clearance and longer duration of action than vecuronium, has about 80% of the potency of the parent drug, and accumulates in patients with renal failure.[2] Liver disease will predictably reduce the elimination of vecuronium and prolong the duration of neuromuscular blockade, especially after repeated doses or the use of prolonged infusions.[3,4]

Amikacin, an aminoglycoside, has been in use for decades and remains an important therapeutic against aerobic gram-negative bacterial infections. In this case it was being used for double coverage against *Pseudomonas aeruginosa*. Amikacin, like other aminoglycosides, increases sensitivity to vecuronium and other nondepolarizing neuromuscular blocking agents. The mechanism is twofold. The aminoglycosides decrease presynaptic quantal release of acetylcholine and they decrease postjunctional sensitivity to acetylcholine.[5]

This case represents an unfortunate confluence of factors leading to prolonged neuromuscular blockade: a drug–drug interaction, poor renal function, poor hepatic function, hypothermia (which prolongs recovery from neuromuscular blocking agents), and a long continuous infusion which promotes build-up of parent drug and active metabolites. The patient in this case was subjected to a preventable complication of ICU care: iatrogenic muscle paralysis in the absence of adequate sedation. Mr. Johnson eventually recovered fully and luckily did not remember the night he spent paralyzed without sedation.

Take-Home Points

- Administration of neuromuscular blocking agents in critically ill patients requires a high level of vigilance to avoid drug–drug interactions or other adverse effects.
- When critically ill patients are on antibiotics, we must be cognizant of the potentially detrimental drug–drug interactions that they might cause.
- When an aminoglycoside is in use and other patient factors might lead to enhanced neuromuscular blockade, we should consider opting for agents that do not require normal organ function for breakdown and elimination. Atracurium and cisatracurium are examples of agents with predictable offset even in the setting of renal and hepatic dysfunction.
- Using peripheral nerve stimulation (eg, train-of-four) and titration to effect, even in cases where extubation is unlikely, might prevent situational overdose of neuromuscular blocking agents.
- Intraoperative overdose of drugs has important postoperative consequences.
- Physicians must minimize factors that contribute to prolonged neuromuscular blockade, such as hypothermia.

Summary

Interaction: pharmacodynamic (complex)
Substrate: vecuronium and amikacin
Receptor site: undetermined
Agonist/Antagonist: undetermined
Clinical effect: increased effect of vecuronium

References

1. Pino RM, Ali HH. Monitoring and Managing Neuromuscular Blockade. In: Longnecker DE, editor. Anesthesiology. New York: McGraw Hill Professional; 2008.
2. Naguib M, Lien C. Pharmacology of Muscle Relaxants and their Antagonists. In: Miller RD, editor. Miller's anesthesia. 6th ed. Philadelphia: Elsevier Churchill Livingstone; 2005.

3. Shanks AB, Long T, Aitkenhead AR. Prolonged neuromuscular blockade following vecuronium. A case report. Br J Anaesth. 1985;57(8):807–10.
4. Kronenfeld MA, Thomas SJ, Turndorf H. Recurrence of neuromuscular blockade after reversal of vecuronium in a patient receiving polymyxin/amikacin sternal irrigation. Anesthesiology. 1986;65(1):93–4.
5. Singh YN, Marshall IG, Harvey AL. Pre- and postjunctional effects of aminoglycoside, polymyxin, tetracycline and lincosamide antibiotics. Br J Anaesth. 1982;54(12):1295–306.

The Patient Who Could Not Raise Her Head

99

Vecuronium, gentamicin

Nicole L. Varela MD, Toby N. Weingarten MD, and Juraj Sprung MD, PhD

Abstract
This case discusses a synergistic pharmacodynamic interaction between vecuronium and gentamicin.

Case

A thin, 63-year-old woman was transferred from the nursing home to the hospital, with a report of abdominal pain and fever. She had a past history of diverticulitis and stroke that resulted in permanent and profound right-sided weakness. A working diagnosis of diverticulitis was made and she was started on metronidazole (500 mg 98 h intravenously) and gentamicin (4 mg/kg intravenously once daily), given the patient's history of penicillin allergy. A left hemicolectomy was recommended after additional workup was concerning for bowel microperforation.

The patient presented to the operating room immediately after completion of her morning doses of gentamicin and metronidazole. The anesthesiologist decided to avoid succinylcholine and use vecuronium to facilitate intubation, given her profound right-side weakness from her prior stroke. The patient received vecuronium for muscle relaxation during the case. At skin closure, train-of-four (TOF) stimuli to the left facial nerve showed two of four twitches. Neostigmine and glycopyrrolate were given to reverse residual effects of the neuromuscular blockade. She was extubated ten minutes later, after breathing spontaneously, opening her eyes, and squeezing her left hand.

N.L. Varela MD (✉)
Department of Anesthesiology, Winona Health, Winona, MN, USA
e-mail: nicole@varela.net

T.N. Weingarten MD • J. Sprung MD, PhD
Department of Anesthesiology, Mayo Clinic, Rochester, MN, USA

C. Marcucci et al. (eds.), *A Case Approach to Perioperative Drug-Drug Interactions*, DOI 10.1007/978-1-4614-7495-1_99

In the recovery room, the patient had labored respirations. Her oxygen saturation on pulse oximetry showed a decrease from 95% to 85%. She still was able to grasp weakly with her left hand but was unable to sustain a head lift for longer than 1 second. She was started on bilevel positive airway pressure via a closed mask to assist her respiratory effort. Over the next 60 minutes, her oxygenation levels improved and her strength returned to her baseline level.

Discussion

This is an example of a synergistic pharmacodynamic interaction.

More specifically, this is an example of gentamicin potentiating the neuromuscular blockade of vecuronium, resulting in prolonged muscle weakness.

Aminoglycosides are known to have neuromuscular blocking effects that can manifest as muscle weakness.[1,2] These antibiotics inhibit both presynaptic and postsynaptic transmissions, but the presynaptic activity predominates.[3,4] Traditionally, it was thought that aminoglycosides directly inhibited the presynaptic, voltage-activated calcium channels, but direct inhibition of these channels occurs at very high concentrations only.[2] It is now believed that the primary mechanism is mediated by aminoglycoside activation with presynaptic calcium ion–sensing receptors (CaSRs). When the CaSR is activated by calcium, it inhibits voltage-dependent nonselective cation channels (Fig. 99.1). These channels allow the fusion of acetylcholine-containing vesicles with the terminal membrane, permitting acetylcholine release. At normal calcium concentrations, CaSR is not fully activated, allowing acetylcholine release in response to an action potential. However, when exposed to calcium and an aminoglycoside, the CaSR becomes fully activated and inhibits the nonselective cation channels, preventing acetylcholine release.[2] Aminoglycoside activity at both the presynaptic CaSRs and the presynaptic voltage-activated calcium channels results in a decrease in acetylcholine release at the neuromuscular junction, in response to presynaptic action potentials.

The neuromuscular effects of aminoglycosides typically result in mild generalized weakness of little clinical significance. However, more severe weakness may manifest in patients with underlying neuromuscular disease, such as myasthenia gravis. Aminoglycosides and neuromuscular blockers, when used in conjunction, have synergistic effects at the neuromuscular end plate: 1) inhibition of acetylcholine release at the neuromuscular synapse by the aminoglycoside, and 2) competitive antagonism of acetylcholine at the motor end plate receptors by the neuromuscular blocking agent. Prolonged neuromuscular blockade has been reported in patients who simultaneously receive gentamicin and vecuronium, as was the case with the present patient.[5,6]

The synergism between neuromuscular blocking agents and aminoglycosides appears to be more profound with vecuronium than other muscle relaxants, such as

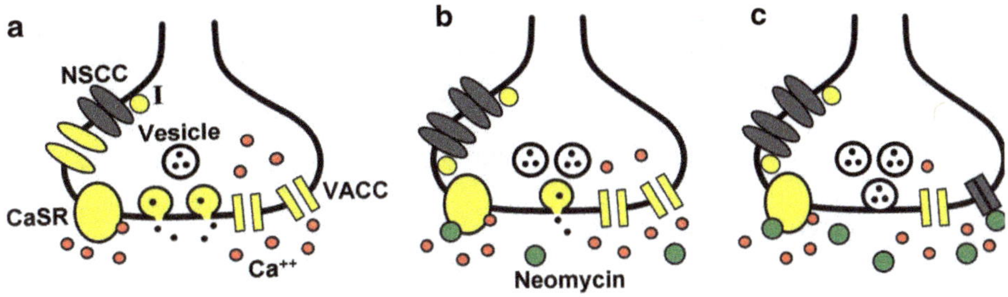

Fig. 99.1 Diagram of proposed model for aminoglycoside inhibition of acetylcholine release at the presynaptic motor nerve terminal. A, Under normal physiologic conditions, the presynaptic calcium ion (Ca^{++})–sensing receptor (CaSR) (yellow oval) is partially activated by extracellular Ca^{++} (red circles). When activated by Ca^{++}, the CaSR inhibits voltage-dependent nonselective cation channels (NSCCs) (black ovals), which impedes the fusion of acetylcholine-containing vesicles with the terminal membrane and prevents release of acetylcholine (black circles). At physiologic concentrations of Ca^{++}, CaSR is not fully activated and acetylcholine is released in response to an action potential. I indicates inhibition; VACC, voltage-activated calcium channel. B, During low concentration of the aminoglycoside neomycin (green circles), the CaSR binds to both neomycin and Ca^{++} and becomes fully activated, reducing acetylcholine release. C, During high concentration of neomycin, the CaSR is fully activated, plus neomycin blocks the VACCs, further attenuating acetylcholine release. Active molecules are colored yellow and inactive molecules are colored gray. The second messenger-mediating signaling between NSCC and CaSR has not been identified and is denoted by a small, yellow, intracellular circle [Adapted from Harnett MT, Chen W, Smith SM. Calcium-sensing receptor: a high-affinity presynaptic target for aminoglycoside-induced weakness. *Neuropharmacology* 2009;57:502-505. With permission from Elsevier.]

atracurium.[6] Compared with divided doses, once-daily dosing of gentamicin may enhance the synergistic activity of vecuronium between these two medications, but this observation is not consistent.[5,6] The prolonged neuromuscular blockade between gentamicin and vecuronium may not always be easily reversed with anticholinesterases.[4,6] It has been suggested that calcium administration may facilitate the reversal of the neuromuscular blockade induced by aminoglycosides.[4]

The potential for prolonged neuromuscular blockade of patients receiving both gentamicin and vecuronium should be monitored closely. In addition, the anesthesiologist should be aware that prolonged neuromuscular blockade may persist in the recovery room, despite use of reversal agents. Ideally in this case, clinical signs of strength (adequate head lift) would have been assessed before extubation, given the patient's history of underlying muscle weakness secondary to a previous stroke.

Take-Home Points

- Aminoglycosides can inhibit acetylcholine release at the neuromuscular junction, resulting in generalized muscle weakness. Fortunately, this effect is usually mild. However, it can be clinically significant for patients with neuromuscular dysfunction.

- The simultaneous use of gentamicin and vecuronium can lead to prolonged neuromuscular blockade, and this blockade may not be reversed easily with neostigmine.

- The mechanism for prolonged neuromuscular blockade is due to the combination of prejunctional effects by aminoglycosides and the motor end plate receptor blockade by nondepolarizing neuromuscular blockers.

Summary

Interaction: pharmacodynamic (synergism)
Substrates: vecuronium and gentamicin
Mechanism/site of action: inhibition of acetylcholine release at the neuromuscular synapse by the aminoglycoside and competitive antagonism of acetylcholine at the motor end-plate receptors by the neuromuscular blocking agent
Clinical effect: enhanced neuromuscular weakness

References

1. Molgo J, Lemeignan M, Uchiyama T, et al. Inhibitory effect of kanamycin on evoked transmitter release: reversal by 3,4-diaminopyridine. Eur J Pharmacol. 1979;57:93–7.
2. Harnett MT, Chen W, Smith SM. Calcium-sensing receptor: a high-affinity presynaptic target for aminoglycoside-induced weakness. Neuropharmacology. 2009;57:502–5.
3. Fiekers JF. Effects of the aminoglycoside antibiotics, streptomycin and neomycin, on neuromuscular transmission. I Presynaptic considerations. J Pharmacol Exp Ther. 1983;225: 487–95.
4. Paradelis AG, Triantaphyllidis C, Giala MM. Neuromuscular blocking activity of aminoglycoside antibiotics. Methods Find Exp Clin Pharmacol. 1980;2:45–51.
5. Dotan ZA, Hana R, Simon D, et al. The effect of vecuronium is enhanced by a large rather than a modest dose of gentamicin as compared with no preoperative gentamicin. Anesth Analg. 2003;96:750–4.
6. Dupuis JY, Martin R, Tetrault JP. Atracurium and vecuronium interaction with gentamicin and tobramycin. Can J Anaesth. 1989;36:407–11.

An Unexpected Wait

100

Pancuronium, mivacurium

Michael W. Best MD and Shawn T. Beaman MD

Abstract
This case discusses a pharmacodynamic interaction between pancuronium and mivacurium. Pancuronium administered before mivacurium can result in prolonged muscular blockade.

Case

A 54-year-old man with a history of type 2 diabetes and chronic obstructive pulmonary disease (COPD) arrived for a wedge resection of his right upper lobe after being diagnosed with lung cancer. He had no previous adverse reactions to anesthesia while undergoing an appendectomy at age 15 and a right knee repair at age 52. He took only metformin, and denied any use of illicit drugs or alcohol.

He underwent an uncomplicated general anesthetic. He was given succinylcholine for intubation and pancuronium was administered after return of train-of-four (TOF) upon peripheral nerve stimulation. Towards the end of the case, the surgeons requested "brief but heavy" neuromuscular blockade to help close the chest. In an effort to facilitate extubation immediately postoperatively, a dose of mivacurium was administered to provide paralysis for the remainder of the procedure. At the conclusion of the procedure 20 minutes later, the patient did not have any detectable twitches and the neuromuscular blockade was unable to be reversed. The patient remained under anesthesia in the operating room for another 30 minutes before he recovered adequate twitch height to be reversed. The patient was then extubated and transferred to the postanesthesia care unit. No adverse reactions were otherwise noted, and the patient was later discharged to home.

M.W. Best MD (✉)
Department of Anesthesiology, University of Pittsburgh Medical Center, Pittsburgh, PA, USA
e-mail: bestmw@upmc.edu

S.T. Beaman MD
Department of Anesthesiology, University of Pittsburgh School of Medicine, Pittsburgh, PA, USA

C. Marcucci et al. (eds.), *A Case Approach to Perioperative Drug-Drug Interactions*, DOI 10.1007/978-1-4614-7495-1_100

Discussion

This is an example of a complex synergistic pharmacodynamic interaction.

Nondepolarizing neuromuscular blocking agents (NMBA) bind to one of the two α subunits of the nicotinic acetylcholine receptor at the neuromuscular junction. They act as reversible competitive inhibitors of acetylcholine, preventing propagation of action potentials from the neuron to the muscle. These drugs are often described by the length of their duration as short, intermediate, or long-acting.

Mivacurium, a short-acting NMBA, is predominantly metabolized by plasma pseudocholinesterase. This results in only a small portion of the administered dose reaching its site of action at the neuromuscular junction.[1] Although no longer manufactured in North America, the drug is still used in much of the world and maintains some popularity for neuromuscular blockade in pediatric cases. It can be administered in boluses or as a continuous infusion. Pancuronium, on the other hand, is a long-acting NMBA with duration of action of approximately 1.5 to 2 hours.[2] It has an active metabolite whose potency is about one-half of pancuronium itself. Unlike other NMBAs, it has been shown to increase heart rate, blood pressure, and cardiac output, making it a popular choice for cardiac surgery often in combination with high-dose fentanyl regimens.[2]

It has been shown that the combined use of structurally different NMBAs results in a synergistic effect.[1,3–5] Structurally different molecules may have different prejunctional and postjunctional effects, leading to a greater number of occupied receptors. *In vitro* studies have confirmed synergistic interactions with combinations of cisatracurium and rocuronium, as well as cisatracurium and vecuronium.[4,5] However, when structurally similar NMBAs are combined, such as two aminosteroids (eg, rocuronium and vecuronium) or two benzylisoquinolines (eg, cisatracurium and atracurium), the effect has been shown only to be additive.[4,5] In the case described above, mivacurium is a benzylisoquinoline and pancuronium is an aminosteroid. Their structural dissimilarity likely contributed partially, although not fully, to the unexpectedly prolonged neuromuscular block.

Beyond structural dissimilarity, prior administration of pancuronium further potentiated the effects of mivacurium. This is due to a reduction in pancuronium pseudocholinesterase levels after administration of pancuronium. It has been shown that pancuronium transiently decreases pseudocholinesterase by approximately 25%, which can lead to clinically significant prolongations of action for both succinylcholine and mivacurium.[1–3,6] In the case of mivacurium, it is believed that the decrease in pseudocholinesterase not only results in a delay of metabolism, but it also allows more of the administered dose to initially reach the site of action.[1] The end result is a more effective and prolonged neuromuscular blockade.

Take-Home Points

- The administration of mivacurium after pancuronium can result in prolonged paralysis as a result of mivacurium behaving more like an intermediate-acting, rather than short-acting NMBA. This prolonged effect is from decreased plasma pseudocholinesterase activity caused by pancuronium and from the use of structurally different NMBAs.
- The use of structurally different NMBAs in combination has been shown to have synergistic effects. Specifically, this includes the use of benzylisoquinolines (eg, atracurium, cisatracurium) with aminosteroids (eg, rocuronium, vecuronium).
- The use of structurally similar NMBAs in combination has been shown only to have additive effects.

Summary

Interaction: pharmacodynamic (synergism)
Substrates: pancuronium and mivacurium
Mechanisms/sites of action: increased binding at the α subunit of nicotinic acetylcholine receptor at neuromuscular junction, decreased levels of plasma cholinesterase
Clinical effects: prolonged neuromuscular blockade

References

1. Motamed C, Menad R, Farinotti R, et al. Potentiation of mivacurium blockade by low dose of pancuronium. Anesthesiology. 2003;98:1057–62.
2. Dubois MY, Fleming NW, Lea DE. Effects of succinylcholine on the pharmacodynamics of pipecuronium and pancuronium. Anesth Analg. 1991;72:364–8.
3. Motamed C, Kirov K, Combes X, et al. Interaction between mivacurium and pancuronium: impact of the order of administration. Eur J Clin Pharmacol. 2005;61:175–7.
4. Kim KS, Chun YS, Chon SU, et al. Neuromuscular interaction between cisatracurium and mivacurium, atracurium, vecuronium or rocuronium administered in combination. Anaesthesia. 1998;53:872–8.
5. Naguib M, Samarkandi AH, Bakhamees HS, et al. Comparative potency of steroidal neuromuscular blocking drugs and isobolographic analysis of the interaction between rocuronium and other aminosteroids. Br J Anaesth. 1995;75:73–42.
6. Erkola O, Rautoma P, Meretoja O. Mivacurium when preceded by pancuronium becomes a long-acting muscle relaxant. Anesthesiology. 1996;84(3):562–5.

Diabolical Cough Syrup

101

Rocuronium, pholcodine

Melisa N. Weingarten RN, MS, Juraj Sprung MD, PhD, and Toby N. Weingarten MD

Abstract
This case discusses IgE sensitization by pholcodine resulting in cross-sensitization to rocuronium bromide.

Case

A 70 kg, 23-year-old Norwegian man who was a graduate student in the United States presented to the operating room for laparoscopic abdominal exploration for suspected appendicitis. He had been nauseated, so the anesthesiologist decided to use rapid sequence induction for intubation. General anesthesia was induced with fentanyl (100 mcg) given intravenously (IV), propofol (150 mg IV) and rocuronium (80 mg IV).

Shortly after induction the patient became profoundly hypotensive, tachycardic, and hypoxic. Urticaria developed across his face, torso, and limbs. Ventilation of his lungs was difficult. The anesthesiologist suspected anaphylactic reaction and administered epinephrine (0.5 mg), diphenhydramine (50 mg), and hydrocortisone (100 mg), all intravenously. After 45 minutes of aggressive treatment, the blood pressure, ventilation, and oxygenation normalized. The appendix appeared to be perforated and the surgery continued with an open technique. The patient was extubated at the end of the case, and he was transferred to the intensive care unit for observation. Six hours later, a tryptase level was 67 ng/mL (normal <11 ng/mL). Consultation was sought with an allergist, and skin prick test performed 6 weeks later disclosed a positive response to rocuronium. On questioning, the patient

M.N. Weingarten RN, MS (✉)
Patient Education, Mayo Clinic, Rochester, MN, USA
e-mail: Weingarten.melisa@mayo.edu

J. Sprung MD, PhD • T.N. Weingarten MD
Department of Anesthesiology, Mayo Clinic, Rochester, MN, USA

C. Marcucci et al. (eds.), *A Case Approach to Perioperative Drug-Drug Interactions*, DOI 10.1007/978-1-4614-7495-1_101

reported that on a visit home to Norway 3 months prior to surgery he had developed a severe cough. He had self-medicated with an old bottle of the cough syrup Tuxi® which he had found in his father's medicine cabinet.

Discussion

This is an example of a pharmacodynamic (immunologic) drug interaction.

More specifically, this is an example of IgE sensitization by pholcodine resulting in cross-sensitization to rocuronium bromide.

Severe intraoperative anaphylactic reactions are rare but associated with substantial morbidity and mortality. Several large epidemiological studies from Europe have reported that neuromuscular blocking agents (NMBA) are the most frequent cause for perioperative anaphylactic reactions.[1–3] However, a recent study that reported intraoperative allergic reactions from the Mayo Clinic practice found that NMBA were rarely associated with anaphylactic reactions.[4] Furthermore, even within Europe, regional discrepancies have also been noted. For example, compared with Sweden, a 10-fold greater incidence of anaphylactic reactions to NMBA drugs were observed in Norway.[5] Analysis of sera from Norwegians and Swedes found that Norwegians had higher rates of IgE antibodies to morphine and succinylcholine.[5,6]

The IgE antibody-binding site of antigens may contain quaternary ammonium ions (QAI). Studies have found that common QAIs may exist on unrelated substances, which serve as common allergenic epitopes on different antigens.[7] Thus, a patient who has been previously sensitized to another environmental antigen with a similar QAI may experience an anaphylactic reaction following exposure to an unrelated drug event after the first time this drug is administered. For example, QAIs are found on compounds used in cosmetics, toiletries, and household cleaners and disinfectants. A study of a British patient who had suffered a near-fatal reaction to succinylcholine showed IgE antibody cross-reactivity to three common ingredients of cosmetics and two commonly used disinfectants.[10]

In regards to the differences observed in Scandinavia, it was found that there was widespread use of the cough suppressant, pholcodine (marked as Tuxi®) in Norway, but not in Sweden. It was estimated that at the time when pholcodine was on the market about 40% of the population were taking the drug, and about 5% to 10% of population became IgE sensitized to pholcodine, indicating that this drug is a potent sensitizer.[8] Pholcodine is thought to share a QAI with NMBAs and morphine. A previously pholcodine IgE-sensitized individual after a 7-day exposure to pholcodine had a 60-fold increase in overall serum IgE levels and 60-fold to 85-fold

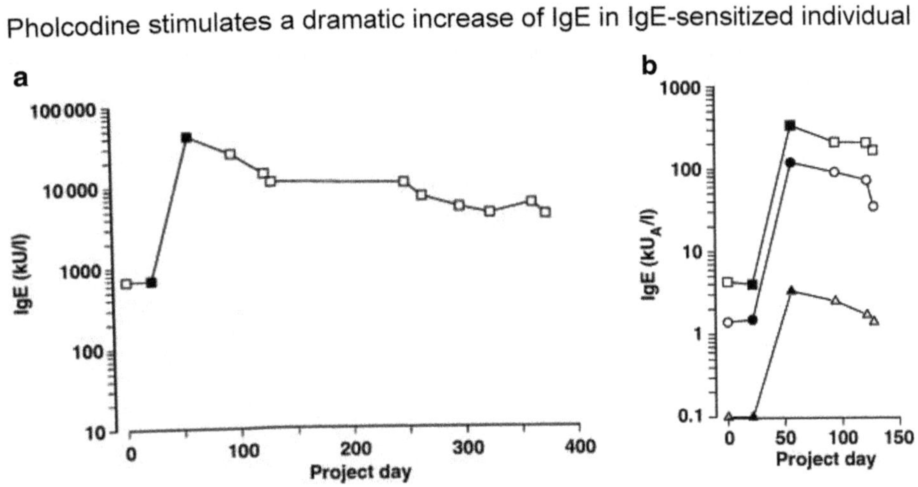

Fig. 101.1 An individual previously sensitized to pholcodine was exposed to 20 mg pholcodine daily for 7 days. Serum levels of IgE increased by 60 fold and remained elevated for more than 1 year (Panel A). Levels of IgE antibodies to pholcodine, morphine, and succinylcholine increased between 60-fold and 85- fold from baseline values (Panel B) [Modified from Florvaag E, Johansson SG, Irgens A et al. IgE-sensitization to the cough suppressant pholcodine and the effects of its withdrawal from the Norwegian market. Allergy. 2011; 66:955-960. With permission from John Wiley & Sons.]

increase in IgE antibodies to pholcodine, morphine, and succinylcholine (Fig. 101.1).[9] In that individual, serum IgE levels remained elevated for more than 1 year. Pholcodine was withdrawn from the Norwegian market in 2007. Subsequently, there has been a decrease in the rate of Norwegians with detectable IgE antibodies to succinylcholine as well as a significant (45%) decline in the total number of suspected anaphylactic reactions attributed to NMBAs between 2005 and 2009.[8]

Take-Home Points

- In many countries, neuromuscular blocking agents were reported to be a primary cause of intraoperative anaphylactic reactions.
- Numerous antigens contain common quaternary ammonium ions that serve as binding sites to IgE antibodies, which can result in cross sensitization between unrelated substances.
- A cough suppressant, pholcodine, which was widely used in Europe, was found to cause sensitization to neuromuscular blocking agents and morphine. This resulted in increased rates of anaphylactic reactions related to these drugs during anesthesia in Europe.

- Withdrawal of pholcodine from the Norwegian market resulted in a dramatic reduction of allergic reactions to neuromuscular blocking agents in that country.

- It has been suggested that cosmetics, shampoos, and cleaning agents that have additives with quaternary ammonium ion sites have also caused clinically significant immunologic reactions to succinylcholine.

- New substances—drugs with quaternary (as well as tertiary) ammonium ion epitopes—need to be closely monitored for potential for inducing cross-sensitization against NMBAs.

Summary

Interaction: immunologic
Cross-reactants: pholcodine and rocuronium bromide
Mechanism: quaternary ammonium ions serve as common allergenic epitopes on different antigens leading to cross-reactivity and IgE-sensitivity
Clinical effects: allergic reaction or anaphylaxis when a patient is exposed to unrelated compound with a common quaternary ammonium ion moiety

References

1. Mertes PM, Laxenaire MC, Alla F. Anaphylactic and anaphylactoid reactions occurring during anesthesia in France in 1999-2000. Anesthesiology. 2003;99:536–45.
2. Laxenaire MC, Mertes PM. Anaphylaxis during anaesthesia. Results of a two-year survey in France. Br J Anaesth. 2001;87:549–58.
3. Harboe T, Guttormsen AB, Irgens A, et al. Anaphylaxis during anesthesia in Norway: a 6-year single-center follow-up study. Anesthesiology. 2005;102:897–903.
4. Gurrieri C, Weingarten TN, Martin DP, et al. Allergic reactions during anesthesia at a large United States referral center. Anesth Analg. 2011;113:1202–12.
5. Florvaag E, Johansson SG, Oman H, et al. Prevalence of IgE antibodies to morphine. Relation to the high and low incidences of NMBA anaphylaxis in Norway and Sweden, respectively. Acta Anaesthesiol Scand. 2005;49:437–44.
6. Fisher MM, Baldo BA. Immunoassays in the diagnosis of anaphylaxis to neuromuscular blocking drugs: the value of morphine for the detection of IgE antibodies in allergic subjects. Anaesth Intensive Care. 2000;28:167–70.
7. Baldo BA, Fisher MM. Substituted ammonium ions as allergenic determinants in drug allergy. Nature. 1983;306:262–4.
8. Florvaag E, Johansson SG, Irgens A, et al. IgE-sensitization to the cough suppressant pholcodine and the effects of its withdrawal from the Norwegian market. Allergy. 2011;66:955–60.
9. Florvaag E, Johansson SG, Oman H, et al. Pholcodine stimulates a dramatic increase of IgE in IgE-sensitized individuals. A pilot study. Allergy. 2006;61:49–55.
10. Weston A, Assem ES. Possible link between anaphylactoid reactions to anaesthetics and chemicals in cosmetics and biocides. Agents Actions. 1994;41 Spec. No:C138–9.

Drug–Drug Interactions Involving Antibiotics and Antifungals

XI

Introduction 102

Catherine Marcucci MD

Abstract
This section introduces drug–drug interactions involving antibiotics and antifungals.

The drug–drug interactions in this section are well worth the reader's time and attention. It is a sad fact that antibiotics and antifungals, although in ubiquitous use, are very far from being benign drugs. It is notable the **Fatal Forty** has not just three individual drugs from these related drugs classes, but three *families* of drugs—the azole antifungals, the macrolides, and the quinolones, plus the solo agent rifampin. What is more, these drugs exist in our informal "**Perpetrators**" subclass of the Fatal Forty drug list. The azole antifungals are potent cytochrome P450 (CYP) 3A4 inhibitors, ketoconazole being the worst actor in a family of drug–drug interaction troublemakers. Remember that the CYP3A4 enzyme is the "workhorse" enzyme—there are no inborn poor metabolizers of CYP3A4 as it is not consistent with life and/or evolutionary advantage. Macrolide antibiotics are also 3A4 inhibitors and inhibit P-glycoprotein as well. The quinolones are QT prolongers and, of this drug class, ciprofloxacin, ofloxacin, and norfloxacin are CYP1A2 and CYP3A4 inhibitors. Rifampin is somewhat of an outlier in the antibiotic class as it is a P450 pan-inducer as well as being a P-glycoprotein inducer. Anesthesiologists working in the intensive care unit will frequently encounter some or many of these drugs. Likewise, pain physicians may see patients on rifampin, as of course, neither chronic nor tuberculosis has ever been conquered as a public health issue, and comorbidities abound in every patient cohort.

To summarize in list form:

Azole antifungals (ketoconazole, itraconazole): strong CYP3A4 inhibitors

Macrolide antibiotics (azithromycin, clarithromycin, erythromycin): inhibit CYP3A4 and P-glycoprotein

C. Marcucci MD
Anesthesia Services Department, Philadelphia Veterans Affairs Medical Center, Philadelphia, PA, USA
e-mail: sandson.marcucci@comcast.net

C. Marcucci et al. (eds.), *A Case Approach to Perioperative Drug-Drug Interactions*, DOI 10.1007/978-1-4614-7495-1_102

Quinolones: QT prolongers (ciprofloxacin, ofloxacin, and norfloxacin are CYP1A2 and CYP3A4 inhibitors)

Rifampin: paninducer of P450 and P-glycoprotein

Full Stop

103

Ceftriaxone, calcium

Norah Janosy MD

Abstract
This case discusses the physicochemical interaction between calcium and ceftriaxone and the potentially fatal consequences in neonates.

Case

It was late in the day when the pediatric anesthesia fellow finished her last case. As she was packing up her things, the attending anesthesiologist asked her to do one more case. The patient was a 7-day-old, 3 kg term male baby delivered by normal spontaneous vaginal delivery who had just been added to the operating room (OR) schedule for an emergency exploratory laparotomy. Three days ago, the mother of the infant noticed his stomach was getting bigger and rounder, but she did not bring him to the hospital until the infant started vomiting his breast milk feedings. The abdominal x-ray had been read as distended loops of bowel with possible free air in the abdomen. His only preoperative laboratory abnormality was hypocalcemia.

General anesthesia was induced using a 22-gauge peripheral intravenous (IV) line in place in the left antecubital fossa, which was dispensing a D10 1/4NS solution at maintenance rate. After the infant was successfully intubated, the fellow noted that the heart rate and blood pressure were low. Fluids and a dose of calcium were administered to treat the neonate's depressed cardiac output. The surgeon requested that the neonate be given an appropriate dose of ceftriaxone prior to incision. The fellow mixed the antibiotic and just as she was about to give it as an IV bolus, the attending walked back into the room and asked which antibiotic had been chosen. The fellow responded and the attending yelled: "STOP!" The fellow, startled by the outburst, stepped back from the OR table, antibiotic still in hand.

N. Janosy MD
Department of Anesthesiology, The Children's Hospital, Aurora, CO, USA
e-mail: norah.janosy@childrenscolorado.org; janosyn@ohsu.edu

C. Marcucci et al. (eds.), *A Case Approach to Perioperative Drug-Drug Interactions*, DOI 10.1007/978-1-4614-7495-1_103

Discussion

This is an example of a physicochemical drug–drug interaction (DDI).

More specifically, this is an example of the physical incompatibility of calcium and ceftriaxone. Concurrent use of these drugs is contraindicated in neonates.

Ceftriaxone is a third-generation cephalosporin. Current indications for the use of third generation cephalosporins in neonates include suspected meningitis, and initial empiric therapy of other neonatal infections including pneumonia, nosocomial bacteremia (as in this infant), and urinary tract infections.

When calcium, or any calcium-containing solution, is mixed with ceftriaxone, there is a risk for precipitation of a ceftriaxone-calcium salt. This drug interaction has been the probable cause of seven reported deaths in neonates. All died of cardiopulmonary arrest. On autopsy, a precipitate, or white crystalline material, was found in the vascular beds, most often the lungs, of the neonates.[1] This drug-drug interaction came to the attention of the Food and Drug Administration (FDA) via international case reports, thus leading to a change in the package insert of ceftriaxone.[2] The current recommendation is that ceftriaxone sodium should never be reconstituted with any solution containing calcium, such as Ringer's Lactate, because of the risk for precipitate formation. Neonates (infants <28 days old) should not receive concomitant IV ceftriaxone and calcium even if they are given using different IV tubing or at different times. At no time should a neonate receive ceftriaxone if he is receiving total parenteral nutrition containing calcium, or is on an IV calcium infusion.[2] The FDA has modified its September 2007 recommendations (which recommended that no age group should receive these medications within 48 hours of each other) in April, 2009. The relaxation of the 2007 recommendation was based results of testing for precipitation in adult and neonatal serum done by Roche at the FDA's request. Neonates remain a special risk group in the 2009 alert. This particular DDI appears to be limited to neonates as there have been no reports of cardiopulmonary arrest from this interaction in adults. However, the recommendation is to verify that the IV line is fully flushed prior to giving these two drugs in succession to an adult. The reports of cardiopulmonary arrest are limited to the IV forms of ceftriaxone and calcium.[3] Bradley et al. suggest that the increased risk for death in neonates could be due to a variety of factors including, a higher dose of ceftriaxone being given than is recommended by the FDA, the antibiotic being administered as an IV push, or the entire daily dose being administered as one infusion.

Many medical centers have instituted policies that mandate an automatic substitution (by the pharmacy) of cefotaxime (another third generation cephalosporin) for ceftriaxone in neonates. This is an effective safeguard outside of the OR environment and should be adopted in the surgical suite. We recommend substitution of cefotaxime for ceftriaxone in this vulnerable population. All anesthesia providers need to know of the potential fatal outcome of coadministering calcium and ceftriaxone to neonates.

Take-Home Points

- It is contraindicated to give a neonate calcium and ceftriaxone.
- Drug–drug interactions may be different for different patient populations. This interaction can be fatal in neonates, but has not been shown to be fatal in adults.
- If when administering drugs to patients, a precipitate forms in the intravenous line, do not push the precipitate into the patient.

Summary

Interaction: physicochemical
Substrates: ceftriaxone and calcium
Mechanism: chemical precipitation
Clinical effect: cardiopulmonary arrest

References

1. Bradley JS, Wassel RT, Lee L, et al. Intravenous ceftriaxone and calcium in the neonate: assessing the risk for cardiopulmonary adverse events. Pediatrics. 2009;123:609–13.
2. The FDA alert 9/2007, update 4/2009. http://www.fda.gov/Drugs/DrugSafety/PostmarketDrugSafetyInformationforPatientsandProviders/DrugSafetyInformationforHeathcareProfessionals/ucm084263.ht. Last accessed Sept 15 2009.
3. Product information: ROCEPHIN. Nutley: Roche Laboratories Inc.; 2009.

Flummoxed by the FLOX 104

Fatal Forty DDI: ciprofloxacin, tizanidine, CYP1A2

Janice Kim MD

Abstract
This case discusses the pharmacokinetic interaction between tizanidine and ciprofloxacin. Tizanidine is a cytochrome P450 1A2 substrate and ciprofloxacin is a 1A2 inhibitor.

Case

A 16-year-old girl was scheduled for an outpatient cystoscopy as part of a workup for recurrent urinary tract infections. She reported a history only of idiopathic scoliosis for which she took tizanidine (Zanaflex®) to help alleviate muscle spasms and back pain; her last dose was the morning of her procedure. She took no other medications aside from ibuprofen as needed for back pain. The nurse practitioner in the preoperative clinic consulted the urology service standing orders and prescribed ciprofloxacin (400 mg orally BID) for 4 days as the patient's preoperative antibiotic, as she was allergic to sulfa.

In the preoperative area, the anesthesiologist encountered a patient that appeared very different from the healthy teen she was expecting. The patient was very drowsy and failed to arouse to the anesthesiologist's voice alone. When she finally did arouse to a sharp shake of her shoulder, she complained of being dizzy. Her blood pressure was 88/50 mm Hg with a heart rate of 59 beats per minute, both of these vital signs were decreased from the patient's preoperative vital signs of 112/63 mm Hg and 70 beats per minute. Suspecting a drug–drug interaction (DDI), the anesthesiologist immediately opened up the patient's intravenous fluids to administer a fluid bolus. The surgical case was postponed and the nurse practitioner and her

J. Kim MD
Department of Anesthesiology, Children's Hospital Colorado,
University of Colorado School of Medicine, Aurora, CO, USA
e-mail: Janice.kim@childrenscolorado.org; jankim17@gmail.com

C. Marcucci et al. (eds.), *A Case Approach to Perioperative Drug-Drug Interactions*, DOI 10.1007/978-1-4614-7495-1_104

supervising physician met later in the day to discuss the case and it was agreed that ciprofloxacin would not be automatically prescribed on a standing basis for preoperative patients without a specific review of the medication list for possible DDIs.

Discussion

This is an example of an inhibitor added to a substrate.

Tizanidine is an α-adrenergic agonist and a centrally acting skeletal muscle relaxant. It has a narrow therapeutic index. The adverse side effects of tizanidine—including a decrease in heart rate and blood pressure as well as symptoms of drowsiness, dizziness, and dry mouth—occur in a dose-dependent manner. Studies have shown that plasma tizanidine concentrations are linearly related to dose. Metabolism occurs mainly by cytochrome P450 (CYP) 1A2 and undergoes extensive first-pass metabolism such that the oral bioavailability is only 21%.[1,2] Ciprofloxacin, a fluoroquinolone, is a potent inhibitor of 1A2.[3] The concurrent administration of tizanidine and ciprofloxacin will therefore increase tizanidine's plasma concentration by inhibition of its metabolism.[4,5] In this patient, the ciprofloxacin increased the concentration-dependent adverse effects of tizanidine.

Take-Home Points

- Tizanidine is principally metabolized by CYP1A2. Thus, this medication is very susceptible to the effects of 1A2 inhibition and induction.
- The side effects of tizanidine occur in a dose-dependent manner.
- Ciprofloxacin is an inhibitor of the 1A2 enzyme.
- Both tizanidine and ciprofloxacin are commonly used medications. The astute provider should be aware of the drug–drug interaction between them.

Summary

Interaction: pharmacokinetic
Substrate: tizanidine
Enzyme: CYP1A2
Inhibitor: ciprofloxacin
Clinical effects: sedation, hypotension

References

1. Granfors MT, Backman JT, Laitila J, et al. Tizanidine is mainly metabolized by cytochrome P450 1A2 in vitro. Br J Clin Pharmacol. 2004;57:349–53.
2. Henney III HR, Runyan JK. A clinically relevant review of tizanidine hydrochloride dose relationships to pharmacokinetics, drug safety and effectiveness in healthy subjects and patients. Int J Clin Pract. 2008;62:314–24.
3. Karjalainen MJ, Neuvonen PJ, Backman JT. *In vitro* inhibition of CYP1A2 by model inhibitors, anti-inflammatory analgesics, and female sex steroids: predictability of *in vivo* interactions. Basic Clin Pharmacol Toxicol. 2008;103:157–65.
4. Granfors MT, Backman JT, Neuvonene M, et al. Ciprofloxacin greatly increases concentrations and hypotensive effect of tizanidine by inhibiting its cytochrome P450 1A2-mediated presystemic metabolism. Clin Pharmacol Ther. 2004;76:598–606.
5. Momo K, Ohkoshi N, Yoshizawa T, et al. Drug interaction of tizanidine and ciprofloxacin: case report. Clin Pharmacol Ther. 2006;80:715–20.

Tales of Terror

Fatal Forty DDI: ciprofloxacin, simvastatin, CYP3A4

105

Arun Subramanian MBBS and Juraj Sprung MD, PhD

Abstract
This case discusses the pharmacokinetic interaction between simvastatin and ciprofloxacin, resulting in statin toxicity and rhabdomyolysis. Simvastatin is a cytochrome P450 3A4 substrate and ciprofloxacin is a 3A4 inhibitor.

Case

After an outbreak of anthrax due to a bioterrorism attack using the US Postal Service, the US Department of Health and Human Services identified all persons who had suspected contact with anthrax spores and instructed them to seek post-exposure prophylaxis. As part of this initiative, a 50-year-old male postal worker was sent to his primary care physician for initiation of antibiotic prophylaxis. His past medical history included hypertension managed with metoprolol (50 mg BID) and hyperlipidemia managed with simvastatin (40 mg every night). He began a 2-month treatment of oval ciprofloxacin (500 mg BID).

Three days after starting the treatment, the patient had severe muscle aches and generalized weakness. He also noted that his urine was dark red. He presented to the local emergency department. There, he was found to have increased erythrocyte sedimentation rate and creatine kinase level, and his urine was positive for myoglobin. Rhabdomyolysis was diagnosed, and he was admitted to an intensive care unit (ICU) for treatment.

In an extensive search for the etiologic factors of the patient's rhabdomyolysis, most of the common causes were excluded. His medications also were carefully reviewed. It was noted that he had been taking a stable dose of simvastatin, which he was tolerating well, and ciprofloxacin was a newly added therapy. A quick search of the

A. Subramanian MBBS (✉) • J. Sprung MD, PhD
Department of Anesthesiology, Mayo Clinic, Rochester, MN, USA
e-mail: Subramanian.arun@mayo.edu

C. Marcucci et al. (eds.), *A Case Approach to Perioperative Drug-Drug Interactions*, DOI 10.1007/978-1-4614-7495-1_105

medical literature by the diligent ICU pharmacist confirmed rhabdomyolysis as an adverse effect of the combination of ciprofloxacin and simvastatin. Ciprofloxacin therapy was changed to doxycycline treatment, and supportive management and physical therapy were instituted. The patient was discharged to a rehabilitation facility 5 days later.

Discussion

This is an example of an inhibitor added to a substrate.

Simvastatin belongs to the statins, a class of drugs that lower serum cholesterol levels by decreasing cholesterol synthesis. Simvastatin decreases the synthesis of cholesterol by inhibiting 3-hydroxy-3-methylglutaryl coenzyme A (HMG-CoA) reductase, which catalyzes the first step in the cholesterol synthesis pathway. Simvastatin is a prodrug and is hydrolyzed extensively in the liver during first-pass metabolism to the β-hydroxy acid derivative, its active form.

Metabolism of simvastatin is through the cytochrome P450 (CYP) system in the liver: 80% by CYP3A4 and 20% by CYP2C8.[1] P-glycoproteins and multidrug resistance–associated proteins, members of the adenosine triphosphatase–binding cassette (ABC) drug efflux transport family, also may have a role in the excretion of statins. The functioning of these proteins is subject to inhibition by many drugs, including simvastatin and ciprofloxacin.

Statin use has two major adverse effects: myopathy and elevated liver transaminase levels. Myopathy is present in 0.1% to 0.2% of cases of statin monotherapy, although the presence of myalgias is substantially greater.[2] These adverse effects are thought to be a direct result of HMG-CoA inhibition, and the increase is dose-dependent.[3] The incidence of myopathy increases more than 10-fold when simvastatin is administered in combination with drugs that increase its blood level.[2]

Ciprofloxacin is a second-generation fluoroquinolone antibiotic with bactericidal activity against gram-positive and gram-negative organisms. It acts by specifically binding to and inhibiting bacterial DNA gyrase, thus inhibiting relaxation of supercoiled DNA and promoting breakage of double-stranded DNA. Ciprofloxacin is metabolized primarily in the liver, where it strongly inhibits CYP1A2 and CYP3A4 (the isozyme responsible for simvastatin metabolism). The coadministration of simvastatin and ciprofloxacin leads to increased blood levels of simvastatin through inhibition of 3A4 by ciprofloxacin, producing increased blood levels of simvastatin and resulting in simvastatin toxicity.[4]

Take-Home Points

- Simvastatin, an HMG-CoA reductase inhibitor, is an effective lipid-lowering agent used widely in clinical practice; its use has been shown to cause a dose-dependent increase in the incidence of myopathy.
- Simvastatin is metabolized in the liver by CYP3A4 (80%) and CYP2C8 (20%).
- Ciprofloxacin strongly inhibits CYP3A4, the isozyme responsible for simvastatin metabolism.
- The combined use of ciprofloxacin and simvastatin may lead to increased risk of myopathy and rhabdomyolysis, and this fact should be taken into account when a combination of these drugs is prescribed.

Summary

Interaction: pharmacokinetic
Substrate: simvastatin
Enzyme: CYP3A4
Inhibitor: ciprofloxacin
Clinical effect: simvastatin toxicity

References

1. Prueksaritanont T, Ma B, Yu N. The human hepatic metabolism of simvastatin hydroxy acid is mediated primarily by CYP3A, and not CYP2D6. Br J Clin Pharmacol. 2003;56:120–4.
2. Pedersen TR, Berg K, Cook TJ, et al. Safety and tolerability of cholesterol lowering with simvastatin during 5 years in the Scandinavian Simvastatin Survival Study. Arch Intern Med. 1996;156:2085–92.
3. Ucar M, Mjorndal T, Dahlqvist R. HMG-CoA reductase inhibitors and myotoxicity. Drug Saf. 2000;22:441–57.
4. Sawant RD. Rhabdomyolysis due to an uncommon interaction of ciprofloxacin with simvastatin. Can J Clin Pharmacol. 2009;16:e78–9.

Too Low To Go

106

Fatal Forty DDI: erythromycin, nifedipine, CYP3A4

Catherine Marcucci MD and Neil B. Sandson MD

Abstract
This case discusses a pharmacokinetic interaction between erythromycin and nifedipine resulting in postinduction hypotension. Nifedipine is a cytochrome P450 3A4 substrate and erythromycin is a 3A4 inhibitor.

Case

At 8:10 AM one morning, the intensive care unit (ICU) resident received a call that the first case in room 5 was being cancelled and the patient was coming over intubated and on a phenylephrine drip. The patient that arrived was a 64-year-old man who had been scheduled for a cystectomy for bladder cancer. He had completed an at-home bowel prep regimen.

The operating room (OR) anesthesia team reported that the patient had a history of asthma, chronic stable angina, and a remote history of seizures while a heavy drinker many years earlier. His standing medications were nifedipine (Procardia® 20 mg three times daily), an asthma inhaler as needed, and a multivitamin. On arrival in the preoperative area, the patient reported that he had taken his nifedipine that morning as instructed. His blood pressure was 92/49 mm Hg. He had complained of being "dry as a chip" and a "little dizzy coming in from the car" and was given a fluid bolus of 1000 cc of Ringer's Lactate at the time of intravenous line insertion. The first blood pressure in the operating room was 101/57 mm Hg and the attending mentioned to the resident that the patient was "probably a little dry, so a light hand

C. Marcucci MD (✉)
Anesthesia Services Department, Philadelphia Veterans Affairs Medical Center, Philadelphia, PA, USA
e-mail: sandson.marcucci@comcast.net

N.B. Sandson MD
Department of Psychiatry, University of Maryland Medical System, Baltimore, MD, USA

Department of Psychiatry, VA Maryland Health Care System, Baltimore, MD, USA

C. Marcucci et al. (eds.), *A Case Approach to Perioperative Drug-Drug Interactions*, DOI 10.1007/978-1-4614-7495-1_106

with the propofol, please." After intubation, the first blood pressure reading was 47/37 mm Hg. Thinking this was the typical drop in blood pressure seen after induction in a bowel-prepped patient, the anesthesia team continued to give fluids and began administering increasing boluses of both ephedrine and phenylephrine. They were unsuccessful in maintaining a sustained blood pressure greater than 90/50 mmHg without wide-open fluids and continuous sympathomimetics and the case was cancelled.

The patient's blood pressure stabilized in the ICU and the pressors were slowly weaned over the next 15 hours. The ICU resident was assigned to present the case in the next week's cancellation conference. She found an important clue pertaining to the patient's severe postinduction hypotension when she thought to check the patient's bowel prep regimen and found that it specified multiple large doses of erythromycin.

Discussion

This is an example of an inhibitor added to a substrate.

This is an especially interesting example of inhibition of cytochrome P450 (CYP) 3A4-mediated nifedipine metabolism. Nifedipine is a CYP3A4 substrate.[1] Erythromycin is recognized as an irreversible "suicide" 3A4 inhibitor—that is, it binds irreversibly to the enzyme, rendering the protein permanently incapable of enzymatic action.[2] Symptomatic hypotension has been described when CYP3A4 inhibitors are administered with dihydropyridine calcium antagonists, such as nifedipine. This interaction, coupled with volume depletion due to the bowel prep, accounted for the patient's somewhat hypotensive state on arrival to the OR. When he received propofol for induction (on first look, not an unreasonable choice, given his history of asthma and seizures), the hypotensive effects were compounded. In this example, the pharmacokinetic interaction had the clinical effect of making nifedipine a longer-acting drug, so treatment required both supportive measures and time.

It is important for perioperative clinicians to recognize that antibiotic bowel preps that include erythromycin typically involve large doses. For most indications the usual adult dose of erythromycin is 250 mg every 6 hours. If given for Legionnaire's Disease, the recommended dose is 500 mg every 12 hours. However, an antibiotic bowel prep contains multiple doses of erythromycin 1 g in the 1 to 2 days prior to surgery. Due to the covalent binding capabilities of erythromycin to the CYP3A4 enzyme, this almost certainly results in meaningful inhibition of 3A4-mediated metabolism.

This patient had a number of reasons to become hypotensive after induction, including volume depletion and the hemodynamic effects of propofol. However, most patients induced with propofol, even those who undergo bowel preps, do not have their cases cancelled before the surgery begins. As supporting evidence, when she presented in conference, the resident took with her a copy of the bowel prep order sheet used by the urologists and literature citing clinical effects (such as orthostasis) resulting from the interaction between nifedipine and fluoxetine (another CYP3A4 inhibitor).[3–5]

Take-Home Points

- The antibiotic bowel prep can pose a significant drug–drug interaction risk if it includes erythromycin.
- Erythromycin is a "suicide" inhibitor of CYP3A4—it irreversibly binds to the enzyme molecule. This is also known as mechanism-based inhibition. In order for "full-strength" metabolism to take place again, the inactivated enzyme must be replaced by newly synthesized enzyme proteins.

Summary

Interaction: pharmacokinetic
Substrate: nifedipine
Enzyme: CYP3A4
Inhibitor: erythromycin
Clinical effects: exaggerated nifedipine effects and persistent hypotension in the setting of volume depletion

References

1. Iribane C, Dreano Y, Bardou LG, et al. Interaction of methadone with substrates of human hepatic cytochrome P450 3A4. Toxicology. 1997;117:13–23.
2. Zhou S, Chan E, Lim LY, et al. Therapeutic drugs that behave as mechanism-based inhibitors of cytochrome P450 3A4. Curr Drug Metab. 2004;5(5):415–42.
3. Greenblatt DJ, von Moltke LL, Harmatz JS, et al. Human cytochromes and some newer antidepressants: kinetics, metabolism, and drug interactions. J Clin Psychopharmacol. 1999;19(5 Suppl 1):23S–35.
4. von Moltke LL, Greenblatt DJ, Court MH, et al. Inhibition of alprazolam and desipramine hydroxylation in vitro by paroxetine and fluvoxamine: comparison with other selective serotonin reuptake inhibitor antidepressants. J Clin Psychopharmacol. 1995;15(2):125–31.
5. Azaz-Livshits TL, Danenberg HD. Tachycardia, orthostatic hypotension and profound weakness due to concomitant use of fluoxetine and nifedipine. Pharmacopsychiatry. 1997;30(6):274–5.

A Fungal Story

Fatal Forty DDI: fluconazole, phenytoin, CYP2C9, CYP2C19

107

Jerusha Taylor PharmD, BCPS
and Ansgar M. Brambrink MD, PhD

Abstract
This cases discusses a pharmacokinetic interaction between phenytoin and fluconazole, resulting in phenytoin toxicity. Phenytoin is a cytochrome P450 2C9 and 2C19 substrate and fluconazole is a 2C9 and 2C19 inhibitor.

Case

A 35-year-old woman with metastatic breast cancer was admitted to the neurointensive care unit (ICU) after suffering several serious seizures at home from new brain metastases. She had an indwelling chemotherapy catheter. The ICU team decided to start anticonvulsant therapy with intravenous (IV) phenytoin. She was given a loading dose of fosphenytoin (15 mg PE/kg, 1200 mg PE IV once) and then started on a maintenance dose of oral phenytoin extended release (ER) capsules (200 mg/12h). Her baseline albumin level was 3.1 grams/dl and all of her laboratories were within normal limits, including renal and hepatic function.

On hospital day 7, the patient developed fevers and an elevated white blood cell count. Blood cultures were drawn from the porta-catheter which grew *Candida albicans*. Fluconazole was started at 800 mg IV once followed by 400 mg by mouth daily. Four days later, the patient became more drowsy. Upon neurologic evaluation, she had nystagmus and ataxia. An urgent free phenytoin level came back at 3.8 mg/dL.

J. Taylor PharmD, BCPS (✉)
Department of Pharmacy, Oregon Health and Science University, Portland, OR, USA
e-mail: taylorje@ohsu.edu

A.M. Brambrink MD, PhD
Department of Anesthesiology and Perioperative Medicine, Oregon Health and Science University, Portland, OR, USA

C. Marcucci et al. (eds.), *A Case Approach to Perioperative Drug-Drug Interactions*, DOI 10.1007/978-1-4614-7495-1_107

An astute anesthesiology resident recognized a drug interaction between fluconazole and phenytoin. Further doses of phenytoin were held until the patient's free phenytoin level was < 2 mg/dL. She was restarted on oral phenytoin ER capsules at a lower dosage (200 mg every evening). Her symptoms of dizziness, ataxia, and nystagmus diminished over the next few days as her phenytoin level decreased. The patient finished a 14-day course of fluconazole for the *C. albicans* fungemia and her porta-cath was removed. She was discharged home shortly after on phenytoin 200 mg ER at bedtime and her follow-up level in clinic 1 week later was 0.7. Her dose was then increased back to 200 mg ER every 12 hours.

Discussion

This is an example of an inhibitor added to a substrate.

Fluconazole is an azole antifungal and a potent inhibitor of the cytochrome P450 (CYP) enzyme 2C9.[1] It is a less potent inhibitor of CYP2C19 and CYP3A4. Phenytoin is metabolized via 2C9 and 2C19.[2] Fluconazole inhibits the metabolism of phenytoin and patients can experience elevations in phenytoin concentrations with concomitant therapy. Phenytoin toxicity can occur as early soon as 2 days after the addition of fluconazole.[3,4] Therefore, when a patient is taking both fluconazole and phenytoin, phenytoin serum concentrations must be monitored due to the risk for phenytoin toxicity.

Take-Home Points

- Phenytoin is a CYP2C9 and 2C19 substrate.
- Fluconazole is a potent inhibitor of CYP2C9.
- Phenytoin and the azole antifungals are both implicated in clinically significant drug–drug interactions.
- Remember that inhibition happens in a matter of days, as opposed to induction, which happens in a matter of weeks.
- Patients must have phenytoin serum concentrations monitored while on fluconazole due to inhibition of phenytoin metabolism.

Summary

Interaction: pharmacokinetic
Substrate: phenytoin
Enzyme: CYP2C9 and 2C19
Inhibitor: fluconazole
Clinical effect: phenytoin toxicity

References

1. Niemi M, Backman JT, Neuvonen M, et al. Effects of fluconazole and fluvoxamine on the pharmacokinetics and pharmacodynamics of glimepiride. Clin Pharmacol Ther. 2001;69(4): 194–200.
2. Mamiya K, Ieiri I, Shimamoto J, et al. The effects of genetic polymorphism of CYP2C9 and CYP2C19 on phenytoin metabolism in Japanese adult patients with epilepsy: studies in stereoselective hydroxylation and population pharmacokinetics. Epilepsia. 1998;39(12):1317–23.
3. Blum RA, Wilton JH, Hilligoss DM, et al. Effect of fluconazole on the disposition of phenytoin. Clin Pharmacol Ther. 1991;49(4):420–5.
4. Cadle RM, Zenon 3rd GJ, Rodriguez-Barradas MC, et al. Fluconazole-induced symptomatic phenytoin toxicity. Ann Pharmacother. 1994;28(2):191–5.

Rejection Protection Turned Kidney Killer

108

Fatal Forty DDI: voriconazole, tacrolimus, CYP3A4, P-glycoprotein

Erica D. Wittwer MD, PhD, Juraj Sprung MD, PhD, and Christine M. Formea PharmD, BCPS

Abstract
This case discusses a pharmacokinetic interaction between tacrolimus and voriconazole, resulting in elevated tacrolimus plasma levels. Tacrolimus is a cytochrome P450 3A4 and P-glycoprotein substrate and voriconazole is a cytochrome P450 3A4 and P-glycoprotein inhibitor.

Case

A 55-year-old, 91 kg man was admitted to the intensive care unit (ICU) with an apparently seriously infected right groin angiogram access site. He had a history of hypertension, diabetes mellitus, and kidney failure and had undergone cadaveric kidney transplant 1 year earlier. His medications were tacrolimus (5 mg orally BID), mycophenolate mofetil (1 g orally BID), prednisone (2.5 mg orally daily), oral extended-release metoprolol (200 mg orally daily), and regular human insulin (as directed). His baseline serum creatinine concentration was stable at 1.0 mg/dL since his renal transplant and his baseline tacrolimus level was 7 ng/mL.

Preliminary culture results indicated the presence of *Candida albicans*. Treatment was started with broad-spectrum antibiotics and a loading dose of voriconazole (550 mg intravenously once every 12 h over 24 h). He then received maintenance

E.D. Wittwer MD, PhD (✉) • J. Sprung MD, PhD
Department of Anesthesiology, Mayo Clinic, Rochester, MN, USA
e-mail: Wittwer.erica@mayo.edu

C.M. Formea PharmD, BCPS
Pharmacy Research, College of Medicine, Mayo Clinic, Rochester, MN, USA

C. Marcucci et al. (eds.), *A Case Approach to Perioperative Drug-Drug Interactions*, DOI 10.1007/978-1-4614-7495-1_108

doses of IV voriconazole (360 mg 912 h) because of his immunosuppressive drug regimen and his clinically threatening situation. His urine output was low initially, but improved after fluid administration.

On hospital day 3, the patient's urine output was noted to be slowly decreasing and his serum creatinine had increased to 2.1 mg/dL from 1.5 mg/dL the previous day and 1.2 mg/dL at admission. Tacrolimus toxicity was suspected when the tacrolimus level was discovered to be 18 ng/mL and the drug was stopped immediately. A tacrolimus trough level was obtained the following morning and tacrolimus therapy was restarted at 33% of his normal dose and for 14 days while he continued to take voriconazole to treat the candidemia. His urine output improved and his serum creatinine concentration began to decrease toward his baseline level during the next several days. He resumed his baseline tacrolimus dosing and instituted closer renal surveillance after discharge from the hospital.

Discussion

This is an example of an inhibitor added to a substrate.

Tacrolimus and cyclosporine are calcineurin inhibitors used as immunosuppressive agents to prevent transplant allograft rejection. The therapeutic index of these medications is narrow, and both tacrolimus and cyclosporine can cause significant nephrotoxicity when their blood concentrations become supratherapeutic.[1]

Also, tacrolimus and cyclosporine are substrates that are metabolized and cleared from the human body through the combined activities of cytochrome P450 (CYP) isozyme 3A4 in the liver and gut and the P-glycoprotein pump on the intestinal mucosa.[1,2] P-glycoprotein works to actively transport substances out of the body and reduce plasma concentrations of many drugs, including tacrolimus and cyclosporine.[1–3]

Transplant patients are at increased risk for fungal infection, and the mortality of these infections is high. Azole antifungals—including fluconazole, itraconazole, ketoconazole, posaconazole, and voriconazole—inhibit the metabolism of CYP3A4 substrates and result in increased plasma concentrations of the antifungal.[3,4] In addition, the azole antifungals inhibit P-glycoprotein transporter activity, which increases drug absorption in the gut and ultimately results in increased plasma concentrations.[3,4] The azole antifungals increase tacrolimus and cyclosporine plasma concentrations through these two mechanisms.[1] This response is of particular concern because of the narrow therapeutic windows of cyclosporine and tacrolimus, since supratherapeutic plasma concentrations of these two drugs can result in nephrotoxicity. Dose adjustments and frequent drug level monitoring are necessary when azole antifungals are administered concomitantly with either tacrolimus or cyclosporine.[1,3]

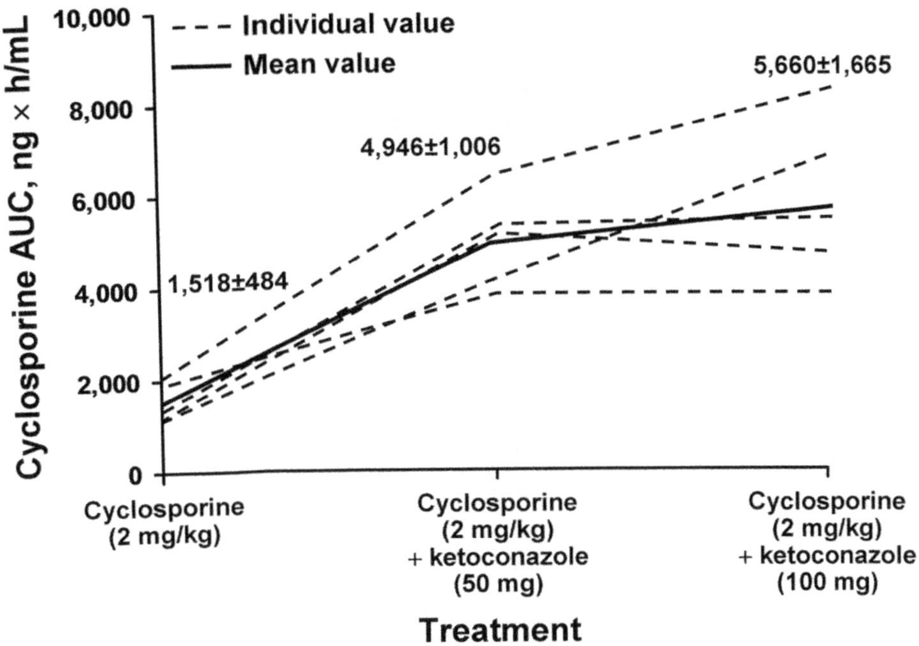

Fig. 108.1 Augmentation of area under the time concentration curve (AUC) of cyclosporine with addition of 50 mg of ketoconazole. With addition of 100 mg of ketoconazole, the mean rise of AUC of cyclosporine did not increase further significantly [Adapted from Abraham MA, Thomas PP, John GT et al. Efficacy and safety of low-dose ketoconazole (50 mg) to reduce the cost of cyclosporine in renal allograft recipients. Transplant Proc 2003;35:215–216. With permission from Elsevier.]

All azole antifungals increase levels of cyclosporine and tacrolimus and thus require dose reductions of immunosuppressants during coadministration.[3] Orally administered ketoconazole has been shown to increase by two fold the bioavailability of orally and intravenously administered tacrolimus, from 14% to 30%.[5] Ketoconazole at a dose of 50 mg increases the area under the concentration curve of cyclosporine by almost three-fold [(6)] (Fig. 108.1). Itraconazole increases cyclosporine trough concentrations, and this effect lasts several weeks because of the long half-life of itraconazole.[7,8] When itraconazole is administered with tacrolimus, the pharmacokinetics of tacrolimus are altered, an effect that lasts for a prolonged period also and requires a tacrolimus dose reduction of approximately 50%.[9] A dose reduction of 40% has been recommended when oral tacrolimus is given concomitantly with oral fluconazole.[10]

In the present case, the iatrogenic administration of an antifungal agent caused rapid elevation of serum creatinine level, which signaled acute nephrotoxicity due to supratherapeutic tacrolimus plasma concentrations.

Take-Home Points

- Tacrolimus and cyclosporine are commonly used immunosuppressants that are metabolized through CYP3A4 and whose absorption is mediated by P-glycoprotein.
- Azole antifungals, including fluconazole, itraconazole, ketoconazole, posaconazole, and voriconazole, inhibit the CYP3A4 isozyme and the P-glycoprotein transporter.
- Patients taking immunosuppressant drugs are at risk for infection and may need treatment with azole antifungals. When an immunosuppressant agent is administered concomitantly with an azole antifungal, the plasma concentrations of either drug may become dangerously increased unless the dose of that drug is reduced appropriately.
- Interactions between immunosuppressants and CYP3A4 inhibitors need to be monitored closely and dose reductions, evaluation of immunosuppressant levels, and further dose adjustments must be made on the basis of the patient's response.

Summary

Interaction: pharmacokinetic
Substrate: tacrolimus
Enzyme/transporter: CYP3A4 and P-glycoprotein
Inhibitor: voriconazole
Clinical Effect: renal failure

References

1. Quan DJ, Winter ME. Immunosuppressants: cyclosporine, tacrolimus, and sirolimus. In: Troy DB, editor. Basic clinical pharmacokinetics. 4th ed. Philadelphia: Lippincott Williams & Wilkins; 2004. p. 228–50.
2. Nowack R. Review article: cytochrome P450 enzyme, and transport protein mediated herb-drug interactions in renal transplant patients: grapefruit juice, St John's Wort—and beyond! Nephrology (Carlton). 2008;13:337–47.
3. Saad AH, DePestel DD, Carver PL. Factors influencing the magnitude and clinical significance of drug interactions between azole antifungals and select immunosuppressants. Pharmacotherapy. 2006;26:1730–44.
4. Venkatakrishnan K, von Moltke LL, Greenblatt DJ. Effects of the antifungal agents on oxidative drug metabolism: clinical relevance. Clin Pharmacokinet. 2000;38:111–80.
5. Floren LC, Bekersky I, Benet LZ, et al. Tacrolimus oral bioavailability doubles with coadministration of ketoconazole. Clin Pharmacol Ther. 1997;62:41–9.

6. Abraham MA, Thomas PP, John GT, et al. Efficacy and safety of low-dose ketoconazole (50 mg) to reduce the cost of cyclosporine in renal allograft recipients. Transplant Proc. 2003;35:215–6.
7. Isoherranen N, Kunze KL, Allen KE, et al. Role of itraconazole metabolites in CYP3A4 inhibition. Drug Metab Dispos. 2004;32:1121–31.
8. Gubbins PO, Amsden JR. Drug-drug interactions of antifungal agents and implications for patient care. Expert Opin Pharmacother. 2005;6:2231–43.
9. Banerjee R, Leaver N, Lyster H, et al. Coadministration of itraconazole and tacrolimus after thoracic organ transplantation. Transplant Proc. 2001;33:1600–2.
10. Toda F, Tanabe K, Ito S, et al. Tacrolimus trough level adjustment after administration of fluconazole to kidney recipients. Transplant Proc. 2002;34:1733–5.

Can't Get Well

109

Fatal Forty DDI: itraconazole, budesonide, CYP3A4

Michael J. Sikora MD, Barbara Jericho MD,
and Randal O. Dull MD, PhD

Abstract
This case discusses a pharmacokinetic interaction between budesonide and itraconazole, resulting in Cushing's disease. Budesonide is a cytochrome P450 3A4 substrate and itraconazole is a 3A4 inhibitor.

Case

A 46-year-old male with a 50 pack-year smoking history presented to his primary care physician with tinea corporis. The patient's past medical history was significant for a worsening chronic cough, fatigue, and unintentional weight loss over the past 2 months. A chest radiograph revealed a 2 cm right upper lobe lung mass. The patient was started on inhaled budesonide (200 mcg BID) for his pulmonary symptoms and oral itraconazole for his fungal skin infection.

Thoracic surgery was consulted for the evaluation of the lung mass and the patient underwent a video-assisted thoracoscopy. The intraoperative biopsy revealed non-small cell carcinoma, and his surgeon performed an upper lobe resection of the lung. The patient's postoperative course was notable for moderate hypertension, weight gain, a rounded face, and easy bruising. A dexamethasone suppression test was

M.J. Sikora MD (✉)
Department of Anesthesiology, Cincinnati Children's Hospital Medical Center, Cincinnati, OH, USA
e-mail: Michael.Sikora@cchmc.org

B. Jericho MD
Department of Anesthesiology, University of Illinois Hospital and Health Sciences System, University of Illinois-Chicago, Chicago, IL, USA

R.O. Dull MD, PhD
Department of Anesthesiology, University of Illinois at Chicago, Chicago, IL, USA

C. Marcucci et al. (eds.), *A Case Approach to Perioperative Drug-Drug Interactions*, DOI 10.1007/978-1-4614-7495-1_109

ordered and revealed that the morning cortisol level was elevated and did not respond to intravenous steroid, leading to a diagnosis of iatrogenic Cushing's syndrome. His symptoms resolved after the patient discontinued itraconazole and budesonide. The patient then restarted only the inhaled budesonide without the return of Cushing's syndrome.

Discussion

This is an example of an inhibitor added to a substrate.

The oral antifungals, ketoconazole and itraconazole, both inhibit cytochrome P450 (CYP) 3A4, while steroids are substrates of CYP3A4.[1] This clinical vignette illustrated how adding itraconazole to budesonide over a relatively short period of time resulted in increased levels of the substrate, budesonide.[1] In this case, elevated budesonide translated into elevated cortisol, manifesting clinically as exogenous Cushing's syndrome. Not only brief courses of steroids but also longer courses of steroids administered with CYP3A4 inhibitors may cause secondary adrenal insufficiency. For example, the chronic administration of steroids along with a nefazodone (a CYP3A4 inhibitor) was reported by Hagan et al.[2] They presented a case in which a woman medicated for depression with nefazodone underwent triamcinolone injections secondary to chronic back pain.[2] One month later, she displayed undetectable cortisol levels.[2] This observation becomes clinically relevant to the anesthesiologist when deciding whether to administer a stress dose of steroids intraoperatively. Patients remotely treated with steroids but chronically treated with CYP3A4 inhibitors may be at increased risk for secondary adrenal insufficiency during an operation. In addition to oral antifungals and nefazodone, case reports of CYP3A4 inhibition also exist for diltiazem and the protease inhibitor ritonavir.[3,4]

Take-Home Points

- Itraconazole is a CYP3A4 inhibitor and budesonide is a substrate of CYP3A4.
- This clinical vignette illustrates how adding itraconazole to the inhaled steroid budesonide can result in increased levels of budesonide.[3]
- In this case, increased budesonide manifests as iatrogenic Cushing's syndrome.
- Case reports discussing CYP3A4 inhibition also exist for diltiazem and the protease inhibitor ritonavir.[4,5]

Summary

Interaction: pharmacokinetic
Substrate: budesonide
Enzyme: CYP3A4
Inhibitor: itraconazole
Clinical effects: Cushing's syndrome

References

1. De Wachter E, Malfroot A, De Schutter I, et al. Inhaled budesonide induced Cushing's syndrome in cystic fibrosis patients, due to drug inhibition of cytochrome P450. J Cyst Fibros. 2003;2(2):72–5.
2. Hagan JB, Erickson D, Singh RJ. Triamcinolone acetonide induced secondary adrenal insufficiency related to impaired CYP3A4 metabolism by coadministration of nefazodone. Pain Med. 2010;11(7):1132–5. Epub 2010 Apr 29.
3. Levin TT, Bakr MH, Nikolova T. Case report: delirium due to a diltiazem-fentanyl CYP3A4 drug interaction. Gen Hosp Psychiatry. 2010;32(6):648.e9–648.e10. Epub 2010 Sep 22.
4. Mahlab-Guri K, Asher I, Gradstein S, et al. Inhaled fluticasone causes iatrogenic cushing's syndrome in patients treated with Ritonavir. J Asthma. 2011;48(8):860–3. Epub 2011 Aug 22.

Linezolid (I): Be "VREy" Careful

110

Fatal Forty DDI: linezolid, bupropion

Bruce T. Dumser MD

Abstract
This case discusses the interaction of linezolid and bupropion resulting in hypertension.

Case

A 54-year-old man with history of depression and a 40 pack-year history of smoking was readmitted to the vascular surgery service with a graft infection on postoperative day 7 after a femoral-popliteal bypass. One year earlier, the patient had been placed on bupropion (Wellbutrin®) by his primary care provider, to help with smoking cessation. This medication was continued in the hospital. Over the next several days, there was little improvement in his status from antibiotic therapy and blood cultures revealed vancomycin-resistant *Enterococcus faecium* (VRE). The patient was started on linezolid and scheduled for graft removal the next day.

The next day, the anesthesiologist reviewed the patient's previous anesthetic record from two weeks earlier and noted that the patient was hemodynamically stable during an anesthetic performed with 0.8% isoflurane, 50% nitrous oxide, and minimal opioids. Her anesthetic plan was to repeat the prior anesthetic. Following an uneventful induction, however, the patient had multiple severe elevations in blood pressure, including one reading as high as 250/130 mm Hg. With the unexpected hemodynamic lability, the anesthesiologist placed an arterial line and started a nitroprusside infusion. Upon reviewing the chart again, she noted that the only difference in this patient's management from the last anesthetic was the introduction of linezolid. The patient was admitted

B.T. Dumser MD
Anesthesiology Consultants of Walla Walla, Walla Walla, WA, USA
e-mail: bruce.medicine@gmail.com

C. Marcucci et al. (eds.), *A Case Approach to Perioperative Drug-Drug Interactions*, DOI 10.1007/978-1-4614-7495-1_110

to the intensive care unit (ICU) following surgery, and the psychiatry and infectious disease services were consulted. Upon full review of his history and a discussion with the patient on risks and benefits, the ICU team proceeded to discontinue his Wellbutrin® while continuing the linezolid with close hemodynamic monitoring. No further episodes of acute hypertension were noted, the patient finished his linezolid course without additional episodes of extreme hypertension, and was ultimately discharged to home.

Discussion

This is an example of a two-stage pharmacodynamic interaction at the neurotransmitter level.

Bupropion is an antidepressant that is also a non-nicotine aid to smoking cessation and is chemically unrelated to tricyclic antidepressants (TCAs), selective serotonin reuptake inhibitors (SSRIs), or other antidepressants. Along with one of its metabolites (hydroxybupropion), bupropion is a relatively weak inhibitor of neuronal uptake of norepinephrine and dopamine, which are monoamines. Bupropion and hydroxybupropion are also inhibitors of cytochrome P450 (CYP) 2D6.[1]

Linezolid is an oxazolidinone with potent antimicrobial effects against gram-positive bacteria, including methicillin-resistant *Staphylococcus aureus* (MRSA), penicillin-resistant pneumococci, macrolide-resistant streptococci, and VRE. It is equally potent as an oral or parenteral agent. Because of these desirable characteristics, linezolid is increasingly being prescribed.[2]

Interestingly, linezolid was originally developed as an antidepressant. In addition to its antimicrobial properties, linezolid is a reversible, relatively weak nonselective monoamine oxidase inhibitor (MAOI). Despite this, no linezolid-SSRI interactions were noted in Phase I, II, or III studies prior to its 2000 FDA approval.[2] However, since its release, linezolid has been implicated in multiple drug interactions consistent with its MAOI qualities. On most occasions, this has been with the serotonin syndrome, but as can be seen with this case presentation, it may lead to severe hypertensive events.[3–6]

In this case, the MAOI (linezolid) was added to bupropion, a norepinephrine and dopamine reuptake inhibitor. With the inhibition of MAO, there were increasing amounts of norepinephrine and dopamine, leading to the severe hypertensive episodes similar to the adrenergic crises seen with pheochromocytoma.[4]

Management of the severe hypertensive episodes should include cessation of the inciting agents, placement of an arterial line for beat-to-beat monitoring, and aggressive treatment of the blood pressure with anti-hypertensive agents. Recommended therapies include phentolamine or nitroprusside with β-blockers. It may be prudent to avoid β-blockers as a first-line therapy, as there is a risk for paradoxically increased blood pressure from unopposed α effects.[7,8]

There is debate in the literature about the best way to prescribe linezolid for patients already taking antidepressants. At present, all antidepressants exert their effects through biogenic amine pathways, and the MAOI properties of linezolid may lead to excessive accumulation of those substrates. At present, the literature suggests the most frequent interaction is with the SSRIs leading to serotonin syndrome.[3,5,6] However, linezolid is a *weak* MAOI and a study demonstrated that even when a patient concomitantly took an SSRI and linezolid, only 3% developed the serotonin syndrome.[6] For this reason, the authors suggest simply adding linezolid to the antidepressant therapy with close monitoring for the serotonin syndrome. At the other end of the spectrum, several sources (including the manufacturer) espouse a 14-day "washout" of the antidepressant before starting linezolid and another 14 day "washout" before restarting antidepressant therapy.[2] Psychotherapy and electroconvulsive therapy (ECT) may be utilized to help treat the depression while on linezolid.

Curiously, although this is a pharmacodynamic interaction, it is still meaningful to refer to substrates and inhibitors in this interaction. However, the substrate in question is not a drug, rather, the substrates are the neurotransmitters norepinephrine and dopamine.

Take-Home Points

- Linezolid is a reversible, weak nonselective MAOI. One must be careful when adding this antibiotic to patients on antidepressants, as all current antidepressants exert effects through biogenic amine pathways. Drug interactions may include central serotonin syndrome or hypertensive crises, depending on the antidepressant. Both conditions are possibly life threatening.

- If linezolid is required, providers may consider the use of psychotherapy or electroconvulsive therapy in lieu of pharmacologic antidepressants.

- There is debate about how to best introduce linezolid to patients on antidepressants, ranging from simply adding the linezolid with close monitoring to 14-day "washouts" before and after antibiotic therapy.

- Beware the use of β-blockers as a first-line agent in treating MAOI-induced severe hypertension, as it may lead to unopposed α effects and paradoxically increased blood pressure.

- Bupropion and hydroxybupropion are also inhibitors of CYP2D6. Care should be taken when this medication is prescribed to ensure no other prescribed medications utilize that pathway.

Summary

Interaction: pharmacodynamic
Substrates: norepinephrine and dopamine (levels are increased because neuronal reuptake is blocked by bupropion)
Mechanism/sites of action: cathecholaminergic receptors
Inhibitor: linezolid (inhibits monoamine oxidase and the metabolism of neurotransmitters)
Clinical effect: hypertension

References

1. Zyban [package insert]. Research Triangle Park: GlaxoSmithKline; 2008.
2. Zyvox [package insert]. New York: Pharmacia and Upjohn Company; 2008.
3. Lawrence KR, Adra M, Gillman PK. Serotonin toxicity associated with the use of linezolid: a review of postmarketing data. Clin Infect Dis. 2006;42:1578–83.
4. Marcucci C, Sandson NB, Dunlap JA. Linezolid-bupropion interaction as possible etiology of severe intermittent intraoperative hypertension? [letter]. Anesthesiology. 2004;101:1487–8.
5. Sola CL, Bostwick JM, Hart DA, et al. Anticipating potential linezolid-SSRI interactions in the general hospital setting: an MAOI in disguise. Mayo Clin Proc. 2006;81:330–4.
6. Taylor JJ, Wilson JW, Estes LL. Linezolid and serotonergic drug interactions: a retrospective survey. Clin Infect Dis. 2006;43:180–7.
7. Feldstein C. Management of hypertensive crises. Am J Ther. 2007;14:135–9.
8. Marik PE, Varon J. Hypertensive crises. Chest. 2007;131:1949–62.

Linezolid (II): Hyper and Hot

111

Linezolid, meperidine, serotonin syndrome

Erica D. Wittwer MD, PhD, Toby N. Weingarten MD, and Juraj Sprung MD, PhD

Abstract
This case discusses the pharmacodynamic interaction between linezolid and meperidine, resulting in serotonin syndrome.

Case

A 58-year-old man was in the hospital after a radical retropubic prostatectomy for prostate cancer. His postoperative course was complicated with a surgical wound infection, for which he was receiving appropriate antibiotic therapy. He was scheduled to return to surgery for wound irrigation and débridement. Two nights prior to surgery, he had a fever. Blood cultures grew an *Enterococcus* resistant to vancomycin, and his antibiotic therapy was changed to linezolid.

The patient had been healthy previously and was taking no medications before his hospitalization. He tolerated his previous anesthetic well and was intubated without difficulty. Aside from antibiotics, he was receiving meperidine via a patient-controlled intravenous pump. The morning of surgery, the nurse in the preoperative holding area mentioned that the patient was irritable and confused, which was in contrast to his usually intact mental status noted on multiple surgical progress notes. He had reported incisional pain, and the surgical team had encouraged him to use his patient-controlled analgesia more often.

E.D. Wittwer MD, PhD (✉) • T.N. Weingarten MD • J. Sprung MD, PhD
Department of Anesthesiology, Mayo Clinic, Rochester, MN, USA
e-mail: Wittwer.erica@mayo.edu

C. Marcucci et al. (eds.), *A Case Approach to Perioperative Drug-Drug Interactions*, DOI 10.1007/978-1-4614-7495-1_111

The consultant anesthesiologist evaluated the patient and found him to be agitated and confused. He was tachycardic, diaphoretic, and febrile (40 °C). The surgical procedure was canceled, and the patient was transferred to the intensive care unit for further evaluation and monitoring. There, the patient was found to have clonus. A diagnosis of serotonin syndrome was made, and both the linezolid and meperidine were discontinued.

Discussion

This is an example of a pharmacodynamic interaction.

Serotonin syndrome, also referred to as *serotonin toxicity*, is the result of an increased intrasynaptic serotonin concentration, elevated to a level at which symptoms occur. Serotonin syndrome manifests as three categories of excitatory symptoms: neuromuscular, autonomic, and mental status alterations, which include hyperreflexia, clonus, myoclonus, diaphoresis, tachycardia, fever, excitement, confusion, and agitation.[1] The severity of the serotonin toxicity is directly related to the amount of serotonin. Normally, serotonin is released in the nerve synapse and is cleared through reuptake or through metabolism with monoamine oxidase (MAO). Its levels can increase with serotonin reuptake inhibition or the inhibition of MAO.

Linezolid is both a synthetic antibacterial agent used to treat vancomycin-resistant enterococcus, pneumonia, and various other infections and a reversible, nonselective inhibitor of monoamine oxidase.[2] Meperidine is an opioid medication that blocks the reuptake of serotonin by nerve endings and that is therefore contraindicated in patients receiving monoamine oxidase inhibitors (MAOi). Meperidine has been reported to also cause serotonin syndrome when used with selective serotonin reuptake inhibitors, including citalopram, and in one report caused serotonin syndrome without the administration of another drug that influenced serotonin levels.[3,4] Linezolid used in combination with serotonin reuptake inhibitors has caused serotonin syndrome, but recently a case was described in which the simultaneous use of linezolid and meperidine caused serotonin syndrome.[5,6] The combination of decreased metabolism of serotonin due to linezolid administration and the decreased reuptake of serotonin due to meperidine therapy can lead to elevated levels of serotonin and thus cause toxicity.

Successful treatment of serotonin syndrome relies on recognition of the syndrome and discontinuation of the inciting agents (Table 111.1). Serotonin syndrome is potentially fatal, and although supportive care may be adequate for recovery, consideration may be given to the use of serotonin antagonists, such as methysergide and cyproheptadine.[7] Health care providers should be familiar with the various drugs that can cause serotonin syndrome and avoid the use of multiple agents that influence serotonin level (metabolism or uptake) in a sole patient.[8]

Table 111.1 Medications Associated With Serotonin Toxicity

Monoamine oxidase inhibitors	Linezolid, moclobemide, selegiline hydrochloride, phenelzine sulfate, isoniazid, procarbazine hydrochloride, toloxatone, tranylcypromine sulfate
Selective serotonin reuptake inhibitors	Paroxetine hydrochloride, sertraline hydrochloride, fluoxetine hydrochloride, citalopram hydrobromide, venlafaxine hydrochloride, fluvoxamine maleate, duloxetine hydrochloride
Serotonin reuptake inhibitors	Clomipramine hydrochloride, imipramine pamoate, chlorpheniramine maleate, brompheniramine maleate
Opioids	Meperidine hydrochloride, tramadol hydrochloride, methadone hydrochloride, dextromethorphan hydrobromide
Illicit drugs	Methylenedioxymethamphetamine, amphetamine sulfate, cocaine hydrochloride
Direct serotonin receptor agonists	Carbamazepine, buspirone hydrochloride, lithium carbonate
Increased serotonin formation	Tryptophan

[Based on data from refs 1, 2, 6, 8]

Take-Home Points

- Serotonin syndrome (also called *serotonin toxicity*) is a potentially fatal condition caused by abnormally elevated levels of serotonin in the nerve synapse.
- Symptoms of serotonin syndrome are neuromuscular excitation, autonomic stimulation, and altered mental status.
- Serotonin syndrome has been associated with the use of monoamine oxidase inhibitors and selective serotonin reuptake inhibitors, as well as such other medications as linezolid.
- Treatment of serotonin syndrome involves the discontinued use of the inciting drugs, supportive treatment, and, possibly, use of serotonin antagonists.

Summary

Interaction: pharmacodynamic
Substrates: linezolid and meperidine
Sites of action/enzyme: serotonin reuptake transporter and monoamine oxidase
Clinical effect: serotonin syndrome

References

1. Gillman PK. Monoamine oxidase inhibitors, opioid analgesics and serotonin toxicity. Br J Anaesth. 2005;95:434–41.
2. Zyvox (linezolid) [package insert] [Internet]. Peapack: Pharmacia & Upjohn. [cited 2009 Dec]. Available from: http://www.zyvox.com/pdfs/zyvox_full_prescribe_012001.pdf.
3. Altman EM, Manos GH. Serotonin syndrome associated with citalopram and meperidine. Psychosomatics. 2007;48:361–3.
4. Guo SL, Wu TJ, Liu CC, et al. Meperidine-induced serotonin syndrome in a susceptible patient. Br J Anaesth. 2009;103:369–70.
5. Das PK, Warkentin DI, Hewko R, et al. Serotonin syndrome after concomitant treatment with linezolid and meperidine. Clin Infect Dis. 2008;46:264–5.
6. Taylor JJ, Wilson JW, Estes LL. Linezolid and serotonergic drug interactions: a retrospective survey. Clin Infect Dis. 2006;43:180–7.
7. Sporer KA. The serotonin syndrome: implicated drugs, pathophysiology and management. Drug Saf. 1995;13:94–104.
8. Isbister GK, Buckley NA, Whyte IM. Serotonin toxicity: a practical approach to diagnosis and treatment. Med J Aust. 2007;187:361–5.

Not Sweet At All

112

Fatal Forty DDI: trimethoprim/sulfamethoxazole, glipizide, CYP2C9

Mayumi Horibe MD and Michael J. Bishop MD

Abstract
This case discusses the pharmacokinetic interaction between glipizide and trimethoprim-sulfamethoxazole (TMP/SMX), resulting in hypoglycemia. Glipizide is a cytochrome P450 2C9 substrate and TMP/SMX is a 2C9 inhibitor.

Case

A 79-year-old woman was posted for exploratory laparotomy because of severe abdominal pain. She had type 2 diabetes mellitus and a history of heavy alcohol use in the past. Her diabetes was under fair control on glipizide (10 mg BID). Five days prior to her admission through the Emergency Department (ED), she had visited her primary care provider (PCP) and complained of urinary frequency and dysuria. She was found to have a urinary tract infection with a strain of *Escherichia coli* that was susceptible to trimethoprim-sulfamethoxazole (TMP/SMX) and her PCP had initiated a one-week course of therapy with TMP/SMX (160/800 mg) twice a day. In the ED, an X-ray revealed a ureteral stone and the patient was brought to the operating room (OR) for stent placement.

On arrival in the OR, the patient appeared anxious, diaphoretic, and confused. Although the ED had attributed this to her age and illness, the anesthesiologist drew

M. Horibe MD (✉)
Department of Anesthesiology and Pain Medicine, University of Washington, Seattle, Washington, USA
e-mail: mayumi.horibe@va.gov

M.J. Bishop MD
Department of Anesthesiology, University of Washington School of Medicine, Seattle, WA, USA

C. Marcucci et al. (eds.), *A Case Approach to Perioperative Drug-Drug Interactions*, DOI 10.1007/978-1-4614-7495-1_112

a blood glucose and a chemistry panel. Her blood glucose level was 38 mg/dL and the serum creatinine was 1.98 with calculated creatinine clearance of 23 mL/min. The remainder of the laboratory tests were within the normal range. An intravenous bolus of dextrose (50% dextrose, 50 ml) rapidly improved her mental status and she became alert and oriented. The case was completed uneventfully. The next morning, however, she became again unresponsive. Her blood glucose level was again very low. Her insulin level was 30 mU/L (normal range 5–20 mU/L) and C-peptide level was 2.2 nmol/L (normal range 0.3–1.32 nmol/L). Growth hormone, adrenocorticotropic hormone, and serum cortisol were all within the normal range. TMP/SMX was discontinued. The patient required repeated boluses of 50% dextrose and continuous dextrose infusion to maintain adequate blood glucose levels. The next day, the dextrose infusion was discontinued and she was discharged home.[1]

Discussion

This is an example of an inhibitor added to a substrate.

Glipizide is an oral hypoglycemic of the sulfonylurea class used to control blood glucose in patients with type 2 diabetes mellitus. The mechanism action is stimulation of insulin release from the pancreas and increased tissue sensitivity to insulin.

Trimethoprim-sulfamethoxazole (TMP/SMX) is one of the most commonly prescribed antimicrobial agents in clinical practice, especially as a first-line agent for the treatment of urinary tract infection, bronchitis, and *Pneumocystis carinii* pneumonia in patients with AIDS. One of the rare, but serious adverse reactions of TMP/SMX is hypoglycemia. The mechanism of hypoglycemia with sulfamethoxazole is likely due to its structural similarity to the sulfonylureas.[2–4] Elevated or non-suppressed insulin and C-peptide concentrations observed during a hypoglycemic episode indicate that hypoglycemia resulted from increased endogenous insulin secretion.[3,4] Some patients can develop protracted hypoglycemia for more than 8 hours despite intravenous glucose infusion.[2]

Hypoglycemia secondary to the addition of TMP/SMX to sulfonylurea therapy has been a previously recognized drug–drug interaction.[4,5] The mechanism of the interaction is probably inhibition of hepatic metabolism of glipizide by TMP/SMX.

Cytochrome P450 (CYP) 2C9 is the principal enzyme responsible for the metabolism of numerous drugs, such as phenytoin, warfarin, glipizide, and tolbutamide.[6] Although trimethoprim is mainly excreted unchanged in urine, 20% of the dose is metabolized by the cytochrome P450 system (CYP2C8 and CYP2C9).[7] Sulfamethoxazole is eliminated mainly by metabolism and 2C9 plays an important role in its N4-hydroxylation.[7] It has been suggested that competitive inhibition of 2C9 activity by TMP/SMX is the mechanism involved in the drug–drug interactions between TMP/SMX and glipizide.[7,8]

The risk factors predisposing to the development of TMP/SMX induced hypoglycemia include renal insufficiency, prolonged fasting conditions, malnutrition, the use of excessive doses, age, history of alcohol abuse and liver dysfunction.[2,3,8] When prescribing TMP/SMX to patients who are on glipizide, patients should be closely monitored and dose adjustment should be considered, especially for patients with renal dysfunction.

Take-Home Points

- Drug–drug interactions are an important type of adverse drug event and the possible mechanisms for symptomatic hypoglycemia. Hypoglycemia is a serious, potentially life-threatening complication and needs prompt treatment.
- Hypoglycemia resulting from the combination of sulfonylureas and sulfonamides is a recognized drug interaction.
- Cytochrome P450 (CYP) 2C9 is the main enzyme catalyzing the biotransformation of sulfonylureas (tolbutamide, glibenclamide, glyburide, glimepiride, glipizide). TMP/SMX is an inhibitor of CYP2C9. Hypoglycemia is secondary to a TMP/SMX-induced reduction of glipizide metabolism.
- Patients receiving glipizide or other sulfonylureas, especially with decreased drug metabolism, should be monitored closely for signs and symptoms of hypoglycemia when TMP/SMX is added to their regimen. Patients with renal dysfunction need to adjust the dose depending on the renal function.

Summary

Interaction: pharmacokinetic
Substrate: glipizide
Enzyme: CYP2C9
Inhibitor: trimethoprim-sulfamethoxazole
Clinical effect: hypoglycemia

References

1. Sandson NB. Drug-drug interaction primer: a compendium of case vignettes for the practicing clinician. Washington, DC: American Psychiatric Press, Inc; 2007. p. 178–9.
2. Lee AJ, Maddix DS. Trimethoprim/sulfamethoxazole-induced hypoglycemia in a patient with acute renal failure. Ann Pharmacother. 1997;31:727–32.
3. Strevel EL, Kuper A, Gold WL. Severe and protracted hypoglycaemia associated with co-trimoxazole use. Lancet Infect Dis. 2006;6:178–82.

4. Hekimsoy Z, Biberoğlu S, Cömlekçi A, et al. Trimethoprim/sulfamethoxazole – induced hypoglycemia in a malnourished patient with severe infection. Eur J Endocrinol. 1997;136:304–6.
5. Johnson JF, Dobmeier ME. Symptomatic hypoglycemia secondary to a glipizide – trimethoprim/sulfamethoxazole drug interaction. DICP. 1990;24:250–1.
6. Kirchheiner J, Roots I, Goldammer M, et al. Effect of genetic polymorphisms in cytochrome p450 (CYP) 2C9 and CYP2C8 on the pharmacokinetics of oral antidiabetic drugs: clinical relevance. Clin Pharmacokinet. 2005;44:1209–25.
7. Wen X, Wang JS, Backman JT, et al. Trimethoprim and sulfamethoxazole are selective inhibitors of CYP2C8 and CYP2C9, respectively. Drug Metab Dispos. 2002;30:631–5.
8. Juurlink DN, Mamdani M, Kopp A, et al. Drug-drug interactions among elderly patients hospitalized for drug toxicity. JAMA. 2003;289:1652–8.

Where Did All the Sugar Go?

113

Fatal Forty DDI: levofloxacin, glyburide, complex interaction

Nicole L. Varela MD, Federica Scavonetto MD, Toby N. Weingarten MD, and Juraj Sprung MD, PhD

Abstract
This case discusses the potentiation of hypoglycemic effect with the coadministration of levofloxacin and glyburide.

Case

An 82-year-old woman presented to the preoperative clinic for evaluation before an operation scheduled for the following week. She recently had a productive cough and had been seen by her primary care provider the previous day. At that time, she started therapy with levofloxacin (250 mg orally QOD) for a 10-day antibiotic course to treat a presumed bronchitis. She now reported feeling weak, light-headed, and diaphoretic. Her daughter reported that the patient did not seem herself that morning and her speech appeared slowed. Her daughter thought it was due to the haste needed to make their early morning appointment.

Review of the patient's past medical history was notable for congestive heart failure (ejection fraction, 45%), type 2 diabetes mellitus, and chronic kidney disease (glomerular filtration rate, 45 mL/min/1.73 m^2). Home medications included lisinopril, carvedilol, and glyburide. Her finger-stick glucose value was 41 mg/dL. The patient

N.L. Varela MD (✉)
Department of Anesthesiology, Winona Health, Winona, MN, USA
e-mail: nicole@varela.net

F. Scavonetto MD • T.N. Weingarten MD • J. Sprung MD, PhD
Department of Anesthesiology, Mayo Clinic, Rochester, MN, USA

C. Marcucci et al. (eds.), *A Case Approach to Perioperative Drug-Drug Interactions*, DOI 10.1007/978-1-4614-7495-1_113

was given orange juice, which she sipped slowly. Dextrose and glucagon were given. The patient's finger-stick glucose evaluation was repeated 30 minutes later and continued to be low, at 48 mg/dL. Subsequently, this level was confirmed with a serum glucose result of 42 mg/dL. An infusion of 10% dextrose with 0.45 normal saline was started. The patient was hospitalized for ongoing medical management of persistent hypoglycemia.

Discussion

This is an example of a multifactorial interaction between levofloxacin and glyburide.

More specifically, this is an example of potentiated hypoglycemic effect by antibiotic fluoroquinolones in a patient receiving an oral hypoglycemic drug (glyburide).

Dysregulation of glucose homeostasis is more common with fluoroquinolone use than with any other antibiotic agent. Studies comparing episodes of hypoglycemia have reported an increased incidence in patients receiving fluoroquinolones when compared with patients receiving antibiotics such as ceftriaxone.[1] Several case studies also have reported considerable hyperinsulinar hypoglycemia, not only with gatifloxacin, which has been subsequently withdrawn from the market, but also with other fluoroquinolones, such as ciprofloxacin hydrochloride and levofloxacin.[2–6] The mechanism of fluoroquinolone-induced hypoglycemia is not completely understood, but these drugs are believed to inhibit adenosine triphosphate–sensitive potassium channels in the pancreatic ß-cells which subsequently increases insulin secretion.[7] However, levofloxacin has less effect than gatifloxacin on these channels. In reported cases, sequelae have varied from prolonged hospitalization to the devastating effects of anoxic brain injury.[3] These episodes of hypoglycemia are often persistent and are at times refractory.[2,3,5]

Several risk factors have been identified in case-controlled studies.[4] Risk factors include older age, female gender, sepsis, renal insufficiency, hepatic dysfunction, hypoalbuminemia, and type 2 diabetes with oral hypoglycemic drug therapy.[3–5] However, patients with renal insufficiency who are taking oral hypoglycemic drugs appear to be most at risk.

Sulfonylurea type drugs such as glyburide also increases endogenous insulin secretion through inhibition of the pancreatic β-cell adenosine triphosphate–sensitive potassium channels. The combination of a sulfonylurea (glyburide) with a fluoroquinolone (levofloxacin) can result in a synergistic reaction of increased insulin secretion and predispose the patient to severe hypoglycemia.[2]

For patients taking oral hypoglycemic drug therapy, renal insufficiency poses an increased risk. Decreased renal clearance can often lead to elevated blood levels of glyburide.[2] This drug combination, with elevated levels of glyburide along with the increased insulin secretion effect of levofloxacin, further increases the risk for hypoglycemia.[5]

The timing of hypoglycemia usually occurs within 72 to 96 hours of starting a fluoroquinolone regimen.[5] However, case studies have reported episodes of hypoglycemia after only one dose of a fluoroquinolone.[2,8] The hypoglycemia may occur in 1.1% of hospitalized patients receiving levofloxacin.[1,4,5] Nevertheless, hypoglycemia can be refractory and life threatening.[2,3,5,9]

Current recommendations include close monitoring of glucose for patients concurrently taking an oral hypoglycemic agent and a fluoroquinolone. Consideration should be given for an alternative antibiotic, particularly for those patients who have renal insufficiency and take oral hypoglycemic drug therapy.

Take-Home Points

- Irregularities in glucose homeostasis have been reported with the use of fluoroquinolones, resulting in hypoglycemia.
- Sulfonylureas and fluoroquinolones independently increase insulin secretion from pancreatic beta cells, and the hypoglycemia is believed to be mediated through this mechanism.
- Close glucose monitoring should be implemented when patients start taking a fluoroquinolone, such as levofloxacin, particularly for patients who take oral hypoglycemic medications, such as glyburide.
- The presence of renal insufficiency may increase the risk for hypoglycemia further for patients who take sulfonylureas and fluoroquinolones simultaneously.

Summary

Interaction: pharmacodynamic
Substrates: glyburide and levofloxacin
Mechanism/site of action: increase in insulin secretion by both levofloxacin and glyburide
Clinical effects: potentiated hypoglycemia effect

References

1. Mohr JF, McKinnon PS, Peymann PJ, et al. A retrospective, comparative evaluation of dysglycemias in hospitalized patients receiving gatifloxacin, levofloxacin, ciprofloxacin, or ceftriaxone. Pharmacotherapy. 2005;25:1303–9.
2. Lin G, Hays DP, Spillane L. Refractory hypoglycemia from ciprofloxacin and glyburide interaction. J Toxicol Clin Toxicol. 2004;42:295–7.
3. Lawrence KR, Adra M, Keir C. Hypoglycemia-induced anoxic brain injury possibly associated with levofloxacin. J Infect. 2006;52:e177–80.
4. Graumlich JF, Habis S, Avelino RR, et al. Hypoglycemia in inpatients after gatifloxacin or levofloxacin therapy: nested case-control study. Pharmacotherapy. 2005;25:1296–302.
5. Garber SM, Pound MW, Miller SM. Hypoglycemia associated with the use of levofloxacin. Am J Health Syst Pharm. 2009;66:1014–9.
6. Park-Wyllie LY, Juurlink DN, Kopp A, et al. Outpatient gatifloxacin therapy and dysglycemia in older adults. N Engl J Med. 2006;354:1352–61.
7. Saraya A, Yokokura M, Gonoi T, et al. Effects of fluoroquinolones on insulin secretion and β-cell ATP-sensitive K^+ channels. Eur J Pharmacol. 2004;497:111–7.
8. Kelesidis T, Canseco E. Levofloxacin-induced hypoglycemia: a rare but life-threatening side effect of a widely used antibiotic. Am J Med. 2009;122:e3–4.
9. Singh M, Jacob JJ, Kapoor R, et al. Fatal hypoglycemia with levofloxacin use in an elderly patient in the post-operative period. Langenbecks Arch Surg. 2008;393:235–8.

Exposed! (Part 1)

114

Fatal Forty DDI: rifampin, buspirone, CYP3A4

L. Michele Noles MD and Catherine Marcucci MD

Abstract
This case discusses the pharmacokinetic interaction between buspirone and rifampin, leading to decreased anti-anxiety effect of buspirone. Buspirone is a cytochrome P450 3A4 substrate and rifampin is a 3A4 inducer.

Case

A surgical house officer who had been exposed to a trauma patient with active tuberculosis (TB) developed a positive purified protein derivative (PPD) skin test a few weeks after the exposure. The strain was determined to be resistant to isoniazid. His chest X-ray was deemed negative for active disease. He was thus placed on a 4-month course of rifampin (300 mg orally twice a day) for latent TB. Prior to the TB exposure he had been relatively healthy. His only other medical issue was a diagnosis of generalized anxiety disorder (GAD) for which he had been taking buspirone (30 mg orally BID) with great success for two years.

He initially experienced no side effects with the rifampin, but after a couple of weeks noticed he was feeling increasingly anxious. Thinking that the stress of the recent TB exposure coupled with worsened sleep deprivation due to a new baby at home was causing more strain than usual, he tried to use some of the stress-reduction coping strategies that had served him well in the past. However, he continued to feel increasingly anxious and in fact developed gastrointestinal symptoms including nausea, loss of appetite, disrupted sleep, and decreased libido. As things worsened,

L.M. Noles MD (✉)
Department of Anesthesiology and Perioperative Medicine, Oregon Health and Science University, Portland, OR, USA
e-mail: nolesl@ohsu.edu

C. Marcucci MD
Anesthesia Services Department, Philadelphia Veterans Affairs Medical Center, Philadelphia, PA, USA

C. Marcucci et al. (eds.), *A Case Approach to Perioperative Drug-Drug Interactions*, DOI 10.1007/978-1-4614-7495-1_114

he began to feel like he had before starting the buspirone, and made an appointment with his psychiatrist. After reviewing his medications, the psychiatrist decided to discontinue the buspirone and replace it with clonazepam.

Discussion

This is an example of an inducer added to a substrate.

Rifampin is an antibiotic drug used primarily in the treatment of tuberculosis. It is a classic "pan-inducer" of the cytochrome P450 (CYP) enzyme system, including the 3A4 enzyme.[1] Buspirone, a non-benzodiazepine anxiolytic medication that belongs to the azapirone group, is metabolized primarily by the CYP3A4 enzyme.[1] In the presence of rifampin, there is an increased amount of 3A4 enzyme which then proceeds to more quickly metabolize its substrates—in this case, buspirone. The significant drop in blood levels of buspirone due to its increased metabolism is usually seen within 1 to 3 weeks of starting rifampin, and can be dramatic. Studies have shown that in the presence of rifampin, buspirone peak plasma concentration (C_{max}) is decreased by 84% compared with buspirone levels in the absence of rifampin.[2] Additionally, the total area under the plasma concentration-time curve (AUC) of buspirone in the presence of rifampin averaged only 10% of the baseline AUC in the absence of rifampin. The dramatically decreased plasma levels of buspirone can easily explain the recurrence of GAD symptoms in our subject.

Take-Home Points

- Rifampin is a "pan-inducer" of many cytochrome P450 enzymes, including the CYP3A4 enzyme.
- Buspirone is a CYP3A4 substrate.
- This drug–drug interaction can lead to a clinically significant drop in buspirone blood levels with loss of clinical efficacy of buspirone.

Summary

Interaction: pharmacokinetic
Substrate: buspirone
Enzyme: CYP3A4
Inducer: rifampin
Clinical effect: decreased anti-anxiety efficacy of buspirone

References

1. Sandson NB. Drug-drug interaction primer: a compendium of case vignettes for the practicing clinician. Arlington: American Psychiatric Publishing, Inc.; 2007.
2. Lamberg TS, et al. Concentrations and effects of buspirone are considerably reduced by rifampicin. Br J Clin Pharmacol. 1998;45:381–5.

Exposed! (Part 2)

115

Fatal Forty DDI: rifampin, ondansetron, CYP3A4

L. Michele Noles MD and Catherine Marcucci MD

Abstract
This case discusses the pharmacokinetic interaction between ondansetron and rifampin, resulting in decreased anti-emetic effect of ondansetron. Ondansetron is a cytochrome P450 3A4 substrate and rifampin is a 3A4 inducer.

Case

As the resident in the previous scenario switched to clonazepam for symptom control, he gradually began to feel less anxious, but his nausea and GI upset continued. Having learned his lessons well from his postoperative patients, he promptly obtained a prescription for oral ondansetron. However, he did not obtain the relief that he had anticipated.

Discussion

This is an example of a substrate added to an inducer.

As noted above, rifampin is a powerful pan-inducer of the cytochrome P450 (CYP) P450 enzymes.[1,2] Ondansetron is a selective 5-HT3-receptor antagonist used as an antiemetic agent. It is primarily metabolized by P450 enzymes, with CYP3A4

L.M. Noles MD (✉)
Department of Anesthesiology & Perioperative Medicine, Oregon Health and Science University, Portland, OR, USA
e-mail: nolesl@ohsu.edu

C. Marcucci MD
Anesthesia Services Department, Philadelphia Veterans Affairs Medical Center, Philadelphia, PA, USA

C. Marcucci et al. (eds.), *A Case Approach to Perioperative Drug-Drug Interactions*, DOI 10.1007/978-1-4614-7495-1_115

playing an important role. Similar to the interaction between rifampin and buspirone, the presence of rifampin considerably lowers the plasma concentration of ondansetron. In the presence of rifampin, the mean Area Under the Curve (AUC) (0-∞) of orally administered ondansetron is decreased by 65% and the maximum plasma concentration (C_{max}) is decreased by 50%. Intravenous ondansetron showed a similar pattern when given in the presence of rifampin: the AUC (0-∞) decreased by 48%.[3] The efficacy of ondansetron is directly related to its plasma concentration, so it follows that one would see a reduced antiemetic effect with decreased plasma concentrations.

Take-Home Points

- Rifampin is a "pan-inducer" of many cytochrome P450 enzymes, including the CYP3A4 enzyme and interacts with many other medications.
- Ondansetron is a CYP3A4 substrate.
- Induction of P450 enzymes by rifampin can lead to loss of efficacy of buspirone, ondansetron, and many other medications.
- Important perioperative medications (in addition to ondansetron) which may be affected by rifampin include dexamethasone, haloperidol, ibuprofen, midazolam, and methadone, as well as many others.

Summary

Interaction: pharmacokinetic
Substrate: ondansetron
Enzyme: CYP3A4
Inducer: rifampin
Clinical effect: decreased anti-emetic effect of ondansetron

References

1. Sandson NB. Drug-drug interaction primer: a compendium of case vignettes for the practicing clinician. Arlington: American Psychiatric Publishing, Inc.; 2007.
2. Lamberg TS, et al. Concentrations and effects of buspirone are considerably reduced by rifampicin. Br J Clin Pharmacol. 1998;45:381–5.
3. Villikka K, et al. The effect of rifampin on the pharmacokinetics of oral and intravenous ondansetron. Clin Pharmacol Ther. 1999;65:377–81.

Seizures on 5 West

116

Carbapenem, valproic acid,
P-glycoprotein, UGT

Elizabeth Duggan MD and Nabil M. Elkassabany MD

Abstract
This case discusses a complex interaction between valproic acid and carbapenem, resulting in decreased seizure threshold.

Case

A 60-year-old Vietnam veteran was admitted for revascularization of his right lower extremity. His past medical history included a chronic right heel ulcer with dry gangrenous margins, diabetes mellitus, and a seizure disorder due to a traumatic head injury he sustained in combat. He had been maintained on valproate (750 mg BID). The patient had been seizure-free for six years and his current dosage was continued upon admission to the hospital. A serum valproic acid (VPA) level was checked and noted to be 80.6 mcg/mL (normal therapeutic levels are between 50–100 mcg/mL).

Although the femoral-popliteal bypass procedure was successful, on the third postoperative day the patient was found to have a softly necrotic ulcer with dry eschar overlying the ulcer. The eschar was removed and the necrotic tissue was debrided at the bedside. Afterward, wound cultures show a *Pseudomonas* species sensitive to carbapenem antibiotics. The infectious disease service recommended imipenem (500 mg 98 h for 10 days). Four days later, the patient suffered a grand mal seizure and was admitted to the intensive care unit. His valproate level at that time was discovered to be 24.7 mcg/mL.

E. Duggan MD (✉)
Department of Anesthesiology, Emory University School of Medicine, Atlanta, GA, USA
e-mail: ejw323cu@gmail.com

N.M. Elkassabany MD
Section of Orthopedic Anesthesiology, Department of Anesthesiology and Critical Care, University of Pennsylvania, Wayne, PA, USA

C. Marcucci et al. (eds.), *A Case Approach to Perioperative Drug-Drug Interactions*, DOI 10.1007/978-1-4614-7495-1_116

Discussion

This is an example of a complex pharmacokinetic interaction in which multiple synergistic mechanisms produce increased clearance of a substrate.

Carbapenems are a class of ß-lactam antibiotics with a broad spectrum of antibacterial activity. They have a structure that renders them highly resistant to ß-lactamases. When they are prescribed for patients taking valproic acid for seizure treatment or prophylaxis, serum VPA can decrease to subtherapeutic levels, increasing the likelihood of seizure recurrence.

As early as 1997, case reports documented decreases in the levels of serum valproic acid in patients during treatment with carbapenem antibiotics.[1] Since then, several further case reports have documented incidents in which patients treated with both drugs experienced epileptic seizures.[2–4] A retrospective study of an 18-month period, looking at 39 patients treated simultaneously with valproic acid and meropenem, revealed a drop in serum valproic acid levels by an average of 66% within 24 hours of initiation of the antibiotic. Similarly, a Japanese case series of seven patients revealed that VPA serum levels were decreased by 70.4% when patients were started on carbapenem therapy.[3]

The pharmacokinetic interaction between valproic acid and carbapenem antibiotics has been studied in several animal models to elucidate the mechanism of decreased VPA concentration. To date however, the mechanism of interaction is not completely understood. Valproic acid is excreted from the kidney, after conjugation by UDP-glucuronosyltransferase (UGT) into a glucuronide conjugate (VPA-Glu).[4] Proposed mechanisms for the decreased serum levels of VPA in the presence of carbapenems, include an increase in the hepatic metabolism of valproic acid to the glucuronide conjugate (VPA-Glu) through an increase in UGT activity.[5,6] Other researchers have suggested that decreasing serum levels of VPA are due to increased renal clearance of VPA-Glu in the presence of carbapenems.[7] It has also been reported that the decrease in plasma VPA may be partially due to carbapenems enhancing the accumulation of VPA in erythrocytes by inhibiting the activity of multidrug resistance proteins (MRPs). MRPs are ATP-dependent proteins that use inside-out vesicles to transport VPA; when inhibited by carbapenems, as demonstrated to occur *in vivo*, erythrocyte distribution of VPA is increased and plasma levels are decreased.[8] The P-glycoprotein transporter is one of the better-elucidated MRPs. Finally, oral valproic acid has been shown to undergo decreased intestinal absorption during coadministration of carbapenems. Torii et al. demonstrated that carbapenems inhibit valproic acid transport from apical to basal cell membranes when carbapenem antibiotics are added to the basolateral side, by inhibiting VPA movement across cell layers.[9] Although this mechanism is less likely because of the small concentration of carbapenem antibiotics in the intestine during intravenous (vs. oral) administration, it may still play a role in decreased serum VPA levels.

Take-Home Points

- Patients receiving treatment with valproic acid should be carefully monitored if carbapenem antibiotics are to be coadministered. The FDA recommends that "serum valproic acid concentrations should be monitored frequently after initiating carbapenem therapy."
- The specific mechanisms by which serum valproic acid levels may be lowered after carbapenem drug therapy include decrease in absorption by P-glycoprotein inhibition and increase in by metabolism due to increase in UGT activity.
- Given the evidence suggesting that a drug interaction between carbapenems and valproic acid can produce subtherapeutic VPA levels and increased seizure risk, choosing an alternative antibiotic may be advisable.

Summary

Interaction: pharmacokinetic (complex)
Substrate: valproic acid
Enzymes/transporters/sites of action: UGT and P-glycoprotein; possible renal involvement
Inducer: carbapenem (of UGT)
Inhibitor: carbapenem (of P-glycoprotein)
Clinical effect: decreased serum valproic acid levels and decreased seizure threshold

References

1. Nagai K, Shimizu T, Togo A, et al. Decrease in serum levels of valproic acid during treatment with a new carbapenem, panipaenem/betamipron. J Antimicob Chemother. 1997;39:295–6.
2. Llinares F, Bosacoma N, Hernandez C, et al. Pharmacokinetic interaction between valproic acid and carbapenem-like antibiotics. A discussion of three cases. Farm Hosp. 2003;27:258–63.
3. Lee SG, Kim JH, Joo JY, et al. Seven cases of decreased serum valproic acid concentration during concomitant use of carbapenem antibiotics. Korean J Lab Med. 2007;27(5):338–43.
4. Radomynska-Pandya A, Czernik PJ, Little JM, et al. Structural and functional studies of UDP-glucuronosyltransferases. Drug Metab Rev. 1999;31:817–99.
5. Yamamura N, Imura-Miyoshi K, Naganuma H. Panipenem, a carbapenem antibiotic, enhances the glucouronidation of intravenously administered valproic acid in rats. Drug Meta Dispos. 2000;27:724–30.
6. Mori H, Takahashi K, Mitzutani T. Interaction between valproic acid and carbapenem antibiotics. Drug Metab Rev. 2007;39:647–57.

7. Yokogawa K, Iwashita S, Kubota A, et al. Effect of meropenem on disposition kinetics of valproate and its metabolites in rabbits. Pharm Res. 2001;18:1320–6.
8. Ogawa K, Yumoto R, Hamada N, et al. Interaction of valproic acid and carbapenam antibiotics with multidrug resistance-associated proteins in rat erythrocyte membranes. Epilepsy Res. 2006;71:76–87.
9. Torii M, Takiguchi Y, Izumi M, et al. Carbapenem antibiotics inhibit valproic acid transport in Caco-2 cell monolayers. Int J Pharm. 2002;233:253–6.

Drug–Drug Interactions Involving Cardiovascular Medications

XII

Introduction

117

Michael P. Hutchens MD

Abstract
This section introduces drug–drug interactions involving cardiovascular medications.

Cardiovascular medications transmit, support, or interfere with the basic processes of life. They receive our respect in the perioperative environment, but practitioners of other specialties often see our frequent use of bolus pressors and antihypertensives as appallingly blithe. Yet in our hands, the 18-year-old who is hypotensive after induction is safer when appropriately treated with a single bolus of fast-acting vasoconstrictor; this is a fundamental lesson of early training in anesthesiology.

The medications in this section are also bedrocks of perioperative management. Patients come to the operating room on antihypertensives, receive pressors in the operating room and intensive care unit, develop and have their heart failure treated with inotropes, and all too frequently require antiarrhythmia drugs for perioperative atrial fibrillation.

Put another way, powerful cardiovascular medications are ubiquitous and well-understood in our environment. Yet their interactions with other medications are poorly understood—witness the current controversy over perioperative use of angiotensin-converting enzyme (ACE) inhibitors and perioperative hypotension. In my own practice and teaching in the cardiothoracic intensive care unit, a formative step for learners is understanding the pharmacodynamic interaction between epinephrine, glucose, insulin, and potassium. Although the anesthesiology residents may give these medications every day on the cardiac anesthesia rotation, they do not understand without having it explained that the potassium will predictably rise when insulin and epinephrine are taken away at the same time. It's basic physiology,

M.P. Hutchens MD
Department of Anesthesiology and Perioperative Medicine, Oregon Health and Science University, Portland, OR, USA
e-mail: hutchenm@ohsu.edu

C. Marcucci et al. (eds.), *A Case Approach to Perioperative Drug-Drug Interactions*, DOI 10.1007/978-1-4614-7495-1_117

but the observation lies, as so many drug interactions do, at the border between specialties and phases of care.

I hope that this section, which is full of complex interactions of ubiquitous medications, offers you a passport to that borderland, opening a vista in which "pressure up" and "pressure down" are informed by the fullness of the landscape of our patients.

Riding the Rollercoaster

118

Nitroglycerine, sodium nitroprusside, propofol

Catherine Marcucci MD, Erica D. Wittwer MD, PhD, and Juraj Sprung MD, PhD

Abstract
This case discusses a pharmacodynamic interaction between propofol, nitroglycerin, and sodium nitroprusside, resulting in severe hypotension.

Case

An anesthesia attending and the new resident on the vascular anesthesia rotation were walking over to the operating room to start the anesthetic for a carotid endarterectomy. The patient was 65-year-old man with a history of smoking, hypertension, transient ischemic attacks, and coronary artery disease. The coronary lesions were not amenable to bypass. The patient suffered from unstable angina and frequently used nitroglycerin paste. The attending asked her resident to make up nitroglycerin and nitroprusside infusions and to draw up syringes of both drugs as well.

Anesthesia was induced with propofol and maintained with isoflurane. The patient had a high carotid bifurcation and the operative case proved to be technically difficult. The surgeons were concerned about the integrity of patch, and they asked the anesthesia team for a smooth emergence and tracheal extubation. As the patient emerged from general anesthesia his electrocardiogram revealed ST segment depression and a nitroglycerin infusion was started. Just as the surgeons were closing the neck, the patient began to swallow. A few seconds later he coughed and the surgical field rapidly filled with blood. The blood pressure was recorded as 209/123 mm Hg. The surgeons put pressure on the wound and yelled for the patient "to go back to

C. Marcucci MD (✉)
Anesthesia Services Department, Philadelphia Veterans Affairs Medical Center, Philadelphia, PA, USA
e-mail: sandson.marcucci@comcast.net

E.D. Wittwer MD, PhD • J. Sprung MD, PhD
Department of Anesthesiology, Mayo Clinic, Rochester, MN, USA

C. Marcucci et al. (eds.), *A Case Approach to Perioperative Drug-Drug Interactions*, DOI 10.1007/978-1-4614-7495-1_118

sleep." The resident, who in the stress of the moment had forgotten that the nitroglycerin infusion was on, grabbed the propofol and nitroglycerin syringes and delivered a bolus of each into an open port of the line where the nitroglycerin infusion was being infused. Several seconds later the blood pressure sank like a stone with an immediate deepening of ST segment depression. Fluids and phenylephrine were administered, which caused a mild overshoot of the blood pressure. The patient received an additional (but smaller!) bolus of propofol and nitroprusside, as well as fentanyl. The propofol infusion was restarted. An hour later the patient and resident were in the step-down unit. The patient was calm and at ease, the resident was not.

Discussion

This is an example of multiple pharmacodynamic interactions at both the cellular messenger and end-organ level.

This unfortunate clinical scenario has happened, in one version or another, to every anesthesia provider! The goal, having brought a patient and yourself through a case like this, is to do everything you can so that it doesn't happen again. Experience helps guide the administration of such potent drugs, but understanding the pharmacology and realizing the cumulative, and potentially profound, pharmacodynamic effects when drugs are given in close succession is key.

Medical nitroglycerin is a glyceryl trinitrate that has been in clinical use for patients with coronary artery disease for many years. It is now understood that nitroglycerine is not a direct dilator of the vasculature (Fig. 118.1). Instead, organic nitrates act *via* mitochondrial aldehyde dehydrogenase to initiate a series of steps involving several interim compounds that result in increased nitric oxide levels.[1] Nitric oxide is a natural and potent dilator of the vasculature. Although administration of nitroglycerin will dilate both arteries and veins, it is preferentially a venodilator and causes a decrease in cardiac output primarily by decrease in preload. Decreases in preload are advantageous in the treatment of myocardial ischemia by reducing diastolic wall stress and increasing subendocardial blood flow, which ultimately results in improved oxygen delivery. However, decreases in preload will also decrease cardiac output and blood pressure *via* decreases in stroke volume.

Sodium nitroprusside is an intravenous-only, short-acting inorganic nitrate compound that will release nitric oxide spontaneously. Unlike nitroglycerin, it acts primarily as a vasodilator or preferential dilator of the arterial vasculature. Sodium nitroprusside is extremely potent and rapid in onset and can be used in cases of true hypertensive emergency to decrease cardiac afterload and systolic blood pressure.

In addition to the robust nature of the pharmacodynamic interaction between nitroglycerine and sodium nitroprusside, the propofol also contributed to the precipitous decline in blood pressure. Even normotensive and normovolemic patients can

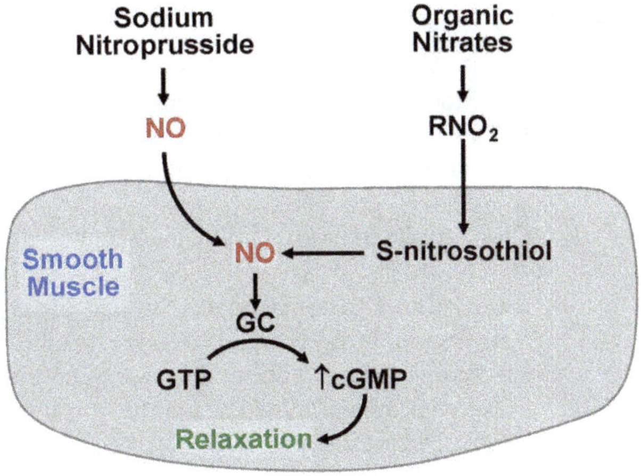

Fig. 118.1 Illustration showing the two basic types of nitrodilators: those that release nitric oxide spontaneously such as sodium nitroprusside, and organic nitrates that require and enzymatic process to for nitric oxide [Figure used with kind permission from Richard E. Klabunde, PhD http://cvpharmacology.com/vasodilator/nitro.htm]

exhibit a moderate decrease in blood pressure with the administration of propofol. Propofol decreases afterload by decreasing systemic vascular resistance. The mechanism is probably associated with inhibition of the sympathetic nervous system and its attendant vasoconstrictor actions.

Finally, our patient suffered severe hypotension after the resident gave boluses of propofol and nitroprusside through the side port of a running nitroglycerin infusion. Remember that there is a considerable dose of drug contained in the volume of those lines!

Take-Home Points

- Nitroglycerin is an organic nitrate that decreases blood pressure by indirectly initiating release of nitric oxide. It causes hypotension mainly through venodilation.
- Sodium nitroprusside in an inorganic nitrate that directly increases nitric oxide. It causes hypotension chiefly through vasodilation (arterial dilation). Its rapid blood pressure-lowering effects can be profound.
- Whenever administering nitroglycerin or sodium nitroprusside as bolus wait and observe hemodynamic response before administering a second bolus or a bolus of a second potent vasodilator.
- Propofol lowers blood pressure by decreasing systemic vasculature resistance.
- When given simultaneously, these drugs can have a profound pharmacologic hemodynamic effect.

Summary

Interaction 1: pharmacodynamic (cellular messenger)
Substrates: nitroglycerin and sodium nitroprusside
Mechanism/site of action: direct and indirection stimulation of nitric oxide release
Clinical effects: profound hypotension

Interaction 2: pharmacodynamic (end-organ)
Substrates: nitroglycerine, sodium nitroprusside, and propofol
Mechanism/site of action: decrease of cardiac preload and afterload leading to decrease in cardiac output
Clinical effects: hypotension

Reference

1. Chen Z, Foster MW, Zhang J, et al. An essential role for mitochondrial aldehyde dehydrogenase in nitroglycerin bioactivation. Proc Natl Acad Sci U S A. 2005;102:12159–64.

A Pressing Need for Vasopressin!

119

ACE-Is, general anesthesia

Erin B. Payne MD and Anna Dubovoy MD

Abstract

This case discusses the pharmacodynamic interaction between angiotensin-converting enzyme inhibitors (ACE-Is) and general anesthesia, resulting in profound hypotension. Preoperative recommendations and treatment of the hypotension is also discussed.

Case

A 78-year-old, 75 kg woman presented for total thyroidectomy as part of a surgical preparation for an upcoming thoracic aneurysm repair. She had a history of hypertension (treated with captopril and hydrochlorothiazide), atrial fibrillation, and syncopal episodes of unclear etiology. After induction of general anesthesia with fentanyl (150 mcg), lidocaine (40 mg), 140 propofol (140 mg), cisatracurium (16 mg) and endotracheal intubation, the patient became hypotensive, with a noninvasive systolic blood pressure ranging from 50 mm Hg to 70 mm Hg, decreased from a baseline of 125 mm Hg. A radial arterial catheter was placed. Initially, the patient's treatment included fluid resuscitation, as well as administration of phenylephrine and ephedrine. She was unresponsive to resuscitation efforts and ultimately required discontinuation of inhalational anesthesia; the patient received one dose of scopolamine for amnesic effect as the surgery continued. An urgent transesophageal echocardiogram exam was performed to assess for stability of the thoracic aneurysm, hypovolemia, and any wall motion abnormalities; the findings were unremarkable. An arterial blood gas

E.B. Payne MD (✉)
Department of Anesthesiology, Preoperative Assessment Clinic, University of Michigan Health System, Plymouth, MI, USA
e-mail: ebosher@umich.edu

A. Dubovoy MD
Department of Anesthesiology, University of Michigan Hospital Center, Ann Arbor, MI, USA

C. Marcucci et al. (eds.), *A Case Approach to Perioperative Drug-Drug Interactions*, DOI 10.1007/978-1-4614-7495-1_119

analysis did not reveal any acidosis, hypoxemia, or electrolyte abnormalities that would account for profound hypotension. The patient eventually responded to incremental boluses of 1 unit vasopressin (5 units total), intravenous (IV) fluid boluses of Lactated Ringers, and an infusion of vasopressin. Following completion of the surgery, the patient remained intubated and was subsequently transferred to the intensive care unit where she was ruled out for myocardial infarction.

Discussion

This is an example of a pharmacodynamic interaction.

There are three separate mechanisms that regulate vascular tone, in order to ensure adequate blood pressure, preserve cardiac output, and perfuse all vital organs. These include: the sympathetic nervous system, the renin-angiotensin system (RAS), and the vasopressin system. Each system acts individually and as compensatory mechanisms for the other two, especially when one system has been functionally compromised.

The RAS is a biochemical cascade that regulates "effective" blood volume, the blood volume adequate to maintain ample cardiac output. An important enzyme in the cascade, angiotensin-converting enzyme (ACE), acts to convert angiotensin I to angiotensin II and also inactivates central opioids, enkephalins, and bradykinin. The final product of this cascade, angiotensin II, is involved in maintaining blood pressure via vasoconstriction, increasing aldosterone secretion for sodium and water reabsorption, and stimulating catecholamine release, central pressor release and thirst.[1]

Angiotensin-converting enzyme inhibitors (ACE-Is, eg, captopril, ramipril) block the production of angiotensin II, thereby impeding blood pressure regulation by the RAS. ACE inhibitors cause arterial and venous dilation, resulting in decreased systemic vascular resistance and reduced cardiac output adaptation to ventricular loading, respectively. In addition, ACE inhibitors interfere with the degradation of bradykinin, a potent vasodilator.[2] Cardiac baroreflex response is "reset" with ACE inhibition, tending toward an increase in parasympathetic tone, but sympathetic response is intact in awake, euvolemic patients. Blockade of the RAS via ACE inhibition allows the vasopressin and sympathetic systems to be active in the maintenance of blood pressure during hypovolemia.[1]

The induction of anesthesia is associated with the suppression of the sympathetic nervous system via the effects of inhalational anesthetics, sedative-hypnotics, and opioids. Under general anesthesia, patients not chronically treated with ACE-I can compensate via RAS and vasopressin arms to maintain hemodynamic stability. Profound hypotension under general anesthesia is observed in patients on chronic ACE-I therapy, when the RAS is blocked and only the vasopressin system is left to compensate. It has been shown that the incidence of hypotension in this population is close to 75% to 100% if the ACE-I is continued until the day of surgery and is reduced to less than 20% if the medication is withheld the day prior to surgery.[3] Moreover, Kheterpal et al. demonstrated that patients on chronic diuretic therapy in addition to ACE-I had more frequent episodes of hypotension in the perioperative period.[2]

The treatment for ACE-I/general anesthesia induced hypotension is multimodal. Resuscitation with fluid (either crystalloid or colloid) may help expand the intravascular volume and improve cardiac output and systolic blood pressure. Sympathetic agonists, such as ephedrine, phenylephrine, and epinephrine should be administered concomitantly with fluid resuscitation. However, the drug of choice for ACE-I induced hypotension remains a V1-receptor agonist like vasopressin, in 1 unit bolus increments (with repeated doses until systolic artery pressure is restored) with an infusion of vasopressin as necessary to restore the blood pressure to within 30% of baseline.[3] In 2010, Papadopoulos et al. showed that low-dose infusion of vasopressin is beneficial to coronary artery bypass graft patients who are hemodynamically unstable because of vasodilatory vasoplegic syndrome secondary to ACE-I and low ejection fraction.[4] Terlipressin, a long-acting synthetic analog of vasopressin, has been studied for treatment of ACE-I induced hypotension. However, it was found to be less optimal than norepinephrine because of intense vasoconstriction, a reflex decrease in cardiac output with accompanying decrease in splanchnic blood flow resulting in significant decrease in gastric mucosal perfusion.[5]

To best avoid perioperative hypotension secondary to chronic ACE-I therapy, the current recommendation is to discontinue the medication the day prior to surgery, or for minimum of 10 hours.[6] As suggested by Augoustides, future studies should focus on strategies to minimize the risk for perioperative hypotension associated with angiotensin blockade and whether extension of the preoperative discontinuation period is necessary.[7]

Take-Home Points

- Intraoperative hypotension in patients chronically treated with ACE inhibitors presents the anesthesiologist with a potentially challenging problem when conventional methods of regulating blood pressure are unsuccessful.

- The final product of the RAS cascade, angiotensin II, is involved in maintaining blood pressure via vasoconstriction, increasing aldosterone secretion for sodium and water reabsorption, and stimulating catecholamine release.

- Patients on chronic ACE-I therapy presenting for general anesthesia are more prone to developing profound hypotension, particularly if they have concomitant use of diuretics.
- Given that the vasopressin is the only compensatory mechanism left to maintain hemodynamics in this population, small vasopressin boluses with or without infusion is the treatment of choice for ACE-I induced hypotension.

Summary

Interaction: pharmacodynamic
Substrates: captopril and general anesthesia
Mechanism/site of action: depression of sympathetic nervous system by general anesthesia and depression of the renin-angiotensin system by the ACE-I, loss of compensatory mechanism
Clinical effects: profound, refractory hypotension

References

1. Colson P, Ryckwaert F, et al. Renin-angiotensin system antagonists and anesthesia. Anesth Analg. 1999;89:1143–55.
2. Kheterpal S, et al. Chronic angiotensin-converting enzyme inhibitor or angiotensin receptor blocker therapy combined with diuretic therapy is associated with increased episodes of hypotension in noncardiac surgery. J Cardiothorac Vasc Anesth. 2008;22(2):180–6.
3. Brabant S, Bertrand M, et al. The hemodynamic effects of anesthetic induction in vascular surgical patients chronically treated with angiotensin II receptor antagonists. Anesth Analg. 1999;89(6):1388–92.
4. Papadopoulos G, Sintou E, et al. Perioperative infusion of low-dose of vasopressin for prevention and management of vasodilatory vasoplegic syndrome in patients undergoing coronary artery bypass grafting – a double-blind randomized study. J Cardiothorac Surg. 2010;5:17.
5. Morelli A, Tritapepe L, et al. Terlipressin versus norepinephrine to counteract anesthesia-induced hypotension in patients treated with renin-angiotensin system inhibitors: effects on systemic and regional hemodynamics. Anesthesiology. 2005;102:12–9.
6. Coriat P, Richer C, et al. Incidence of chronic angiotensin-converting enzyme inhibition on anesthetic induction. Anesthesiology. 1994;81:299–307.
7. Augoustides J. Angiotensin blockade and general anesthesia: so little known, so far to go. J Cardiothorac Vasc Anesth. 2008;22(2):177–9.

Too Young to Die

120

Fatal Forty DDI: bupropion, pseudoephedrine, pharmacodynamic interaction

Catherine Marcucci MD

Abstract
This case discusses the pharmacodynamic interaction between bupropion and pseudoephedrine, resulting in myocardial ischemia and infarction.

Case

A 27-year-old male Jehovah's Witness presented to the operating room for repair of multiple injuries after sustaining a left open femoral fracture, a severe scalp laceration, and a severe tongue laceration when he bit through his tongue after jumping down a steep ravine to join some friends at a beach party. He had a history of depression and childhood asthma. His medications were bupropion 100 mg twice a day. He received prehospital fluid resuscitation of unknown type and volume. His toxicology screen was negative for cocaine, opioids, and marijuana. His last known hemoglobin was 8.1 g/dL. His patient directive stated that he refused packed red blood cells under all circumstances.

The surgeons called into the room to make sure the anesthesia team realized that a nasal endotracheal tube would be required. He was placed on the operating room table and his heart rate was noted to be 122 beats per minute and his blood pressure was 88/42 mm Hg. He was reassured, sedated with midazolam, and a small fluid bolus was given. Post sedation, his blood pressure was noted to be 78/40 mm Hg. The anesthesia attending asked the resident to give a small amount of phenylephrine and to topicalize the patient's nose with pseudoephedrine, stating, "That should get his blood pressure up a little and spare him a little fluid administration."

C. Marcucci MD
Anesthesia Services Department, Philadelphia Veterans Affairs Medical Center, Philadelphia, PA, USA
e-mail: sandson.marcucci@comcast.net

C. Marcucci et al. (eds.), *A Case Approach to Perioperative Drug-Drug Interactions*, DOI 10.1007/978-1-4614-7495-1_120

Five minutes later, the patient began complaining of chest pain. He became diaphoretic and nauseated. The monitor showed significant ST-segment elevations and the hemoglobin was now 5.9 g/dL. The patient's family confirmed that the anesthesia team should abide by the patient's wishes that he not be transfused. The patient was intubated with difficulty and transferred to the intensive care unit where he expired 2 days later.

This is an example of a pharmacodynamic interaction.

Bupropion is an antitypical antidepressant that is a norepinephrine and dopamine reuptake inhibitor. It also stimulates the release of both catecholamines. It is one of the few antidepressants that does not cause sexual dysfunction, so is commonly prescribed for young adults.

Pseudoephedrine is a commonly used decongestant, both in the outpatient setting and by otolaryngologists. It is a sympathomimetic drug, chemically related to the phenethylamine and amphetamine chemical classes.

There have been a number of reports of myocardial ischemia and myocardial infarction with coadministration of bupropion and pseudoephedrine in young adults presumably through sympathetic-mediated coronary vasospasm.[1–3] This patient's poor oxygen-carrying capacity due to his acute anemia was a potentiating factor in his cardiac decompensation.

Take-Home Points

- Take time to ascertain which of your patient's outpatient medications are sympathomimetic. Have a healthy respect for the catecholamine reuptake blockers.
- Coadministration of sympathomimetics can have severe consequences, even in young adults with good cardiovascular health.

Summary

Interaction: pharmacodynamic
Substrates: bupropion and pseudoephedrine
Mechanism/site of action: combined effect of catecholamine reuptake inhibition and sympathomimetic effects
Clinical effect: myocardia ischemia and myocardial infarction

References

1. Pederson KJ, Kuntz DH, Garbe GJ. Acute myocardial ischemia associated with ingestion of bupropion and pseudoephedrine in a 21-year-old man. Can J Cardiol. 2001;17(5):599–601.
2. Manini AF, Kabrhel C, Thomsen TW. Acute myocardial infarction after over-the-counter use of pseudoephedrine. Ann Emerg Med. 2005;45(2):213–6.
3. Wiener I, Tilkian AG, Palazzolo M. Coronary artery spasm and myocardial infarction in a patient with normal coronary arteries: temporal relationship to pseudoephedrine ingestion. Cathet Cardiovasc Diagn. 1990;20(1):51–3.

A Widening Gyre

Epinephrine, phosphorus, insulin

121

Edward A. Kahl MD and Michael P. Hutchens MD

Turning and turning in the widening gyre
The falcon cannot hear the falconer;
Things fall apart; the centre cannot hold

-W.B. Yeats

Abstract
This case discusses the pharmacodynamic interactions of epinephrine, insulin, and phosphorus in the post-cardiopulmonary bypass patient.

Case

An otherwise healthy 64-year-old woman underwent mitral valve replacement requiring a prolonged cardiopulmonary bypass run. She arrived in the intensive care unit (ICU) late in the afternoon suffering from combined cardiogenic and vasodilatory shock. She was on epinephrine at 0.08 mcg/kg/min and high-dose vasoconstrictors as well as an insulin infusion, running at 20 units an hour. Her admission blood sugar was very elevated despite the insulin infusion and remained difficult to control. On admission labs, her serum phosphate was critically low, and was replaced, per protocol, over 6 hours.

During the night, the patient's cardiogenic shock remained critical, despite the addition of a milrinone infusion. The early morning serum phosphate was again critically low. The night call physician ordered a higher dose of potassium phosphate repletion, given over 2 rather than 6 hours. The ICU nurse noted that after the first hour, the patient's cardiac index had significantly improved, and over the ensuing hours

E.A. Kahl MD (✉) • M.P. Hutchens MD
Department of Anesthesiology and Perioperative Medicine, Oregon Health and Science University, Portland, OR, USA
e-mail: kahle@ohsu.edu

C. Marcucci et al. (eds.), *A Case Approach to Perioperative Drug-Drug Interactions*, DOI 10.1007/978-1-4614-7495-1_121

before morning rounds, the epinephrine, milrinone, and vasoconstrictors were rapidly weaned down, with maintenance of hemodynamic stability. Insulin requirements also declined.

On morning rounds, the patient was noted to be greatly improved, and orders were written to titrate the insulin, epinephrine, and vasoconstrictor infusions off in the early hours. Potassium was again supplemented. Renal and electrolyte assessment were ordered for the early afternoon.

In the mid-afternoon, the ICU physician was paged by the lab to report a serum potassium of 6.0. The patient was given insulin, dextrose, and enteral sodium polystyrene; and the hyperkalemia had completely resolved by evening without any sequelae. In fact, overnight, further potassium supplementation was required.

Discussion

This is an example of a complex pharmacodynamic interaction between epinephrine, insulin, and electrolytes, administered in the situation of hypophosphatemia and cardiogenic shock.

Epinephrine is a pleiotropic catecholamine hormone, which is released in times of stress and frequently administered for the treatment of cardiogenic shock. It is a β-adrenergic receptor agonist that increases myocardial contractility. Effects on other organ systems include reduced insulin secretion, increased glycogenolysis, hypokalemia, hyperlactatemia, and hypophosphatemia.[1]

In this case, the patient's initial hypophosphatemia likely contributed to her postcardiopulmonary bypass cardiogenic shock, increasing her requirements for epinephrine and inotropic support. The increase in epinephrine, in turn, worsened her hypophosphatemia and hyperglycemia. The worsening hypophosphatemia contributed to worsening cardiogenic shock; and the worsening hyperglycemia contributed to worsening hypophosphatemia.[2,3] Like the falcon leaving the falconer, the epinephrine, despite controlled and appropriate administration, became the vehicle of a chaotic, destructive cascade. When this cascade was interrupted with aggressive phosphate repletion, and with time to recover from the insult of bypass, the patient's cardiac function rapidly improved.

The ICU providers correctly responded to this improvement in cardiac function by rapidly and successfully weaning inotropes and vasoconstrictors. Removing epinephrine reduced insulin requirements. At the same time, however, removing the epinephrine increased serum potassium by allowing its release from skeletal muscle stores, and coupled with the withdrawal of insulin, this effect was exaggerated.

Although the patient's serum potassium was transiently elevated, it was rapidly cleared in the presence of normal renal function, and probably would have been even without medical treatment.

It is not uncommon for patients to present to the ICU with cardiogenic and/or vasodilatory shock after cardiac surgery. There are many causes for these hemodynamic derangements. As illustrated in this case, prolonged cardiopulmonary bypass with a cardioplegic and arrested heart, and electrolyte disturbances, were the primary etiologies. It is extremely important that all physicians who care for critically ill patients be aware of the side effects of epinephrine. As seen here, epinephrine is used to treat cardiogenic shock, but its side effects of hypophosphatemia (and hyperglycemia leading to hypophosphatemia) can also exacerbate the very condition it is intended to treat.[4] Additionally, rapid weaning of epinephrine and insulin together can result in hyperkalemia if the epinephrine and insulin are significantly contributing to lowering of potassium.

Take-Home Points

- Cardiac surgery patients may frequently present with cardiogenic and/or vasodilatory shock requiring treatment with epinephrine.
- Hypophosphatemia may worsen cardiogenic shock and increase the need for pressor and inotropic support.
- Epinephrine can cause side effects of hypophosphatemia (and hyperglycemia leading to hypophosphatemia) that can exaggerate the conditions the epinephrine was intended to treat.
- Phosphorus deficiencies should be promptly identified and treated.
- Rapid weaning of epinephrine and insulin can result in hyperkalemia.

Summary

Interaction: pharmacodynamic (complex)
Substrates: epinephrine, insulin, phosphorus
Mechanism: reduced insulin secretion, exacerbation of shock through epinephrine-mediated hypophosphatemia, rapid weaning of epinephrine and insulin
Clinical effects: persistent cardiogenic shock, hypophosphatemia, and hyperglycemia

References

1. Body J, Cryer PE, Offord KP, Heath III H. Epinephrine is a hypophosphatemic hormone in man. Physiological effects of circulating epinephrine on plasma calcium, magnesium, phosphorus, parathyroid hormone, and calcitonin. J Clin Invest. 1983;71(3):572–8.
2. Swaminathan R, Morgan DB, Ionescu M, et al. Hypophosphataemia and its consequences in patients following open heart surgery. Anaesthesia. 1978;33(7):601–5.
3. Daniel A, Geerse DA, Alexander J, Bindels AJ, Michael A, Kuiper MA, et al. Treatment of hypophosphatemia in the intensive care unit: a review. Crit Care. 2010;14(4):R147.
4. Betro MG, Pain RW. Hypophosphataemia and hyperphosphataemia in a hospital population. Br Med J. 1972;1(5795):273–6.

Misusing Mom's Meds

122

Chronic amphetamine, indirect-acting sympathomimetics

Pulsar Li DO and Steven L. Orebaugh MD

Abstract

This case discusses the pharmacodynamic interaction seen with catecholamine depletion seen with chronic amphetamine and indirect acting sympathomimetics.

Case

A 20-year-old otherwise healthy man was seen in the preoperative holding area in preparation for an elective inguinal herniorrhaphy. He admitted to slight anxiety and drinking a few beers the day before to calm himself down. He denied other licit and illicit drug use. His vital signs were remarkable for a persistent heart rate of 95 beats per minute (bpm) and mildly elevated blood pressure of 137/89 mm Hg. He had surprisingly bad dentition for a young man and slightly decreased skin turgor. He received midazolam (2 mg) for preoperative sedation.

After an uneventful induction of anesthesia, the patient received sevoflurane, fentanyl, and vecuronium. After incision, the patient's blood pressure gradually drifted to a range of 100 s/40 s mm Hg with a heart rate of about 70 bpm. The hypotension persisted despite a 500 mL fluid and two doses of ephedrine (10 mg) each were provided, and the blood pressure drifted to 90/40 mm Hg. The patient finally responded to two divided doses of 200 mcg phenylephrine but required this every 20 minutes of the procedure to maintain a systolic pressure of 130 mm Hg. A phenylephrine drip was started and normotension was restored and maintained.

P. Li DO (✉)
Department of Anesthesiology, University of Pittsburgh Medical Center, Pittsburgh, PA, USA
e-mail: lip3@upmc.edu

S.L. Orebaugh MD
Department of Anesthesiology & Critical Care, University of Pittsburgh School of Medicine, Pittsburgh, PA, USA

C. Marcucci et al. (eds.), *A Case Approach to Perioperative Drug-Drug Interactions*, DOI 10.1007/978-1-4614-7495-1_122

Postoperatively, the patient remained normotensive on the phenylephrine drip. He was asked once again if he utilized any illicit drugs and he then admitted a 2-year history of methamphetamine abuse, supplied by his mother's prescription for narcolepsy. A urine drug screen was positive for cannabinoids and amphetamines. The patient was admitted to the intensive care unit and the phenylephrine was weaned. He was referred to the endocrinology service to rule out adrenal insufficiency, referred to an outpatient addiction program, and advised of the common and life-threatening withdrawal symptoms associated with amphetamine use.

Discussion

This is an example of an antagonistic pharmacodynamic interaction at the transmitter level.

Careful intraoperative blood pressure control is important to optimize perfusion to vital organs. Maintaining a mean arterial pressure within the cerebral autoregulation range (between 50 mm Hg and 140 mm Hg) helps to ensure adequate cerebral perfusion pressure. Blood pressure can be controlled in a number of different ways. Before immediately administering large doses of pressor agents, a thoughtful analysis of a potential underlying cause should take place. These considerations include obstruction to cardiac output, such as embolism or tension pneumothorax, and widespread vasodilation occurring with sepsis or systemic inflammatory conditions. Volume status, potentially affected by surgical blood loss, other fluid losses, or NPO status should also be considered. In a patient with adequate cardiac reserve, fluid boluses can be helpful in diagnosing and treating hypovolemia. Perhaps most commonly in anesthesia, vasodilatory drugs are the cause of hypotension. In this case, pressors such as ephedrine, phenylephrine, and vasopressin may then be used to increase arterial pressure.

Patients actively abusing cocaine and amphetamines are at risk for intraoperative hemodynamic instability. A thorough preoperative assessment evaluating for substance use should be performed. Some symptoms and signs of amphetamine use include paranoia, increased wakefulness, "meth mouth" (extensive tooth decay due to drug-induced psychological and physiological changes resulting in dry mouth and long periods of poor oral hygiene), pupil dilation, hallucinations, seizures, and violent behavior.[1] If abuse is suspected, urine testing can be helpful to ensure the absence of these substances before proceeding. Because inadequate analgesia can potentially activate addiction, optimization of analgesia with nonopioids and regional techniques should be considered and discussed with the patient.

In this case, the patient's history of chronic methamphetamine abuse caused hypotension refractory to ephedrine administration. Methamphetamine's active metabolite, amphetamine, is a sympathomimetic amine that stimulates the release of norepinephrine, directly stimulating α and β-receptors. This results in increased arterial pressure, tachycardia, cardiac arrhythmias, weak bronchodilatation, mydriasis, and bladder sphincter contraction.[1] Long term use may lead to ventricular hypertrophy, myocardial necrosis, and nasal septal perforation.[1] At higher doses, the drug stimulates release of dopamine, which can result in behavioral changes. At even higher doses, amphetamine stimulates the release of 5-hydroxytryptamine (5-HT), which can result in psychotic behavior seen in some heavy users.

As an indirect agonist, methamphetamine is associated with tachyphylaxis due to the decreasing supply of endogenous neurotransmitter. As a result, chronic abusers of methamphetamine may become catecholamine-depleted and further, may have poor responses to the usual doses of other indirect-acting sympathomimetics.[2] For example, ephedrine is an indirect-acting sympathomimetic that releases norepinephrine and is commonly used in the hypotensive parturient, or in mild hypotension associated with bradycardia. Repeat administration of this drug in addition to the patient's chronic abuse of methamphetamine contributed to its poor effect in the case described. Phenylephrine, which is not subject to tachyphylaxis since it is a direct-acting α_1-agonist, was utilized more effectively to raise the blood pressure to an acceptable range. In summary, this case highlights the importance of eliciting a substance abuse history in every adult patient, even if it is not necessarily suspected. Hemodynamic instability due to chronic methamphetamine abuse is best treated with phenylephrine or other direct-acting sympathomimetics.

Take-Home Points

- Both methamphetamines and ephedrine are indirect sympathomimetics, exerting their effects through the release of catecholamines from secretory granules of preganglionic sympathetic neurons.
- Chronic use of methamphetamine can deplete these intracellular stores of catecholamines, causing tachyphylaxis and ineffectiveness of other indirect sympathomimetics such as ephedrine.
- Use of direct-acting sympathomimetics to maintain sympathetic tone is recommended, since it directly stimulates postganglionic receptors.
- A complete preoperative assessment requires an understanding of the patient's elicit substance use. If the patient is not forthcoming, subtle physical signs such as "meth mouth," restlessness, and paranoia may build suspicion to guide the anesthetic management.

Summary

Interaction: pharmacodynamic (antagonism)
Substrates: amphetamines and indirectly acting sympathomimetic agents
Mechanism/site of action: preganglionic sympathetic neurons
Clinical effect: loss of efficacy of indirectly acting sympathomimetic agents

References

1. Cruickshank CC, Dyer KR. A review of the clinical pharmacology of methamphetamine. Addiction. 2009;104(7):1085–99. Epub 2009 Apr 29.
2. Johnston RR, Way WL, Miller RD. Alteration of anesthetic requirement by amphetamine. Anesthesiology. 1972;36(4):357–63.

If the Patient Has No Renal Failure, Why Is Her Potassium So High?

123

Candesartan, spironolactone

Jennifer A. Rabbitts MB, ChB,
Wayne T. Nicholson MD, PharmD, MSc,
and Juraj Sprung MD, PhD

Abstract
This case discusses the pharmacodynamic interaction between candesartan and spironolactone, resulting in hyperkalemia. Candesartan is angiotensin II receptor blocker and spironolactone is a potassium-sparing diuretic.

Case

A 52-year-old woman presented to the preoperative area before a scheduled cholecystectomy for chronic cholecystitis. Her symptoms consisted of biliary colic and nausea but no vomiting. She had a history of hypertension and mild congestive heart failure and was taking spironolactone (25 mg once daily), amlodipine (5 mg once daily), metoprolol (25 mg BID), and candesartan (8 mg once daily). Six weeks ago, she had the second of two monthly follow-up visits with her physician after starting candesartan therapy 2 months earlier. At that follow-up, she was in good health and her test results showed normal electrolyte values, a creatinine value of 1.0 mg/dL, a

J.A. Rabbitts MB, ChB (✉)
Department of Anesthesiology, Seattle Children's Hospital and University of Washington, Seattle, WA, USA
e-mail: jennifer.rabbitts@seattlechildrens.org

W.T. Nicholson MD, PharmD, MSc • J. Sprung MD, PhD
Department of Anesthesiology, Mayo Clinic, Rochester, MN, USA

C. Marcucci et al. (eds.), *A Case Approach to Perioperative Drug-Drug Interactions*, DOI 10.1007/978-1-4614-7495-1_123

normal complete blood cell count, and echocardiogram results unchanged from the previous study. No further testing was undertaken before her operation, in accordance with the American Society of Anesthesiologists Task Force on Preanesthesia Evaluation, which states that test results within 6 months of surgery are adequate if no substantial changes in medical history have occurred since the testing.[1] The only additional concern during the preoperative assessment was that the patient was obese; although the result of her airway examination was reassuring, the anesthesiologist decided to administer succinylcholine in case difficulty arose with airway management.

In the operating room, while waiting for the patient's initial blood pressure reading on the monitor before administering anesthesia induction drugs, the anesthesiologist noticed that the QRS complex appeared widened, the T waves were peaked, and P waves were absent on the echocardiogram tracings. He called for a 12-lead echocardiogram and asked for immediate electrolyte testing. The echocardiogram appeared suspicious for hyperkalemia, and the electrolyte values showed a potassium level of 7.6 mEq/L. The procedure was cancelled, and the patient was admitted to the hospital for emergency treatment of hyperkalemia.

While in the operating room, the patient initially received calcium gluconate intravenously and albuterol by continuous nebulizer, as well as insulin with dextrose to shift potassium from the extracellular to the intracellular space until definitive treatment could be given. Subsequently, she received furosemide and sodium polystyrene sulfonate to promote excretion of potassium through the kidneys and the gastrointestinal tract, respectively. Two days later, the patient underwent an uncomplicated cholecystectomy after her potassium level had normalized (4.2 mEq/L) and was discharged to home with amlodipine, metoprolol, candesartan, and furosemide.

Discussion

This is an example of a complex synergistic pharmacodynamic interaction.

The combination of spironolactone and an angiotensin II receptor blocker (ARB) can cause life-threatening hyperkalemia.[2,3] In this clinical setting, administration of succinylcholine, which causes an additional increase in potassium (approximately 0.5 mEq/L), can lead to cardiovascular arrest. The timing of risk for hyperkalemia after starting or adding therapy with these medications is uncertain. There have been case reports of normal potassium levels for several months after addition of one of these medications, with subsequent severe hyperkalemia.[3] The hyperkalemia may occur at any dose; however, the risk increases with greater-than-normal doses, dose escalation, and longer-acting medications. The risk increases further with β-blockers or nonsteroidal anti-inflammatory drugs and decreases with thiazides or a loop diuretics. Risk for hyperkalemia also increases with advanced age, poorly controlled diabetes mellitus (severe hyperglycemia can osmotically shift potassium extracellularly), renal insufficiency (creatinine, >2.0 mg/dL), and acute illness or dehydration.[2]

The Candesartan in Heart Failure: Assessment of Reduction in Mortality and Morbidity (CHARM) trial, which established the role of candesartan for heart failure treatment, was analyzed separately for incidence and predictors of clinically important hyperkalemia.[2,4] The data showed positive interaction between spironolactone and candesartan in the development of clinically important hyperkalemia, defined as hyperkalemic events either requiring dose reduction, drug discontinuation, or hospitalization or resulting in death. The incidence of clinically significant hyperkalemia increased mildly with spironolactone, moderately with candesartan, and markedly (to 9.2%) with a candesartan and spironolactone combination (Table 123.1).

Patients who take a combination of these medications likely will be seen more commonly because ARBs, spironolactone, angiotensin-converting enzyme inhibitors, and β-blockers have been shown to reduce left ventricular systolic dysfunction and mortality in heart failure in a large, diverse patient population.[4] Therefore, it is essential that anesthesiologists are aware of this potentially serious complication.

The mechanisms of hyperkalemia caused by ARBs and aldosterone antagonists when used alone are well known. Spironolactone is a pharmacologic antagonist of aldosterone, primarily through competitive binding of mineralocorticoid receptors at the aldosterone-dependent sodium-potassium exchange site in the late distal renal tubule and collecting duct. Aldosterone antagonism causes increased excretion of sodium and water while potassium is retained. Spironolactone acts as both a diuretic and an antihypertensive through this mechanism.[5] Candesartan blocks the vasocon-

Table 123.1 Incidence of Clinically Significant Hyperkalemia in Heart Failure Patients in the CHARM Trial

	Spironolactone		
Candesartan		No	Yes
	No	1.8%	1.9%
	Yes	4.4%	**9.2%**

[Based on data from ref. 2]
Abbreviation: CHARM, Candesartan in Heart Failure: Assessment of Reduction in Mortality and Morbidity.

strictor and aldosterone-secreting effects of angiotensin II by selectively blocking the binding of angiotensin II to the angiotensin AT_1-receptor in many tissues, including vascular smooth muscle and adrenal gland. Additionally, angiotensin-converting enzyme inhibitors have identical potential for hyperkalemia through decreased angiotensin II production. With prevention of angiotensin II–induced stimulation of aldosterone release, increased amounts of sodium and water are excreted and potassium is retained. Potassium needs to be considered when these agents are used concomitantly, especially since the expected effects of candesartan and spironolactone on potassium are inadequate to explain the extent of the synergistic interaction shown in CHARM trial analysis.

β-Blockers may increase the risk for hyperkalemia by β_2-receptor blockade, thereby decreasing skeletal muscle uptake of potassium or inhibiting renin secretion from the juxtaglomerular apparatus.[2,6] Nonsteroidal anti-inflammatory drugs may increase potassium through inhibition of renin secretion. Other medications to consider in combination with these drugs include other potassium-sparing diuretics (eg, amiloride hydrochloride, triamterene, eplerenone), aliskiren (competitive inhibitor of renin), sotalol hydrochloride (β-blocking effects), and potassium supplements. Additionally, in drug-induced hyperkalemia, succinylcholine administration may result in cardiac arrest. Succinylcholine causes a potassium increase of 0.3 to 0.5 mEq/L in patients with normal muscle. This response is caused through binding of acetylcholine receptors, resulting in increased permeability at the acetylcholine receptor during depolarization and thereby causing potassium efflux.[7] Table 123.2 summarizes important agents that can result in hyperkalemia.

Table 123.2 Agents That May Cause Hyperkalemia

Agents	Mechanism and Comments
Amiloride (Midamor) and triamterene (Dyrenium)	Diminishes potassium secretion by reducing the electrical gradient between the intracellular space and the renal tubule, causing potassium to leave the cells
Amino acids[a]	Lysine, arginine, or epsilon-aminocaproic acid enters cells in exchange for potassium, causing hyperkalemia
ARBs and ACE inhibitors	Decreases aldosterone synthesis; hyperkalemia often can be reduced by concomitant diuretic use; ARBs less likely to cause hyperkalemia than ACE inhibitors
Azole antifungals	Inhibits adrenal steroid synthesis, which can lead to aldosterone deficiency
β-blockers	Decreases sodium-potassium adenosine triphosphatase (ATPase) activity; β_2 agonists decrease potassium levels
Cyclosporine (Sandimmune)	Suppresses renin release, leading to decreased aldosterone synthesis, decreased potassium secretion in collecting duct
Digoxin at toxic levels	Decreases sodium-potassium ATPase activity
Eplerenone (Inspra)	Blocks aldosterone binding at mineralocorticoid receptors

(continued)

Table 123.2 (continued)

Agents	Mechanism and Comments
Ethinyl estradiol/drospirenone (Yasmin)	Spironolactone analogue
Fluoride toxicity	Decrease aldosterone synthesis; most common in patients on dialysis who drink water with high fluoride levels
Glucose infusions or insulin deficiency	Hypertonicity caused by hyperglycemia from glucose infusions can drive potassium out of the intracellular space, leading to hyperkalemia. Hyperkalemia may occur with continuous infusions or with boluses of hypertonic glucose. May be present with hypertonicity caused by other agents such as mannitol (Osmitrol) as well
Heparins	Can cause hyperkalemia in patients with decreased renal function; inhibits adrenal aldosterone synthesis
Herbal remedies with digitalis-like effect	Specific agents include milkweed, lily of the valley, Siberian ginseng, Hawthorn berries, or preparations from dried toad skin (Bufo, Chan'su, Senso). All these agents act by decreasing sodium-potassium ATPase activity, leading to elevated extracellular potassium
NSAIDs	Decreased prostaglandin production leads to decreased afferent arteriolar flow, suppressing renin and aldosterone secretion. Typical of NSAIDs as well as cyclooxygenases-2 selective inhibitor drugs
Nutritional and herbal supplements	Herbs containing high potassium levels (eg, Noni juice, alfalfa, dandelion, horsetail, nettle)
Packed red blood cells	Stored cells can partially hemolyze and release potassium when infused
Penicillin G potassium	Can cause hyperkalemia in patients with impaired renal function caused by increased potassium load; can be administered orally or intravenously
Potassium supplements or salt substitutes	Ingestion of potassium can lead to hyperkalemia, particularly if renal function is impaired; dietary sources include bananas, melon, and orange juice
Spironolactone (Aldactone)	Inhibits binding of aldosterone to receptors in the renal tubule
Succinylcholine (Anectine)	Increases nicotinic acetylcholine receptors in damaged skeletal muscle (eg, trauma or burn patients)
Tacrolimus (Prograf)	Suppresses renin release, leading to decreased aldosterone synthesis and decreased potassium secretion in collecting duct
Trimethoprim (Proloprim) and pentamidine (Pentam 300)	Diminishes potassium secretion by reducing the electrical gradient between the intracellular space and the renal tubule, causing potassium to leave the cells

ARB = angiotensin receptor blockers; ACE-angiotensin-converting enzymes; NSAID = nonsteroidal anti-inflammatory drug

[a]Hyperkalemia can occur in the setting of amino acids administered intravenously as part of total parenteral nutrition. It is unknown whether oral dietary amino acid supplements cause hyperkalemia

[Reprinted from Hollander-Rodriguez JC, Calvert Jr. JF. Hyperkalemia. American Family Physician 2006;283-290 with permission from American Academy of Family Physicians.]

Take-Home Points

- The CHARM trial reported a 4.4% incidence of clinically significant hyperkalemia in patients taking candesartan and a 9.2% incidence in patients taking both candesartan and spironolactone. It is important that clinicians be vigilant for this drug combination and ask the patient about recent drug addition or dosage change.

- Patients may have hyperkalemia, after having normal potassium levels for several months, since 1) starting treatment with these medications, 2) having one of these medications added, or 3) having a dose escalation several months prior, despite no recent change. Therefore, electrolyte levels should be rechecked in these patients even when recent test results have been normal.

- Additional risk factors for hyperkalemia in patients taking these medications include greater-than-normal drug doses, dose escalation, longer-acting medications, concomitant β-blockers or nonsteroidal anti-inflammatory drugs, advanced age, diabetes, renal insufficiency (creatinine, >2.0 mg/mL), and acute illness or dehydration. These factors are commonly present in patients coming for surgery.

- In patients at risk for acute hyperkalemia, a review of the electrocardiogram on the operating room monitor before anesthetic induction may help to detect features of this potentially severe electrolyte disturbance.

Summary

Interaction: pharmacodynamic
Substrates: candesartan (and other angiotensin II receptor blockers) and spironolactone, (and other potassium-sparing diuretics), and metoprolol (and other β-blockers)
Mechanism/sites of action: competitive binding of mineralocorticoid receptors at the aldosterone-dependent sodium-potassium exchange site in the late distal renal tubule and collecting duct, selective blockade of the binding of angiotensin II to the angiotensin AT_1-receptor in many tissues, including vascular smooth muscle and adrenal gland, blockade of β_2 receptors
Clinical effects: hyperkalemia

References

1. American Society of Anesthesiologists Task Force on Preanesthesia Evaluation. Practice advisory for preanesthesia evaluation: a report by the American Society of Anesthesiologists Task Force on Preanesthesia Evaluation. Anesthesiology. 2002;96:485–96.
2. Desai AS, Swedberg K, McMurray JJ, et al. CHARM Program Investigators: Incidence and predictors of hyperkalemia in patients with heart failure: an analysis of the CHARM Program. J Am Coll Cardiol. 2007;50:1959–66.
3. Fujii H, Nakahama H, Yoshihara F, et al. Life-threatening hyperkalemia during a combined therapy with the angiotensin receptor blocker candesartan and spironolactone. Kobe J Med Sci. 2005;51:1–6.
4. Bhakta S, Dunlap ME. Angiotensin-receptor blockers in heart failure: evidence from the CHARM trial. Cleve Clin J Med. 2004;71:665–73.
5. Aldactone [package insert]. New York: G. D. Searle LLC; 2008.
6. Saito M, Nakayama D, Takada M, et al. Carvedilol accelerate elevation of serum potassium in chronic heart failure patients administered spironolactone plus furosemide and either enalapril maleate or candesartan cilexetil. J Clin Pharm Ther. 2006;31:535–40.
7. Gronert GA, Theye RA. Pathophysiology of hyperkalemia induced by succinylcholine. Anesthesiology. 1975;43:89–99.

Prazosin and the PTSD Paratrooper

124

Prazosin, tadalafil

Allen N. Gustin MD, FCCP and Michael J. Bishop MD

Abstract

This case discusses α_1-adrenergic blockade by prazosin and PDE 5-mediated hypotension by tadalafil in the presence of local anesthetic-induced sympathectomy

Case

A 54-year-old male veteran with a history of posttraumatic stress disorder (PTSD) arrived at the preoperative holding area for bilateral knee replacements after suffering injuries to both knees while serving as a paratrooper in Desert Storm. He was taking prazosin to alleviate PTSD-associated nightmares and insomnia, his knee pain was treated with occasional hydrocodone/acetaminophen, and he used tadalafil for sexual dysfunction. Preoperatively, a lumbar epidural catheter was place for both the intraoperative anesthetic management and for the postoperative pain management. The patient's blood pressure remained between 110/60 mm Hg and 125/81 mm Hg during the insertion of the lumbar epidural catheter. A lidocaine test dose was given to the patient and was assessed negative when the patient reported no heart rate change and no other symptoms.

In the operating room, a bolus dose of 10 cc of lidocaine 2% was administered into the lumbar epidural catheter with a subsequent decrease in blood pressure to

A.N. Gustin MD, FCCP (✉)
Department of Anesthesia and Critical Care, University of Chicago Pritzker School of Medicine, Chicago, IL, USA
e-mail: agustin@dacc.uchicago.edu

M.J. Bishop MD
Department of Anesthesiology, University of Washington School of Medicine, Seattle, WA, USA

C. Marcucci et al. (eds.), *A Case Approach to Perioperative Drug-Drug Interactions*, DOI 10.1007/978-1-4614-7495-1_124

60/40 mm Hg. The patient was resuscitated with multiple fluid and phenylephrine boluses, but the blood pressure remained 60/40 mm Hg. The patient became somnolent and more difficult to arouse and required intubation. A radial artery line was placed and the patient was given boluses of epinephrine and vasopressin. A blood pressure of 80/58 mm Hg was finally achieved and sustained. The operative case was cancelled and the patient went to the ICU with a central venous catheter and an epinephrine infusion. Over the next 90 minutes, the patient's blood pressure stabilized and the epinephrine infusion was weaned and the patient aroused and was extubated without difficulty.

Discussion

This is an example of a pharmacodynamic interaction involving multiple individual drug effects leading to a cumulative effect at the end-organ (vascular) level.

The exact mechanism of action of the hypotensive action of prazosin is unknown. Prazosin causes a decrease in total peripheral resistance and recent studies have suggested that the vasodilator effect of prazosin is also related to blockade of postsynaptic α_1-adrenoceptors. Unlike conventional α_1-blockers, the antihypertensive action of prazosin is usually not accompanied by a reflex tachycardia. Hemodynamic studies have been carried out in patients following single dose administration and during the course of long-term maintenance therapy using prazosin. The results confirm that the therapeutic effect is a fall in blood pressure unaccompanied by any clinically significant change in cardiac output, heart rate, renal blood flow, or glomerular filtration rate. Following oral administration, human plasma concentrations reach a peak at about 3 hours with a plasma half-life of 2 to 3 hours. The drug is highly bound to plasma protein. Bioavailability studies have demonstrated that the total absorption relative to the drug is 90%. Excretion of the drug occurs via hepatic metabolism.[1]

Prazosin is being used increasingly for the treatment of PTSD. PTSD is a disabling anxiety disorder seen in 25% to 30% of individuals experiencing a traumatic event.[2] An estimated 70-87% of patients who suffer from posttraumatic stress experience sleep disruption – difficulty falling asleep and staying asleep, as well as distressing nightmares where the traumatic event is reexperienced.[3] Selective serotonin reuptake inhibitors are the usual pharmaceutical treatment for PTSD, but they are often ineffective or only partially effective for sleep problems. Some sedative-hypnotics (tranquilizers, barbiturates, etc) may be helpful in the short term but are associated with tolerance and addiction. In the central nervous system, α_1-adrenergic receptors are known to be important in both the startle and sleep responses. Stimulation of these receptors may contribute to PTSD-related trauma-content nightmares. The α_1-blocker prazosin has been shown to decrease trauma nightmares in both combat veterans and patients with non-combat-related PTSD.[3] The available data, although mostly from open-label trials, suggest that prazosin improves sleep quality, sense of well-being, and ability to function in daily activities in those patients with PTSD.[3] Orthostatic hypotension following initiation of prazosin is a known hazard and is monitored when the drug is started in patients with PTSD.

Tadalafil (Cialis®) is used in the treatment of sexual dysfunction. The physiologic mechanism of erection of the penis involves release of nitric oxide (NO) in the corpus cavernosum during sexual stimulation. NO then activates the enzyme guanylate cyclase, producing smooth muscle relaxation in the corpus cavernosum and allowing inflow of blood.

Tadalafil (itself) has no direct relaxant effect on isolated human corpus cavernosum, but enhances the effect of (NO) by inhibiting phosphodiesterase type 5 (PDE 5). When sexual stimulation causes local release of NO, inhibition of PDE 5 by tadalafil causes increased levels of cyclic guanosine monophosphate (cGMP) in the corpus cavernosum, resulting in smooth muscle relaxation and inflow of blood to the corpus cavernosum. Tadalafil at recommended doses has no effect in the absence of sexual stimulation.[4]

After one oral dose, tadalafil reaches peak plasma concentrations around 2 hours and has an average elimination half-life of 17.5 hours.[4] Thus, tadalafil has the longest duration of action of any of the oral PDE 5 inhibitors. Tadalafil's pharmacokinetics are dose proportional over the recommended dose range. It is eliminated predominantly by hepatic metabolism and is converted to an active metabolite with properties similar to the parent molecule. The concomitant use of cytochrome P450 (CYP) 3A4 inhibitors (eg, erythromycin, ketoconazole, itraconazole) can increase plasma levels of tadalafil well beyond the already long half-life of 17.5 hours.

Studies have shown small additive drops in blood pressure when PDE 5 inhibitors were given to patients already taking α or β blockers, calcium blockers, angiotensin converting enzyme inhibitors, angiotensin receptor blockers, and diuretics. An exception to these findings can be the α or β-blockers, which in some patients may be associated with an increase in orthostatic hypotension when administered with PDE 5 inhibitors. α-blockers may be used for treating hypertension, benign prostatic hypertrophy, PTSD sleep disturbances, or all of the above. When used together, PDE 5 inhibitors and α_1-blockers are associated with hypotension (systolic blood pressure < 85 mm Hg).[5]

As of June 2006, a change occurred in the labeling bringing the precaution for sildenafil and α_1-blockers in line with that of the other PDE 5 inhibitors. The wording for the precaution is now: "Caution is advised when PDE 5 inhibitors are coadministered with $\alpha_1$blockers." PDE5 inhibitors (tadalafil) and α_1-adrenergic blocking agents (prazosin) are both vasodilators with blood pressure-lowering effects.[5] When vasodilators are used in combination, an additive effect on blood pressure may be anticipated. In some patients, concomitant use of these two drug classes can lower blood pressure significantly; leading to symptomatic hypotension (eg, dizziness, light headedness, fainting).

The precaution goes on to suggest that patients should be on stable α_1-blocker therapy before PDE 5 inhibitors are started and that lowest doses of the PDE 5 inhibitor be used to initiate therapy. Conversely, if a patient is already taking an optimal dose of a PDE 5 inhibitor and an α_1-blocker needs to be started, the α_1-blocker should be started at the lowest dose. Other variables such as intravascular volume status and use of other antihypertensives should be considered when using a combination of both a PDE 5 inhibitor and an α_1-blocker.[5]

Thus, all three PDE 5 inhibitors now carry precautions regarding the use of α_1-blockers, warning of the possible development of orthostatic hypotension with drug combination, but no longer are the PDE 5 inhibitors contraindicated with α_1-blockers.[5]

α-blockers in combination with PDE 5 inhibitors increase risk for hypotension with anesthesia. Each α_1-blocker and each oral PDE 5 inhibitor have warnings regarding the risk for hypotension when added together. Either agent has the ability to interact with one another to produce orthostatic hypotension. Awake and unanesthetized patients might tolerate the drug combination well. When both drugs are present during anesthetics that provide sympathetic blockade (epidural, spinal, or other anesthetic agents), the potential for hypotension can be high. Patients should be educated to avoid the use of PDE 5 inhibitors during the immediate preoperative period. Given the increasing proportion of combat veterans with diagnosed PTSD and given the benefits of α_1-blockers/PDE 5 inhibitors in PTSD symptom control, more patients may present to the operating room with combinations of both of these agents. It is necessary for anesthesiologists to be aware of this potential interaction and be prepared for the potential hypotension that may arise in the operating room when these patients are exposed to anesthesia.

Take-Home Points

- Patients with PTSD show alleviation of symptoms of nocturnal symptoms when prescribed the α_1-blocker prazosin.
- Prazosin is an α_1-adrenergic receptor blocker used primarily for the treatment of hypertension, symptoms of PTSD, and benign prostatic hypertrophy.
- Patients with sexual dysfunction have improvement in their symptoms with the use of PDE 5 inhibitors.

- Tadalafil is a PDE 5 inhibitor used to treat sexual dysfunction and has a long duration of action.

- Patients taking both α_1-blockers and PDE 5 inhibitors are cautioned of the risks of orthostatic hypotension.

- Patients taking both α_1-blockers and PDE 5 inhibitors may develop severe hypotension under anesthesia, during which sympathetic blockade may occur.

- Anesthesia providers should be aware of the potential risks of hypotension and should make preparations to minimize the impact/treat the symptoms of any observed hypotension.

Summary

Interaction: pharmacodynamic (end-organ)
Substrates: prazosin, tadalafil, lidocaine
Mechanism/site of action: α_1-adrenergic blockade by prazosin and PDE 5-mediated hypotension by tadalafil in the presence of local anesthetic-induced sympathectomy
Clinical effects: severe, refractory hypotension

References

1. Prazosin [package insert]. New York: Pfizer Inc; 2004.
2. Hildago RB, Davidson JR. Posttraumatic stress disorder: epidemiology and health related considerations. J Clin Psychiatry. 2006;61 Suppl 7:5–13.
3. Miller LJ. Prazosin for the treatment of post traumatic stress disorder sleep disturbances. Pharmacotherapy. 2008;28(5):656–66.
4. Tadalafil [package insert]. New York: Elli Lilly Inc.; 2005.
5. Klover RA. Pharmacology and drug interaction effects of the PDE 5 inhibitors: focus on alpha blocker interaction. Am J Cardiol. 2005;96 Suppl 2:42–6.

Nicardipine Notes

125

Fatal Forty DDI: nicardipine, tacrolimus, CYP3A4

Nenna Nwazota MD and Randal O. Dull MD, PhD

Abstract
This case discusses an interaction between tacrolimus and nicardipine. Tacrolimus is a cytochrome P450 3A4 substrate and nicardipine is a 3A4 inhibitor. The interaction resulted in tacrolimus toxicity. The pharmacokinetics of nicardipine are also discussed.

Case

A 20-year-old, 72 kg Caucasian man underwent uncomplicated living-related kidney transplantation for end-stage renal disease caused by obstructive uropathy following a failed, primary kidney transplantation, due to chronic allograft nephropathy. The evening prior to surgery he received a 5 mg dose of tacrolimus, and he did not receive any the next morning

In the immediate postoperative period, adequate urine output was noted and maintenance immunosuppression was started with tacrolimus (5 mg BID), mycophenolate mofetil and prednisone. The patient was noted to be hypertensive. A nicardipine infusion at a rate of 1 mcg/kg/min was started and was quickly increased to 3 mcg/kg/min for improved blood pressure control. He also received extended release nifedipine (60 mg orally) and oral labetalol overnight. On postoperative day 1, his initial tacrolimus trough level was 16.3 ng/mL (target range 12-18 ng/mL). He was maintained on the nicardipine infusion and oral extended release nifedipine. The tacrolimus dose was adjusted to 2.5 mg that evening and 4.0 mg the next morning. His

N. Nwazota MD (✉)
Department of Anethesiology, Baylor College of Medicine, Houston, TX, USA
e-mail: Nenna.nwazota@gmail.com

R.O. Dull MD, PhD
Department of Anesthesiology, University of Illinois at Chicago, Chicago, IL, USA

C. Marcucci et al. (eds.), *A Case Approach to Perioperative Drug-Drug Interactions*, DOI 10.1007/978-1-4614-7495-1_125

urine output decreased from 850 mL/h to 50 mL/h despite careful fluid management and a stable creatinine of 1.7 mg/dL for 24 hours.

The nicardipine infusion was discontinued after 33 hours. The 12-hour tacrolimus trough level drawn on the morning of postoperative day 2 was markedly elevated at 50 ng/mL and the trough level drawn that evening was severely elevated 84.8 ng/mL. Tacrolimus was held until trough levels fell to 9.6 ng/mL on postoperative day 5, at which time tacrolimus was reinstated at 2 mg twice daily. At this point, urine output had increased and creatinine had fallen to 1.5 mg/dL. Over the next 2 days tacrolimus dosing was increased to 6 mg twice daily to achieve trough levels around 10 ng/mL despite continued therapy with oral extended release nifedipine at 120 mg BID.[2]

Discussion

This is an example of an inhibitor added to a substrate.

The clinical scenario above is a good example of the potential for adverse drug reactions among compounds with known cytochrome activity. In this case elevated plasma concentrations of tacrolimus, a known cytochrome P450 (CYP) 3A4 substrate, were observed in the setting of coadministration with a 3A4 inhibitor (nicardipine).

Both nicardipine and tacrolimus have been shown to have dual roles as inhibitors and substrates for cytochrome activity. Nifedipine is also a substrate of 3A4, but it generally does not act as a competitive inhibitor of 3A4. Nicardipine is a dihydropyridine calcium channel antagonist used to treat many cardiac conditions including hypertension. It has well-documented interactions with 3A4.[3,6] Recent studies suggest additional inhibition of CYP2B6, CYP2C9, and CYP2D6.[3] Tacrolimus, a calcineurin inhibitor commonly used in the management of solid organ transplant, has demonstrated inhibitory effects on 3A4 and 3A5. however, the clinical significance of this is questionable given this effect was only seen at concentrations above 1 micromole.[1,4]

Several factors predispose the inhibition of the hepatic cytochrome system by nicardipine, namely its amine functional group and ability to produce reactive metabolites.[7] More studies are needed to investigate the potential for adverse drug interactions between nicardipine and other compounds. However, it is important to use caution when coadministering nicardipine with the following anesthetic drugs, which are known P450 substrates: benzodiazepines, propofol, and certain narcotics (hydrocodone, oxycodone, codeine).[5]

Take-Home Points

- Tacrolimus is metabolized mainly by CYP3A4.
- Nicardipine is a potent inhibitor of CYP3A4 and has milder inhibitory effects on CYP2B, CYP2C9, and CYP2D6.
- Vigilance in the form of therapeutic drug monitoring is very important when coadministering cytochrome substrates with significant metabolic inhibitors.

Summary

Interaction: pharmacokinetic
Substrate: tacrolimus
Enzyme: CYP3A4
Inhibitor: nicardipine
Clinical effects: tacrolimus toxicity

References

1. Amundsen R, Asberg A, Ohm I, et al. Cyclosporine A and tacrolimus mediated inhibition of cytochrome P450 3A4 and 3A5 in vitro. Drug Metab Dispos. 2011. [Epub ahead of print].
2. Hooper D, Carle A, Schuchter J, et al. Interaction between tacrolimus and intravenous nicardipine in the treatment of post-kidney transplant hypertension at pediatric hospitals. Pediatr Transplant. 2011;15:88–95.
3. Katoh M, Nakajima M, Shimada N, et al. Inhibition of human cytochrome P450 enzymes by 1,4-dihydropyridine calcium antagonists: prediction of in vivo drug-drug interactions. Eur J Clin Pharmacol. 2000;55:843–52.
4. LeCointre K, Furlan V, Taburet A. *In vitro* effects of tacrolimus on human cytochrome P450. Fundam Clin Pharm. 2022;16:455–60.
5. Roth S, Munoz R, Schmitt C, et al. Vasodilators. In: Munoz R, Schmitt C, Roth S, editors. Handbook of pediatric cardiovascular drugs. London: Springer; 2008. p. 77–119.
6. Zangar R, Okita J, Kim H, et al. Effect of calcium channel antagonists nifedipine and nicardipine on rat cytochrome P-450 2B and 3A Forms. J Pharmacol Exp Ther. 1999;290:1436–41.
7. Zhou S, Xue C, Yu X, et al. Clinically important drug interactions potentially involving mechanism-based inhibition of cytochrome P450 3A4 and the role of therapeutic drug monitoring. Ther Drug Monit. 2007;29:687–710.

Hypotension Harry

126

Fatal Forty DDI: nicardipine, clarithromycin, CYP3A4

Matthew Hart MSN, CRNA, Bryan J. Read MSN, CRNA, Wayne T. Nicholson MD, PharmD, MSc, and Toby N. Weingarten MD

Abstract

This case discusses a pharmacokinetic interaction between nifedipine and clarithromycin resulting in hypotension. Nifedipine is a cytochrome P450 3A4 substrate and clarithromycin is a 3A4 inhibitor.

Case

Harry was a 55-year-old physically active construction worker who enjoyed relatively good health except for hypertension and recurrent sinus infections. He woke up one morning with a sensation of pain and pressure over his right maxilla and green purulent drainage from his right nostril. He went to an urgent care center where he was diagnosed with a sinus infection and prescribed a 7-day course of extended-release clarithromycin. After 3 days he felt lightheaded upon waking. He fainted at work and was taken to the emergency room of the community hospital where he was found to be bradycardic and hypotensive. He was admitted to the intensive care unit (ICU), resuscitated with intravenous fluids, and placed on a dopamine infusion to support his hemodynamics.

M. Hart MSN, CRNA (✉) • B.J. Read MSN, CRNA
Department of Anesthesiology & Perioperative Medicine, Oregon Health and Science University, Portland, OR, USA
e-mail: hartma@ohsu.edu

W.T. Nicholson MD, PharmD, MSc
Department of Anesthesiology, Mayo Clinic, Rochester, MN, USA

T.N. Weingarten MD
Patient Education, Mayo Clinic, Rochester, MN, USA

C. Marcucci et al. (eds.), *A Case Approach to Perioperative Drug-Drug Interactions*, DOI 10.1007/978-1-4614-7495-1_126

Fortunately for the patient, the intensivist had very recently trained at an academic center with a robust didactic program on drug–drug interactions (DDIs). The ICU physician also had taken the time during training to discuss with the SICU pharmacologist the importance of reviewing the medication list for DDIs at the time of admission. Thus, our well-trained young ICU doctor was not surprised to discover on review of Harry's medications that he was on extended release nifedipine to treat hypertension and he immediately recognized a significant DDI with clarithromycin. He was administered intravenous calcium chloride which resulted in normalization of his hemodynamic instability. The clarithromycin was discontinued and Harry made a full recovery.

Discussion

This is an example of an inhibitor added to a substrate.

Nifedipine is a dihydropyridine calcium channel antagonist that is commonly used to treat cardiovascular disorders including hypertension. Nifedipine undergoes extensive oxidative biotransformation in the hepatic microsomes into pharmacologically inactive metabolites.[1] The cytochrome P450 (CYP) 3A subfamily (ie, CYP3A4, 3A5, and 3A7) all have a role in oxidative metabolism with CYP3A4 providing the greatest contribution to nifedipine clearance.[2] Although oral nifedipine is well absorbed, due to extensive first pass-metabolism the oral bioavailability of nifedipine is approximately 50%.[1] In addition to hepatic metabolism, intestinal CYP3A4 may contribute to the first pass-metabolism of nifedipine, however studies are mixed as to the degree.[3] Other commonly used calcium channel blockers both dihydropyridine (eg, amlodipine) and non-dihydropyridine (diltiazem and verapamil) are also substrates of the 3A subfamily.[4]

Clarithromycin is a macrolide antibiotic used to treat upper respiratory infections that is metabolized by the cytochrome P450 3A subfamily and primarily by CYP3A4.[2,5] Clarithromycin is also a potent inhibitor of CYP3A, and it has been shown to inhibit metabolism of nifedipine in both *in vitro* and *in situ* animal models.[5,6] Clinically relevant inhibition of metabolism caused by clarithromycin is known to occur with many CYP3A substrates.[4,5] Additionally, the combination of nifedipine and clarithromycin has been reported to result in hypotension and cardiac instability, which are signs of calcium channel antagonist overdose.[6,7]

Take-Home Points

1. Nifedipine and other calcium channel blockers are extensively metabolized by CYP3A4.

2. Clarithromycin is also metabolized by CYP3A4, but also inhibits its activity that can affect the pharmacokinetics of other drugs dependent on CYP3A4 metabolism.

3. Inhibition of CYP3A4 can result in increased plasma levels of nifedipine and lead to nifedipine toxicity.

4. Drugs undergoing a large first-pass metabolism may result in serious adverse drug reactions following inhibition of their metabolism.

5. Knowledge of and surveillance for DDIs should begin in training. The ICU pharmacologists are there to help!

Summary

Interaction: pharmacokinetic
Substrate: nifedipine
Enzyme: CYP3A4
Inhibitor: clarithromycin
Clinical effects: prolonged and enhanced effect of nicardipine leading to hypotension

References

1. Kleinbloesem CH, van Brummelen P, van de Linde JA, et al. Nifedipine: kinetics and dynamics in healthy subjects. Clin Pharmacol Ther. 1984;35(6):742–9.
2. Williams JA, Ring BJ, Cantrell VE, et al. Comparative metabolic capabilities of CYP3A4, CYP3A5, and CYP3A7. Drug Metab Dispos. 2002;30(8):883–91.
3. Lin JH, Chiba M, Baillie TA. Is the role of the small intestine in first-pass metabolism overemphasized? Pharmacol Rev. 1999;51(2):135–58.
4. Flockhart DA. Drug Interactions: Cytochrome P450 Drug Interaction Table. Indiana University School of Medicine. 2007. http://medicine.iupui.edu/clinpharm/ddis/table.aspx. Accessed 30 May 2012.
5. Rodrigues AD, Roberts EM, Mulford DJ, et al. Oxidative metabolism of clarithromycin in the presence of human liver microsomes. Major role for the cytochrome P4503A (CYP3A) subfamily. Drug Metab Dispos. 1997;25:623–30.
6. Tsuruta S, Nakamura K, Arimori K, et al. Effects of erythromycin, clarithromycin and rokitamycin on nifedipine metabolism in rats. Biol Pharm Bull. 1997;20:411–6.
7. Geronimo-Pardo M, Cuartero-del-Pozo AB, Jimenez-Vizuete JM, et al. Clarithromycin-nifedipine interaction as possible cause of vasodilatory shock. Ann Pharmacother. 2005;39:538–42.

Too Slow to Flow

CYP2D6 ultraslow metabolism of metoprolol

127

Scott W. Cantwell MD, Toby N. Weingarten MD, and Juraj Sprung MD, PhD

Abstract
This case discusses a drug–gene interaction involving and ultraslow metabolism of metoprolol by a cytochrome P450 (CYP) 2D6 allele, leading to excessive bradycardia in the clinical setting of a high dermatomal level of spinal anesthetic.

Case

A 72-year-old man with a history of hypertension, diabetes mellitus, and coronary artery presented to the operating room for a right total-knee arthroplasty. Two weeks before surgery, his primary care physician initiated therapy with metoprolol (25 mg orally BID) to reduce the risk for perioperative myocardial ischemia.

In the preoperative holding area, the anesthesiologist noted that the patient had a heart rate of 45 beats per minute (bpm). However, the patient was normotensive and denied symptoms of orthostatic hypotension. Because the patient's previous total knee arthroplasty under spinal anesthesia had gone well, spinal anesthesia was planned for this procedure as well. After a one liter fluid bolus an uncomplicated spinal anesthesia of bupivacaine (15 mg) and preservative-free morphine (0.5 mg) was given.

Ten minutes later, the patient complained of feeling light-headed and had moderate hypotension that resolved with phenylephrine (100 mcg). However, over the next 20 minutes, the patient's heart rate gradually declined to 30 bpm, he vomited and lost

S.W. Cantwell MD (✉)
Kansas Professional Anesthesia & Pain Management Specialists, Wichita, KS, USA
e-mail: Cantwell.scott@gmail.com

T.N. Weingarten MD • J. Sprung MD, PhD
Department of Anesthesiology, Mayo Clinic, Rochester, MN, USA

C. Marcucci et al. (eds.), *A Case Approach to Perioperative Drug-Drug Interactions*, DOI 10.1007/978-1-4614-7495-1_127

consciousness. Asystole was observed on the cardiac monitor. Appropriate resuscitation was administered including intubation, chest compressions, and intravenous epinephrine (1 mg). His heart rate returned to sinus tachycardia, followed by normal sinus rhythm, and he became normotensive. The case was cancelled and the patient was transferred to the ICU, where he was extubated and had no further adverse sequelae.

The cardiology service was consulted. During the interview with the cardiologist, the patient reported that several years ago he had a very slow heart rate when he tried metoprolol therapy, which had been discontinued at that time. Following this consultation, the current metoprolol therapy was discontinued. After a night on the telemetry ward, the patient was discharged home. Two weeks later he returned and underwent total knee arthroplasty under spinal anesthetic without incident.

Discussion

This is an example of a drug–gene interaction.

Metoprolol is a lipophilic, β_1-selective adrenergic receptor antagonist regularly used in the management of cardiovascular diseases. It undergoes 50% metabolism on first pass through the liver, during which cytochrome P450 (CYP) 2D6 is the major enzyme, to the inactive metabolites α-hydroxymetoprolol and *O*-demethylmetoprolol.[1–3] A small percentage (<10%) of metoprolol is excreted unchanged in the urine.

The *CYP2D6* gene is polymorphic with approximately 80 alleles and allele variants. Five specific phenotypes of CYP2D6 have been identified and have varying abilities to metabolize medications: ultrarapid metabolizers, extensive metabolizers, extensive metabolizers with reduced activity, intermediate metabolizers, and poor metabolizers. Individuals with poor 2D6 metabolism have two nonfunctioning alleles. Approximately 7% to 10% of the caucasian population has the poor 2D6 metabolizer phenotype.[4] In persons with poor 2D6 metabolism, the elimination half-life of metoprolol is increased from 2.8 hours to 7.5 hours compared with patients who have extensive 2D6 metabolism.[1]

In a prospective double-blind study, Rau et al showed that study participants who were poor CYP2D6 metabolizers had metoprolol plasma concentrations 4.9-fold greater than participants who did not have poor metabolism (Fig. 127.1).[5] This difference resulted in a more marked reduction in heart rate and blood pressure.

In the present case, the patient most probably had poor 2D6 metabolism, as evidenced by his bradycardic response to a modest dose of metoprolol, as well as his previous history of intolerance to metoprolol. Even though he tolerated this medication preoperatively, the β-adrenergic antagonism produced through the metoprolol therapy inhibited a normal cardiac response to the vasodilatation from the spinal anesthetic

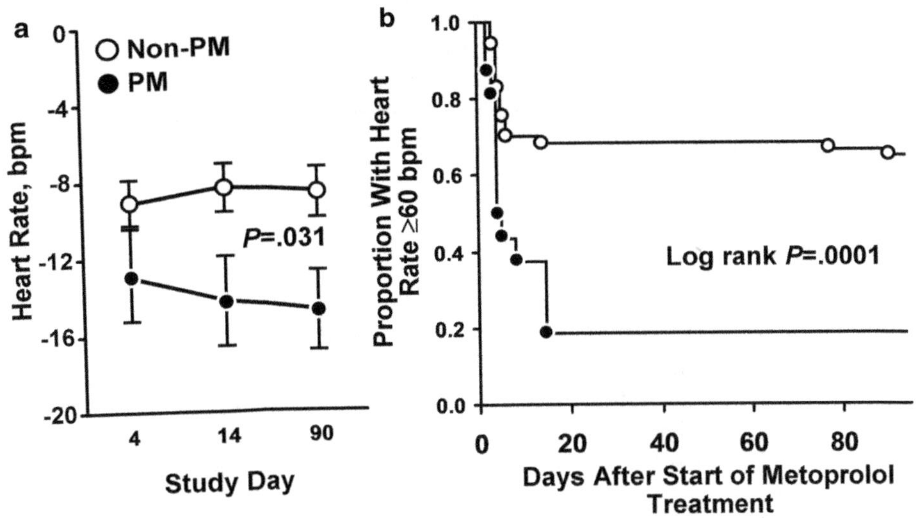

Fig. 127.1 Effect of the *CYP2D6* genotype on metoprolol-evoked heart rate reduction. A, Change in heart rate from baseline at study time points according to *CYP2D6* genotype. Heart rate changes were more pronounced in persons with poor CYP2D6 metabolism (PMs) than persons without the poor metabolism (non-PMs). B, Kaplan-Meier analysis of the time elapsed between the start of metoprolol treatment and the first occurrence of a heart rate less than 60 bpm (as determined by electrocardiogram). bpm indicates beats per minute. Error bars represent the standard error of the mean [Adapted from Rau T, Wuttke H, Michels LM et al. Impact of the CYP2D6 genotype on the clinical effects of metoprolol: a prospective longitudinal study. *Clin Pharmacol Ther.* 2009;85: 269–272. With permission from Nature Publishing Group.]

and he became hypotensive. When the nurse anesthetist placed the patient in Trendelenburg position in response to hypotension, the bupivacaine was allowed to spread cephalad, where it inhibited the cardiac acceleration fibers (T1-4). The combination of profound β-adrenergic antagonism and high spinal anesthetic resulted in the development of asystole.

Take-Home Points

- Metoprolol is metabolized in the liver by CYP2D6.
- The *CYP2D6* gene has many alleles and five specific phenotypes that affect medication metabolism. One of these phenotypes is termed *poor metabolizer* and makes up a considerable proportion (7%-10%) of the caucasian population.
- Persons with poor CYP2D6 metabolism have an increased plasma concentration of metoprolol compared with other phenotypes, and consequently they are more likely to have an increased clinical response.

- When bupivacaine in a dextrose solution is used for spinal anesthetic, the anesthesia provider must be aware that changes in patient position affect the spread of the local anesthetic. In such circumstances, Trendelenburg position results in a more cephalad spread and increases the possibility of a high spinal response.

Summary

Interaction: pharmacogenomic (drug–gene)
Substrate: metoprolol
Enzyme: CYP2D6
Polymorphism: poor CYP2D6 metabolizer
Clinical effect: poor metabolism of metoprolol causing bradycardia further complicating a high dermatomal level of spinal anesthetic

References

1. Lennard MS, Silas JH, Freestone S, et al. Oxidation phenotype: a major determinant of metoprolol metabolism and response. N Engl J Med. 1982;307:1558–60.
2. McGourty JC, Silas JH, Lennard MS, et al. Metoprolol metabolism and debrisoquine oxidation polymorphism: population and family studies. Br J Clin Pharmacol. 1985;20:555–66.
3. Kendall MJ, Maxwell SR, Sandberg A, et al. Controlled release metoprolol: clinical pharmacokinetic and therapeutic implications. Clin Pharmacokinet. 1991;21:319–30.
4. Sachse C, Brockmoller J, Bauer S, et al. Cytochrome P450 2D6 variants in a Caucasian population: allele frequencies and phenotypic consequences. Am J Hum Genet. 1997;60:284–95.
5. Rau T, Wuttke H, Michels LM, et al. Impact of the CYP2D6 genotype on the clinical effects of metoprolol: a prospective longitudinal study. Clin Pharmacol Ther. 2009;85:269–72.

Better Sleep but Slower Heart

128

Metoprolol, diphenhydramine, CYP2D6

Erica D. Wittwer MD, PhD and Juraj Sprung MD, PhD

Abstract
This case discusses the pharmacokinetic interaction between metoprolol and diphenhydramine. Metoprolol is a cytochrome P450 2D6 substrate. Diphenhydramine is a 2D6 inhibitor. Coadministration results in metoprolol toxicity.

Case

A 55-year-old woman presented for a right breast mastectomy for breast cancer. Three days earlier she had an open breast biopsy under general anesthesia in a small rural medical center. She had a history of hypertension for which she was taking metoprolol (50 mg BID). After finding out the results of her biopsy and that she needed to undergo radical mastectomy with possible axillary lymph node dissection, she decided to have the procedure done in a larger medical center. Her husband reported that the patient's elderly mother used Tylenol PM® (acetaminophen 500 mg and diphenhydramine 25 mg) for joint pain and as a mild soporific and the patient had been taking three of her mother's Tylenol PM capsules per day to alleviate pain from the breast biopsy site and get some sleep. The patient had even been able to sleep a little bit during the day when she felt drowsy.

In the preoperative holding area, the patient reported feeling lightheaded and fatigued and appeared tired. Her heart rate was 30 beats per minute (bpm) and blood pressure was 85/50 mm Hg. The electrocardiogram (ECG) showed sinus bradycardia. Although the patient insisted that she had not changed her regimen for taking metoprolol lately, the anesthesiologist was concerned that her hemodynamic parameters were indicative of excessive ß-receptor blockade with metoprolol. Her husband had

E.D. Wittwer MD, PhD (✉) • J. Sprung MD, PhD
Department of Anesthesiology, Mayo Clinic, Rochester, MN, USA
e-mail: Wittwer.erica@mayo.edu

C. Marcucci et al. (eds.), *A Case Approach to Perioperative Drug-Drug Interactions*, DOI 10.1007/978-1-4614-7495-1_128

her medical records from her local hospital with him that revealed that during the biopsy procedure the patient's heart rates was 55 bpm and her blood pressure was 125/85 mm Hg. The mastectomy was canceled and she was admitted to a monitored care ward overnight where she was treated with glycopyrrolate and ephedrine, and the regular evening dose of metoprolol was withheld. Over the next 12 hours, her heart rate and blood pressure increased and she felt better subjectively. She underwent the planned surgical procedure the following day.

Discussion

This is an example of an inhibitor added to a substrate.

More specifically, this is an example of metoprolol toxicity associated with concomitant use of diphenhydramine.

Metoprolol blocks β_1-adrenergic receptors and is commonly used in the treatment of hypertension, angina, and congestive heart failure. It is metabolized via the cytochrome P450 2D6 enzyme (CYP2D6), which is responsible for approximately 25% of all biotransformation by cytochromes, including antidepressants, antipsychotics, antiemetics, codeine, dextromethorphan, H_1-antihistamines, and some cardiac drugs. With respect to CYP2D6, individuals can be described as poor metabolizers, with no active copies of the *CYP2D6* allele, extensive metabolizers, with at least one active copy of the allele, or ultra-rapid metabolizers, with three or more copies of the allele. Extensive metabolizers metabolize drugs normally, while poor metabolizers and ultra-rapid metabolizers have decreased and increased metabolism, respectively.

Diphenhydramine, an over-the-counter H_1-antihistamine drug, is metabolized primarily by CYP2D6 and has also been shown to inhibit the 2D6 enzyme in a concentration-dependent fashion.[1] Concurrent diphenhydramine administration can slow metoprolol metabolism, increase serum metoprolol levels and therefore potentiate negative chronotropic activity.[2] The pharmacokinetics and pharmacodynamics of metoprolol and its interaction with diphenhydramine were examined in a randomized, double-blind, crossover, placebo-controlled manner in healthy, premenopausal extensive and poor metabolizers.[2] Diphenhydramine coadministration in extensive metabolizers caused a 2.2- to 3.2-fold decrease in total clearance of metoprolol enantiomers with a resulting 21% increase in area under the effect curve (AUEC) and shifted the pharmacokinetic profile of extensive metabolizers towards that of poor metabolizers.[2] The maximum concentration of metoprolol achieved (C_{max}) in extensive metabolizers was increased by 30% after administration of diphenhydramine and the area under the concentration versus time curve (AUC) was increased two-fold. However, diphenhydramine did not alter the disposition of metoprolol or α-hydroxymetoprolol in women that were poor metabolizers beyond the effects resulting from their genetic constellation (Fig. 128.1).

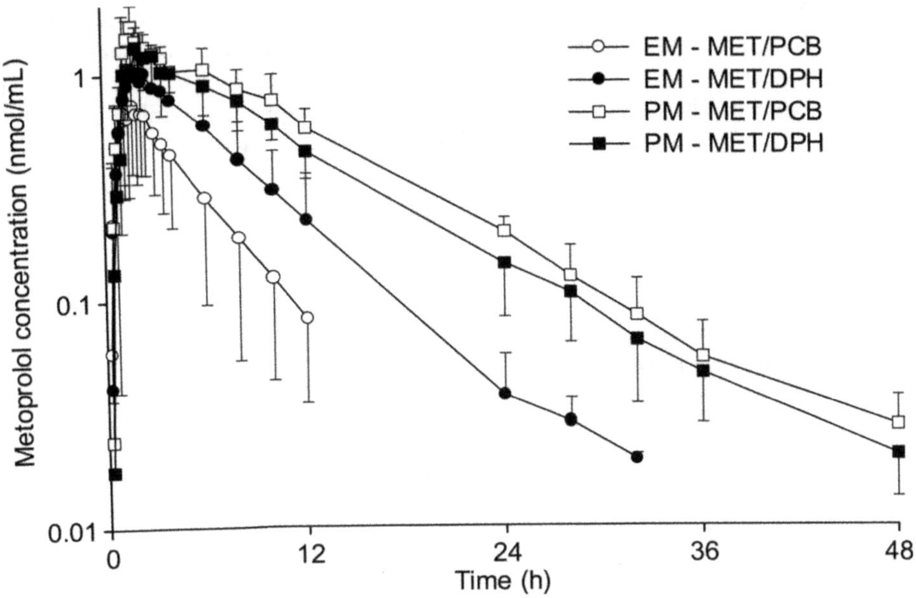

Fig. 128.1 Pharmacokinetic profile of racemic metoprolol in 16 extensive and 4 poor metabolizer women after the administration of a single oral dose of 100 mg of metoprolol tartrate with or without concomitant administration of diphenhydramine or placebo to steady state. Results presented as mean ± SD, MET, metoprolol; PCB, placebo; DPH, diphenhydramine [Reprinted from Sharma A, Pibarot P, Pilote S et al. Modulation of metoprolol pharmacokinetics and hemodynamics by diphenhydramine coadministration during exercise testing in healthy premenopausal women. *J Pharmacol Exp Ther*. 2005;313:1172–81. With permission from American Society for Pharmacology and Experimental Therapeutics]

Women are particularly vulnerable to this effect and have been shown to have a greater decrease in heart rate when diphenhydramine is administered with metoprolol.[2,3] When our patient repeatedly took Tylenol PM® at home to treat her pain (acetaminophen) and insomnia (diphenhydramine) she induced an alteration in metoprolol pharmacokinetics and pharmacodynamics by diphenhydramine, leading to an increase in serum metoprolol concentrations, resulting in bradycardia and hypotension.

Take-Home Points

- Over-the-counter diphenhydramine and the other H_1-antihistamines are metabolized by CYP2D6 and also can inhibit this enzyme.
- Individuals who are CYP2D6 extensive metabolizers (90% of population) may have increased side effects or toxicity from other medications metabolized via the CYP2D6 enzyme during coadministration.

- Metoprolol is a frequently prescribed cardiac medication and its metabolism is predominantly mediated by the CYP2D6 system, the same system that can be inhibited by diphenhydramine. This effect is more prominent in women. Therefore, caution is required when diphenhydramine is repeatedly administered to patients receiving metoprolol therapy.

Summary

Interaction: pharmacokinetic
Substrate: metoprolol
Enzyme: CYP2D6
Inhibitor: diphenhydramine
Clinical effects: bradycardia and hypotension due to metoprolol toxicity

References

1. He N, Zhang WQ, Shockley D, Edeki T. Inhibitory effects of H1-antihistamines on CYP2D6- and CYP2C9-mediated drug metabolic reactions in human liver microsomes. Eur J Clin Pharmacol. 2002;57:847–51.
2. Sharma A, Pibarot P, Pilote S, et al. Modulation of metoprolol pharmacokinetics and hemodynamics by diphenhydramine coadministration during exercise testing in healthy premenopausal women. J Pharmacol Exp Ther. 2005;313:1172–81.
3. Sharma A, Pibarot P, Pilote S, et al. Toward optimal treatment in women: the effect of sex on metoprolol-diphenhydramine interaction. J Clin Pharmacol. 2010;50:214–25.

Extreme Blood Pressure After Ephedrine: Should We Rule Out Pheochromocytoma?

129

Ephedrine, selegiline

Erica D. Wittwer MD, PhD, Juraj Sprung MD, PhD, and Wayne T. Nicholson MD, PharmD, MSc

Abstract

This case discusses a pharmacokinetic interaction between selegiline and ephedrine-induced norepinephrine resulting in hypertension.

Case

A 54-year-old morbidly obese man was scheduled for gastric bypass surgery. He had a history of type 2 diabetes treated with rosiglitazone, depression treated with selegiline (12-mg transdermal patch daily), and obstructive sleep apnea managed with nightly continuous positive airway pressure. The patient took no medications for hypertension.

After an uneventful induction and intubation, the resident tried to place a radial artery catheter while the attending placed a second intravenous line. The resident had not placed many arterial lines and tried for several minutes without success. At this point, the resident reported that she no longer felt a strong pulse. The patient's noninvasive blood pressure was 70/35 mm Hg, and ephedrine (10 mg) was administered. The subsequent blood pressure was 81/45 mm Hg, and again ephedrine (20 mg) was administered. Two minutes later, the resident reported detecting an improved radial pulse, and she successfully cannulated the artery. After the arterial

E.D. Wittwer MD, PhD (✉) • J. Sprung MD, PhD • W.T. Nicholson MD, PharmD, MSc
Department of Anesthesiology, Mayo Clinic, Rochester, MN, USA
e-mail: Wittwer.erica@mayo.edu

C. Marcucci et al. (eds.), *A Case Approach to Perioperative Drug-Drug Interactions*, DOI 10.1007/978-1-4614-7495-1_129

line was transduced, the resident and the consultant were surprised to see a blood pressure of 210/100 mm Hg and a heart rate of 140 beats per minute.

After treating with labetalol, the anesthesia team discussed whether the patient could have an undiagnosed pheochromocytoma and recommended that the case be postponed. The patient's blood pressure stabilized at 140/75 mm Hg and heart rate at 90 beats per minute in the recovery room, and he was sent to the step-down unit. Work-up results for a pheochromocytoma were negative. The next day, the operating room pharmacist mentioned to the resident that the patient was taking selegiline for depression and suggested that the excessive hypertension after ephedrine was administered in the operating room would be a good topic for the residents' conference that week.

Discussion

This is an example of a pharmacodynamic drug–drug interaction.

More specifically, this is an example of a pharmacodynamic interaction of a monoamine oxidase inhibitor (selegiline) interfering with the metabolism of norepinephrine, released because of ephedrine administration.

Selegiline is a monoamine oxidase B (MAO-B) inhibitor used to treat Parkinson's disease and depression. It binds irreversibly to inhibit the enzyme responsible for dopamine metabolism, through which it treats Parkinson's disease. Although selegiline is considered to selectively inhibit MAO-B enzyme, there is evidence that it also inhibits monoamine oxidase A (MAO-A), particularly at higher dosages.[1,2] MAO-A metabolizes norepinephrine and serotonin, along with dopamine. Inhibition of MAO-A may lead to serotonin syndrome because of inhibition of serotonin metabolism, as well as hypertension secondary to the inhibition of norepinephrine metabolism.[3,4]

Ephedrine is both an α- and β-agonist that also acts by triggering the release of norepinephrine, increasing heart rate and blood pressure through action on α_1 and β_1 receptors and making ephedrine a medication with direct-indirect sympathomimetic effects. This drug is frequently used by anesthesiologists to treat hypotension; however, it also may be used by individuals for its stimulant properties, such as a weight loss supplement.

The combination of ephedrine, a drug that increases the release of norepinephrine, with a drug that decreases norepinephrine metabolism through inhibition of the enzyme MAO-A, may lead to dangerously elevated heart rate and blood pressure. One case has been reported in which the patient presented with elevated blood pressure and was believed to have a pheochromocytoma.[5] On further investigation, it was noted that the patient had elevated levels of norepinephrine but not of epinephrine and had only slightly increased urinary vanillylmandelic acid concentrations. A computed tomographic scan of the adrenal glands showed normal results. The elevated levels of norepinephrine were believed to be caused by interaction between selegiline, ephedrine, and a tricyclic antidepressant.

Investigators also have questioned the safety of common cold medications, such as pseudoephedrine and dextromethorphan, used by patients taking selegiline.[6] A recent study showed that the pharmacokinetics and pharmacodynamics of pseudoephedrine and phenylpropanolamine were not significantly altered by administration of selegiline (6 mg/24 h) in a transdermal system.[7] Although the pharmacologic parameters of these sympathomimetics were not significantly affected, the study investigators concluded that it was still prudent to avoid concomitant use of a selegiline transdermal system and sympathomimetics. Despite the findings of that study, this conclusion maintains clinical relevance. Since MAO-A inhibition caused by selegiline appears to be dose related, it may be likely that this interaction gains greater importance when an increased dose (eg, 9 mg or 12 mg/24 h) is administered.

Take-Home Points

- Selegiline is an MAO-B inhibitor used to treat Parkinson's disease that also is used to treat depression.
- Selegiline has the potential to inhibit MAO-A, particularly when given in greater doses, and may reduce the metabolism of norepinephrine or serotonin. Therefore, levels of norepinephrine and serotonin may be increased in patients taking selegiline.
- Ephedrine acts indirectly as a sympathomimetic by increasing the release of norepinephrine at the nerve terminals.
- Medications that impact norepinephrine and serotonin levels, such as ephedrine, should be used with caution in patients taking selegiline.

Summary

Interaction: pharmacodynamic
Substrates: selegiline and ephedrine
Enzyme: monoamine oxidase B
Clinical effect: hypertension

References

1. Dingemanse J, Kneer J, Wallnofer A, et al. Pharmacokinetic-pharmacodynamic interactions between two selective monoamine oxidase inhibitors: moclobemide and selegiline. Clin Neuropharmacol. 1996;19:399–414.
2. Korn A, Wagner B, Moritz E, et al. Tyramine pressor sensitivity in healthy subjects during combined treatment with moclobemide and selegiline. Eur J Clin Pharmacol. 1996;49:273–8.
3. Hinds NP, Hillier CE, Wiles CM. Possible serotonin syndrome arising from an interaction between nortriptyline and selegiline in a lady with parkinsonism. J Neurol. 2000;247:811.
4. McGrath PJ, Stewart JW, Quitkin FM. A possible L-deprenyl induced hypertensive reaction. J Clin Psychopharmacol. 1989;9:310–1.
5. Lefebvre H, Noblet C, Moore N. Pseudo-phaeochromocytoma after multiple drug interactions involving the selective monoamine oxidase inhibitor selegiline. Clin Endocrinol (Oxf). 1995;42:95–8.
6. Jacob JE, Wagner ML, Sage JI. Safety of selegiline with cold medications. Ann Pharmacother. 2003;37:438–41.
7. Azzaro AJ, VanDenBerg CM, Ziemniak J, et al. Evaluation of the potential for pharmacodynamic and pharmacokinetic drug interactions between selegiline transdermal system and two sympathomimetic agents (pseudoephedrine and phenylpropanolamine) in healthy volunteers. J Clin Pharmacol. 2007;47:978–90.

Heart-Stopping Treatment 130

Fatal Forty DDI: verapamil, erythromycin, CYP3A4

Erica D. Wittwer MD, PhD, Toby N. Weingarten MD, and Juraj Sprung MD, PhD

Abstract
This case discusses a pharmacokinetic interaction between verapamil and erythromycin, leading to AV nodal blockade and prolongation of QTc interval. Verapamil is a cytochrome P450 3A4 substrate and erythromycin is a 3A4 inhibitor.

Case

A second-year anesthesia resident called her attending one night to discuss the preoperative evaluations she had done for their patients having surgery the following day. Chief among her concerns was a 68-year-old man scheduled for elective shoulder replacement surgery, who had reported a worrisome history of an intensive care unit (ICU) admission for "heart block" 3 months earlier. The patient reported that he had a history of hypertension, treated with verapamil (480 mg daily in divided doses) and had a bout of pneumonia at that time, but could give no other details.

The case was moved to the end of the day and the records were obtained from the outside hospital. These revealed that the patient been brought to that hospital after collapsing when arising from a chair. At that time, he was being treated with erythromycin (500 mg/6 h) for pneumonia and had felt initial improvement before feeling ill again. The electrocardiogram (ECG) from the emergency room of the previous hospital showed bradycardia with a heart rate of 35 beats per minute, third-degree atrioventricular conduction blockade, and a prolonged QTc interval. The patient had received atropine and a temporary venous pacemaker was placed.

E.D. Wittwer MD, PhD (✉) • T.N. Weingarten MD • J. Sprung MD, PhD
Department of Anesthesiology, Mayo Clinic, Rochester, MN, USA
e-mail: Wittwer.erica@mayo.edu

C. Marcucci et al. (eds.), *A Case Approach to Perioperative Drug-Drug Interactions*, DOI 10.1007/978-1-4614-7495-1_130

The anesthesia team noted that the ICU pharmacist at the outside hospital recommended that patient's usual dose of verapamil be held until discharge and that pneumonia treatment be changed to cefuroxime and azithromycin.

After reviewing these records, the anesthesia attending approved the case to proceed as scheduled and asked the resident to read up on the hepatic cytochrome P450 (CYP) 3A4 enzyme.

Discussion

This is an example of an inhibitor added to a substrate.

More specifically, this is an example of an inhibitor (erythromycin) added to a substrate (verapamil), resulting in AV nodal blockade and prolongation of QTc interval.

Erythromycin is a commonly prescribed macrolide antibiotic that has been associated with QT-interval prolongation and sudden cardiac death, especially when administered intravenously.[1] The mechanism by which erythromycin causes arrhythmias may be its inhibition of the delayed rectifier potassium current at clinical concentrations.[2] Additionally, erythromycin is metabolized by the cytochrome P450 (CYP) 3A4 isozyme.[3] It also competitively and irreversibly inhibits CYP3A4. Erythromycin administration can reduce the metabolism of drugs that are also metabolized by 3A4, leading to increased levels of those drugs.

One study reviewed the risk for sudden cardiac death and found that the rate of sudden cardiac death was twice as high for patients taking erythromycin as for those who did not take the medication.[4] Additionally, the rate of sudden cardiac death was more than five times higher in patients who took erythromycin (considered now as a 3A4 substrate) and other, more potent, 3A4 inhibitors at the same time (Table 130.1). No increase in risk was found in patients who took amoxicillin or who had taken erythromycin in the past.

Verapamil blocks L-type calcium channels, leading to both reduced contractility and conduction in cardiac muscle and, to a lesser degree, vascular smooth muscle relaxation.[5] Verapamil is metabolized by and inhibits CYP3A4. Coadministration of verapamil and other medications that inhibit 3A4, such as erythromycin, can result in elevated plasma levels of verapamil. Prolongation and complete blockade of atrioventricular conduction were reported in a patient prescribed erythromycin who also was taking verapamil.[6]

Table 130.1 Sudden Cardiac Death Among Patients Currently Taking Medications

Current Drug Use	Person-years, No.[a]	Deaths, No.	Incidence-Rate Ratio (95% CI)[b]
Use of CYP3A4 inhibitor			
Erythromycin	194	3	5.35 (1.72-16.64)
Amoxicillin	254	0	NA
No antibiotic	36,518	116	0.93 (0.76-1.13)
No use of CYP3A4 inhibitor[c]			
Erythromycin	4,874	7	1.79 (0.85-3.76)
Amoxicillin	6,304	8	1.48 (0.74-2.97)
No antibiotic	1,163,087	1,235	1.00

Abbreviations: CI, confidence interval; NA, not applicable
[a]The total number of person-years with current use of erythromycin (5,304) differs from the total in the study (5,305) because of rounding
[b]Incidence-rate ratios were adjusted with Poisson regression for the following variables: calendar year; age, sex, and race; type of Medicaid enrollment; low frequency of outpatient medical encounters; score for the risk for cardiovascular disease; dose of antipsychotic and tricyclic antidepressant medications; and hospital admission or visit to the emergency department for noncardiovascular disease. Incidence-rate ratios and 95% CIs were calculated directly from the regression model
[c]Patients with no use of a CYP3A4 inhibitor and no antibiotic use were the reference group
[Adapted from Ray WA, Murray KT, Meredith S et al: Oral erythromycin and the risk of sudden death from cardiac causes. N Engl J Med 2004;351: 1089–1096. With permission from Massachusetts Medical Society]

When using two or more medications that are meaningful competitive inhibitors (and therefore substrates) of the same enzyme, it is not necessarily determinable in advance which one will, by virtue of binding avidity for the metabolizing enzyme and hepatic concentrations, behave as the "inhibitor" in relation to the other drug as the "substrate." Indeed, depending on the specific dosages involved, these relationships can vary from individual to individual, and often the drugs reciprocally act as competitive inhibitors of each others metabolism, leading to elevations in the levels of both drugs.

Other medications have the potential to cause cardiac toxicity when coadministered with erythromycin. Coadministration of cisapride (a gastroprokinetic agent that is now available only in "compassionate use" protocols) and a macrolide antibiotic has been associated with electrocardiographic changes, including QT prolongation and torsades de pointes. However, the similar prokinetic agent mosapride has not been found to be associated with QT prolongation when administered with a macrolide antibiotic.[7] Terfenadine is an antihistamine that was removed from the market because of QT prolongation and subsequent cardiac arrhythmias. When erythromycin was used concurrently with terfenadine, the risk for QT prolongation and cardiac arrhythmias was increased.[8]

Take-Home Points

- Erythromycin is a CYP3A4 inhibitor and can cause increased levels of medications that are metabolized by CYP3A4.
- Erythromycin has been associated with increased risk for sudden cardiac death. When combined with other CYP3A4 inhibitors, such as verapamil, this risk is increased further.
- Coadministration of erythromycin and verapamil has been shown to cause cardiac toxicity.

Summary

Interaction: pharmacokinetic
Substrate: verapamil
Enzyme: CYP3A4
Inhibitor: erythromycin
Clinical effects: AV node blockade and QTc interval prolongation

References

1. Tschida SJ, Guay DR, Straka RJ, et al. QTc-interval prolongation associated with slow intravenous erythromycin lactobionate infusions in critically ill patients: a prospective evaluation and review of the literature. Pharmacotherapy. 1996;16:663–74.
2. Stanat SJ, Carlton CG, Crumb Jr WJ, et al. Characterization of the inhibitory effects of erythromycin and clarithromycin on the HERG potassium channel. Mol Cell Biochem. 2003;254:1–7.
3. Zhou S, Yung Chan S, Cher Goh B, et al. Mechanism-based inhibition of cytochrome P450 3A4 by therapeutic drugs. Clin Pharmacokinet. 2005;44:279–304.
4. Ray WA, Murray KT, Meredith S, et al. Oral erythromycin and the risk of sudden death from cardiac causes. N Engl J Med. 2004;351:1089–96.
5. Katzung BG, Chatterjee K. Vasodilators & the treatment of angina pectoris: pharmacodynamics. In: Katzung BG, editor. Basic and clinical pharmacology. 10th ed. New York: McGraw-Hill Medical; 2007. p. 191–3.
6. Goldschmidt N, Azaz-Livshits T, Gotsman I, et al. Compound cardiac toxicity of oral erythromycin and verapamil. Ann Pharmacother. 2001;35:1396–9.
7. Piquette RK. Torsade de pointes induced by cisapride/clarithromycin interaction. Ann Pharmacother. 1999;33:22–6.
8. Hanrahan JP, Choo PW, Carlson W, et al. Terfenadine-associated ventricular arrhythmias and QTc interval prolongation: a retrospective cohort comparison with other antihistamines among members of a health maintenance organization. Ann Epidemiol. 1995;5:201–9.

Induction Crashes: Are There Clues in the Ashes?

131

Fatal Forty DDI: theophylline, smoked tobacco, CYP1A2

Dawn L. Baker MD, MS and L. Lazarre Ogden MD

Abstract
This case discusses an interaction between smoked tobacco and theophylline. Theophylline is a cytochrome P450 1A2 substrate and smoked tobacco is a 1A2 inducer. Cessation of smoking will cause reversal of induction.

Case

A 60-year-old man was involved in a car accident on a remote highway. He presented to the Emergency Room with multiple orthopedic injuries and a small subdural hematoma. Medical information gathered by the emergency response team was limited to a history of hypertension treated with amlodipine and asthma managed with theophylline. The trauma service elected to admit him to the intensive care unit (ICU) for close observation given the subdural hematoma. After exhibiting stable vital signs and neurologic examinations in the ICU, and he was transferred to the intermediate care unit and on day 6 of his hospital stay, he was taken to the operating room for definitive repair of his femur. Upon induction of general anesthesia, the patient became severely hypotensive and developed a supraventricular tachycardia. The anesthesiologist had difficulty converting his heart rhythm with adenosine but was eventually successful with intravenous esmolol. In an effort to investigate the cause of these events, the anesthesiologist checked a theophylline level and found that it was significantly elevated at 37 mcg/mL. After further discussion with the patient's wife, it was revealed that he smoked two packs of cigarettes per day for 30 years.

D.L. Baker MD, MS (✉) • L.L. Ogden MD
Department of Anesthesiology, University of Utah, Salt Lake City, UT, USA
e-mail: dawn.baker@hsc.utah.edu

C. Marcucci et al. (eds.), *A Case Approach to Perioperative Drug-Drug Interactions*, DOI 10.1007/978-1-4614-7495-1_131

Discussion

This is an example of reversal of induction.

More specifically, it is an example of the reversal of an induction interaction between cigarette smoking and theophylline when a patient abruptly ceases smoking.

The patient above suffered from theophylline toxicity, resulting in an intraoperative episode of supraventricular tachycardia refractory to adenosine therapy. Theophylline is a methylxanthine that structurally resembles caffeine. Traditionally used to treat asthma and chronic obstructive pulmonary disease (COPD), it undergoes a predictable metabolism via the cytochrome P450 (CYP) 1A2 enzyme. Therapeutic levels in adults occur between 10 mcg/mL and 20 mcg/mL. While the drug is considered to be second-line due to a large side-effect profile, it is still used for COPD treatment regimes when cost is a significant issue and is used in an IV form (aminophylline) for acute bronchodilation in the ICU and pediatric settings.

It has been well documented that cigarette smoking induces the CYP1A2 enzyme, thus requiring higher substrate levels to achieve a desired therapeutic effect (although it is not pertinent to this clinical case, smoking tobacco products also induces CYP2E1). Lee et al found that theophylline clearance was increased by 58% to 100% with a corresponding reduction in half-life for smokers vs. nonsmokers.[1] With abstinence from smoking for one week, they also observed a 37.6% decrease in clearance and a 35.8% increase in half-life. Faber and Fuhr also reported that CYP1A2 reductions after smoking cessation were highest at 1 week.[2] While thousands of particulate and gaseous compounds are present in tobacco smoke, it is thought that polycyclic aromatic hydrocarbons (PAHs) are responsible for the enzymatic induction.[3,4] Thus, substituting a nicotine patch during abrupt smoking cessation will not ameliorate the reversal of induction.

This reversal of induction can be an especially significant factor when dosing drugs with narrow therapeutic windows, such as theophylline. With abrupt smoking cessation, the induction mechanism is reversed, resulting in higher levels of the previously induced substrate present in the body. The result can be potential toxicity, as is the case for theophylline. Symptoms of acute theophylline toxicity include tachyarrhythmias, nausea, vomiting, abdominal pain, electrolyte disturbances, and rarely seizures. Treatment of theophylline toxicity normally involves activated charcoal and supportive care measures. Esmolol is commonly successful for treatment of unstable SVT in theophylline overdose; the purinergic agonist adenosine was not helpful in the clinical situation above. Theophylline is also a purine receptor antagonist, and thus high levels in the body may result in refractory response to adenosine therapy.[5]

As demonstrated in this clinical vignette, documentation of patient smoking status can be of vital importance in the perioperative setting. This tenet applies to inpatient and outpatient scenarios as well. Screening patients who smoke or have recently quit for whatever reason may be of vital importance in preventing potentially harmful drug interactions.

Take-Home Points

- Smoking induces CYP1A2 enzymes, resulting in the need for higher drug levels to achieve the desired effect. This can complicate drug dosing regimens, especially for those drugs that have narrow therapeutic windows.
- Conversely, abrupt smoking cessation (as short as 5 to 7 days) can reverse this enzymatic induction and lead to buildup of toxic drug levels.
- Theophylline is metabolized via the CYP1A2 pathway and may produce dangerous toxic effects such as arrhythmia in cases of altered metabolism and decreased clearance.
- Polycyclic aromatic hydrocarbons produced in cigarette smoke are responsible for its effects on CYP1A2; thus, nicotine patch substitution during periods of smoking cessation will not prevent the impending reversal of enzymatic induction and potential drug toxicity.
- Awareness of patients' smoking status is crucial for achieving both safe and therapeutic drug-dosing regimens.

Summary

Interaction: pharmacokinetic
Substrate: theophylline
Enzyme: CYP1A2
Inducer: smoked tobacco

References

1. Lee BL, Benowitz NL, Jacob 3rd P. Cigarette abstinence, nicotine gum, and theophylline disposition. Ann Intern Med. 1987;106(4):553–5.
2. Faber MS, Fuhr U. Time response of cytochrome P450 1A2 activity on cessation of heavy smoking. Clin Pharmacol Ther. 2004;76(2):178–84.
3. Kroon LA. Clinical review: drug interactions with smoking. Am J Health Syst Pharm. 2007;64:1917–21.
4. Schaffer SD, Yoon S, Zadezensky I. A review of smoking cessation: potentially risky effects on prescribed medications. J Clin Nurs. 2009;18:1533–40.
5. Anderson PO, Knoben JE. Handbook of clinical drug data. 8th ed. Stamford: Appleton & Lange; 1997. p. 227.

The Wakeup Call: 2AM Trauma

132

β-blockers, cocaine

Devin C. Tang MD and Nabil M. Elkassabany MD

Abstract
The case discusses the pharmacodynamic interaction between ß-blockers and cocaine. ß-blockade of cocaine-induced tachycardia can lead to unopposed action at the α-receptor and myocardial ischemia.

Case

After a restful Saturday, the sleeping anesthesia resident on call received a page at 2AM from the trauma team about a 37-year-old man who was being transported by helicopter to the trauma center. The patient, who was driving a truck across the country, had also unfortunately gone to sleep and crashed into another car earlier that evening. The patient was unconscious at the scene. He was extricated from the vehicle and intubated in the field.

Upon arrival to the trauma bay, the patient was still unresponsive. His heart rate was 120 beats per minute, blood pressure was 169/ 99 mm Hg, and respiratory rate was 22 breaths per minute. Past medical history, as obtained by from a friend, was unremarkable. The secondary trauma survey revealed a closed fracture of his left tibial plateau. A computed tomography scan of the brain showed a subdural hematoma with mild to moderate midline shift. Laboratory work was unremarkable except for a urine toxicology screen positive for cocaine and alcohol.

D.C. Tang MD (✉)
MedStar Harbor Hospital, Baltimore, MD, USA
e-mail: devintang@hotmail.com

N.M. Elkassabany MD
Section of Orthopedic Anesthesiology, Department of Anesthesiology and Critical Care, University of Pennsylvania, Wayne, PA, USA

C. Marcucci et al. (eds.), *A Case Approach to Perioperative Drug-Drug Interactions*, DOI 10.1007/978-1-4614-7495-1_132

The patient was taken emergently to the operating room for evacuation of the subdural hematoma. As the case proceeded the patient remained hypertensive (blood pressure 185/107 mm Hg) and tachycardic in spite of an adequate depth of anesthesia. He was then given metoprolol (5 mg in 1 mg increments). There was minimal change in blood pressure, however, his heart rate slowed in response to the ß-blocker therapy. Unfortunately, ST segment elevation of more than 2 mm from the baseline was noted on the monitor. Intravenous nitroglycerine was used to decrease the blood pressure and help with the new onset myocardial ischemia with limited response. Postoperatively, serial cardiac enzymes were positive, and a 12-lead electrocardiogram (ECG) showed ST elevations in anterolateral leads. The diagnosis of myocardial ischemia was confirmed by the cardiology service.

Discussion

This is an example of a complex pharmacodynamic interaction.

This case is an example of an intraoperative pharmacodynamic interaction between cocaine and ß-blockers. The mechanism of cocaine-induced myocardial ischemia can be attributed to the exaggerated sympathetic response associated with cocaine abuse.[1] Cocaine blocks the reuptake of norepinephrine and dopamine at the presynaptic adrenergic terminals, causing an accumulation of catecholamines at the postsynaptic receptor.[2] The resulting sympathomimetic response leads to an increase in heart rate, blood pressure, and contractility. These effects are augmented by alcohol and cigarette smoking.[3] The direct effect on the coronary vessels results in coronary artery vasospasm.[4]

In addition, there is evidence that cocaine activates platelets, increases platelet aggregation, and promotes thrombus formation.[5] The use of ß-blockers for treatment of cocaine-induced myocardial ischemia may leave the sympathetic effect mediated through the α-receptors unopposed which can exacerbate coronary artery vasoconstriction. Lang et al. demonstrated, in the cardiac catheterization lab, a decrease in coronary sinus blood flow and an increase in coronary vascular resistance with cocaine administration. Subsequent administration of propranolol caused a further decrease in coronary sinus blood flow and increase in coronary vascular resistance.[6]

Esmolol has been used in the treatment of cocaine-induced myocardial ischemia with some success in few case reports. The short half-life of esmolol and the ability to titrate the infusion rate against a target heart rate and possibly changes in ST segments were the principal reasons for the reported success with esmolol.[7] Labetolol has been shown to decrease the mean arterial pressure in the setting of cocaine use, but it does not reverse the effect of cocaine-induced vasoconstriction.[8] Moreover, in animal models, labetolol has been shown to increase risk of seizure and death in the setting of cocaine toxicity.[9] The current statement from the American Heart Association (AHA) states that ß-blockers with some alpha adrenergic blocking effect do not offer any advantage over traditional ß-blockers in the treatment of myocardial ischemia in the setting of acute cocaine toxicity. The results of a recent study by Dattilo and colleagues challenged these concepts.[10] The authors concluded that ß-blockers may reduce the risk for myocardial infarction after cocaine use. They also conclude that the benefit of ß-blockers on myocardial function may offset the risk for coronary artery spasm.

The current AHA recommendation for treatment of chest pain and myocardial infarction associated with acute cocaine toxicity is to use nitroglycerin and aspirin as a first-line therapy.[11] ß-blockers should not be used for that purpose. The anesthesiologist should keep these considerations in mind when administering ß-blockers to patients positive for cocaine and individualize treatment by weighing risks and benefits of ß-blockade for patients at higher risk for cardiac complications.

Take-Home Points

- ß-blockers are first-line treatment intraoperatively for elevated blood pressure with or without tachycardia. However, in the setting of cocaine use, a vasodilator, such as nitroglycerin might be a better choice.

- Treatment should be tailored to each individual while weighing the risks and benefits of ß-blockade for higher risk cardiac patients vs the potential for worsening of myocardial ischemia.

Summary

Interaction: pharmacodynamic (complex)
Substrates: cocaine and metoprolol
Mechanism/sites of action: ß-blockade combined with unopposed α agonism of coronary artery receptors
Clinical effects: coronary artery vasoconstriction and myocardial ischemia

References

1. Lange RA, Hillis LD. Cardiovascular complications of cocaine use. N Engl J Med. 2001;345(5):351–8.
2. Whitby LG, Hertting G, Axelrod J. Effect of cocaine on the disposition of noradrenaline labelled with tritium. Nature. 1960;187:604–5.

3. Foltin RW, Fischman MW. Ethanol and cocaine interactions in humans: cardiovascular consequences. Pharmacol Biochem Behav. 1988;31:877–83.
4. Lange RA, Cigarroa RG, Yancy Jr CW, et al. Cocaine-induced coronary-artery vasoconstriction. N Engl J Med. 1989;321:1557–62.
5. Stenberg RG, Winniford MD, Hillis LD, et al. Simultaneous acute thrombosis of two major coronary arteries following intravenous cocaine use. Arch Pathol Lab Med. 1989;113:521–4.
6. Lange RA, Cigarroa RG, Flores ED, et al. Potentiation of cocaine-induced coronary vasoconstriction by ß-adrenergic blockade. Ann Intern Med. 1990;112:897–903.
7. Sand IC, Brody SL, Wrenn KD, et al. Experience with esmolol for the treatment of cocaine-associated cardiovascular complications. Am J Emerg Med. 1991;9(2):161–3.
8. Boehrer JD, Moliterno DJ, Willard JE, et al. Influence of labetolol on cocaine-induced coronary vasoconstriction in humans. Am J Med. 1993;94:608–10.
9. Smith M, Garner D, Niemann JT. Pharmacologic interventions after an LD50 cocaine insult in a chronically instrumented rat model: are ß-blockers contraindicated? Ann Emerg Med. 1991;20:768–71.
10. Dattilo PB, Hailpern SM, Fearon K, et al. Beta-blockers are associated with reduced risk of myocardial infarction after cocaine use. Ann Emerg Med. 2008;51:117–25.
11. McCord J, Jneid H, Hollander JE, et al. American Heart Association Acute Cardiac Care Committee of the Council on Clinical Cardiology. Management of cocaine-associated chest pain and myocardial infarction: a scientific statement from the American Heart Association Acute Cardiac Care Committee of the Council on Clinical Cardiology. Circulation. 2008;17(4):1897–907.

Falling Down

133

Fatal Forty DDI: nifedipine, fluoxetine, CYP3A4

Scott Kennedy MD and Norman A. Cohen MD

Abstract

This case discusses the pharmacokinetic interaction between nifedipine and fluoxetine. Nifedipine is a cytochrome P450 3A4 substrate and fluoxetine is a 3A4 inhibitor.

Case

The anesthesiologist covering the postanesthesia care unit (PACU) was paged STAT after a post-spinal patient suffered near-syncope and a fall. He was a 63-year-old man who had undergone a urological procedure under uneventful subarachnoid block (SAB) that afternoon. The PACU nurse had assessed that the block resolved and then assisted the patient to standing, on which he complained of lightheadedness and fell to his knees. The anesthesiologist found that the patient's blood pressure had been 96/50 mm Hg on arrival to PACU, for which he had received 500 mL of normal saline. While in the supine position the patient had been without complaint. The anesthesiologist agreed that the SAB had completely resolved with no motor or sensory deficits and after an additional hour's wait, returned to PACU to help the nurse assist the patient to the standing position. On rising, the patient stated "I don't feel so good," and started to fall again. Fortunately, the fall was prevented.

A chart review showed that 8 weeks before surgery, the patient visited his primary care physician (PCP) for urinary obstruction and sleep problems. That physician correctly documented the patient's history of hypertension, which had been well

S. Kennedy MD (✉)
Columbia Anesthesia Group, Vancouver, WA, USA
e-mail: scottkmd@gmail.com

N.A. Cohen MD
Department of Anesthesiology and Perioperative Medicine, Oregon Health & Science University, Portland, OR, USA

C. Marcucci et al. (eds.), *A Case Approach to Perioperative Drug-Drug Interactions*, DOI 10.1007/978-1-4614-7495-1_133

controlled for years with nifedipine, his only medication, and he also diagnosed depression, initiating treatment with fluoxetine. The PCP also referred the patient to a urologist. On further interviewing, the patient reported that although he had not fallen prior to surgery, he had noticed that it had become necessary to rise slowly to avoid lightheadedness in the past 4 weeks.

The blood pressure was checked in the supine and standing positions, and the patient experienced a symptomatic change from 105/62 mm Hg to 83/49 mm Hg. The anesthesiologist informed the surgeon that his patient required admission due to the near-syncopal episode and orthostatic hypotension. He recommended that the patient's nifedipine be held and contacted the patient's PCP to discuss his findings.

Discussion

This is an example of an inhibitor added to a substrate.

Fluoxetine is a widely used selective serotonin reuptake inhibitor (SSRI). It is approved for use in the treatment of adult and pediatric major depressive and obsessive-compulsive disorder, eating disorders, panic disorders and premenstrual dysphoric disorder.

Fluoxetine, through its metabolite norfluoxetine, is a cytochrome P450 (CYP) 3A4 inhibitor.[1–3] Nifedipine is a 3A4 substrate. Orthostatic hypotension attributed to drug–drug interaction (DDI) with fluoxetine has been reported.[4] The administration of fluoxetine to this patient inhibited nifedipine metabolism through inhibition of 3A4 activity. Decreased metabolism resulted in an increased plasma level of nifedipine. These elevated nifedipine levels resulted in orthostatic hypotension, near syncope, and the two falls. Coadministration of several dihydropyridine calcium channel blockers (such as felodipine, nicardipine, and nimodipine), has been associated with clinically significant DDIs due to elevations in calcium channel blocker blood levels.[5–7]

This case demonstrates the importance of looking for possible DDIs in the preoperative evaluation. Such an evaluation may have identified the patient's complaint of light-headedness, tied that finding to a nifedipine-fluoxetine interaction, and led to a delay in this elective case to allow for either replacing nifedipine with an alternative agent not affected by 3A4 inhibition, or significantly reducing the nifedipine dose. Alternatively, the consultant anesthesiologist might have chosen an alternative anesthetic plan which carried less risk for perioperative hypotension than the SAB.

CYP 3A4 is a common site of DDIs that have specific implications for anesthesia care.[8]

Take-Home Points

- Fluoxetine is a commonly administered SSRI antidepressant with a host of other approved applications
- Fluoxetine can significantly inhibit the cytochrome P450 3A4 metabolic pathway. Because it is approved for the number of conditions, it is important for practitioners to recognize it on medication lists.
- Drugs dependent on CYP3A4 for metabolism may have markedly elevated plasma levels when 3A4 has been inhibited.
- Hypertensive patients on dihydropyridine calcium channel blockers such as nifedipine who are also receiving fluoxetine may benefit from preoperative screening for orthostatic hypotension.
- Anesthetic evaluation should consider the possibility of this common DDI in depressed, hypertensive patients. The anesthetic plan may require alteration to minimize the impact of this DDI.
- CYP3A4 inhibition also impairs the metabolism of other drugs commonly used by anesthesiologists, such as certain benzodiazepines (diazepam and midazolam, but not lorazepam) and opioids (fentanyl, alfentanil, and methadone).

Summary

Interaction: pharmacokinetic
Substrate: nifedipine
Enzyme: CYP3A4
Inhibitor: fluoxetine
Clinical effect: exaggerated antihypertensive effect; orthostatic hypertension

References

1. Greenblatt DJ, von Moltke LL, Harmatz JS, et al. Human cytochromes and some newer antidepressants: kinetics, metabolism, and drug interactions. J Clin Psychopharmacol. 1999;19:23–35.
2. Ring BJ, Binkley SN, Roskos L, et al. Effect of fluoxetine, norfluoxetine, sertraline and desmethyl sertraline on human CYP3A catalyzed 19-hydroxy midazolam formation in vitro. J Pharmacol Exp Ther. 1995;275:1131–5.

3. Von Moltke LL, Greenblatt DJ, Cotreau-Bibbo MM, et al. Inhibitors of alpralozam metabolism in vitro: effect of serotonin-reuptake-inhibitor antidepressants, ketoconazole and quinidine. Br J Clin Pharmacol. 1994;38:23–31.
4. Azaz-Livshits T, Danenberg H. Tachycardia, orthostatic hypotension, and profound weakness due to concomitant use of fluoxetine and nifedipine. Pharmacopsychiatry. 1997;30:274–5.
5. Nicardipine hydrochloride [package insert]. Toronto: Genpharm Inc.; 2006.
6. Nimodipine [package insert]. Detroit: Caraco Pharmaceutical Laboratories, Ltd.; 2012.
7. Felodipine [package insert]. North Las Vegas: Med-Health Pharma, LLC; 2011.
8. Fahmi OA, Hurst S, Plowchalk D, et al. Comparison of different algorithms for predicting clinical drug-drug interactions, based on the use of CYP3A4 in vitro data: predictions of compounds as precipitants of interaction. Drug Metab Dispos. 2009;37:1658–66.

A Hidden Drug

134

Fatal Forty DDI: diltiazem, sildenafil, CYP3A4 and sildenafil, nitroglycerin

Helga Komen MD, Toby N. Weingarten MD, and Juraj Sprung MD, PhD

Abstract

This case discusses both a pharmacokinetic and a pharmacodynamic interaction between sildenafil and diltiazem. Sildenafil is a cytochrome P450 3A4 substrate. Diltiazem is a 3A4 inhibitor. In addition, the coadministration of sildenafil and diltiazem can result in severe hypotension.

Case

A 63-year-old man presented for angiography of the coronary arteries. He had chronic hypertension, hypercholesterolemia, and a 15-year history of mild angina. His medications were diltiazem, atenolol, atorvastatin calcium, and nitroglycerin sublingually as needed. His episodes of angina were rare, occurred mostly during exercise, and were responsive to sublingual nitroglycerin. However, he recently had suffered several anginal episodes at rest, so his cardiologist decided to perform a diagnostic coronary angiogram. The anesthesia team was asked to cover the case and provide sedation if necessary.

On the morning of the angiogram, the patient felt well and denied chest pain, nausea, or palpitations. He took his medications as prescribed, and his blood pressure was 110/70 mm Hg. After the coronary artery was cannulated, the patient began to report chest pain and nausea. His blood pressure was 115/75 mm Hg.

H. Komen MD (✉)
Department of Anesthesiology and Critical Care Medicine, University Hospital Rijeka, Rijeka, Croatia
e-mail: helga.komen@ri.t-com.hr

T.N. Weingarten MD • J. Sprung, MD, PhD
Department of Anesthesiology, Mayo Clinic, Rochester, MN, USA

C. Marcucci et al. (eds.), *A Case Approach to Perioperative Drug-Drug Interactions*, DOI 10.1007/978-1-4614-7495-1_134

The electrocardiogram monitor showed normal sinus rhythm but with ST-segment depression. The anesthesiologist administered sublingual nitroglycerin, after which the chest pain and nausea resolved and the ST segments normalized.

However, shortly afterward, the patient's blood pressure acutely declined to 60/40 mm Hg and he reported lightheadedness and chest pain again. The anesthesiologist administered phenylephrine. The patient's blood pressure increased to 95/70 mm Hg, and he reported that the chest pain had subsided and he was comfortable. The angiogram was completed without further complications. Afterwards, it was determined that the patient had taken an unprescribed 50-mg dose of sildenafil the night before the procedure.

Discussion

This is an example of the coadministration of a substrate and an inhibitor. It is also an example of pharmacodynamic potentiation.

More specifically, this case involves inhibition of the cytochrome P450 (CYP) 3A4-mediated metabolism of sildenafil and potentiation of nitric oxide–mediated vasodilatation by both sildenafil and nitroglycerin.

Diltiazem is an inhibitor of calcium ion influx during membrane depolarization of cardiac and vascular smooth muscle. Diltiazem is indicated for management of chronic stable angina and angina due to coronary artery spasm. Its antianginal actions are due to dilatation of coronary arteries, as well as reduction of myocardial oxygen demand. This reduction is accomplished through decreases in heart rate and systemic blood pressure. Diltiazem undergoes extensive hepatic biotransformation through *N*-demethylation by CYP3A4, and it is also a clinically significant competitive inhibitor of this isozyme.[1]

Sildenafil enhances the effect of nitric oxide by inhibiting phosphodiesterase type 5 in both the corpus cavernosum of the penis and the smooth muscles of the pulmonary vasculature. Nitric oxide increases cyclic guanosine monophosphate in the smooth muscle cells of the vasculature, resulting in vasodilatation. Phosphodiesterase type 5 contributes to the breakdown of cyclic guanosine monophosphate, thereby terminating the effects of nitric oxide. Thus, its inhibition results in vasodilation and increased inflow of blood to the corpus cavernosum. Sildenafil undergoes hepatic metabolism, mainly by CYP3A4. The duration of action is up to 4 hours. Hepatic and renal function impairment, as well as advanced age, may be associated with increased sildenafil plasma level.[1,2]

Because diltiazem slows the metabolism of sildenafil through inhibition of CYP3A4, coadministration of these drugs elevates the plasma concentrations of sildenafil and increases the risk of hypotension.[1,2] In addition, precaution is suggested in the presence of other potent CYP3A inhibitors, such as the azole antifungals, antiretroviral protease inhibitors, or macrolide antibiotics (except azithromycin) (Table 134.1).[2] However, a large study showed that sildenafil can be well tolerated by patients taking one or more antihypertensives, although an initial dose of 25 mg should be considered.[3]

Sildenafil use is contraindicated in patients taking organic nitrates because of a high risk of marked vasodilation when the drugs are used together. Sildenafil substantially enhances the relaxant effects of a vasodilator with a nitric oxide donor property (ie, isosorbide dinitrate, sodium nitroprusside, nicorandil, and nipradilol). Recent studies show that in men with angina, there is an interaction between sildenafil and nitroglycerin which reduces blood pressure for 8 hours or longer after sildenafil administration (Fig. 134.1).[4,5] These observations have been made in the absence of CYP3A4 inhibition.[4,5] There has been a report of profound hypotension in a man on diltiazem therapy for stable angina who used sildenafil and was later administered nitrates for angina.[6]

In the this case, diltiazem inhibited the function of CYP3A4, resulting in inhibition of sildenafil metabolism and high plasma sildenafil levels. The increased plasma levels of sildenafil resulted in profound hypotension after administration of nitroglycerin, which potentiated nitric oxide–mediated vasodilatation.

Table 134.1 Drugs with major interactions when taken simultaneously with sildenafil

Diltiazem hydrochloride
Amoxicillin
Clarithromycin
Erythromycin
Isosorbide dinitrate
Isosorbide mononitrate
Itraconazole
Ketoconazole
Lansoprazole
Lopinavir
Nitroglycerin
Nitroprusside sodium
Ritonavir
Voriconazole

[Based on data from Corona G, Razzoli E, Forti G et al. The use of phosphodiesterase 5 inhibitors with concomitant medications. *J Endocrinol Invest*. 2008;31:799–808]

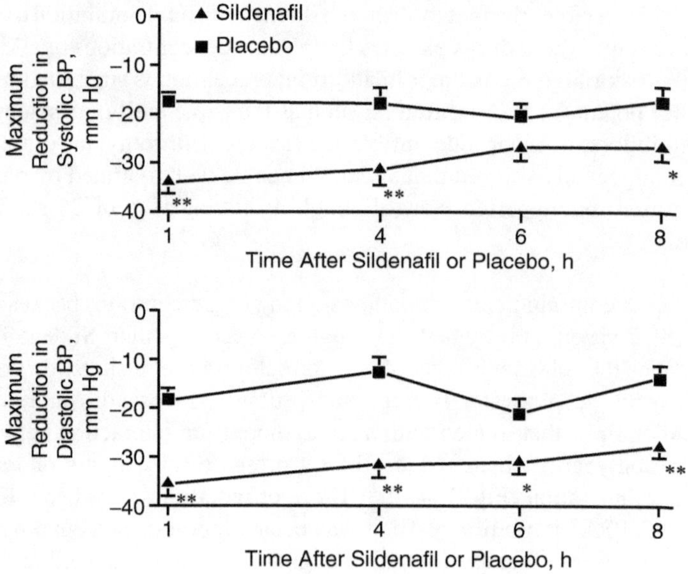

Fig. 134.1 Duration of hypotensive effect of sildenafil when taken with nitroglycerin. Mean maximum changes in sitting blood pressure (BP) with nitroglycerin given after sildenafil and after placebo in patients with angina. Changes are from baseline recordings taken before sildenafil or placebo administration. Error bars represent standard error of mean. *$P<.05$; **$P<.01$ [Adapted from Oliver JJ, Kerr DM, Webb DJ. Time-dependent interactions of the hypotensive effects of sildenafil citrate and sublingual glyceryl trinitrate. Br J Clin Pharmacol 2009;67: 403–412. With permission from John Wiley & Sons, Inc.]

Take-Home Points

- The coadministration of diltiazem and sildenafil may increase the risk for such adverse reactions as hypotension because of the inhibition of CYP3A4 metabolism and increased plasma concentrations of sildenafil.
- Other potent inhibitors of CYP3A4 metabolism also can increase plasma concentrations of sildenafil.
- Sildenafil is contraindicated in patients taking any type of organic nitrates because this drug combination can potentiate nitric oxide–induced vasodilation.

Summary

Interaction 1: pharmacokinetic and pharmacodynamic
Substrate: (pharmacokinetic): sildenafil
Enzyme: CYP3A4
Inhibitor: diltiazem

Interaction 2: pharmacodynamic
Substrate: (pharmacodynamic): sildenafil and diltiazem
Mechanism/site of action: nitric oxide mediated-vasodilatation
Clinical effect: severe hypotension

References

1. Maenpaa J, Ruskoaho H, Pelkonen O. Inhibition of hepatic microsomal drug metabolism in rats by five calcium antagonists. Pharmacol Toxicol. 1989;64:446–50.
2. Corona G, Razzoli E, Forti G, et al. The use of phosphodiesterase 5 inhibitors with concomitant medications. J Endocrinol Invest. 2008;31:799–808.
3. Bohm M, Burkart M, Baumann G. Sildenafil is well tolerated by erectile dysfunction patients taking antihypertensive medications, including those on multidrug regimens. Curr Drug Saf. 2007;2:5–8.
4. Oliver JJ, Kerr DM, Webb DJ. Time-dependent interactions of the hypotensive effects of sildenafil citrate and sublingual glyceryl trinitrate. Br J Clin Pharmacol. 2009;67:403–12.
5. Sakuma I, Akaishi Y, Tomioka H, et al. Interactions of sildenafil with various coronary vasodilators in isolated porcine coronary artery. Eur J Pharmacol. 2002;437:155–63.
6. Khoury V, Kritharides L. Diltiazem-mediated inhibition of sildenafil metabolism may promote nitrate-induced hypotension. Aust N Z J Med. 2000;30:641–2.

I'm Listening, I'm Listening 135

Fatal Forty DDI: diltiazem, carbamazepine, CYP3A4

Catherine Marcucci MD, Jerusha Taylor PharmD, BCPS, Ansgar M. Brambrink MD, PhD, and Neil B. Sandson MD

Abstract
This case discusses a complex pharmacokinetic interaction between carbamazepine and diltiazem, resulting in carbamazepine toxicity and decreased efficacy of diltiazem. Carbamazepine is both a cytochrome P450 3A4 substrate and inducer and diltiazem is a 3A4 inhibitor and substrate.

Case

A 65-year-old man was admitted for craniotomy and resection of recurrent left temporal recurrent meningioma. He had a past medical history of seizure disorder, hyperlipidemia, hypertension, and benign prostatic hypertrophy. Medications included carbamazepine (400 mg BID), lisinopril, aspirin, and metoprolol (25 mg daily). All laboratories were within normal limits upon admission; serum carbamazepine level was 8.2 mcg/L (therapeutic range 4–12 mcg/dL).

Postoperatively, the patient developed difficult-to-control atrial fibrillation with rapid ventricular rate and altered mental status. Over the next 12 hours the

C. Marcucci MD (✉)
Anesthesia Services Department, Philadelphia Veterans Affairs Medical Center, Philadelphia, PA, USA
e-mail: sandson.marcucci@comcast.net

J. Taylor PharmD, BCPS
Department of Pharmacy, Oregon Health and Science University, Portland, OR, USA

A.M. Brambrink MD, PhD
Department of Anesthesiology and Perioperative Medicine, Oregon Health and Science University, Portland, OR, USA

N.B. Sandson MD
Department of Psychiatry, University of Maryland Medical System, Baltimore, MD, USA

Department of Psychiatry, VA Maryland Health Care System, Baltimore, MD, USA

C. Marcucci et al. (eds.), *A Case Approach to Perioperative Drug-Drug Interactions*, DOI 10.1007/978-1-4614-7495-1_135

patient required a diltiazem bolus and a steadily increasing diltiazem rate. Finally, the patient's heart rate was controlled at 110 beats per minute with a diltiazem infusion rate of 20 mg/hr. His mental status improved and he was generally hemodynamically stable. He was eventually transitioned to diltiazem (180 mg orally/8h).

Three days later, Dr. Julio Novartis rotated onto the service. Julio had been his wife's audience after dinner one evening recently for a practice presentation of her upcoming psychiatry grand rounds entitled "Review of Antiepileptic Mood Stabilizers." Dr. Novartis reassured his spouse that, *yes*, he was interested her talk and, *yes*, he was paying attention.

The following day, the craniotomy patient developed altered mental status, dizziness, tremors, and was noted to have mild nystagmus.

Because Dr. Novartis had told his wife the truth, he was able to quickly recommend checking a serum carbamazepine level, which was found to be elevated at 18.2 mcg/dL. The patient's carbamazepine doses were held for the next 48 hours until his serum level was back within therapeutic range. Diltiazem was discontinued and he was restarted on his metoprolol. He remained rate controlled on oral metoprolol 25 mg BID. His mental status improved over the next few days as his carbamazepine level returned to therapeutic range, and he was discharged home the following week.

This is an example of both an inhibitor (diltiazem) added to a substrate (carbamazepine) and also of a substrate (diltiazem) added to an inducer (carbamazepine).

Carbamazepine (CBZ) is an anticonvulsant medication that is extensively metabolized via the cytochrome P450 (CYP) 3A4 enzyme system. Diltiazem inhibits carbamazepine metabolism by inhibiting hepatic and intestinal CYP3A4. The inhibition of carbamazepine metabolism can lead to increased levels of carbamazepine and result in toxicity. Toxic symptoms are likely to occur two to three days after starting diltiazem.[1–3] Symptoms of carbamazepine toxicity include dizziness, ataxia, tremor, nystagmus, urinary retention, dysrhythmias, coma, respiratory depression, and neuromuscular disturbances.

There are several case reports illustrating carbamazepine toxicity with concurrent diltiazem use. In these cases, toxicity resolved when CBZ dose was decreased.

A less overtly important, but potentially quite significant reciprocal interaction, is that in the presence of carbamazepine, it is much more difficult to give enough diltiazem to produce desired clinical effects. Diltiazem, as is the case with most calcium channel blockers, is a substrate of CYP3A4.[4] Carbamazepine is a potent inducer of 3A4.[5–7] Although the combination of CBZ with a notably 3A4-inhibiting calcium channel blocker first and most strikingly produces increases in carbamazepine levels, it is no less true that the levels of most calcium channel blockers decrease or are much lower than expected in the presence of carbamazepine, thus the need for much higher than expected dosages of diltiazem in the scenario above.[8,9]

Finally, verapamil, another calcium channel blocker, also inhibits CYP3A4 and can also increase serum levels of carbamazepine. There is little evidence that coadministration of felodipine and nifedipine with carbamazepine results in toxicity. However, felodipine is metabolized extensively by the liver and is highly susceptible to enzyme induction. Since carbamazepine is a paninducer of CYP enzymes, felodipine concentrations are shown to be lower when given concomitantly with carbamazepine.

Take-Home Points

- Carbamazepine is a CYP3A4 substrate
- Diltiazem is a CYP3A4 inhibitor.
- A clinically relevant drug–drug interaction (DDI) resulting in carbamazepine toxicity has been documented when diltiazem is added to steady-state carbamazepine therapy. Toxicity will result in several days.
- Carbamazepine is a pan-inducer of CYP enzymes, including 3A4.
- Diltiazem is a CYP3A4 substrate. Carbamazepine will induce the metabolism of diltiazem
- Remember that inhibition is faster than induction.The first effect of the addition of diltiazem to carbamazepine will be inhibition of carbamazepine and toxicity. Then, as the 3A4 enzyme is induced, metabolism of diltiazem will increase, requiring higher drug doses.
- It is imperative to monitor CBZ serum levels when a patient is receiving concomitant diltiazem. CBZ doses may need to be decreased in order to prevent toxicity.
- The "cardiovascular" drugs and the "psychiatry" drugs run into each other quite a lot in the DDI world. One of the main street corners for this sizeable neighborhood group is CYP3A4. Review it often!

Summary

Interaction 1: pharmacokinetic
Substrate: carbamazepine
Inhibitor: diltiazem
Enzyme: CYP3A4
Clinical effect: carbamazepine toxicity

Interaction 2: pharmacokinetic
Substrate: diltiazem
Inducer: carbamazepine
Enzyme: CYP3A4
Clinical effect: decreased diltiazem levels and decreased efficacy

References

1. Ahmad S. Diltiazem-carbamezapine interaction. Am Heart J. 1990;120:1485.
2. Bahls F, et al. Interactions between calcium channel blockers and the anticonvulsants carbamazepine and phenytoin. Neurology. 1991;41:740.
3. Hansten P, Horn J. Drug interactions analysis and management. St Louis: Wolters Kluwer Health, Inc.; 2007. p. 294–5.
4. DeVane CL, Markowitz JS. Avoiding psychotropic drug interactions in the cardiovascular patient. Bull Menninger Clin. 2000;64(1):49–59.
5. Spina E, Pisani F, Perucca E. Clinically significant pharmacokinetic drug interactions with carbamazepine. An update. Clin Pharmacokinet. 1996;31(3):198–214.
6. Crawford P, Chadwick DJ, Martin C, et al. The interaction of phenytoin and carbamazepine with combined oral contraceptive steroids. Br J Clin Pharmacol. 1990;30(6):892–6.
7. Ogg MS, Williams JM, Tarbit M, et al. A reporter gene assay to assess the molecular mechanisms of xenobiotic-dependent induction of the human CYP3A4 gene in vitro. Xenobiotica. 1999;29(3):269–79.
8. Mück W, Ahr G, Kuhlmann J. Nimodipine. Potential for drug-drug interactions in the elderly. Drugs Aging. 1995;6(3):229–42.
9. Yasui-Furukori N, Tateishi T. Carbamazepine decreases antihypertensive effect of nilvadipine. J Clin Pharmacol. 2002;42(1):100–3.

Jump Start My Heart

136

Fatal Forty DDI: metoprolol, amiodarone, CYP2D6, CYP1A2

Katarina Bojanić MD, Juraj Sprung MD, PhD, and Toby N. Weingarten MD

Abstract
This case discusses the pharmacokinetic interaction between metoprolol and amiodarone, resulting in bradycardia. Metoprolol is a cytochrome P450 1A2 and 2D6 substrate and amiodarone is a cytochrome P450 1A2 and 2D6 inhibitor.

Case

A 70-year-old, 65 kg man presented to the emergency department with a report of crushing substernal chest pain, shortness of breath, and nausea. A 12-lead electrocardiogram (ECG) showed sinus tachycardia, ST-segment elevation in leads V_1 through V_4, and frequent, multifocal premature ventricular contractions. A presumptive diagnosis of myocardial infarction was made and the patient received appropriate measures including intravenous metoprolol (15 mg) was administered in divided doses to control the patient's heart rate and reduce myocardia oxygen demand. Emergent cardiac catheterization showed a 90% occlusion of the distal left anterior descending coronary artery and a drug-eluting stent was inserted.

Orders written for the coronary care unit called for administration of oral metoprolol (50 mg) every 6 hours. Twelve hours after catheterization, the patient again had multifocal premature ventricular contractions, as well as an episode of nonsustained ventricular tachycardia. He received intravenous amiodarone (150 mg) over 10 minutes, followed by an infusion (1 mg/min) for the initial 6 hours. The infusion was reduced to 0.5 mg/min thereafter. The ventricular ectopy resolved after the loading dose of amiodarone.

K. Bojanić MD (✉)
Division of Neonatology, Clinical Hospital Merkur, Zagreb, Croatia
e-mail: sprungkatarina@hotmail.com

J. Sprung MD, PhD • T.N. Weingarten MD
Department of Anesthesiology, Mayo Clinic, Rochester, MN, USA

C. Marcucci et al. (eds.), *A Case Approach to Perioperative Drug-Drug Interactions*, DOI 10.1007/978-1-4614-7495-1_136

One hour after his third dose of oral metoprolol, the patient had bradycardia with a heart rate of 36 beats per minute (bpm). An ECG showed third-degree heart block. The bradycardia did not resolve after 0.5 mg of intravenous atropine. A temporary venous pacemaker was inserted and the heart was paced at a rate of 80 bpm. The amiodarone infusion and the oral metoprolol were discontinued. After 12 hours, the third-degree heart block resolved and the patient no longer required pacing.

Discussion

This is an example of an inhibitor added to a substrate.

Metoprolol is a selective β_1-receptor antagonist and is also a Class II antiarrhythmic commonly used for unstable coronary artery syndromes and for tachyarrhythmias. Approximately 80% of metoprolol is metabolized by the cytochrome P450 (CYP) isozyme 2D6, with the remainder metabolized by the isozyme CYP1A2.[1] Amiodarone is a class III antiarrhythmic that has been used in both the treatment of acute, life-threatening arrhythmias and the suppression of supraventricular and ventricular dysrhythmias.[2] It has pharmacokinetic interactions with various therapeutic drugs, including warfarin, phenytoin, flecainide, cyclosporine, and, as in this case, metoprolol.[3] Amiodarone is extensively metabolized to desethylamiodarone in the liver by CYP3A4 and CYP2C8.[3] Desethylamiodarone has a marked inhibitory effect on CYP2D6. Therefore, continuous therapy with amiodarone further inhibits the metabolism of metoprolol. On average, the plasma concentration of metoprolol doubles after an amiodarone loading dose (Fig. 136.1).[3]

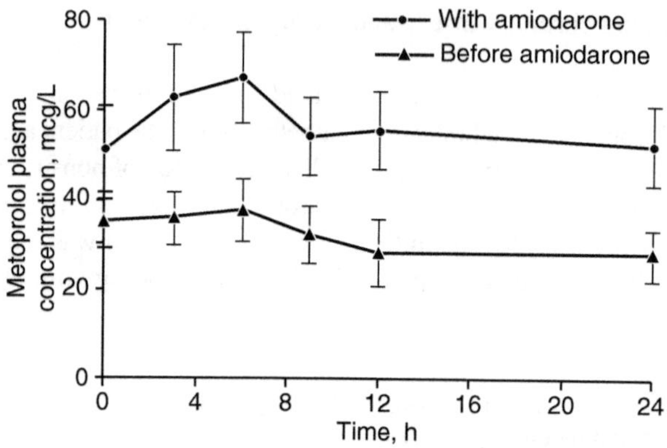

Fig. 136.1 Metoprolol plasma concentration over time before and after an amiodarone loading dose. Error bars indicate standard error of mean [Adapted from Werner D, Wuttke H, Fromm MF et al. Effect of amiodarone on the plasma levels of metoprolol. Am J Cardiol. 2004;94:1319–1321. with permission from Elsevier]

Combination amiodarone and metoprolol therapy has been associated with development of severe bradyarrhythmias resistant to atropine administration.[4] Treatment of such bradyarrhythmias may require pharmacologic heart rate augmentation using isoproterenol hydrochloride or temporary pacing. Although β-blockers and amiodarone are frequently used in combination, the clinician should be aware that amiodarone can potentiate the effects of β-blockers. Further, the clinician should use caution when providing β-blockers to patients taking medications that inhibit the CYP2D6 system.

Take-Home Points

- Amiodarone inhibits the metabolism of metoprolol (and other β-blockers), and a reduced dose of β-blocker should be used for patients treated with amiodarone.
- On average, plasma concentration of metoprolol nearly doubles after an amiodarone loading dose.
- For patients medicated with amiodarone and β-blockers, close monitoring of excessive effects of β-blockade (bradycardia and/or hypotension) should be exercised.
- Bradyarrhythmias associated with β-blocker toxicity may be atropine resistant and require more aggressive treatment.

Summary

Interaction: pharmacokinetic
Substrate: metoprolol
Enzymes: CYP1A2 and CYP2D6
Inhibitor: amiodarone
Clinical effect: increased effect of metoprolol (bradycardia)

References

1. Johnson JA, Burlew BS. Metoprolol metabolism via cytochrome P4502D6 in ethnic populations. Drug Metab Dispos. 1996;24:350–5.
2. Fukumoto K, Kobayashi T, Tachibana K, et al. Effect of amiodarone on the serum concentration/dose ratio of metoprolol in patients with cardiac arrhythmia. Drug Metab Pharmacokinet. 2006;21:501–5.
3. Werner D, Wuttke H, Fromm MF, et al. Effect of amiodarone on the plasma levels of metoprolol. Am J Cardiol. 2004;94:1319–21.
4. Leor J, Levartowsky D, Sharon C, et al. Amiodarone and beta-adrenergic blockers: an interaction with metoprolol but not with atenolol. Am Heart J. 1988;116:206–7.

The Statin Trilogy (I): 'Statin' from the Beginning

137

Fatal Forty DDI: simvastatin, cimetidine, diltiazem, CYP3A4

Brian Mitchell MD

Abstract
This case discusses a pharmacokinetic interaction between simvastatin, cimetidine, and diltiazem, resulting in increased incidence of rhabdomyolysis. Simvastatin is a cytochrome P450 3A4 substrate and cimetidine and diltiazem are 3A4 inhibitors.

Case

A 68-year-old woman with a history of gastroesophageal reflux disease (GERD) and hypertension was admitted to the hospital with intermittent left-sided chest pain. The admitting intern, on the Cardiology service for one more week before starting his anesthesiology residency, noted that the patient was on cimetidine for her GERD and diltiazem for blood pressure control. The intern filled out the standard "rule out MI" order set, which included a ß-blocker, nitroglycerin, aspirin, and simvastatin. He was not sure of the appropriate starting dose for the ß-blocker since the patient was already on diltiazem, so he contacted the on-call clinical pharmacist for some help on dosing.

The pharmacist suggested that the intern start with a low dosage and asked if he wanted her to check for any drug interactions while they were on the phone. She soon discovered a potential problem—the new statin order. The intern interrupted the pharmacist and said that he already made sure that the patient did not drink grapefruit juice. The pharmacist then went on to explain that, while grapefruit juice

B. Mitchell MD
Department of Anesthesiology and Perioperative Medicine,
Oregon Health and Science University, Portland, OR, USA
e-mail: brianmitchell@gmail.com

C. Marcucci et al. (eds.), *A Case Approach to Perioperative Drug-Drug Interactions*, DOI 10.1007/978-1-4614-7495-1_137

is a known inhibitor of the cytochrome P450 (CYP) 3A4 isoenzyme that metabolizes simvastatin, the patient's two other home medications, cimetidine and diltiazem, also inhibit this isoenzyme. The pharmacist suggested that the intern instead order fluvastatin which is metabolized by a different cytochrome P450 isoenzyme (CYP2C9). She commented that it was a good drug–drug interaction to learn early in his career and he would be one drug interaction "ahead of the pack" come July 1.

Discussion

This is an example of a substrate (almost) added to an inhibitor.

This case illustrates the significant disconnect between the one major statin drug–drug interaction (DDI) commonly taught in medical school and the many interactions that are potentially present in clinical practice. There are two major classes of DDIs that the perioperative practitioner should be aware of when prescribing and reviewing statins. These interactions are summarized in Table 137.1. Drugs most commonly seen in the perioperative period are highlighted in bold in the table.

The first step in understanding statin drug–drug interactions is recognizing that most statins are metabolized by cytochrome p450 enzymes within the liver. The exception to the P450-dependent metabolism of statins is pravastatin.[1,2] Over 90% of rosuvastatin is eliminated unchanged but the remaining drug is metabolized by the CYP2C9 isoenzyme.[3] The first major interaction to be aware of is the combination of a statin with an enzyme inhibitor. An enzyme inhibitor will decrease the enzyme's ability to metabolize the substrate drug. The P450 enzyme inhibitors, when combined with a statin, will increase the circulating statin levels by a factor of 2- to 20-fold.[3] The second major interaction to be aware of is the combination of statin with an enzyme inducer. The combination of the statin with an enzyme

Table 137.1 Statins

	Cytochrome P450 Isoenzyme	
	CYP3A4	**CYP2C9**
Statin Substrates	Lovastatin, simvastatin, atorvastatin	Fluvastatin, rosuvastatin[a]
Enzyme Inhibitor	**amiodarone**, ketoconazole, itraconazole, fluconazole, protease inhibitors, **erythromycin**, **verapamil**, **diltiazem**, clarithromycin, cimetidine, **grapefruit juice**, nefazodone	ketoconazole, fluconazole, **amiodarone**, gemfibrozil
Enzyme Inducer	**dexamethasone**, **barbiturates**, phenytoin, rifampin, cyclophosphamide, carbamazepine, St John's wort	rifampin, phenobarbital, phenytoin

[Adapted from refs [1] & [3]]
[a]Minimal metabolism by CYP2C9

inducer will significantly increase the metabolism of the statin and diminish its therapeutic effects. A third type of statin DDI, which occurs much less frequently than the first two, is when a statin serves as an enzymatic inhibitor in relation to another drug. The majority of such statin DDIs occur when fluvastatin, a potent 2C9 inhibitor, is combined with 2C9 substrates that have a narrow therapeutic index, such as phenytoin, warfarin, and sulfonylureas.

Take-Home Points

- Inhibitors of the hepatic P450 isoenzymes responsible for statin metabolism (CYP3A4 and CYP2C9) can significantly increase the circulating levels of statins. Inhibitors commonly seen in the perioperative period include amiodarone, verapamil, and diltiazem.
- Drug–drug interactions involving statins are to be taken seriously as they can lead to serious adverse events, including potentially fatal rhabdomyolysis, and myopathy.
- Pravastatin is not metabolized by the hepatic P450 isoenzymes and it may be a good alternative medication if a patient must remain on a significant enzyme inhibitor (such as the diltiazem in our case above) or inducer.

Summary

Interaction: pharmacokinetic
Substrate: simvastatin
Enzyme: CYP3A4
Inhibitor: cimetidine and diltiazem
Clinical effects: increased incidence of rhabdomyolysis

References

1. Bellosta S, Paoletti R, Corsini A. Safety of statins: focus on clinical pharmakinetics and drug interactions. Circulation. 2004;109:11150–7.
2. Marcucci C, Hutchens MP, Sandson NB. Perioperative statin therapy may be implicated in a wide array of drug-drug interactions. Anesthesiology. 2009;111:205.
3. Bottorff MB. Statin safety and drug interactions. Clinical implications. Am J Cardiol. 2006;97:27C–31.

The Statin Trilogy (II): Tripped and Fell at the Train 'Statin'

138

Fatal Forty DDI: simavastatin, itraconazole, CYP3A4

Brian Mitchell MD

Abstract
This case discusses the pharmacokinetic interaction between simvastatin and ketoconazole resulting in rhabdomyolysis. Simvastatin is a cytochrome P450 3A4 substrate and ketoconazole is a 3A4 inhibitor.

Case

A 57-year-old man with a history of hyperlipidemia and mild coronary artery disease was rushing to catch his train and tripped and fell while running down the steps to the commuter platform. He sustained a closed fracture of his left foot and tibia and was admitted to the orthopedic surgery service, complaining of significant fracture pain. Outpatient medications included simvastatin for hyperlipidemia and ketoconazole, which he began taking a few days prior to admission for *tinea cruris* (jock itch). The intern ordered the home medications and for the patient to be NPO at midnight for possible surgery the following day. Overnight, the patient's nurse called the intern for an order for a Foley catheter and to report significant pain in the patient's bilateral lower extremity. The senior resident was called when the Foley catheter produced dark, cola-colored urine. He was concerned about compartment syndrome, ordered a creatine kinase (CK) level, and notified the anesthesia on-call team of a possible fasciotomy.

B. Mitchell MD
Department of Anesthesiology and Perioperative Medicine, Oregon Health and Science University, Portland, OR, USA
e-mail: brianmitchell@gmail.com

C. Marcucci et al. (eds.), *A Case Approach to Perioperative Drug-Drug Interactions*, DOI 10.1007/978-1-4614-7495-1_138

The anesthesia resident and the staff anesthesiologist, who was also an intensivist in the SICU, saw the patient for a preoperative evaluation. The attending noted that the recent addition of itraconazole in the setting of chronic simvastatin use was a serious drug–drug interaction and a potential risk for rhabdomyolysis. He advised the surgery team to follow the CK levels, begin treatment for rhabdomyolysis with aggressive intravenous hydration, and switch medications to treat the *tinea cruris*. The attending suggested that the orthopedic team measure the compartment pressures to evaluate for compartment syndrome rather than emergently taking the patient to the operating room for a fasciotomy. He argued that the most likely diagnosis was rhabdomyolysis, without compartment syndrome, from the itraconazole and simvastatin drug–drug interaction. The orthopedic surgery resident measured the compartment pressure, which was normal.

Discussion

This is an example of a competitive inhibitor added to a substrate.

This patient's presentation exposes the risks of combining statins with medications that inhibit the biotransformation of statins in the liver. This inhibition can significantly raise the serum statin levels. Simvastatin biotransformation occurs with the cytochrome P450 (CYP) 450 3A4 isoenzyme, which is significantly inhibited by ketoconazole, itraconazole, and a number of the protease inhibitors. This is not a theoretical concern, but rather is based on a number of published case reports of rhabdomyolysis with these drug–drug interactions.[1,2] While these are the most potent of the inhibitors of the 3A4 isoenzyme, other inhibitors include medications more commonly encountered in the perioperative period such as verapamil, diltiazem, erythromycin, and amiodarone. Amiodarone and the azole antifungals are also inhibitors of CYP2C9, the other major P450 isoenzyme that metabolizes statins.[3] The 2C9 isoenzyme metabolizes fluvastatin and, to a small extent, rosuvastatin. If an enzymatic inhibitor must be added to the regimen of a patient who is also taking one of these statins (for example, a patient with atrial fibrillation who needs to be started on amiodarone), the patient can be switched to pravastatin, which does not undergo P450-mediated metabolism.

Another clinically significant inhibitor of statin metabolism is gemfibrozil. Gemfibrozil inhibits conjugation and biliary excretion of stations, and its combination with statins has lead to a significant number of adverse drug reactions.[2] This combination has a 0.12% prevalence of myopathy.[1]

Summary

Interaction: pharmacokinetic
Substrate: simvastatin
Enzyme: CYP3A4
Inhibitor: itraconazole
Clinical effects: rhabdomyolysis

References

1. Bellosta S, Paoletti R, Corsini A. Safety of statins: focus on clinical pharmakinetics and drug interactions. Circulation. 2004;109:11150–7.
2. Bottorff MB. Statin safety and drug interactions: clinical implications. Am J Cardiol. 2006;97:27C–31.
3. Flockhart DA. Drug interactions: cytochrome P450 drug interaction table. Indiana University School of Medicine; 2007. http://medicine.iupui.edu/clinpharm/ddis/table.asp. Accessed 30 Sept 2009.

The Statin Trilogy (III): Welcome to the United 'Statins' of America

139

Fatal Forty DDI: atorvastatin, phenytoin, CYP3A4

Brian Mitchell MD

Abstract
This case discusses the pharmacokinetic interaction of atorvastatin and phenytoin. Atorvastatin is a cytochrome P450 3A4 substrate and phenytoin is a paninducer of multiple cytochrome P450 enzymes including 3A4.

Case

A 61-year-old man, who was a new US citizen, presented to the cardiac intensive care unit (ICU) from an outside hospital team for possible emergent coronary revascularization. He arrived with substernal chest pain and ST-segment elevation myocardial infarction (STEMI) after an all-night celebration. He had a past medical history of hypertension, diabetes, obesity, and grand mal seizures. His home medications included insulin, phenytoin, metoprolol, and aspirin. The admitting physician assistant, who was also a naturalized citizen, used the STEMI order set including a heparin drip and high-dose atorvastatin, and resumed the patient's home medications. The next morning, the attending anesthesiologist-intensivist (who had just obtained his green card) noted that the addition of the atorvastatin in the presence of long-standing phenytoin use was a potential drug–drug interaction and could lead to an adverse drug reaction, decreasing the serum levels and clinical efficacy of the statin. He switched the patient to pravastatin, as its metabolism is not induced by phenytoin. Later that day, the patient's family gave each ICU staff member a tiny American flag.

B. Mitchell MD
Department of Anesthesiology and Perioperative Medicine, Oregon Health and Science University, Portland, OR, USA
e-mail: brianmitchell@gmail.com

C. Marcucci et al. (eds.), *A Case Approach to Perioperative Drug-Drug Interactions*, DOI 10.1007/978-1-4614-7495-1_139

Discussion

This is an example of a substrate added to an inducer.

The presence of an enzyme inducer will increase the metabolism of the substrate drug. In this case, the long-standing use of phenytoin, a cytochrome P450 (CYP) 3A4 inducer, would significantly decrease the levels of the substrate drug, atorvastatin. This would potentially negate the mortality benefit of high-dose statin therapy during management of acute coronary syndrome.[1] There is also emerging evidence that perioperative statin use can reduce postoperative cardiac events and mortality.[2]

If a statin is started in the presence of a known inducer, its effects should be titrated by following the improvement in both high high-density lipoprotein (HDL) and low-density lipoprotein (LDL) levels. This titration may be difficult to accomplish appropriately in the perioperative period. Once an appropriate response to the statin therapy is established in the presence of the enzyme inducer, its dose should be decreased if the inducer is discontinued. If the inducer is abruptly stopped without adjusting the statin dose (for example, a patient is changed from phenytoin to Keppra [levetiracetam] for seizure management), the patient's circulating levels of statin may increase significantly due to the relative drop in its metabolism. This could potentially set up a similar situation to the combination of a statin and and enzyme inhibitor.

Take-Home Points

- Inhibitors of the hepatic P450 isoenzymes responsible for statin metabolism (CYP3A4 and CYP2C9) can significantly increase the circulating levels of statins. Inhibitors commonly seen in the perioperative period include amiodarone, verapamil, and diltiazem.

- Drug–drug interactions involving statins are to be taken seriously as they can lead to serious adverse events, including potentially fatal rhabdomyolysis, and myopathy.

- Inducers of the hepatic isoenzymes CYP3A4 and CYP2C9 can lead to a significant reduction in the level of the statins metabolized by these enzymes. This may negate the improved cardiac outcomes shown to exist with statins.

- Rapid withdrawal of an enzyme inducer, such as phenytoin or rifampin, can significantly increase the circulating levels of the substrate statin drugs, leading to potential adverse drug reactions.

- Pravastatin is not metabolized by the hepatic P450 isoenzymes and it may be a good alternative medication if a patient must remain on a significant enzyme inhibitor or inducer.
- Gemfibrozil inhibits conjugation and biliary excretion of stations, and its combination with statins can lead to an of adverse drug reaction including myopathy.

Summary

Interaction: pharmacokinetic
Substrate: atorvastatin
Enzyme: CYP3A4
Inducer: phenytoin
Clinical effects: possible decrease in mortality benefit and possible loss of efficacy in reduction of in postoperative mortality and cardiovascular events

References

1. Cannon CP, Braunwald E, McCabe CH, et al. Intensive versus moderate lipid lowering with statins after acute coronary syndromes. N Engl J Med. 2004;350:1495–504.
2. Schouten O, Boersma E, Hoeks SE, Dutch Echocardiographic Cardiac Risk Evaluation Applying Stress Echocardiography Study Group, et al. Fluvastatin and perioperative events in patients undergoing vascular surgery. N Engl J Med. 2009;361:980–9.

Be Still, My Beating Heart 140

Fatal Forty DDI: amiodarone, digoxin, P-glycoprotein

Branka Polić MD, MSc, Julije Meštrović MD, PhD, Toby N. Weingarten MD, and Juraj Sprung MD, PhD

Abstract
This case discusses the inhibition of energy-dependent P-glycoprotein transport of digoxin by amiodarone, resulting in toxic digoxin levels.

Case

A 14-year-old, 56 kg boy with tetralogy of Fallot had undergone corrective surgery 2 months ago. After the procedure, he was given digoxin (0.125 mg BID). He felt well after discharge from the hospital but was later readmitted with fever and dyspnea. The chest radiograph showed left-sided pneumonia and a late-occurring wound infection. The patient was started on an antibiotic and an antipyretic. Although the echocardiogram was reassuring, the patient developed recurrent ventricular tachyarrhythmias. His intensivist added amiodarone hydrochloride (200 mg BID). Before amiodarone therapy was started, his serum digoxin concentration was 0.8 ng/mL (normal therapeutic range, 0.5-2.0 ng/mL).

The patient's condition improved, his heart rhythm converted to normal sinus rhythm, and a chest radiograph showed that the pneumonia had resolved. He was discharged to home after 12 days. A week later, an electrocardiogram showed normal sinus rhythm, and his serum digoxin concentration was 1.5 ng/mL. Three weeks after amiodarone was added, the patient was admitted for nausea, vomiting, diarrhea, and confusion. An electrocardiogram showed ventricular tachycardia, and his serum digoxin level was elevated at 4 ng/mL. After successfully treating the patient's shock and ventricular tachycardia, the intensivist suspended digoxin therapy. Over

B. Polić MD, MSc (✉) • J. Meštrović MD, PhD
Pediatric Intensive Care Unit, Department of Pediatrics, University Hospital of Split, Split, Croatia
e-mail: branka.polic1@st.t-com.hr

T.N. Weingarten MD • J. Sprung MD, PhD
Department of Anesthesiology, Mayo Clinic, Rochester, MN, USA

C. Marcucci et al. (eds.), *A Case Approach to Perioperative Drug-Drug Interactions*, DOI 10.1007/978-1-4614-7495-1_140

the next 5 days, the digoxin blood concentration decreased to the therapeutic range and the symptoms of digoxin toxicity resolved.

Discussion

This is an example of a (P-glycoprotein) inhibitor added to a substrate.

More specifically, this is an example of inhibition of energy-dependent P-glycoprotein transport of digoxin by amiodarone, resulting in toxic digoxin levels.

Amiodarone is a Class III antiarrhythmic used to treat atrial fibrillation and ventricular dysrhythmias. Because of its potentially serious adverse effects, use of amiodarone in children is reserved for refractory dysrhythmias and may be in conjunction with digoxin.[1] However, a considerable increase in serum digoxin concentration is often observed after initiation of amiodarone therapy (Fig. 140.1).[2]

Digoxin has a narrow therapeutic window, and toxicity may occur at concentrations only slightly greater than normal. Digoxin toxicity may cause nausea, vomiting, diarrhea, confusion, xanthopsia, atrioventricular conduction blockade, bigeminy,

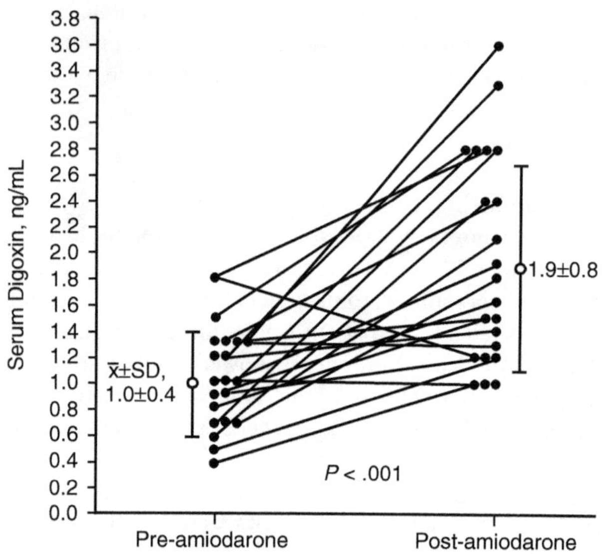

Fig. 140.1 Serum digoxin levels before and after administration of amiodarone for 22 patients [Adapted from Oetgen WJ, Sobol SM, Tri TB et al. Amiodarone-digoxin interaction: clinical and experimental observations. Chest. 1984;86:75–79. With permission from American College of Chest Physicians]

supraventricular nodal tachycardia, and ventricular dysrhythmias and fibrillation. Digoxin bioavailability and excretion are highly dependent on P-glycoprotein (digoxin efflux pump).[3]

P-glycoprotein is an energy-dependent protein that transports digoxin across the apical side of cells (an efflux transporter). It is found along luminal cells and epithelial cells in the intestine, as well as on cell membranes in kidneys and liver. In the intestine, P-glycoprotein limits bioavailability by excreting absorbed digoxin back into the intestinal lumen. In the kidneys and liver, P-glycoprotein facilitates digoxin excretion into urine and bile, respectively (Fig. 140.2).[3] Renal excretion is the primary mechanism of digoxin elimination.

Interaction between amiodarone and digoxin is complex, and several mechanisms have been proposed. First, amiodarone is an important inhibitor of P-glycoprotein.[4] Such inhibition results in increased digoxin levels through both an increase in its bioavailability (through decreasing the amount of digoxin secreted back into the intestinal lumen) and a decrease in elimination (renal and hepatic excretion). Second, an organic anion transporting polypeptide, OATP4C1, recently has been found to be important in digoxin elimination through its facilitation of the uptake of digoxin from the blood and the transport of digoxin across the basolateral membrane in kidney and liver cells.[5,6] OATP4C1 also is inhibited by amiodarone, thus further inhibiting digoxin renal and hepatic elimination.[7] Third, a mechanism unrelated to the inhibition of P-glycoprotein or OATP4C1 was postulated to affect amiodarone-digoxin interaction. Namely, decreased tissue binding of digoxin has been noticed after amiodarone administration, which may lead to an increase in peak serum digoxin levels.[8]

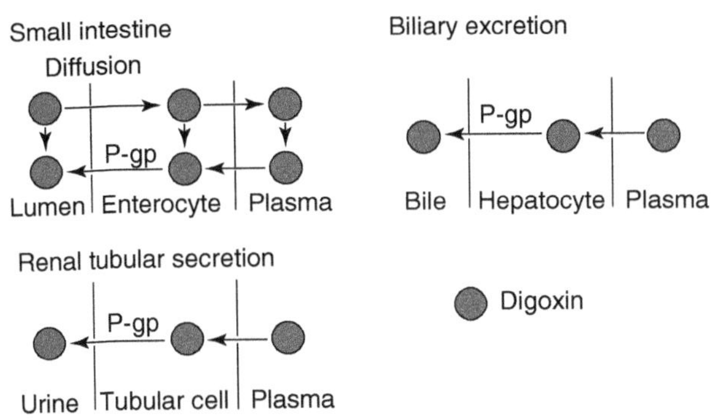

Fig. 140.2 The role of the P-glycoprotein (P-gp) energy-dependent efflux transport system in the elimination of digoxin. P-gp is found in enterocytes, hepatocytes, and renal tubular cells. It pumps digoxin out of cells, resulting in a reduction in digoxin absorption and an increase in its biliary and urinary excretion [Adapted from Horn JR, Hansten PD. Drug interactions with digoxin: the role of P-glycoprotein. Pharmacy Times October 2004;114:. With permission from Intellisphere, LLC]

Interaction between amiodarone and digoxin is more acute and more serious in children than in adults because children are more dependent on drug elimination through renal tubular secretion. The onset of the effect of amiodarone is also more rapid in children than in adults. The terminal half-life of amiodarone is approximately 53 days, and because of this long half-life, the interaction may occur a long time after the cessation of amiodarone treatment.[5] Of note, several frequently used drugs inhibit P-glycoprotein (ie, diltiazem hydrochloride, verapamil hydrochloride, cyclosporine, erythromycin, felodipine, itraconazole, ritonavir, tacrolimus, and sirolimus) and may impact serum levels of drugs dependent on this transport system.

In conclusion, amiodarone-induced inhibition of P-glycoprotein and OATP4C1 increases digoxin bioavailability and decreases digoxin elimination, resulting in clinically significant increases in digoxin serum concentration. When digoxin is used with amiodarone simultaneously, its concentrations need to be monitored and the appropriate dose adjustment (on average, 50%) must be made to avoid digoxin toxicity.[9]

Take-Home Points

- Simultaneous administration of amiodarone and digoxin results in a clinically significant increase in digoxin plasma concentration and may result in digoxin toxicity.
- When digoxin is used in conjunction with amiodarone, its dose needs to be reduced and plasma levels need to be checked.
- Digoxin is a substrate of P-glycoprotein, which is part of the transport system in the membranes of intestines, kidneys, and the biliary system. P-glycoprotein facilitates digoxin secretion into both the intestinal lumen (which decreases bioavailability) and the kidney and biliary canaliculi (which increases elimination).
- Clearance of digoxin from the blood into the cells of the kidneys and liver is facilitated by the organic anion transporting polypeptide OATP4C1.
- Amiodarone alters the bioavailability and elimination of digoxin through inhibition of both the P-glycoprotein and OATP4C1 transporter systems.

Summary

Interaction: pharmacokinetic (uptake and elimination)
Substrate: digoxin
Transporter: P-glycoprotein
Inhibitor: amiodarone
Mechanism/site of action: increased net uptake of digoxin in the intestinal lumen and decreased elimination of digoxin in the kidney leads to greater bioavailability
Clinical effects: digoxin toxicity

References

1. Buck ML. Amiodarone use in children. Pediatric Pharmacotherapy: a monthly newsletter for health care professionals from the Children's Medical Center of the University of Virginia. Charlottesville (VA), University of Virginia Health System, December 2001, vol 7, no 12.
2. Oetgen WJ, Sobol SM, Tri TB, et al. Amiodarone-digoxin interaction: clinical and experimental observations. Chest. 1984;86:75–9.
3. Horn JR, Hansten PD. Drug interactions with digoxin: the role of P-glycoprotein. Pharm Times. 2004;114:45.
4. Katoh M, Nakajima M, Yamazaki H, et al. Inhibitory effects of CYP3A4 substrates and their metabolites on P-glycoprotein-mediated transport. Eur J Pharm Sci. 2001;12:505–13.
5. Mikkaichi T, Suzuki T, Onogawa T, et al. Isolation and characterization of a digoxin transporter and its rat homologue expressed in the kidney. Proc Natl Acad Sci U S A. 2004;101:3569–74.
6. Liu L, Mak E, Tirona RG, et al. Vascular binding, blood flow, transporter, and enzyme interactions on the processing of digoxin in rat liver. J Pharmacol Exp Ther. 2005;315:433–48.
7. Kodawara T, Masuda S, Wakasugi H, et al. Organic anion transporter oatp2-mediated interaction between digoxin and amiodarone in the rat liver. Pharm Res. 2002;19:738–43.
8. DeVore KJ, Hobbs RA. Plasma digoxin concentration fluctuations associated with timing of plasma sampling and amiodarone administration. Pharmacotherapy. 2007;27:472–5.
9. Koren G, Hesslein PS, MacLeod SM. Digoxin toxicity associated with amiodarone therapy in children. J Pediatr. 1984;104:467–70.

The Nice Niece

141

Fatal Forty DDI: Digoxin, St. John's wort, CYP3A4, P-glycoprotein

Michael P. Hutchens MD and Catherine Marcucci MD

Abstract
This case discusses the pharmacokinetic interaction between digoxin and St. John's wort. Digoxin is a cytochrome P450 3A4 substrate and St. John's wort is a 3A4 inducer and also a P-glycoprotein inducer.

Case

A 71-year-old man was evaluated by his anesthesiologist in the coronary care unit on the night before coronary bypass surgery. The history was obtained from the patient and his niece, a naturopathic medicine student. Four days prior, his niece had observed him clutching his chest and becoming diaphoretic after mowing the lawn; work-up had revealed multi-vessel coronary artery disease (CAD). The patient had a 3-month history of progressive dyspnea on exertion, and had become more isolated and frustrated because he was not able to play in his bowling league. His only preoperative medication was St. John's wort extract (*Hypericum perforatum*), which he had been taking for depression, on advice from his niece.

On postoperative day 3, the patient developed atrial fibrillation with rapid ventricular response, and was given an intravenous digoxin load, with gradual control of his heart rate. His digoxin level was therapeutic in the hospital; his recovery was otherwise unremarkable. Discharge medications included a maintenance dose of digoxin, as well as a panel of medications for secondary prevention of CAD.

M.P. Hutchens MD (✉)
Department of Anesthesiology and Perioperative Medicine,
Oregon Health and Science University, Portland, OR, USA
e-mail: hutchenm@ohsu.edu

C. Marcucci MD
Anesthesia Services Department, Philadelphia Veterans Affairs Medical Center,
Philadelphia, PA, USA

C. Marcucci et al. (eds.), *A Case Approach to Perioperative Drug-Drug Interactions*, DOI 10.1007/978-1-4614-7495-1_141

Upon returning to clinic 2 weeks later, the patient denied chest pain and he was eager to get clearance to start bowling again. The nurse noted an irregular, rapid heart beat, and he was found to have atrial fibrillation with rapid ventricular response on an electrocardiogram (ECG). His digoxin level was subtherapeutic, although the patient and the attentive niece insisted he had been taking every medication as scheduled.

Discussion

This is an example of a substrate (digoxin) added to an inducer (St. John's wort extract).

St. John's wort extract is a popular herbal antidepressant that is also used to treat sleep disorders and anxiety. The main constituents of the extract that are believed to have potential central nervous system effects include hypericins, hyperforins, and flavonol glycosides.

Hyperforin increases the activity of the liver enzyme involved with breakdown of digoxin, cytochrome P450 (CYP) 3A4. Similarly, hyperforin induces P-glycoprotein, a transport protein that returns digoxin within enterocytes back into the gut. Because more digoxin is excreted by the higher level of P-glycoprotein triggered by St. John's wort extract, concomitant use of the extract may result in lower digoxin levels. Similarly, digoxin's rate of hepatic metabolism will potentially increase.[1,2] In fact, when healthy volunteers ingesting a constant dose of digoxin began to take extract of St. John's wort daily, digoxin Area-Under-the-Curve (AUC) levels decreased by 26% and maximum digoxin concentration was 38% lower. Another study noted a 33% decrease in digoxin levels after at least 10 days of St. John's wort exposure. In one human study, St. John's wort at a dose of 1800 mg daily for 10 days was associated with an increase of P-glycoprotein expression of 4.2 times.

In the case presented here, a therapeutic level was achieved in the hospital after intravenous loading (which bypasses the increased level of P-glycoprotein on enterocytes), yet a standard oral dose was ineffective in sustaining levels in the goal range, leading to the recurrence of a rapid heart rate.

Take-Home Points

- Anesthesiologists should specifically ask about herbal medications that their patients may be taking during the preoperative assessment, because many patients are either reluctant to report them or are not aware that they are potentially significant.

- To avoid interactions, consider advising patients to discontinue St. John's wort extract 5 days or more before surgery. Patients taking St. John's wort as well as medications with a narrow therapeutic index merit increased vigilance in therapeutic monitoring. In addition to digoxin, other medications relevant to anesthesia that are substrates for CYP3A4 include alfentanil, lidocaine, midazolam, and diltiazem.

- When a patient appears to have unpredictable drug effectiveness despite standard and consistent dosing, consider the possibility of a drug–drug interaction, including one involving herbal medications.

Summary

Interaction: pharmacokinetic
Substrate: digoxin
Enzyme: CYP3A4 and P-glycoprotein
Inducer: St. John's wort
Clinical effect: decreased digoxin levels leading to atrial fibrillation

References

1. Johne A, Brockmöller J, Bauer S, et al. Pharmacokinetic interaction of digoxin with an herbal extract from St John's wort (Hypericum perforatum). Clin Pharmacol Ther. 1999;66(4):338–45.
2. Mueller SC, Uehleke B, Woehling H, et al. Effect of St John's wort dose and preparations on the pharmacokinetics of digoxin. Clin Pharmacol Ther. 2004;75(6):546–57.

Cyclo Killer: Qu'est-ce que c'est?

142

Carvedilol, cyclosporine, P-glycoprotein

Jeff Chen MD, Michael P. Hutchens MD,
and Wayne T. Nicholson MD, PharmD, MSc

Abstract
Addition of carvedilol (a P-glycoprotein inhibitor) to the cyclosporine (a P-glycoprotein substrate) resulted in increased cyclosporine levels and cyclosporine toxicity.

Case

A 47-year-old man with a history of a kidney transplant for polycystic kidney disease and a recent myocardial infarction (MI) was evaluated in preoperative clinic at the request of the vascular surgeon prior to lower extremity bypass. A recent echocardiogram was significant for an ejection fraction of 40%. His medications included lisinopril, aspirin, and pravastatin to treat his coronary artery disease, as well as cyclosporine and prednisone to prevent rejection of his transplanted kidney. Because of the recent MI and upcoming vascular surgery, ß-blocker therapy was started as per hospital protocol. Due to the reduced ejection fraction, the resident selected carvedilol and ordered 12.5 mg BID.

J. Chen MD (✉)
Sierra Anesthesia, Inc., Reno, NV, USA
e-mail: Smartknght@aol.com

M.P. Hutchens MD
Department of Anesthesiology and Perioperative Medicine, Oregon Health and Science University, Portland, OR, USA

W.T. Nicholson MD, PharmD, MSc
Department of Anesthesiology, Mayo Clinic, Rochester, MN, USA

C. Marcucci et al. (eds.), *A Case Approach to Perioperative Drug-Drug Interactions*, DOI 10.1007/978-1-4614-7495-1_142

On the day of surgery 2 weeks later, the patient reported that he had been experiencing fatigue, nausea, and headaches a few days after he started the carvedilol and complained that the Anesthesiology Department was trying to kill him. The blood pressure was 200/120 mm Hg. The anesthesiologist recognized that the symptoms were possibly related to elevated cyclosporine levels. He contacted the patient's nephrologist, who recommended that the preoperative carvedilol be discontinued and metoprolol be initiated. The nephrologist discussed the interaction and that the nephrology service would manage the cyclosporine dose based on levels and anticipated changes. Surgery was postponed. The patient returned 2 weeks later with resolution of symptoms and an acceptable preoperative blood pressure and, and had an uncomplicated perioperative course.

Discussion

This is an example of a P-glycoprotein inhibitor added to a P-glycoprotein substrate.

More specifically, the addition of carvedilol (the inhibitor) to the cyclosporine (the substrate) resulted in increased cyclosporine levels and cyclosporine toxicity.

Cyclosporine is extracted from soil fungus and preferentially suppresses cell-mediated immune reactions, but minimally affects the humoral response. Adverse effects of cyclosporine are dose-dependent. The most serious complication from cyclosporine is renal failure due to nephrotoxicity. Another adverse effect is hypertension. Cyclosporine-induced hypertension is caused by a decrease in endogenous vasodilators (eg, prostacyclin, nitric oxide) and an increase in endogenous vasoconstrictor substances (eg, endothelin, thromboxane).[1] Other adverse reactions that can occur due to elevated levels of cyclosporine include hyperkalemia, tremor, hirsutism, headaches, abdominal discomfort, nausea, glucose intolerance, and gum hyperplasia.

Carvedilol is used in the treatment of hypertension and congestive heart failure. It is a nonselective ß-blocking agent with blocking activity as well, which has been shown to be more effective than metoprolol for the treatment of chronic congestive heart failure.[2] Carvedilol is indicated to reduce cardiovascular mortality in clinically stable patients who have survived the acute phase of a myocardial infarction and have a left ventricular ejection fraction of <40%. Common adverse effects of carvedilol include hypotension, bradyarrhythmias, hyperglycemia, fatigue, and dizziness. Serious side effects include AV block, Stevens-Johnson syndrome, and asthma exacerbation in at-risk patients. It is recommended by the manufacturer that in treatment of heart failure, carvedilol be individualized and started at a very low dose (3.125 mg BID) and slowly up-titrated over weeks based on tolerability.[3]

This vignette considers an example of a transport inhibitor increasing levels of a substrate. P-glycoprotein (P-gp) modulates the absorption of drugs, and its function is unique in that it serves as an *exporter* which *decreases* the amount of systemic absorption. In this clinical situation, cyclosporine is a substrate for the intestinal P-gp transporter and carvedilol is an inhibitor of the transporter.[4] In a small clinical study, effects of P-gp inhibition by carvedilol on cyclosporine levels were highly variable among individual renal transplant patients.[5] Overall, as the carvedilol was increased, the total daily dose of cyclosporine was reduced, demonstrating that P-gp inhibition was dose related.

Consultation with the service managing the immunosuppressant agents was the appropriate action by the attending anesthesiologist. The nephrologist in this case recommended metoprolol as a perioperative ß-blocker since it does not interact with P-gp, thereby removing the interaction while readjusting the cyclosporine. Carvedilol could be used concomitantly if the cyclosporine dose is decreased as the carvedilol is titrated upward, while monitoring plasma levels. Although studies have demonstrated an overall 10% to 20% reduction of the cyclosporine dose when administered with carvedilol due to interpatient variability, different doses used, and other drugs the patient patient may receive concurrently, it can be difficult to clearly predict clinical outcome without close monitoring.[5,6]

Transplant patients ubiquitously present with multiple medications, thus additional interactions should be a consideration. An unintentional increase in the cyclosporine levels may further increase the risk of other drug interactions. In this case, the patient was also receiving pravastatin. Although cyclosporine is known to interact with HMG-CoA reductase inhibitors (statins) and result in possible myopathy or rhabdomyolysis, this combination is still often seen in clinical use. These interactions are well known to transplant teams and adverse effects are closely monitored when changing medication dosages. The interaction depends on the method of statin drug clearance. Because cyclosporine is a cytochrome P450 (CYP) 3A4 inhibitor, statins cleared by this enzymatic pathway (eg, lovastatin, simvastatin, atorvastatin) are more likely to cause myopathy.[7,8] In addition, some statins are cleared by a biliary mechanism (eg, pravastatin) and are reduced in combination with cyclosporine.[8] This is due to the inhibition of OATP, an importer that promotes statin excretion into the bile.[9]

Take-Home Points

- Transplant patients present with multiple medications, thus drug–drug interactions should be a consideration.
- Systemic levels from oral cyclosporine are regulated in part by the P-glycoprotein transport system in the gastrointestinal tract.

- Intestinal P-glycoprotein is an export transporter which decreases the serum level of oral medications.

- Carvedilol is an inhibitor of the P-glycoprotein transporter, which can thus increase the serum level of cyclosporine.

- On average, reductions of cyclosporine doses by 10% to 20% over time may be needed to compensate for the effects of carvedilol. However, due to a large interpatient variability, monitoring is essential.

- Cyclosporine is known to interact with HMG-CoA reductase inhibitors (statins) and may result in myopathy. The mechanism depends on the inherent method of statin drug clearance.

Summary

Interaction: pharmacokinetic
Substrate: cyclosporine
Transporter: P-glycoprotein
Inhibitor: carvedilol
Clinical effects: increased bioavailability of cyclosporine leading to cyclosporine toxicity

References

1. Tedesco D, Haragsim L. Cyclosporine: a review. J Transplant. 2012;2012:230386.
2. Poole-Wilson P, Swedberg K, Cleland J, et al. Comparison of carvedilol and metoprolol on clinical outcomes in patients with chronic heart failure in the Carvedilol or Metoprolol European Trial (COMET): randomized controlled trial. Lancet. 2003;362(9377):7–13.
3. COREG® (carvedilol) tablets Product information. GlaxoSmithKline, Research Triangle Park, NC January 2011.
4. Amioka K, Kuzuya T, Kushihara H, et al. Carvedilol increases ciclosporin bioavailability by inhibiting P-glycoprotein-mediated transport. J Pharm Pharmacol. 2007;59:1383–7.
5. Kaijser M, Johnsson C, Zezina L, et al. Elevation of cyclosporin A blood levels during carvedilol treatment in renal transplant patients. Clin Transplant. 1997;11(6):577–81.
6. Bader F, Hagan M, Crompton J, et al. The Effect of beta-blocker use on cyclosporine level in cardiac transplant recipients. J Heart Lung Transplant. 2005;24(12):2144–7.
7. Gruer PJ, Vega JM, Mercuri MF, et al. Concomitant use of cytochrome P450 3A4 inhibitors and simvastatin. Am J Cardiol. 1999;84(7):811–5.
8. Ballantyne CM, Corsini A, Davidson MH, et al. Risk for myopathy with statin therapy in high-risk patients. Arch Intern Med. 2003;163(5):553–64.
9. Sirtori CR, Mombelli G, Triolo M, et al. Clinical response to statins: mechanism(s) of variable activity and adverse effects. Ann Med. 2011;44(5):419–32 [Epub ahead of print].

Blurry-Eyed with Rapid Heart Beats

143

Fatal Forty DDI: digoxin, hydrochlorothiazide

William A. Shakespeare MD and Juraj Sprung MD, PhD

Abstract
This case discusses the indirect interaction between hydrochlorothiazide and digoxin in the etiology of digoxin toxicity.

Case

A 72-year-old woman scheduled for a thoracoscopy reported visual changes and palpitations in the preoperative area. She had a 10-year history of coronary artery disease and heart failure, normally under therapeutic control with digoxin. Her creatinine level was 1.8 mg/dL. The patient had been admitted to the hospital 2 weeks ago for treatment of pulmonary edema, and during the course of therapy and evaluation was found to have a new right lower-lobe nodule on radiographs. During the inpatient stay, her pulmonary edema had improved gradually with ongoing diuresis, initially with furosemide boluses and more recently with hydrochlorothiazide (12.5 mg/d orally) for maintenance.

Initial evaluation in the preoperative area found the patient sitting in her bed with oxygen administered through nasal cannula; she was slightly tachypneic and short of breath. She stated that her vision had become increasingly unfocused and altered over the past day and the shortness of breath started during transport to the preoperative area. Her heart rate was 151 beats per minute; blood pressure 86/45 mm Hg; and oxyhemoglobin saturation on pulse oximetry, 92%. An electrocardiogram showed accelerated junctional rhythm, which was terminated successfully with a single 6-mg intravenous dose of adenosine. Laboratory results of blood drawn in the preoperative area were remarkable for a digoxin level of 2.3 ng/mL (reference

W.A. Shakespeare MD (✉) • J. Sprung MD, PhD
Department of Anesthesiology, Mayo Clinic, Rochester, MN, USA
e-mail: washakespeare@gmail.edu

C. Marcucci et al. (eds.), *A Case Approach to Perioperative Drug-Drug Interactions*, DOI 10.1007/978-1-4614-7495-1_143

range, 0.5 ng/mL to 2.0 ng/mL) and a serum potassium concentration of 2.6 mEq/L (reference range, 3.0 mEq/L to 6.0 mEq/L). After cardioversion, the patient continued to have sinus rhythm with regular ectopic beats. She was observed overnight in the intensive care unit and received incrementally dosed potassium chloride (total, 40 mEq), with stabilization of cardiac rhythm and resolution of visual disturbance.

Discussion

This is an example of a pharmacodynamic interaction at the level of the sodium-potassium-ATPase pump. It is also an example of a pharmacokinetic (excretion) interaction.

Digoxin was initially described to the western world by William Withering in 1785 and persists as one of the most enduring of modern medical therapies.[1] It operates through binding to the sodium-potassium pump (Na^+-K^+ ATPase) on cardiac myocytes (Fig. 143.1). This binding prevents the pumping of potassium into the cell and the pumping of sodium out of the cell. The disruption has a secondary effect on the sodium-calcium (Na^+-Ca^{++}) exchanger of the myocyte, which has the role of removing calcium from the cell. This apparatus depends on a small intracellular sodium gradient to drive an inward flow of sodium in exchange for an outward flow of calcium. Inhibition of sodium egress by digoxin thereby traps calcium intracellularly.

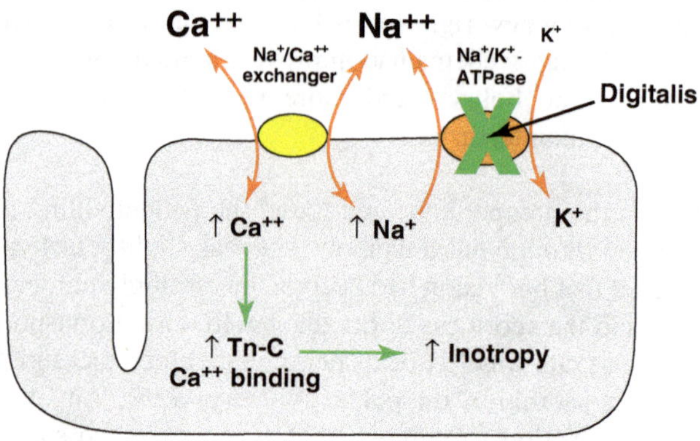

Fig. 143.1 Mechanism of digitalis action. Digitalis blocks the sodium-potassium pump (Na^+/K^+-ATPase), leading to the intracellular accumulation of sodium. The increased intracellular sodium level decreases the gradient that drives the sodium-calcium exchanger. This altered gradient results in decreased removal of calcium ions from the cell (increasing intracellular calcium) and causes increased calcium binding to Tn-C, which increases contractility (inotropy). ATPase indicates adenosine triphosphatase; Ca^{++}, calcium ion; K^+, potassium ion; Na^+, sodium ion; Tn-C, troponin-C [Adapted from Klabunde RE. Cardiovascular Pharmacology Concepts. Available from: http://www.cvpharmacology.com/cardiostimulatory/digitalis.htm. Last Accessed June 4th, 2012. with permission from Richard Klabunde, PhD]

This increased intracellular calcium leads to further increase in calcium from the sarcoplasmic reticulum, which in turn binds to troponin-C leading to increased inotropy. Binding of digoxin on the sodium-potassium transport system (pump) is inhibited by higher levels of potassium, and Na^+-K^+ ATPase activity is increased in the presence of increased magnesium levels. Thus, hypokalemia and hypomagnesemia increase the toxicity of digoxin. In addition, advanced age and renal dysfunction may increase the likelihood of digoxin toxicity.[1]

A narrow therapeutic window has been a nagging challenge to the successful use of digoxin, and studies have shown that toxicity develops in up to 20% of patients taking digoxin.[1] Excessive digoxin levels may lead to symptoms such as anorexia, cardiac arrhythmia, lethargy, muscle cramps, visual disturbance (eg, unfocused vision, changes in color vision), weakness, and hallucinations. Although the incidence of toxicity has improved in recent years, certain populations—especially persons with recent hospitalization—continue to be at high risk.[2,3]

Hypokalemia can complicate the already narrow therapeutic window of digoxin and lead to toxicity within otherwise normal digoxin parameters. Drugs that are known to lead to hypokalemia, such as diuretics, may precipitate symptoms of toxicity. Normally, potassium competes with digoxin at the binding site of the sodium–potassium pump, but in states of low serum potassium levels, the digoxin blockade is more widespread and involves a greater number of blocked sodium–potassium pumps and more toxic adverse effects. Further exacerbating this situation, renal secretion of digoxin decreases once serum potassium levels decrease to less than 3 mEq/L, leading to a prolongation of the drug's half-life.[1]

Take-Home Points

- Digoxin has a narrow therapeutic window.
- Hypokalemia can lead to digoxin toxicity even within normal therapeutic parameters.
- Potassium levels should be monitored closely for patients receiving both digoxin and a diuretic drug, and low serum potassium concentrations should be corrected promptly.

Editor's Note: Look carefully at the medication panels of hospitalized patients, even if they have been on the floor or in the ICU for a significant amount of time! Do not assume that any potential drug–drug interaction will be found and dealt with before the patient gets to the operating room. Remember that one of the guiding principles in diagnosing and managing drug–drug interactions is that drugs are stopped and started in the hospital and perioperative period.

Summary

Interactions: pharmacodynamic and pharmacokinetic
Substrates: digoxin and hydrochlorothiazide
Mechanism/site of action: 1) potentiation of sodium-potassium-ATPase pump activity at multiple sites, and 2) HCTZ-induced hypokalemia leading to decreased renal excretion of digoxin
Clinical effect: digoxin toxicity

References

1. Vivo RP, Krim SR, Perez J, et al. Digoxin: current use and approach to toxicity. Am J Med Sci. 2008;336:423–8.
2. Haynes K, Hennessy S, Localio AR, et al. Increased risk of digoxin toxicity following hospitalization. Pharmacoepidemiol Drug Saf. 2009;18:28–35.
3. Haynes K, Heitjan D, Kanetsky P, et al. Declining public health burden of digoxin toxicity from 1991 to 2004. Clin Pharmacol Ther. 2008;84:90–4.

Drug–Drug Interactions Involving Coagulation Modifiers

XIII

Introduction 144

Catherine Marcucci MD

Abstract
This section introduces drug–drug interactions involving nonopioid pain medications.

Drug–drug interactions (DDIs) involving the coagulation drugs are important clinically and a bit tricky. The coagulation status of both medical and surgical patients is often one of the prime factors in the maintenance of the patient's health. The ability of perioperative providers to reliably predict pertubations in a patient's coagulated, or anticoagulated, state is crucial in planning surgical and other interventions and preventing morbid and even devastating bleeding emergencies. The drugs themselves are not lethal, but there exists the possibility that the DDIs cause seriously morbid or even mortal consequences to the patients.

Two of the drugs in this section are members of the **Fatal Forty**—warfarin and clopidogrel. Clopidogrel is an extremely commonly prescribed drug that is a cytochrome P450 (CYP) 3A4 substrate and also acts as a prodrug substrate for the CYP2C19 isozyme. For some time, omeprazole, a 2C19 inhibitor, was implicated in clinically significant DDIs involving clopidogrel, however, that has recently been called into question. Of greater interest recently has been its action as a 3A4 substrate in DDIs with 3A4 inhibitors such as the calcium channel blockers.

Warfarin fully deserves its place on the **Fatal Forty**. It is a low therapeutic index drug whose use is very common in both the general and surgical patient populations. DDIs involving warfarin have serious clinical sequelae. Warfarin DDIs are also common as warfarin interacts with many drugs including common antibiotics such as the macrolide antibiotics (azithromycin, clarithromycin, erythromycin) and spices such as dong quai and turmeric.

C. Marcucci MD
Anesthesia Services Department, Philadelphia Veterans Affairs Medical Center,
Philadelphia, PA, USA
e-mail: sandson.marcucci@comcast.net

C. Marcucci et al. (eds.), *A Case Approach to Perioperative Drug-Drug Interactions*, DOI 10.1007/978-1-4614-7495-1_144

In learning and reviewing warfarin DDIs, the reader must keep in mind that warfarin is a racemic mixture of two enantiomers, an R-enantiomer and an S-enantiomer. The R-enantiomer (sometimes referred to as R-warfarin) is not as active in anticoagulation and is a CYP1A2 substrate. The more active S-warfarin is a 2C9 substrate. To date, there are several known 2C9 polymorphisms associated with increased warfarin sensitivity.

In short, it is well worth the time of the perioperative clinician to review, study, and master DDIs involving the coagulation drugs, especially because these drugs are both started and stopped by a range of other providers, including both medical and surgical subspecialty providers. We recommend that anesthesiologists and anesthesia providers themselves remain ever-vigilant and on the lookout for the associated DDIs.

Seize the Day

145

Fatal Forty DDI: tranexamic acid, furosemide, ibuprofen

Roman M. Sniecinski MD, Erica D. Wittwer MD, PhD, Kenichi Tanaka MD, MSc, and James Zaidan MD

Abstract
This case discusses a pharmacokinetic reaction involving the decreased elimination of tranexamic acid, resulting in seizures. The patient had renal insufficiency due to coadministration of furosemide and ibuprofen.

Case

A 41-year-old woman with severe mitral regurgitation presented to the operating room for mitral valve repair. She had a strong family history of early coronary artery disease and a personal history of mitral valve prolapse, which had been followed by her cardiologist for more than 2 decades, and she recently decided on surgery due to her increasing shortness of breath. Being a small woman (5' 2", 51 kg), the cardiac surgeon thought she was an excellent candidate for a minimally invasive approach. The length of cardiopulmonary bypass (CPB) required was not felt to be an issue due to her younger age. The patient underwent a preoperative coronary catheterization which ruled out significant coronary disease. She was hypertensive post-procedure which was thought to be due to volume overload. She received intravenous

R.M. Sniecinski MD (✉)
Division of Cardiothoracic Anesthesia, Department of Anesthesiology, Emory University School of Medicine, Atlanta, GA, USA
e-mail: rsnieci@emory.edu

E.D. Wittwer MD, PhD
Department of Anesthesiology, Mayo Clinic, Rochester, MN, USA

K. Tanaka MD, MSc
Department of Anesthesiology, University of Pittsburgh Medical Center, Pittsburgh, PA, USA

J. Zaidan MD
Department of Anesthesiology, Emory University School of Medicine, Stone Mountain, GA, USA

C. Marcucci et al. (eds.), *A Case Approach to Perioperative Drug-Drug Interactions*, DOI 10.1007/978-1-4614-7495-1_145

furosemide (20 mg) and was discharged to home with instructions to take 20 mg orally daily until her mitral valve repair 2 days later.

The morning of surgery she reported that she had taken the furosemide as instructed and reported she had been taking ibuprofen for her menstrual cramps. Intraoperatively, she received heparin and antifibrinolytic therapy per protocol (tranexamic acid 2 g bolus, followed by 1 g/h infusion while on CPB). The repair was difficult with an unacceptable degree of mitral regurgitation on initial wean from CPB, necessitating a second CPB run. She had persistent hypotension postbypass and was taken to the intensive care unit (ICU) intubated, and on vasopressin and propofol infusions.

Initial labs on arrival to the ICU were notable for a creatinine clearance of 55 mL/min, which had been normal 2 weeks prior to surgery. After 4 hours in the ICU, the vasopressin infusion was weaned off and the patient was hemodynamically stable enough for extubation. However, upon discontinuation of the propofol infusion, the patient began to seize violently. She was immediately given midazolam and placed back on the propofol infusion. These events were repeated several hours later during a second attempt at extubation, so the decision was made to keep her intubated overnight. She was extubated the following morning, neurologically intact. Her renal function returned to baseline rapidly and she recovered from her operation uneventfully.

Discussion

This is an example of a pharmacokinetic drug–drug interaction (DDI) involving decreased elimination of a drug.

Antifibrinolytics are commonly used in cardiac surgery to prevent CPB-induced fibrinolysis and reduce blood transfusion requirements. Tranexamic acid belongs to a class of drugs known as the lysine analogs, which reversibly bind to plasminogen (see Fig. 145.1). This blocks the interaction between plasminogen and fibrin, impairing fibrin degradation.[1]

Outside of the operating room, the lysine analogs can be administered orally to treat a variety of bleeding conditions, including hemophilia and excessive menstrual bleeding.[2] Women with hypermenorrhagia may have increased fibrinolysis in utero due to higher levels of endometrium-derived plasminogen activators. The treatment regimen typically consists of 2 to 4.5 g per day during menstruation and it is generally well tolerated, with only occasional nausea.

However, more serious side effects have been reported when tranexamic acid is acutely administered in high dosages. The drug appears to inhibit GABA-A receptors found in the cerebral cortex, lowering the depolarization threshold and enhancing excitability.[3] When injected directly into cerebrospinal fluid, generalized

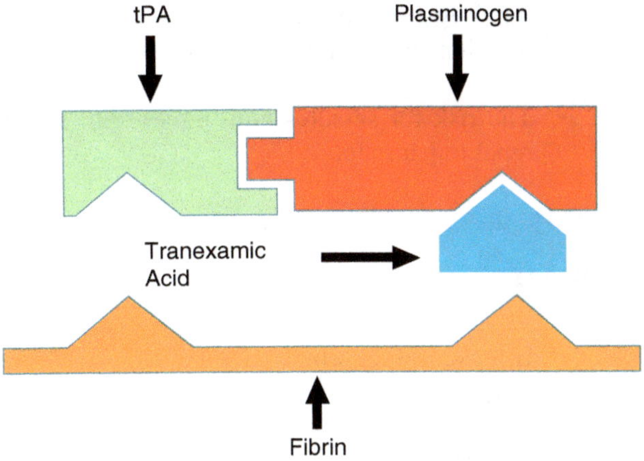

Fig. 145.1 Once activated by tissue plasminogen activating factor (tPA), plasminogen binds to fibrin at the lysine residues and causes its degradation. Lysine analogs, such as tranexamic acid, occupy the lysine-binding site of plasminogen, effectively inhibiting fibrinolysis

seizures have been reported.[4] Patients undergoing cardiac surgery are particularly susceptible to the proconvulsant effect of tranexamic acid, possibly due to an altered blood–brain barrier from the inflammatory effects of CPB. Indeed, a recent study of more than 650 patients reported a 3% incidence of non-ischemic seizures following cardiac surgery with tranexamic acid.[5] In a study of patients undergoing aortic valve replacement receiving tranexamic acid versus ε-aminocaproic acid, seizures occurred in 6.4% of the patients receiving tranexamic acid and 0.6% of those receiving ε-aminocaproic acid. Additional factors that increased the risk for seizure activity were older age, decreased creatinine clearance, and administration of recombinant activated Factor VII.[5]

The proconvulsant effect of tranexamic acid is likely dose-dependent and the presented case illustrates one type of patient at risk for an overdose: a small person who was exposed to a prolonged, high-dose infusion while on CPB complicated by acute renal dysfunction. Our patient's calculated IV dose of tranexamic acid was almost 90 mg/kg, within the dose range associated with seizures in the study by Murkin et al (61–259 mg/kg).[6] Her renal impairment was likely a combination of exposure to contrast dye, over-diuresis via furosemide and ibuprofen use. The drug is minimally bound to plasma proteins and excreted mostly unchanged in the urine.

Take-Home Points

- Lysine analogs, which inhibit plasminogen-dependent fibrin degradation, are commonly utilized in cardiac surgery for antifibrinolytic therapy. They may also be used on an outpatient basis for a variety of bleeding-related conditions.
- One lysine analog in particular, tranexamic acid, is associated with generalized seizures when given in high doses. It seems prudent to administer

the drug using a weight-based regimen. Loading doses of 30 mg/kg and infusions of 15 mg/kg have been used in one multicenter trial.[7]

- The risk for seizures with tranexamic acid is increased in patients with renal impairment.

Summary

Interaction: pharmacokinetic (decreased clearance)
Substrate: tranexamic acid
Inhibitors (of excretion): furosemide and ibuprofen
Mechanism/site of action: decreased clearance through renal impairment
Clinical effects: seizures

References

1. Dunn CJ, Goa KL. Tranexamic acid: a review of its use in surgery and other indications. Drugs. 1999;57:1005–32.
2. Wellington K, Wagstaff AJ. Tranexamic acid: a review of its use in the management of menorrhagia. Drugs. 2003;63:1417–33.
3. Furtmuller R, Schlag MG, Berger M, et al. Tranexamic acid, a widely used antifibrinolytic agent, causes convulsions by a gamma-aminobutyric acid (A) receptor antagonistic effect. J Pharamcol Exp Ther. 2002;301:168–73.
4. Yeh HM, Lau HP, Lin PL, et al. Convulsions and refractory ventricular fibrillation after intrathecal injection of a massive dose of tranexamic acid. Anesthesiology. 2003;98:270–2.
5. Keyl C, Uhl R, Beyersdorf F, et al. High-dose tranexamic acid is related to increased risk of generalized seizures after aortic valve replacement. Eur J Cardiothorac Surg. 2011; 39:e114–21.
6. Murkin JM, Falter F, Granton J, et al. High dose tranexamic acid is associated with nonischemic clinical seizures in cardiac surgical patients. Anesth Analg. 2010;110:350–3.
7. Fergusson DA, Hebert PC, Mazer CD, BART Investigators, et al. A comparison of aprotinin and lysine analogs in high-risk cardiac surgery. N Engl J Med. 2008;358:2319–31.

The Third and Final Complication

146

Fatal Forty DDI: warfarin, nafcillin

Daniel W. Johnson MD

Abstract
This case discusses a pharmacokinetic interaction between warfarin and nafcillin. Nafcillin is an inducer of warfarin metabolism and discontinuation led to reversal of induction and increased anticoagulant effect.

Case

Before leaving for a 3-day break from the orthopedic service, the chief resident decided to see his 72-year-old left hip replacement patient one more time. "She just didn't look right this morning," he recalled. Unfortunately, he was correct as the patient was now febrile, fatigued, and had mild rigors. There was a new superficial wound infection and her left lower leg was swollen. Cultures were sent, broad spectrum antibiotics were started, and the ultrasound diagnosis of a large left popliteal deep vein thrombosis (DVT) prompted the initiation of heparin therapy. The chief felt deflated as he departed for his mini-vacation.

Upon his return, the chief was relieved to learn that cultures had revealed a staphylococcus sensitive to nafcillin and antibiotic therapy had been narrowed to nafcillin alone. Warfarin had also been started, but heparin remained on as the International Normalized Ratio (INR) was subtherapeutic. The next day, the INR was still too low to stop heparin. The medical student on the service remembered that nafcillin and warfarin "have some sort of drug–drug interaction." Satisfied that this explained the

D.W. Johnson MD
Department of Anesthesia, Critical Care & Pain Medicine, Massachusetts General Hospital, Boston, MA, USA
e-mail: DWJOHNSON@PARTNERS.ORG

C. Marcucci et al. (eds.), *A Case Approach to Perioperative Drug-Drug Interactions*, DOI 10.1007/978-1-4614-7495-1_146

slow rise in INR, a resident doubled the dose of warfarin. When the INR remained subtherapeutic 2 days later, the resident doubled the dose again. Finally, 1 week after the diagnosis of the DVT, the INR was in range and the heparin was stopped, allowing the patient to be discharged to an acute rehabilitation center. She was booked for follow up at the anticoagulation clinic and instructed to take the nafcillin for a 2-week course, and the warfarin for 3 months.

After 1 week at the rehabilitation center the patient was discharged home. In her eagerness to get back to her normal schedule, she missed her anticoagulation clinic visits and stopped taking nafcillin because she hadn't felt sick in over a week. Two weeks later, and 1 week before her surgical follow-up visit, she fell while walking through the local park. A jogger ran over to help and found the patient tearful and incoherent. She was rushed back to the hospital and found to have unstable vital signs, a massive intracranial hemorrhage, and an INR of 7. The chief resident was extremely upset when the patient's family was told that the most appropriate course was to pursue palliative care only.

Discussion

This is an example of reversal of induction.

Nafcillin is a common anti-staphylococcal penicillin used for a variety of infections. The patient in this case had culture data that justified narrowing antibiotic coverage to nafcillin alone. Warfarin is the most commonly prescribed oral anticoagulant medication and is appropriate therapy for postoperative DVT. Warfarin is metabolized by the cytochrome P450 (CYP) 2C9, CYP3A4, and CYP1A2.[1] The medical literature contains several case reports in which administration of nafcillin resulted in an increasing warfarin dose requirement to achieve INR consistent with therapeutic anticoagulation. The mechanism that has been proposed, though not proven, is that nafcillin is an inducer of one or more of the P450 enzymes responsible for metabolism of warfarin. In these reports, patients receiving both drugs required warfarin doses in excess of 10 mg daily to achieve an INR greater than 2, and dose requirements returned to baseline (over a period of weeks) when the nafcillin was stopped. In reports where pharmacokinetic data were calculated, enzyme induction by nafcillin was apparent about 1 week after starting the antibiotic and warfarin doses returned to baseline 1 to 4 weeks after stopping nafcillin.[2] Unlike the published case reports, the patient in this case suffered from the *offset* of the enzyme inducer. When the effect of nafcillin subsided, the large dose of warfarin was excessive.

The patient in this case had two common postsurgical complications simultaneously, and both complications were treated appropriately. The potential of this drug–drug interaction (DDI) was not fully appreciated during the hospital stay, although ideally it would have been. Had the patient appropriately followed up in the anticoagulation clinic, the gradual reduction in warfarin dose requirement would have likely been discovered and the supratherapeutic INR could have been avoided. Alternatively, given the complicated postsurgical course and the patient's advanced age, a follow-up appointment with the primary care physician soon after discharge would have been appropriate and might have prevented the lethal outcome. Postoperative patients frequently do not understand the dangers of stopping discharge medications on their own. Perioperative physicians must do all that they can to ensure appropriate medication administration and clinic follow-up after discharge.

Take-Home Points

- Pharmacologic induction of cytochrome P450 enzymes are a frequent cause of increased warfarin metabolism and thus increased dose requirements.
- Increased warfarin requirement in the setting of P450 inducers is commonly recognized. *Decreased* warfarin requirement after the discontinuation of P450 inducers is equally clinically important, yet less readily recognized.
- When a significant (DDI) is recognized, the pharmacologic nature and physiologic consequence of it must be fully elucidated on a case-by-case basis. The plan for prescribing all involved drugs must be carefully made.
- While the responsibility to attend follow-up appointments lies ultimately with the patient, physicians who order drugs with significant drug–drug interactions also bear responsibility to ensure that doses are adjusted properly.

Summary

Interaction: pharmacokinetic
Substrate: warfarin
Enzyme: not as yet determined
Inducer: nafcillin
Clinical effect: reversal of induction led to increased anticoagulant effect of the warfarin

References

1. Kim K, Frey RJ, Epplen K, et al. Interaction between warfarin and nafcillin: case report and review of the literature. Pharmacotherapy. 2007;27(10):1467–70.
2. Cropp JS, Bussey HI. A review of enzyme induction of warfarin metabolism with recommendations for patient management. Pharmacotherapy. 1997;17:917–28.

An Interaction with the Furniture

147

Fatal Forty DDI: warfarin, metronidazole, ciprofloxacin, CYP2C9, CYP1A2

Heather Norvelle PharmD, BCPS
and Ines P. Koerner MD, PhD

Abstract
This case discusses a possible and/or likely pharmacokinetic interaction involving warfarin, metronidazole, and ciprofloxacin, leading to bleeding complications. Warfarin is a cytochrome P450 2C9 and 1A2 substrate. Metronidazole is a 2C9 inhibitor and ciprofloxacin is a 1A2 inhibitor.

Case

A 61-year-old woman presented to the emergency department with abdominal pain, fever, tenderness, and nausea/vomiting. She had a history of diverticulosis and recent deep venous thrombosis (after a knee injury) for which she was on warfarin. Computed tomography (CT) revealed acute diverticulitis within the sigmoid colon without evidence of abscess. Admission labs were unremarkable expect for an elevated white blood cell count of 21 and a therapeutic International Normalized Ratio (INR) of 2.1 (goal 2-3).

General surgery was consulted and recommended antibiotic therapy for diverticulitis. Intravenous ciprofloxacin and metronidazole were initiated and her symptoms rapidly improved. On hospital day 2, she was switched to oral ciprofloxacin and metronidazole in anticipation of discharge. As the patient was getting ready to leave

H. Norvelle PharmD, BCPS (✉)
Department of Infectious Diseases and Critical Care,
Oregon Health and Science University, Portland, OR, USA
e-mail: norvelle@ohsu.edu

I.P. Koerner MD, PhD
Department of Anesthesiology & Perioperative Medicine,
Oregon Health & Science University, Portland, OR, USA

C. Marcucci et al. (eds.), *A Case Approach to Perioperative Drug-Drug Interactions*, DOI 10.1007/978-1-4614-7495-1_147

the hospital, she bent to tie her shoe and accidently hit her head on the bedside table. Over the next 30 minutes, the patient was increasingly obtunded. A head CT demonstrated a large subdural hematoma with mass effect and midline shift. An emergency coagulation panel was significant for an INR of 5. The patient was transferred to the neurointensive care unit for rapid correction of her coagulopathy in preparation for urgent craniotomy and hematoma evacuation. After receiving factor IX complex, factor VIIa, and vitamin K, she underwent uneventful surgical hematoma evacuation. The postoperative course was uneventful, and the patient experienced a full neurologic recovery. The neurointensive care team extensively reviewed the patient's hospital course and hypothesized that potentially significant drug–drug interactions (DDIs) between warfarin and both the ciprofloxacin and metronidazole were the probable cause for the sudden coagulopathy. Antibiotic therapy for the diverticulitis was continued with amoxicillin/clavulanate and warfarin was restarted without additional complications.

Discussion

This is an example of inhibitors added to a substrate.

Both metronidazole and ciprofloxacin are believed to inhibit warfarin metabolism by the liver and increase INR, although the exact mechanism behind each interaction is not completely clear. Warfarin inhibits the vitamin K dependent synthesis of coagulation factors in the liver. It is metabolized and inactivated by the cytochrome P450 (CYP) enzyme family, predominantly by CYP2C9, and to a lesser extent by CYP1A2.[1] Metronidazole has long been thought to be an inhibitor of 2C9, although recent reports question this mechanism.[2,3] Nevertheless, a long list of case series and case reports have described INR elevations and bleeding complications during concurrent warfarin and metronidazole treatment since the initial report of an interaction of metronidazole with warfarin, specifically its S(−) enantiomer, in 1976.[4]

The case is less clear for ciprofloxacin. Experimental data mostly suggest that the effect of CYP1A2 inhibition by ciprofloxacin on coagulation parameters during warfarin therapy should be small, yet case reports and retrospective studies suggest a clinically relevant drug interaction, predominately in the elderly population.[5–8]

While the exact mechanisms of drug interactions between warfarin, metronidazole, and the fluoroquinolones cannot be identified beyond doubt at this time, there is enough clinical concern to warrant careful monitoring of coagulation parameters, and dose adjustments as necessary, when either antibiotic is started for a patient taking warfarin. It has also been recommended to prophylactically reduce the dose of warfarin when metronidazole treatment is initiated.[9] Frequent organisms causing diverticulitis include *Streptococci*, *Escherichia coli*, *Bacteroides*, *Peptostreptococcus*, *clostridium species,* and *fusobacterium*.[10,11] Ciprofloxacin and metronidazole are effective against these bacteria and are appropriate choices for the treatment of acute diverticulitis.[10] Amoxicillin/clavulanate is an alternative treatment option with activity against these bacteria but without the common drug interactions.[10]

Take-Home Points

- Warfarin is metabolized by CYP2C9 and CYP1A2.
- Metronidazole has long been thought to be an inhibitor of 2C9. Ciprofloxacin is a 1A2 inhibitor
- The existing experimental data do not fully elucidate the magnitude of the recognized clinical effects seen with the coadministration of warfarin, metronidazole, and ciprofloxacin.
- Nonetheless, there is enough clinical concern to warrant careful monitoring of coagulation parameters, and dose adjustments as necessary, when either antibiotic is started for a patient taking warfarin.
- Also, the prudent practitioner will consider prophylactically reducing the dose of warfarin when metronidazole treatment is initiated.

Summary

Interaction: pharmacokinetic?
Substrate: warfarin
Enzymes: CYP2C9 and CYP1A2
Inhibitors: metronidazole (CYP2C9) and ciprofloxacin (CYP1A2)
Clinical effects: INR and bleeding complications

References

1. Ogu CC, Maxa JL. Drug interactions due to cytochrome P450. BUMC Proc. 2000;13:421–3.
2. Levy RH. Cytochrome P450 isozymes and antiepileptic drug interactions. Epilepsia. 1995;36 Suppl 5:S8–13.
3. Van Booven D, Marsh S, McLeod H, et al. Cytochrome P450 2C9-CYP2C9. Pharmacogenet Genomics. 2010;20(4):277–81.
4. O'Reilly RA. The stereoselective interaction of warfarin and metronidazole in man. N Engl J Med. 1976;295(7):354–7.
5. Zhang L, Wei MJ, Zhao CY, et al. Determination of the inhibitory potential of 6 fluoroquinolones on CYP1A2 and CYP2C9 in human liver microsomes. Acta Pharmacol Sin. 2008;29(12):1507–14.

6. Israel DS, Stotka J, Rock W, et al. Effect of ciprofloxacin on the pharmacokinetics and pharmacodynamics of warfarin. Clin Infect Dis. 1996;22(2):251–6.
7. Fischer HD, Juurlink DN, Mamdani MM, et al. Hemorrhage during warfarin therapy associated with cotrimoxazole and other urinary tract anti-infective agents: a population-based study. Arch Intern Med. 2010;170(7):617–21.
8. Ellis RJ, Mayo MS, Bodensteiner DM. Ciprofloxacin-warfarin coagulopathy: a case series. Am J Hematol. 2000;63(1):28–31.
9. Holt RK, Anderson EA, Cantrell MA, et al. Preemptive dose reduction of warfarin in patients initiating metronidazole. Drug Metabol Drug Interact. 2010;25(1–4):35–9.
10. Jacobs DO. Diverticulitis. New Eng J Med. 2007;357:2057–66.
11. Brook I, Frazier EH. Aerobic and anaerobic microbiology in intra-abdominal infections associated with diverticulitis. J Med Microbiol. 2000;49:827–30.

Macrolide Mishap for Little Miss Muffett 148

Fatal Forty DDI: warfarin, clarithromycin, CYP2C9

Elizabeth Pedigo MD

Abstract
This case discusses the pharmacokinetic interaction of warfarin and clarithromycin leading to enhanced anticoagulant effect and elevated INR. Warfarin is a cytochrome P450 2C9 substrate and clarithromycin is a 2C9 inhibitor. The use of warfarin for pediatric patients is also discussed.

Case

Midway through her posted ENT cases for the day, the pediatric anesthesiology resident called out to the Day Stay Unit to check on her next patient. The patient was a 3-year-old girl who was having a combined ENT and ophthalmology procedure (ear tubes and strabismus correction). Although she had been seen by the individual surgical clinics preoperatively, no labs had been ordered because each procedure was felt to be of a "minor" nature.

The patient's history included congenital mitral valve insufficiency for which she had undergone initial repair at 7 months of age and replacement 6 months ago. She had been taking warfarin since that time with a target International Normalized Ratio (INR) between 2.5 and 3. The patient's last INR was drawn two weeks ago, and was 2.9. In her review the previous evening of the patient's Electronic Medical Record, the resident had noticed that the patient was completing a 10-day course of clarithromycin (prescribed by a third provider) as therapy for otitis media. The resi-

E. Pedigo MD
Department of Anesthesiology and Perioperative Medicine, Oregon Health and Science University, Portland, OR, USA
e-mail: pedigo@ohsu.edu

C. Marcucci et al. (eds.), *A Case Approach to Perioperative Drug-Drug Interactions*, DOI 10.1007/978-1-4614-7495-1_148

dent knew that erythromycin interacted with warfarin, and was concerned that other macrolide antibiotics could do the same.

The patient was in the Day Stay Unit, and no INR had been sent. The surgical teams agreed to wait for the result before proceeding since this was a potentially important drug–drug interaction (DDI). The blood draw was accomplished and the nurses settled the little patient down with a book of nursery rhymes while the adults waited for the labs. Unfortunately, an INR of 7.2 was returned. The case was cancelled, and the patient was admitted for correction of her excessive anticoagulation.

Discussion

This is an example of an inhibitor added to a substrate.

Warfarin is a drug that was initially marketed as a pesticide against rats and mice and is still popular for this purpose. It is a synthetic derivative of coumarin, a chemical found naturally in many plants, notably woodruff and, at lower levels, in licorice, lavender, and various other species. It is the most widely prescribed oral anticoagulant and the overall 11th most prescribed drug in North America.[1] Despite its effectiveness, treatment with warfarin has several disadvantages. Its activity has to be monitored by frequent blood testing for INR to ensure an adequate yet safe dose is taken, and many commonly used medications interfere with warfarin, as do some foods.

Warfarin is a racemic mixture of R-warfarin (weaker isomer), which is metabolized by the cytochrome P450 (CYP) 1A2 enzyme, and S-warfarin (the more active isomer), which is metabolized by the CYP2C9 enzyme.[2] There are known 2C9 polymorphisms associated with increased warfarin sensitivity.[3] Warfarin works by interfering with the hepatic synthesis of vitamin K sensitive coagulation factors (II, VII, IX, X), and the target of warfarin is vitamin K epoxide reductase. Several common polymorphisms of the complex subunit 1 (VKORC1) have been described that are also associated with increased warfarin sensitivity. In 2007, the US Food and Drug Administration (FDA) modified warfarin labeling to suggest, but not mandate, warfarin pharmacogenetic testing before initiating therapy (commercial kits test for CYP2C9 and VKORC1 polymorphisms).[3] No genetic testing was done in this child prior to the institution of warfarin.

Antibiotics are known to alter the anticoagulation induced by warfarin in adults, but little is known about this interaction in children. In a retrospective review of patients younger than 21 years of age, it was found that antibiotic use was associated with an increase in the mean INR from 2.7 to 3.6, a change that correlated inversely with patient age.[4] Clarithromycin (Biaxin®) is an oral antibiotic used as therapy in uncomplicated bacterial otitis media where the presumed pathogens are *S. pneumoniae*, *H. influenzae*, or *M. catarrhalis*. The macrolides undergo oxidative metabolism by the CYP3A family of isoenzymes and are inhibitors of the CYP1A2, 2C9, and 3A4 isoenzymes. Clarithromycin undergoes activation by CYP enzymes to form inhibitor metabolites, which go on to form stable complexes with the CYPs called metabolic intermediates (MIs). Clarithromycin is also an inhibitor of the P-glycoprotein (p-gp).[2]

In addition to being inhibitors for the CYP isoenzymes, macrolides have been reported to decrease the amount of intestinal flora that produce vitamin K, which can reduce prothrombin production. Patients with impaired vitamin K synthesis or low vitamin K stores, such as those with chronic hepatic disease or malnutrition, may require monitoring of prothrombin time and administration of vitamin K during antibiotic treatment.[5] In addition, fever, a common condition in pediatric infections, may increase the catabolism of vitamin K-dependent coagulation factors and raise the INR.[4] Finally, a patient with an infection will have a stimulated cytokine response, inhibiting the normal ability to metabolize warfarin and possibly cause excessive anticoagulation.[6]

This patient had multiple factors contributing to her elevated INR: CYP2C9 isoenzyme inhibition, youth, reduced intestinal flora, infection, and possibly a predisposing genetic polymorphism.

Take-Home Points

- Warfarin is an anticoagulant whose activity can be severely altered by multiple factors including diet, infection, genetics, and other medications. When caring for patients taking warfarin, it is imperative that INR be closely monitored when any of these variables occur.
- Warfarin exists as a racemic mixture of enantiomers. The R-enantiomer undergoes metabolism by CYP1A2 and the S-enantiomer undergoes metabolism by CYP2C9.
- It is possible and recommended by the FDA to test for 2C9 polymorphisms before initiating warfarin therapy.
- Clarithromycin is a macrolide antibiotic (other macrolide antibiotics are azithromycin and erythromycin)
- The macrolide antibiotics are pan-inhibitors, including inhibition of 2C9. Clarithromycin also binds to CYP enzymes to form stable complexes and is a P-glycoprotein inhibitor as well.

- Warfarin administration and INR variations in children are poorly studied areas, therefore INR surveillance must be increased in this population.
- Pharmacogenetic testing is not yet associated with improved clinical outcomes and does not lessen the requirement for conscientious monitoring.

Summary

Interaction: pharmacokinetic
Substrate: warfarin
Enzyme: CYP2C9
Inhibitor: clarithromycin
Clinical effects: enhanced anticoagulant effect

References

1. Horton JD, Bushwick BM. Warfarin therapy: evolving strategies in anticoagulation. Am Fam Phys. 1999;59(3):635–46.
2. Cozza KL, Armstrong SC, Oesterheld J. Concise guide to drug interaction principles for medical practice: cytochrome P450s, UGTs, P-glycoproteins. 2nd ed. Washington, DC: American Psychiatric Publishing; 2003.
3. Rosove MH, Grody WW. Should we be applying warfarin pharmacogenetics to clinical practice? No, not now. Ann Intern Med. 2009;151:270–3.
4. Johnson MC, Wood M, Vaughn V, et al. Interaction of antibiotics and warfarin in pediatric cardiology patients. Pediatr Cardiol. 2005;26:589–92.
5. Biaxin (R), Clarithromycin Product information. North Chicago: Abbott Laboratories; 2000.
6. Horn JR, Hansten PD. Enhanced warfarin response and antibiotic. Pharm Times. June 2004, 8003. Published Online: June 1, 2004–12:00:00 AM (CDT).

From Asymptomatic to Symptomatic: A Cause of Nosebleed

149

Fatal Forty DDI: warfarin, amiodarone, CYP2C9

Joško Markić MD, MSc, Julije Meštrović MD, PhD, and Juraj Sprung MD, PhD

Abstract

This case discusses amiodarone added to warfarin. Amiodarone is a cytochrome P450 2C9 inhibitor and the more actively anticoagulant S-enantiomer of warfarin is a 2C9 substrate. The interaction results in an enhanced anticoagulant effect.

Case

A 15-year-old boy, who was an otherwise healthy tennis player, went for his preseason physical. Surprisingly, although asymptomatic, the boy was found to have an irregular heart rhythm, and an electrocardiogram showed atrial fibrillation. A 24-hour Holter monitor confirmed atrial fibrillation, two short episodes of supraventricular tachycardia, ventricular extrasystoles, and pauses lasting up to 2 seconds. Transthoracic echocardiography was normal. Treatment with warfarin (6 mg daily) and propafenone (300 mg/12 h) was started, which successfully converted the patient's heart rhythm to sinus. A month later, he was noted to be in atrial fibrillation again with at a heart rate of 90 beats per minute. The patient was instructed to take propafenone (300 mg/12 h). Also, because his International Normalized Ratio (INR) was 1.7, the dose of warfarin was increased (6 mg alternating with 7.5 mg).

J. Markić MD, MSc (✉) • J. Meštrović MD, PhD
Pediatric Intensive Care Unit, Department of Pediatrics, University Hospital of Split, Split, Croatia
e-mail: jmarkic@kbsplit.hr

J. Sprung MD, PhD
Department of Anesthesiology, Mayo Clinic, Rochester, MN, USA

C. Marcucci et al. (eds.), *A Case Approach to Perioperative Drug-Drug Interactions*, DOI 10.1007/978-1-4614-7495-1_149

For the next 6 months, the patient was in sinus rhythm with INR values between 2 and 2.3. However, on the next follow-up visit, atrial fibrillation was noted again. The patient was admitted to the pediatric intensive care unit and the intensivist decided to administer amiodarone hydrochloride (600 mg/d) in two divided doses instead of propafenone. The patient was instructed to return for a follow-up electrocardiogram and INR check the following week.

The patient had to travel abroad because of a family emergency, and he returned for checkup 3 weeks after the originally scheduled appointment. He reported no cardiovascular symptoms; however, he had had 2 episodes of nosebleed during the previous 48 hours. His INR was checked immediately and was 5.1. The warfarin therapy was discontinued, and the patient was readmitted overnight to the step-down unit for observation.

Discussion

This is an example of an inhibitor added to a substrate.

Amiodarone is a Class III antiarrhythmic, meaning that it prolongs the QT interval. Also, it slows the heart rate and atrioventricular nodal conduction, prolongs myocardial refractoriness, and slows intracardiac conduction.[1] Amiodarone is used for the treatment of a wide range of cardiac dysrhythmias, including atrial fibrillation and flutter and ventricular fibrillation. It can be administered intravenously or orally. Its adverse effects are related to the dosage and duration of treatment.[1] The half-life of amiodarone exceeds 50 days. It is metabolized to desethylamiodarone by the cytochrome P450 (CYP) enzyme group, especially the CYP3A4 and CYP2C8 isozymes.[2]

Warfarin is an anticoagulant drug that reduces blood clot formation by inhibiting the formation of vitamin K–dependent clotting factors (ie, factors II, VII, IX, and X) and proteins C and S. After rapid intestinal absorption, warfarin has a half-life of 36 to 42 hours.[3] Warfarin is used to treat venous thrombosis and for prevention and treatment of thromboembolic events in patients with atrial fibrillation and those with prosthetic heart valves. It requires up to 7 days to achieve its full anticoagulant effect.[4] Warfarin is metabolized by the CYP enzyme group, especially the 2C9, 1A2, and 2C19 isozymes. Warfarin is composed of a racemic mixture of R and S isomers, but most of its anticoagulant effect is associated with S-enantiomer, which is predominantly metabolized by 2C9.[2] R-warfarin is primarily metabolized by 1A2 with 3A4 playing a secondary role.[5]

Amiodarone inhibits the activity of several CYP isozymes, including 2C9, 1A2, 2D6, and 3A4.[1] Because of this inhibition, the metabolism of drugs that are substrate to these isozymes is decreased when they are used together with amiodarone, leading to a corresponding increase in substrate blood levels. One of the most clinically important and most frequently encountered interactions is between amiodarone and warfarin, because these drugs often are prescribed concurrently to patients with cardiac dysrhythmias, especially atrial fibrillation.[6] In this drug combination, the anticoagulant effect of warfarin is enhanced, primarily because of slowed metabolism of the S-enantiomer.[7]

To avoid the possible adverse effects of this concurrent treatment, the clinician should monitor the patient's INR closely. The probability of a prolonged INR is highest during the first 12 weeks of combined therapy.[4,8] Although an increase in INR can be evident after 3 or 4 days of concurrent treatment, the peak effects occur 7 weeks after initiation of therapy.[8] For avoidance of an increased risk of hemorrhagic complications, a reduction of 25% to 40% in the warfarin dose is recommended when amiodarone is added to a stable warfarin regimen and then further adjustment of the warfarin dose may be needed in accordance with subsequent INRs.[4,7,8] It has been noticed that the extent of interaction between amiodarone and warfarin seems to be dependent on the maintenance dose of amiodarone (Fig. 149.1).[8]

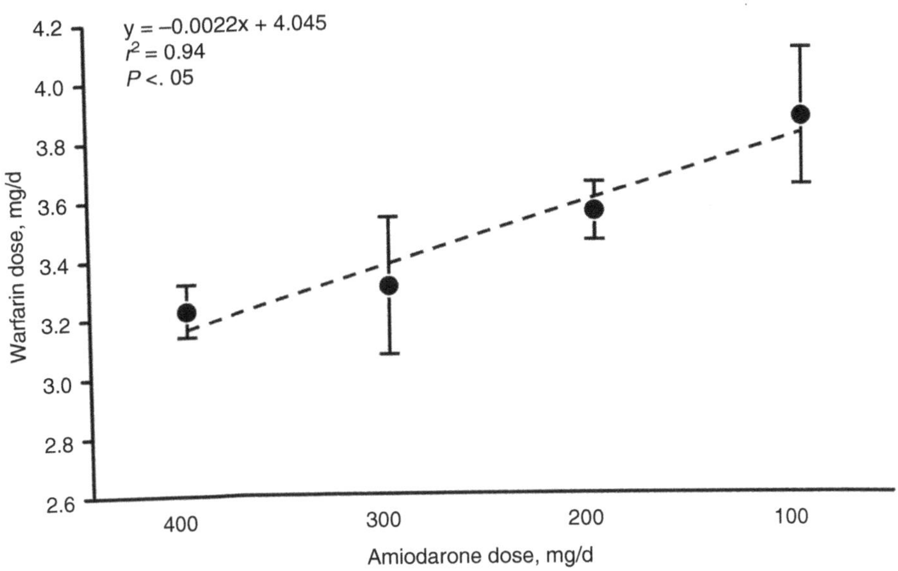

Fig. 149.1 The relationship between amiodarone dose and warfarin dose, showing a strong inverse relationship. As the maintenance dosage of amiodarone is decreased from 400 mg/d to 100 mg/d, the mean daily dose of warfarin correspondingly increased from 3.2 to 3.9 mg. Based on these findings, a reduction of 38%, 36%, 31%, or 25% in the daily warfarin dose was necessary for patients receiving an amiodarone maintenance dosage of 400, 300, 200, or 100 mg/d, respectively. Error bars indicate SD [Adapted from Sanoski CA, Bauman JL. Clinical observations with the amiodarone/warfarin interaction: dosing relationships with long-term therapy. Chest. 2002;121:19–23. With permission from American College of Physicians]

Because of the genetic variability and polymorphism in CYP2C9, patients who have reduced catalytic activity may have a faster onset of interaction.

Of note, several frequently used drugs have an ability similar to that of amiodarone in interfering with warfarin metabolism: fluconazole, sulfamethoxazole-trimethoprim, and metronidazole. These drugs inhibit 2C9 activity and decrease vitamin K production.[3] When a patient is simultaneously taking warfarin and one of these drugs, the patient's INR must be frequently monitored and a warfarin dose reduction of 30% to 50% must be considered.

Take-Home Points

- Warfarin is metabolized by the cytochrome P450 enzyme group. Most of its anticoagulant effect is associated with S-enantiomer, which is predominantly metabolized by CYP2C9.
- Amiodarone inhibits the activity of several CYP isozymes, including CYP2C9. Thus, amiodarone increases the anticoagulant effect of warfarin by inhibiting its metabolism.
- To avoid an increased risk for hemorrhagic complications, a decrease in the warfarin dose is recommended when amiodarone is added to a stable warfarin regimen.
- After initiation of the concurrent amiodarone and warfarin treatment, the INR should be monitored frequently for the first 7 to 10 weeks.
- The extent of interaction between amiodarone and warfarin seems to depend on the maintenance dose of amiodarone.

Summary

Interaction: pharmacokinetic
Substrate: warfarin
Enzyme: primarily CYP2C9
Inhibitor: amiodarone
Clinical effect: enhanced anticoagulant effect

References

1. Siddoway LA. Amiodarone: guidelines for use and monitoring. Am Fam Phys. 2003;68:2189–96.
2. Wilkinson GR. Drug metabolism and variability among patients in drug response. N Engl J Med. 2005;352:2211–21.
3. Thi L, Shaw D, Bird J. Warfarin potentiation: a review of the "FAB-4" significant drug interactions. Consult Pharm. 2009;24:227–30.
4. Lu Y, Won KA, Nelson BJ, et al. Characteristics of the amiodarone-warfarin interaction during long-term follow-up. Am J Health Syst Pharm. 2008;65:947–52.
5. Ansell J, Hirsh J, Hylek E, et al. American College of Chest Physicians: Pharmacology and management of the vitamin K antagonists: American College of Chest Physicians Evidence-Based Clinical Practice Guidelines (8th Edition). Chest. 2008;133:160S–98.
6. Furmaga EM, Good CB. Amiodarone to prevent recurrence of atrial fibrillation. N Engl J Med. 2000;343:579.
7. Kerin NZ, Blevins RD, Goldman L, et al. The incidence, magnitude, and time course of the amiodarone-warfarin interaction. Arch Intern Med. 1988;148:1779–81.
8. Sanoski CA, Bauman JL. Clinical observations with the amiodarone/warfarin interaction: dosing relationships with long-term therapy. Chest. 2002;121:19–23.

The Consequences of Not Following a Cardiac Diet

150

Fatal Forty DDI: clopidogrel, omeprazole, CYP2C19

Kristen B. McCullough PharmD, BCPS, BCOP
and Wayne T. Nicholson MD, PharmD, MSc

Abstract
This case discusses a pharmacokinetic interaction between clopidogrel and omeprazole, resulting in a decreased antiplatelet effect of clopidogrel. Clopidogrel is a cytochrome P450 2C19 substrate and omeprazole is a 2C19 inhibitor.

Case

A 58-year-old, 100 kg man presented to the surgery department for removal of hardware placed during repair of a femoral fracture from a motor vehicle crash. He had a history of hypertension, hyperlipidemia, and a subsequent myocardial infarction 5 months ago, for which he had undergone percutaneous coronary intervention and placement of a drug-eluting stent in the right coronary artery. He consequently took clopidogrel (75 mg once daily) and aspirin (81 mg once daily), with no substantial bleeding events. His hypertension was controlled with metoprolol (25 mg once daily) and his hyperlipidemia was managed with atorvastatin (20 mg once daily).

After his myocardial infarction, the patient had vowed to eat better. However, since the beginning of football season several weeks ago, he spent the weekends watching games and indulging in nachos, hot dogs, buffalo wings, and beer. He had slipped into the habit of spending weekday evenings at the local bar with his friends, dis-

K.B. McCullough PharmD, BCPS, BCOP (✉)
Department of Pharmacy Services, Mayo Clinic, Rochester, MN, USA
e-mail: mccullough.kristen@mayo.edu

W.T. Nicholson MD, PharmD, MSc
Department of Anesthesiology, Mayo Clinic, Rochester, MN, USA

C. Marcucci et al. (eds.), *A Case Approach to Perioperative Drug-Drug Interactions*, DOI 10.1007/978-1-4614-7495-1_150

cussing upcoming games while feasting on burgers, French fries, and beer. Subsequently, he had nighttime heartburn, for which he had been self-medicating with omeprazole each night for the past 18 days.

His cardiologist decided to follow the current guidelines for antiplatelet medications in patients with a drug-eluting stent and recommended that the patient continue taking full antiplatelet therapy perioperatively. The surgeon agreed because the risk for bleeding during the planned operation was minimal. The patient underwent uneventful anesthesia and surgery. While in the recovery room, the patient reported substernal chest pain that radiated to his back and neck and shortness of breath. An electrocardiogram showed ST-segment depression, and cardiac panel testing showed elevated troponin levels. A coronary angiogram showed a clot in the right coronary artery immediately distal to his prior stent placement. Percutaneous coronary intervention was performed and an additional stent placed.

The procedure was successful, and the patient was observed in the hospital over the next 3 days. Omeprazole therapy was switched to ranitidine, and the patient was counseled on lifestyle changes that might reduce his heartburn. At the time of discharge, results of an electrocardiogram and cardiac panel were normal and his blood pressure was within predetermined goals.

Discussion

This is an example of an inhibitor added to a prodrug substrate.

Clopidogrel exhibits an antiplatelet effect by inhibiting adenosine diphosphate from binding to the platelet surface receptor $P2Y_{12}$. In a normal physiologic context, the binding of adenosine diphosphate stimulates activation of the platelet and receptor glycoprotein IIb/IIIa, leading to clot formation. Clopidogrel binds irreversibly to $P2Y_{12}$, thereby preventing adenosine diphosphate binding and subsequent platelet activation.[1]

Clopidogrel is a prodrug that requires metabolism by liver enzymes, including cytochrome P450 (CYP) 2C19.[2] The proposed mechanism of this reaction arises from the ability of proton pump inhibitors (PPIs) to inhibit CYP2C19.[3] It has been suggested that a link may exist that results in decreased activation of clopidogrel and a subsequent decreased antiplatelet effect when a patient takes both medications.

Several studies have investigated this theory. The first of these studies was the Omeprazole, Clopidogrel, Aspirin Study, which found a statistically significant decrease in clopidogrel activity in the presence of omeprazole, as measured by the platelet reactivity index.[3] In a study published in 2009, several PPIs, including rabeprazole sodium, omeprazole, pantoprazole sodium, and lansoprazole, were analyzed in relation to clopidogrel.[4] A subgroup analysis showed a statistically significant risk of a second myocardial infarction for patients taking rabeprazole, omeprazole, and lansoprazole but not for patients taking pantoprazole.

Some hospitals have considered using pantoprazole exclusively, in hopes of avoiding this interaction. Unfortunately, this issue remains unclear, because several other studies surfaced in late 2008 and in 2009 that showed contradicting results. One study showed no interaction between clopidogrel and esomeprazole magnesium or pantoprazole when the platelet reactivity index and adenosine diphosphate aggregation were analyzed.[5] Alternatively, an analysis of patients within the Veterans Affairs hospital system showed an increased risk for rehospitalization, myocardial infarction, and revascularization with nearly all PPIs, with the exception of rabeprazole, which did not have a sufficient population for analysis.[6]

Although pharmacokinetic studies have showed that some PPIs, such as lansoprazole, may undergo more extensive metabolism by CYP2C19, there currently is no clear consensus whether PPIs should be avoided with antiplatelet medications.[7] Pharmacogenomics also may have a role in this interaction, since some patients may have reduced activity of 2C19, and this compounding factor has not been considered a risk factor in current studies. Current guidelines regarding gastrointestinal prophylaxis in patients who take both clopidogrel and aspirin and are at the same increased risk of gastrointestinal bleeding recommend the use of PPIs.[8] However, these guidelines were released in late 2008, before many of these studies were published.

The manufacturers of clopidogrel discourage concomitant use of drugs that inhibit CYP2C19 (eg, omeprazole).[1] They also are working with the US Food and Drug Administration (FDA) to gain additional information. The FDA has recommended that health care providers avoid using clopidogrel and omeprazole together at any time of the day. Additionally, the FDA extends this warning to include esomeprazole but cannot definitively implicate any other PPIs. Its current recommendation is to consider the use of a H_2-antagonist, such as ranitidine or famotidine but excluding cimetidine hydrochloride.[9]

Health care providers need to be aware of this interaction and to consider the consequences for their patients, and they should follow the FDA recommendations. PPIs are indicated for esophagitis, *Helicobacter pylori* infections, gastric and duodenal ulcers, and hypersecretory diseases, such as Zollinger-Ellison syndrome. However, many patients are treated with PPIs for extended periods without an obvious indication or a diagnosis of any of these diseases. In addition, omeprazole may be purchased without a prescription. Therefore, it is important that all medication use is discussed with patients to prevent inappropriate use.

Take-Home Points

- PPIs often are prescribed as part of a gastrointestinal prophylaxis regimen for patients taking dual antiplatelet therapy.
- PPIs may inhibit the metabolism of clopidogrel at a hepatic level, secondary to decreasing the activation of clopidogrel from a prodrug to a therapeutically active compound, presumably through inhibition of CYP2C19.
- Opinions are conflicting about whether inhibition can be considered a PPI class effect. Current evidence suggests that there are some differences among different PPIs in their degree of inhibition.
- Use of a PPI is indicated in some patient categories. However, health care providers should evaluate fully the risk–benefit ratio for their patients and ensure that their patients are not using a PPI wrongfully.
- Further studies need to be completed before enough evidence is available to confidently change the medical recommendations for concomitant use of clopidogrel and a PPI. However, it is prudent that health care providers follow current FDA guidance.

Summary

Interaction: pharmacokinetic
Substrate: clopidogrel (prodrug)
Enzyme: CYP2C19
Inhibitor: omeprazole
Clinical effect: decreased antiplatelet effect of clopidogrel

References

1. Plavix [package insert]. Bridgewater (NJ), Bristol-Myers Squibb/Sanofi Pharmaceutical Partnership; 2009.
2. Ishizaki T, Horai Y. Review article: cytochrome P450 and the metabolism of proton pump inhibitors: emphasis on rabeprazole. Aliment Pharmacol Ther. 1999;13 Suppl 3:27–36.
3. Gilard M, Arnaud B, Le Gal G, et al. Influence of omeprazole on the antiplatelet action of clopidogrel associated to aspirin. J Thromb Haemost. 2006;4:2508–9.
4. Juurlink DN, Gomes T, Ko DT, et al. A population-based study of the drug interaction between proton pump inhibitors and clopidogrel. CMAJ. 2009;180:713–8.
5. Siller-Matula JM, Spiel AO, Lang IM, et al. Effects of pantoprazole and esomeprazole on platelet inhibition by clopidogrel. Am Heart J. 2009;157:148.e1–e5.

6. Ho PM, Maddox TM, Wang L, et al. Risk of adverse outcomes associated with concomitant use of clopidogrel and proton pump inhibitors following acute coronary syndrome. JAMA. 2009;301:937–44.
7. Li XQ, Andersson TB, Ahlstrom M, et al. Comparison of inhibitory effects of the proton pump-inhibiting drugs omeprazole, esomeprazole, lansoprazole, pantoprazole, and rabeprazole on human cytochrome P450 activities. Drug Metab Dispos. 2004;32:821–7.
8. Bhatt DL, Scheiman J, Abraham NS, et al. American College of Cardiology Foundation Task Force on Clinical Expert Consensus Documents: ACCF/ACG/AHA 2008 expert consensus document on reducing the gastrointestinal risks of antiplatelet therapy and NSAID use: a report of the American College of Cardiology Foundation Task Force on Clinical Expert Consensus Documents. Circulation. 2008;118:1894–909.
9. U.S. Food and Drug Administration [Internet]. Follow-up to the January 26, 2009, early communication about an ongoing safety review of clopidogrel bisulfate (marketed as Plavix) and omeprazole (marketed as Prilosec and Prilosec OTC). Rockville (MD), U.S. Department of Health and Human Services. http://www.fda.gov/Drugs/DrugSafety/PostmarketDrugSafetyInformationforPatientsandProviders/DrugSafetyInformationforHeathcareProfessionals/ucm190784.htm. Accessed 19th May 2012.

Clopidogrel (I): Bagel Brunch

151

Fatal Forty DDI: clopidogrel, omeprazole, CYP2C19

Ann Marie Canelas MD and Randal O. Dull MD, PhD

Abstract
This case discusses the interaction between clopidogrel and omeprazole. Clopidogrel is a prodrug metabolized to an intermediate compound by cytochrome P450 2C19. Omeprazole is a 2C19 inhibitor.

Case

An anesthesiologist and internist, married 3 years, were in the habit of sleeping late on Sundays, and then watching the political talk shows while having coffee and bagels (no kids yet!). Talk inevitably strayed from politics to the cases and challenges of the previous week and the couple, who had been medical school classmates, took turns trying to stump each other on medical issues. The husband described a case posted for the previous Friday. The patient was a 67-year-old man scheduled for resection of a massive low-grade abdominal wall sarcoma and abdominal wall reconstruction who had been cancelled when he had gone to the Emergency Department instead of the his preoperative clinic visit complaining of chest pain. He was then found to have ST segment elevations in his anterior leads. The wife, like the good internist she was, asked for the patient's pertinent medical history (hyperlipidemia, new-onset gastroesophageal reflux (CERO), smoking, and hypertension with relatively recent placement of bare metal stent in left anterior descending artery) and medication list (clopidogrel, simvastatin, aspirin, and omeprazole).

"Hmmmm," she said. "Clopidogrel is a 2C19 prodrug. His GERD probably got worse because of the tumor and somebody put him on omeprazole, they probably should have used pantoprazole. We've been hearing about the proton pump inhibi-

A.M. Canelas MD (✉) • R.O. Dull MD, PhD
Department of Anesthesiology, University of Illinois at Chicago, Chicago, IL, USA
e-mail: canelasam@gmail.com

C. Marcucci et al. (eds.), *A Case Approach to Perioperative Drug-Drug Interactions*, DOI 10.1007/978-1-4614-7495-1_151

tors, but the evidence base is evolving on this. Did somebody also put him on an antihypertensive? Mind if I have the poppy seed bagel?"

Discussion

This is an example of inhibitor to a prodrug substrate.

Clopidogrel, a platelet $P2Y_{12}$ adenosine diphosphate receptor inhibitor, is commonly prescribed in combination with aspirin, as part of dual anti-platelet therapy for treatment of coronary atherosclerosis and, specifically, following angioplasty and stent placement. To mitigate gastrointestinal bleeding associated with aspirin, a proton pump inhibitor (PPI), most commonly omeprazole, is frequently prescribed as adjunct therapy. The use of dual anti-platelet therapy in the treatment of unstable angina is supported by randomized trials.[1]

The clinician should be aware of concerns, however, regarding the drug–drug interaction between omeprazole's inhibition of cytochrome P450 (CYP) 2C19, one of the cytochrome P450 isoforms that converts the prodrug clopidogrel to its active form. Clopidogrel is converted to 2-oxo-clopidogrel via several of the P450 isoforms including 2C19, 1A2, and 2B6 and 2-oxo-clopidogrel is then subsequently metabolized to the active compound, R-130964, by 3A4, 2C9, 2C19 and the 2B family of enzymes. Omeprazole is a strong inhibitor of 2C19, thus, inhibiting the initial step in conversion of clopidogrel to its active anti-platelet form. Other proton pump inhibitors including lansoprazole, rabeprazole and esomeprazole have also been shown to inhibit 2C19.

Numerous studies have reported increases in acute coronary events among patients demonstrating clopidogrel resistance and those taking a combination of clopidogrel and proton pump inhibitors.[2–6] Matezky et al were the first to demonstrate clopidogrel resistance, as measured by platelet aggregation assays, in patients who had a myocardial infarction and had been treated with clopidogrel and aspirin.[9] Approximately 25% of study patients demonstrated clopidogrel resistance and this was associated with increased risk for recurrent cardiac events. Ho and colleagues reported a significant increase in combined all-cause mortality and rehospitalization for acute coronary syndrome in patients taking clopidogrel plus a PPI versus those taking clopidogrel alone.[2] The presumed mechanism was inhibition of CYP-dependent clopidogrel metabolism and activation.

Genetics also influence the response to clopidogrel therapy. Genetic polymorphisms of the CYP 2C19 gene can result in 25% to 33% reduction in clopidogrel's anti-platelet activity and this is strongly associated with adverse outcomes including increased myocardial infarction, stent thrombosis and stroke.[5] The CYP 2C19*2 allele was the most frequent, reduced-function allele. Reduced-function polymorphisms are common among Cancasians (30%), persons of African descent (40%) and persons of East Asian descent (55%).[6] At least one study has examined the pharmacogenetic interactions of clopidogrel absorption via the intestinal P-glycoprotein ABCB1 transporter, hepatic cytochrome P450 alleles (CYP 3A4, 3A5, 2C19) and allelic variants in the platelet $P2Y_{12}$ receptor on adverse cardiac outcomes.[7] There was a reported increase in the hazard ratio for patients carrying a variant allele for ABCB1 and either of the two reduced-function alleles for CYP2C19. In fact, patients with two CYP2C19 reduced-function alleles and at least one ABCB1 allele had a cardiac event rate five-fold higher than normal patients.

Induction of CYP 450 enzymes may lead to an enhanced efficacy of clopidogrel, potentially counterbalancing other inhibitory drug–drug interactions. Hyperforin, a constituent of St. John's wort, can induce CYP3A4, although the effect is primarily seen in preparations that contain high hyperforin levels. Likewise, nicotine can induce CYP1A2, which theoretically could enhance clopidogrel metabolism in the setting of 2C19 inhibition. The influence of concurrent enzyme induction has not been shown to alter cardiac outcomes and should not be assumed to provide any clinical benefit. It does highlight, however, the complex influences of food, drugs, and herbal supplement interactions within the P450 system.

In summary, clopidogrel-omeprazole is a demonstration of a prodrug + inhibitor combination, leading to decreased efficacy of the prodrug, due to reduced conversion of the prodrug to an active form. Concurrent genetic influences via r alleles have the potential to accentuate drug–drug interactions and impact clinical outcome. Newer proton pump inhibitors that have much less of a 2C19 inhibitory profile, such as pantoprazole, are currently recommended for use with clopidogrel, as the benefits are thought to outweigh the risks.[8]

Take-Home Points

- Omeprazole and esomeprazole (Nexium®) are strong inhibitors of CYP2C19, the enzyme that converts clopidogrel from a prodrug to an active, antiplatelet drug.
- Inhibition of CYP2C19 reduces the efficacy of clopidogrel therapy and is associated with adverse cardiac outcomes.
- If a patient taking clopidogrel requires treatment with a proton pump inhibitor, it would be prudent to select or switch to an agent other than omeprazole or esomeprazole such as pantoprazole (Protonix®) or lansoprazole (Prevacid®).
- Genetic polymorphisms, including reduced function alleles of the intestinal uptake pump (ABCB1) for clopidogrel and CYP2C19 have superimposed influences on cardiac outcomes.

- Herbal supplements and nicotine may induced specific P450 enzymes and mitigate direct drug-induced inhibition.
- A 2012 report has suggested that higher-quality studies, including the only randomized trial, have not shown any difference concerning adverse cardiovascular events when concomitantly on clopidogrel and PPI or only on clopidogrel.

Summary

Interaction: pharmacokinetic
Substrate: clopidogrel
Inhibitor: omeprazole
Enzyme: CYP2C19
Clinical effect: loss of anticoagulant efficacy

References

1. Yusef S, et al. ;The Clopidogrel in Unstable Angina to Prevent Recurrent Events Trial Investigators. Clopidogrel in unstable angina to prevent recurrent events trail investigators: effects of clopidogrel in addition to aspirin in patients with acute coronary syndrome without ST-segment elevations. N Engl J Med. 2001;345:494–502.
2. Ho PM, Maddox TM, Wang L, et al. Risk of adverse outcomes associated with concomitant use of clopidogrel and proton pump inhibitors following acute coronary syndrome. JAMA. 2009;301(9):937–44.
3. Lau WC, Gurbel PA. The drug-drug interaction between proton pump inhibitors and clopidogrel. CMAJ. 2009;180(7):699–700.
4. Juurlink DN, Gomes T, Ko DT, et al. A population based study of the drug interaction between proton pump inhibitors and clopidogrel. CMAJ. 2009;180:713–8.
5. Mega JL, Close SL, Wiviott SD, et al. Cytochrome P-450 polymorphisms and the response to clopidogrel. N Engl J Med. 2009;360(4):354–62.
6. Desta Z, Zhao X, Shin JG, et al. Clinical significance of the cytochrome P450 2C19 genetic polymorphism. Clin Pharmacokinet. 2002;41:913–58.
7. Simon T, Verstuyft C, Mary-Krause M, et al. Genetic determinant of responses to clopidogrel and cardiovascular events. N Engl J Med. 2009;360(4):363–75.
8. Drepper MD, Spahr L, Frossard JL, et al. Clopidogrel and proton pump inhibitors – where do we stand in 2012? World J Gastroenterol. 2012;18(18):2161–71.
9. Matetzky S, Shenkman B, Guetta V. Clopidogrel resistance is associated with increased risk of recurrent atherothrombotic events in patients with acute myocardial infarction. Circulation. 2004;109(25):3171–5. Epub 2004 Jun 7.

Clopidogrel (II): Conferring over the Kung Pao 152

Clopidogrel, proton pump inhibitors, calcium channel blockers, CYP2C19, CYP3A4

Catherine Marcucci MD and Neil B. Sandson MD

Abstract
This case further discusses the aggregation of risk factors for significant drug–drug interactions involving clopidogrel, proton pump inhibitors, and calcium channel blockers.

Case

The young physician couple in the previous case (an anesthesiologist married to an internist) each worked their way through a hard and busy day at their respective hospitals and decided, on a rainy Tuesday night, to go out for dinner at their favorite Asian restaurant. As the food arrived, the wife mentioned that she had found a couple of papers on clopidogrel metabolism for her favorite handsome anesthesiologist and asked if he would have time later in the week to find out if the patient with the large abdominal wall tumor had been started on an antihypertensive. As luck would have it, her husband had been the attending covering the preoperative center and had asked the nurse practitioners there for the story on the patient. He was able to confirm that the patient had been started on omeprazole for his gastroesophageal reflux disease (GERD). Additionally, as part of the preoperative optimization of the patient's medical status, it had been decided to treat the patient's

C. Marcucci MD (✉)
Anesthesia Services Department, Philadelphia Veterans Affairs Medical Center, Philadelphia, PA, USA
e-mail: sandson.marcucci@comcast.net

N.B. Sandson MD
Department of Psychiatry, University of Maryland Medical System, Baltimore, MD, USA

Department of Psychiatry, VA Maryland Health Care System, Baltimore, MD, USA

C. Marcucci et al. (eds.), *A Case Approach to Perioperative Drug-Drug Interactions*, DOI 10.1007/978-1-4614-7495-1_152

moderate hypertension, and he had been started on verapamil just before he suffered a thrombotic event to his coronary artery stent. Our smart, young couple each popped their phone out of their briefcase and a Kung Pao clopidogrel conference ensued (no kids yet to talk about).[1]

Discussion

This is an example of inhibitors added to a prodrug substrate.

There has been much recent inquiry into both the mechanisms by which clopidogel is converted into an active anticlotting agent, and also what drugs might interfere with this conversion.[1–8] There has been some inconsistency in recent studies. Some studies have suggested that CYP2C19 inhibitors, such as proton pump inhibitors, and CYP3A4 inhibitors, such as diltiazem and verapamil, are implicated in decreasing clopidogrel's anticlotting efficacy.[3–6] However, other studies have called these findings into question.[7,8] Since the conversion from inactive clopidogrel to active anticlotting agent is multiply determined, it is sensible that the most recent studies suggest that an "aggregation of risk factors" approach is more illuminating than evaluating a single, potentially implicated drug–drug interaction. Specifically, one study evaluated three risk factors for poor clopidogrel response: 1) coadministration of a CYP3A4 inhibiting calcium-channel blocker, 2) coadministration of a proton pump inhibitor, and 3) having the CYP2C19 poor metabolizer genotype and corresponding phenotype. The study found that the presence of only one risk factor was not associated with poor clopidogrel response, but that two or more of these risk factors was (although it can be reasonably assumed that using a PPI in someone who was a poor 2C19 metabolizer would be redundant and not create additive risk).[3] This more nuanced approach helps one understand and reconcile the inconsistencies in the previous literature on this topic.

Take-Home Points

- There is an evolving evidence base on drug–drug interactions (DDIs) involving clopidogrel, calcium channel blockers, and proton pump inhibitors.
- A recent compelling study suggested that an aggregation of risk factors is a more reliable approach in assessing clinical risk for clopidogrel DDIs.
- Learn DDIs wherever and whenever you can learn them. Talk to the internists, the oncologists, and the psychiatrists and find out what they know and what drug interactions they deal with. Talk to your spouse if you think they know about a DDI that you don't! Don't be sedate in your knowledge base, follow the evidence base where it goes.

Summary

Interaction: pharmacokinetic
Substrate: clopidogrel (prodrug)
Enzymes: CYP2C19 and CYP3A4
Inhibitors: proton pump inhibitors (CYP2C19) and/or calcium channel blockers (CYP3A4)
Clinic effect: decreased antiplatelet effect leading to stent thrombosis

References

1. Drepper MD, Spahr L, Frossard JL, et al. Clopidogrel and proton pump inhibitors – where do we stand in 2012? World J Gastroenterol. 2012;18(18):2161–71.
2. Gremmel T, Steiner S, Seidinger D, et al. Calcium-channel blockers decrease clopidogrel-mediated platelet inhibition. Heart. 2010;96(3):186–9.
3. Harmsze AM, van Werkum JW, Souverein PC, et al. Combined influence of proton-pump inhibitors, calcium-channel blockers and CYP2C19*2 on on-treatment platelet reactivity and on the occurrence of atherothrombotic events after percutaneous coronary intervention. J Thromb Haemost. 2011;9(10):1892–901.
4. Siller-Matula JM, Lang I, Christ G, et al. Calcium-channel blockers reduce the antiplatelet effect of clopidogrel. J Am Coll Cardiol. 2008;52(19):1557–63.
5. Bhurke SM, Martin BC, Li C, et al. Effect of the clopidogrel-proton pump inhibitor drug interaction on adverse cardiovascular events in patients with acute coronary syndrome. Pharmacotherapy. 2012;32(9):809–18.
6. Fontes-Carvalho R, Albuquerque A, Araújo C, et al. Omeprazole, but not pantoprazole, reduces the antiplatelet effect of clopidogrel: a randomized clinical crossover trial in patients after myocardial infarction evaluating the clopidogrel-PPIs drug interaction. Eur J Gastroenterol Hepatol. 2011;23(5):396–404.
7. Schmidt M, Johansen MB, Robertson DJ, et al. Use of clopidogrel and calcium channel blockers and risk of major adverse cardiovascular events. Eur J Clin Invest. 2012;42(3):266–74. Epub 2011 Aug 11.
8. Kwok CS, Jeevanantham V, Dawn B, et al. No consistent evidence of differential cardiovascular risk amongst proton-pump inhibitors when used with clopidogrel: meta-analysis. Int J Cardiol. 2013;167(3):965–74.

Drug–Drug Interactions Involving Immunosuppressants, Antiemetics, and Chemotherapy

XIV

Introduction 153

Catherine Marcucci MD

Abstract
This section introduces drug–drug interactions involving immunosuppressant and chemotherapy drugs.

The drug–drug interactions (DDIs) discussed in this section are a varied but important lot. Two of the **Fatal Forty** drugs—cimetidine and tamoxifen—reside in these drug classes.

Cimetidine was one of the earlier drugs that was clearly identified as being implicated in clinically significant DDIs—it earns its place on the list by being a paninhibitor of metabolism, including the cytochrome P450 (CYP) isozymes 1A2, 3A4, 2C9, 2C19, 2D6, and 2E1. Although it is not in as widespread use as an H_2 receptor antagonist in the US as previously, it is still used significantly overseas and has multiple other off-label uses, especially in the treatment of serious dermatological conditions.

Tamoxifen, an important and widely used breast cancer treatment, is on the **Fatal Forty** list as a "Victim." The benefits of tamoxifen on the occurrence and survival rates of breast cancer have been well established. However, it is a CYP2D6 prodrug and requires metabolism by that enzyme for it to gain its pharmacologically active and chemotherapeutic effect. CYP2D6 inhibitors are a diverse lot ranging from paroxetine to diphenhydramine. These are not drugs given in the operating room, but this DDI could easily be found by a pain physician or staff member in a preoperative clinic.

Tacrolimus, sirolimus, and cyclosporine are not on the **Fatal Forty** list. Nonetheless, the consequences of missing a deleterious DDI involving these drugs are very serious, considering the scarcity of organ donations and the potentially devastating clinical sequelae of acute or chronic organ rejection.

C. Marcucci MD
Anesthesia Services Department, Philadelphia Veterans Affairs Medical Center, Philadelphia, PA, USA
e-mail: sandson.marcucci@comcast.net

C. Marcucci et al. (eds.), *A Case Approach to Perioperative Drug-Drug Interactions*, DOI 10.1007/978-1-4614-7495-1_153

Beaned

154

Fatal Forty DDI: diltiazem, tacrolimus, CYP3A4, P-glycoprotein

Matthew Hart MSN, CRNA and Michael P. Hutchens MD

Abstract
This case discusses the pharmacokinetic interaction of tacrolimus and diltiazem, including to tacrolimus toxicity. Tacrolimus is a cytochrome P450 3A4 and intestinal P-glycoprotein substrate and diltiazem is an inhibitor.

Case

A 59-year-old woman with a history of cadaveric renal transplant noticed she was feeling lightheaded while picking pole beans in the garden one summer evening. Her transplant had been for membranous glomerulopathy 4 years before. Immunosuppression had been maintained with prednisone, mycophenolate mofetil, and tacrolimus. In the emergency room, she had a blood pressure of 88/40 mm Hg and a heart rate of 155 beats per minute (bpm). An electrocardiogram documented atrial flutter, a diltiazem infusion was started, and the patient was moved to the hospital's small intensive care unit (ICU). The intensivist was an anesthesiologist who had trained at an institution with a cardiac transplant program and he recognized tacrolimus toxicity.

Overnight, the patient's arrhythmia converted to normal sinus rhythm with heart rate in the range of 80 bpm. The following morning the patient was given 90 mg of diltiazem by mouth and the infusion was discontinued. When the arrhythmia had not recurred by early afternoon, the patient was discharged from the hospital with a prescription for diltiazem (90 mg, orally, three times daily) and was scheduled to follow up with the local cardiologist in 1 week.

M. Hart MSN, CRNA (✉) • M.P. Hutchens MD
Department of Anesthesiology and Perioperative Medicine,
Oregon Health and Science University, Portland, OR, USA
e-mail: hartma@ohsu.edu

C. Marcucci et al. (eds.), *A Case Approach to Perioperative Drug-Drug Interactions*, DOI 10.1007/978-1-4614-7495-1_154

During the follow-up with the cardiologist, she denied any further episodes of lightheadedness and had normal vital signs, but complained of 2 days of nausea, diarrhea, headache and tremor, and wondered if it could be the diltiazem. The cardiologist instructed the patient to hold one dose of the tacrolimus while a level was obtained, and discontinued the diltiazem. The tacrolimus level returned the next day at 24.9 ng/mL (reference 6-9 ng/mL). When the cardiologist called the patient at home the following morning, she was out in the garden, already feeling better.

Discussion

This is an example of an inhibitor added to a substrate.

Patients having undergone solid organ transplantation are on a complex regimen of pharmaceutical therapies and it remains a challenge for perioperative and critical care clinicians to juggle all the potential interactions. In this case, the patient's immunosuppression was being managed with oral tacrolimus. Tacrolimus binds with the FK506-binding protein and immunophilins in a complex process that helps to inhibit the early stages of T-cell activation.[1] Tacrolimus has a narrow therapeutic index, poor mean oral bioavailability of 17% to 22% and is highly metabolized by cytochrome P450 (CYP) 3A4 in the liver and small intestine.[1,2] The absorption of tacrolimus is primarily regulated by P-glycoprotein transport in the small intestine through an ATP-dependent efflux pump that reduces intracellular concentrations by pumping it back into the intestinal lumen.[1,2]

The addition of diltiazem, a calcium channel blocker, created an unintended toxic level by both inhibiting the metabolism and increasing the net absorption of tacrolimus.[2–4] Diltiazem competitively binds to the CYP3A4 enzyme, resulting in a decrease in metabolism and increased bioavailability of tacrolimus.[4] Furthermore, diltiazem's properties as a substrate of P-glycoprotein result in a decrease in the amount of tacrolimus extruded back into the intestinal lumen and thus a net increase in absorption of tacrolimus.[3,5]

With the poor oral bioavailability of tacrolimus, this drug–drug interaction may result in a clinically significant toxicity over a relatively short period of time. The most common adverse effects are associated with clinical symptoms of neurotoxicity, nephrotoxicity, and gastrointestinal disturbances.[2] It is recommended that blood therapeutic drug levels of tacrolimus be monitored closely to prevent adverse events and manage unexpected pharmacologic interactions.[6]

Take-Home Points

- The pharmacologic combination of tacrolimus and diltiazem may cause an increase in tacrolimus levels leading to significant toxicity.
- The reliance on the clinical assessment of toxicity in the perioperative environment is often obscured due to the lingering effects of anesthesia, deliberate sedation in the ICU or from the surgical procedure. Therapeutic drug levels should be monitored during the perioperative course on patients receiving tacrolimus.
- When treating acute events on patients receiving tacrolimus, an awareness of the potential interactions needs to be considered along with the risks and benefits of administration for each patient. In this case other calcium channel blockers may have had similar results due to their effects on P-glycoprotein, but the administration of a ß-blocker or other antiarrhythmic might have been a better choice in treating her tachycardia.

Summary

Interaction: pharmacokinetic
Substrate: tacrolimus
Inhibitor: diltiazem
Enzyme/site of action: CYP3A4 and intestinal P-glycoprotein
Clinical effect: tacrolimus toxicity

References

1. Christians U, Jackobson W, Benent L, et al. Mechanisms of clinically relevant drug interactions associated with tacrolimus. Clin Pharmacokinet. 2002;41:813–51.
2. Staatz C, Tett S. Clinical pharmacokinetics and pharmacodynamics of tacrolimus in solid organ transplantation. Clin Pharmacokinet. 2004;43:623–53.
3. Kim R. Drugs as P-Glycoprotein substrates, inhibitors and inducers. Drug Metab Rev. 2002;34:47–54.
4. Li JL, Wang XD, Chen SY, et al. Effects of diltiazem on pharmacokinetics of tacrolimus in relation to CYP3A5 genotype status in renal recipients: from retrospective to prospective. Pharmacogenomics J. 2011;11:300–6.
5. Tachibana T, Kato M, Takano J, et al. Predicting drug-drug interactions involving the inhibition of intestinal CYP3A4 and P-glycoprotein. Curr Drug Metab. 2010;11:762–77.
6. Wallemacq P, Armstrong V, Brunet M, et al. Opportunities to optimize tacrolimus therapy in solid organ transplantation: report of the European consensus conference. Ther Drug Monit. 2009;31:139–52.

Addisonian Adjustment 155

Fatal Forty DDI: prednisone, fluconazole, CYP3A4

Catherine Marcucci MD and Neil B. Sandson MD

Abstract
This case discusses a pharmacokinetic interaction involving prednisone and fluconazole, resulting in adrenal insufficiency. Prednisone is a cytochrome P450 3A4 substrate and fluconazole is a 3A4 inhibitor. Cessation of fluconazole resulted in reversal of inhibition of prednisone.

Case

A 42-year-old man had undergone renal transplantation, which was complicated by an inadvertent bowel perforation. In the subsequent long and complicated intensive care unit (ICU) and hospital course, he was placed on a prednisone regimen for immunosuppressant. Although the medical center did not use prophylactic fluconazole, he eventually developed candidiasis and required ongoing fluconazole therapy. His renal function and other transplant laboratory values were carefully followed in order to titrate his immunosuppression therapy. He eventually developed a severe skin rash that was felt to be associated with the fluconazole therapy, which was discontinued. Over the next several days, he experienced acute onset of fever, vomiting, abdominal pain, delirium, and hypotension. He was quickly given supplementary intravenous cortisol, and an endocrinologist was consulted to address his sudden-onset adrenal insufficiency.

C. Marcucci MD (✉)
Anesthesia Services Department, Philadelphia Veterans Affairs Medical Center, Philadelphia, PA, USA
e-mail: sandson.marcucci@comcast.net

N.B. Sandson MD
Department of Psychiatry, University of Maryland Medical System, Baltimore, MD, USA

Department of Psychiatry, VA Maryland Health Care System, Baltimore, MD, USA

C. Marcucci et al. (eds.), *A Case Approach to Perioperative Drug-Drug Interactions*, DOI 10.1007/978-1-4614-7495-1_155

Discussion

This is an example of reversal of inhibition.

Prednisone is a cytochrome P450 (CYP) 3A4 substrate, and fluconazole is a strong CYP2C9 inhibitor as well as a moderate 3A4 inhibitor.[1–3] The presence of the fluconazole significantly impaired the ability of the CYP3A4 enzyme to metabolize the prednisone. This led to a higher blood level of prednisone than would have existed had the fluconazole not been a part of the patient's regimen. When the fluconazole was discontinued, the isozyme 3A4 returned to its baseline (higher) level of functioning. This led to more efficient metabolism of prednisone by 3A4, with the result that the blood level of prednisone then precipitously declined. This caused the patient to experience an acute Addisonian crisis, requiring emergent administration of additional intravenous cortisol to avert a potential disaster. A similar case involving discontinuation of fluconazole in a patient maintained on prednisone after liver transplant has been reported.[4]

Take-Home Points

- Prednisone is a CYP3A substrate.
- Fluconazole is a moderate CYP3A4 inhibitor as well as a strong CYP2C9 inhibitor.
- The clinical efficacy of the substrate (prednisone) was cotitrated in the presence of coadministration with fluconazole. Cessation of the fluconazole represented the removal of inhibition, which resulted in a decrease in serum substrate levels and a loss of immunosuppressant therapy.

Summary

Interaction: pharmacokinetic
Substrate: prednisone
Enzyme: CYP3A4
Inhibitor: fluconazole
Clinical effects: adrenal insufficiency

References

1. Schwab M, Klotz U. Pharmacokinetic considerations in the treatment of inflammatory bowel disease. Clin Pharmacokinet. 2001;40(10):723–51.
2. Michalets EL, Williams CR. Drug interactions with cisapride: clinical implications. Clin Pharmacokinet. 2000;39(1):49–75.
3. Niemi M, Backman JT, Neuvonen M, et al. Effects of fluconazole and fluvoxamine on the pharmacokinetics and pharmacodynamics of glimepiride. Clin Pharmacol Ther. 2001;69(4):194–200.
4. Tiao GM, Martin J, Weber FL, et al. Addisonian crisis in a liver transplant patient due to fluconazole withdrawal. Clin Transplant. 1999;13(1):62–4.

Tea Time

156

Fatal Forty DDI: St. John's wort, tacrolimus, cyclosporine, CYP3A4, P-glycoprotein

Nikki Jaworski MD

Abstract
This case discusses the pharmacokinetic interaction between cyclosporine and tacrolimus and St. John's wort, resulting in decreased immunosuppression. Tacrolimus and P-glycoprotein are cytochrome P450 3A4 and P-glycoprotein substrates and St. John's wort is a 3A4 and P-glycoprotein inducer.

Case

A 55-year-old man underwent an uneventful cadaveric renal transplantation and was started on cyclosporine and mycophenolate mofetil for immunosuppression. Cyclosporine levels were therapeutic at discharge. He missed his second postoperative visit at the transplant clinic as he was attending a family funeral. Two months later he was seen in clinic and his cyclosporine level was found to be well below the therapeutic level. He required 2 upward adjustments of his dose to maintain an adequate cyclosporine level.

Six months later, he presented for an elective hernia repair and was found to have an elevated serum creatinine. The elective case was postponed and he was referred to the transplant clinic. His cyclosporine levels remained therapeutic but his serum creatinine continued to rise. The transplant team felt the most likely source for his renal dysfunction was calcineurin inhibitor toxicity from his high cyclosporine dose. The cyclosporine was discontinued and the patient was started on tacrolimus,

N. Jaworski MD
Department of Anesthesiology and Perioperative Medicine, Oregon Health and Science University, Portland, OR, USA
e-mail: nikkijaworski@gmail.com

C. Marcucci et al. (eds.), *A Case Approach to Perioperative Drug-Drug Interactions*, DOI 10.1007/978-1-4614-7495-1_156

however, tacrolimus levels were also difficult to titrate and the patient's creatinine continued to rise. A renal biopsy showed acute rejection and pulse steroids were initiated. The patient began complaining of severe depression due to his sister's death and the kidney problems and asked to be put on antidepressant medication. He stated that he was brewing pots of his "mood-elevating" tea all day and that it was no longer working. Upon investigation the transplant discovered that the tea contained St John's wort as the primary ingredient. The patient was instructed to stop drinking the tea as it was likely interacting with his immunosuppressant medications. His tacrolimus dose was subsequently decreased and his episode of rejection responded to antilymphocyte antibody treatment.

Discussion

This is an example of an inducer added to a substrate.

Tacrolimus and cyclosporine are immunosuppressive agents with similar mechanisms of action known as calcineurin inhibitors. Their introduction into standard immunosuppressant regimens for renal transplant has reduced the incidence of acute rejection and improved graft survival. Unfortunately, one side effect of calcineurin inhibitors is renal toxicity as illustrated in the above case with cyclosporine.[1]

Tacrolimus and cyclosporine are substrates for the cytochrome P450 (CYP) 3A4 enzyme and the P-glycoprotein transport protein. Hepatic enzyme CYP3A4 is induced by St John's wort resulting in increased metabolism of both calcineurin inhibitors.[2–4] This increase in metabolism can result in inadequate blood levels of immunosuppressant despite a previously stable regimen. Inadequate blood levels can ultimately resulting in acute rejection of the organ.

In addition, St John's wort increases the expression of duodenal P-glycoprotein transporter.[5,6] P-glycoprotein is an ATP-dependent active transporter on the apical surface of enterocytes that pumps absorbed lipophilic compounds back into the intestinal lumen. Increased expression of the protein eventually results in increased excretion of substrate back into the intestinal lumen. Tacrolimus and cyclosporine are P-glycoprotein substrates and this interaction further contributed to the subtherapeutic drug levels seen in the case.

Take-Home Points

- St John's wort is an herbal supplement that induces both the hepatic enzyme CYP3A4 as well as the duodenal P-glycoprotein transporter, thereby increasing the metabolism and decreasing the absorption of both cyclosporine and tacrolimus.
- St John's wort can be found in many forms and products; therefore it is important to ask patients not only about herbal supplements when taking a thorough history, but to also ask about any product they are using to treat any symptom or problem.

Summary

Interaction: pharmacokinetic
Substrate: cyclosporine and tacrolimus
Enzyme/site of action: CYP3A4 and P-glycoprotein
Inducer: St. John's wort
Clinical effect: decreased immunosuppression

References

1. Gaston R. Current and evolving immunosuppressive regimens in kidney transplantation. Am J Kidney Dis. 2006;47:S3–17.
2. Sandson NB. Drug-drug Interaction primer: a compendium of case vignettes for the practicing clinician. Washington, DC: American Psychiatric Press, Inc; 2007. p. 113–4.
3. Roby CA, Anderson GD, Kantor E, et al. St. John's wort: effect on CYP3A4 activity. Clin Pharmacol Ther. 2000;67:451–7.
4. Hebert M, Park J, Chen Y-L, et al. Effects of St. John's wort (*Hypericum perforatum*) on tacrolimus pharmacokinetics in healthy volunteers. J Clin Pharmacol. 2004;44:89–94.
5. Hennessy M, Kelleher D, Spiers JP, et al. St John's wort increases expression of P-glycoprotein: implications for drug interactions. Br J Clin Pharmacol. 2002;53:75–82.
6. Saeki T, Ueda K, Tanigawara Y, et al. Human P-glycoprotein transports cyclosporine A and FK506. J Biol Chem. 1993;268:6077–80.

157 No Fits at Uffizi

Fatal Forty DDI: phenytoin, cyclosporine, CYP3A4

Michael P. Hutchens MD
and Christine M. Formea PharmD, BCPS

Abstract
This case discusses a pharmacokinetic interaction between cyclosporine and phenytoin, leading to organ rejection. Cyclosporine is a cytochrome P450 3A4 substrate and phenytoin is a 3A4 inducer.

Case

A 45-year-old associate professor of art with a history of orthotopic heart transplant at age 41 was seriously injured in a motor vehicle collision on a mountain road while on vacation near Florence. He had a Glasgow Coma Scale score of 6 T on admission to the intensive care unit (ICU) of the nearby trauma hospital, but fortunately his partner was able to communicate his heart transplant history and the cyclosporine dose, which was given as an intravenous (IV) infusion initially.

On ICU day 1, the patient was loaded with phenytoin (1000 mg IV) and started on phenytoin (150 mg BID) for prophylaxis of early posttraumatic seizures. On hospital day 3, the cyclosporine was transitioned from IV infusion to administration via nasal feeding tube. Despite his serious blunt trauma injuries, the patient made a steady recovery and was extubated on hospital day 5. On hospital day 10, he had several episodes of supraventricular tachycardia associated with hypotension and required reintubation, cardioversion, and a norepinephrine infusion to maintain hemodynamic stability. A transthoracic echocardiogram showed severe left ventricular dysfunction and the ICU team made the provision diagnosis of late sequelae of cardiac contusion, but sent a cyclosporine level "just to make sure." The cyclosporine level came back

M.P. Hutchens MD (✉)
Department of Anesthesiology and Perioperative Medicine,
Oregon Health and Science University, Portland, OR, USA
e-mail: hutchenm@ohsu.edu

C.M. Formea PharmD, BCPS
Pharmacy Research, College of Medicine, Mayo Clinic, Rochester, MN, USA

C. Marcucci et al. (eds.), *A Case Approach to Perioperative Drug-Drug Interactions*, DOI 10.1007/978-1-4614-7495-1_157

the next morning subtherapeutic at 10 ng/mL (therapeutic 150-300 ng/mL) and the diagnosis was revised to acute graft rejection. The patient received a corticosteroid pulse and a cyclosporine loading dose was administered in addition to doubling the maintenance dose. Serial cyclosporine blood trough levels were followed with appropriate adjustment of cyclosporine doses. The prophylactic phenytoin therapy was discontinued, the hemodynamic instability resolved, and the patient was once again extubated within days. He returned home to the United States via air ambulance with follow-up care at his cardiac transplant clinic for the rejection episode and further management of his immunosuppression. He continued to be followed closely for his cyclosporine blood trough levels which resolved approximately 2 weeks after discontinuation of the prophylactic phenytoin therapy.

Discussion

This is an example of an inducer added to a substrate.

Even years after organ transplant, management of even simple medical issues can be complex, and most transplant centers maintain a lifelong relationship with their patients because of this. In this case, this relationship was complicated by foreign travel, and this, as well as the multisystem disease of multitrauma, served to flummox even the highly sophisticated trauma service at a tertiary care facility in a European nation.

Phenytoin is perhaps the best-known inducer of hepatic drug metabolism and is a potent inducer of cytochrome P450 (CYP) 3A4.[1,2] Cyclosporine is a primarily metabolized by 3A4.[3] The trauma team initially exercised commendable diligence in tracking down the patient's immunosuppressive regimen and reinstituting the immunosuppressive medication during his intubation. Unfortunately, the addition of prophylactic phenytoin to the patient's drug regimen resulted in a severe drug–drug interaction (DDI) and caused a rapid increase in the metabolism of cyclosporine, thus resulting in subtherapeutic cyclosporine blood trough levels and the onset of an acute rejection episode.[4–8] Therapeutic options for prophylaxis of early post-traumatic seizure for this postcardiac transplant patient who was on cyclosporine therapy included valproate (which has a complex, non–3A4-mediated metabolic profile), or alternatively, expectant management.

Take-Home Points

- Because of the wide variety of drugs stopped and started there, the ICU is an especially likely place for unintentional DDIs to occur.
- Careful review of a patient's medication regimen is warranted when phenytoin therapy is initiated, as it is a potent inducer of the cytochrome P450 3A4 enzyme family.

- Transplant patients frequently take immunosuppressive drugs that are subject to drug interactions which may result in supra- or subtherapeutic immunosuppressive drug levels that could result in episodes of organ transplant rejection. Careful review and management of immunosuppressive drugs is required and should be managed by the patient's transplant care team.

Summary

Interaction: pharmacokinetic
Substrates: cyclosporine
Enzyme: CYP3A4
Inducer: phenytoin
Clinical effects: subtherapeutic immunosuppressant levels leading to acute organ rejection

References

1. Gibson GG, el-Sankary W, Plant NJ. Receptor-dependent regulation of the CYP3A4 gene. Toxicology. 2002;181–182:199–202.
2. Raucy JL. Regulation of CYP3A4 expression in human hepatocytes by pharmaceuticals and natural products. Drug Metab Dispos. 2003;31:533–9.
3. Kronbach T, Fischer V, Meyer UA. Cyclosporine metabolism in human liver: identification of a cytochrome P-450III gene family as the major cyclosporine-metabolizing enzyme explains interactions of cyclosporine with other drugs. Clin Pharmacol Ther. 1988;43:630–5.
4. D'Souza MJ, Pollock SH, Solomon HM. Cyclosporine-phenytoin interaction. Drug Metab Dispos. 1988;16(1):57–9.
5. Wadhwa NK, Schroeder TJ, Pesce AJ, et al. Cyclosporine drug interactions: a review. Ther Drug Monit. 1987;9(4):399–406.
6. Freeman DJ, Laupacis A, Keown PA, et al. Evaluation of cyclosporin-phenytoin interaction with observations on cyclosporin metabolites. Br J Clin Pharmacol. 1984;18:887–93.
7. Noguchi M, Kiuchi C, Akiyama H, et al. Interaction between cyclosporin A and anticonvulsants. Bone Marrow Transplant. 1992;9(5):391.
8. Keown PA, Laupacis A, Carruthers G, et al. Interaction between phenytoin and cyclosporine following organ transplantation. Transplantation. 1984;38(3):304–6.

Quit Steroids Quit Kidneys 158

Steroids, tacrolimus, CYP3A, P-glycoprotein

Toby N. Weingarten MD,
Wayne T. Nicholson MD, PharmD, MSc,
and Christine M. Formea PharmD, BCPS

Abstract
This case discusses the pharmacokinetic interaction between tacrolimus and prednisone, leading to tacrolimus toxicity.

Case

A 26-year-old woman presented to the intensive care unit (ICU) with hyperkalemia, severe hypertension, tremor, and headache. She was a type 1 diabetic with the sequelae of diabetic nephropathy and had undergone a renal transplant with a living related renal allograft 7 months earlier. The graft had been functioning well, but her ICU admission serum creatinine concentration had increased by 100% from a serum creatinine concentration one month ago. For immunosuppressive therapy, she was maintained on tacrolimus, prednisone, and mycophenolate mofetil. Three weeks ago she decided to self-discontinue prednisone as she felt it was more difficult to control her blood sugar as well as disliking the cosmetic effects of a cushingoid appearance. Her tacrolimus blood trough level was measured and found to be 28 ng/mL(typical target trough levels range from 6 to 15 ng/mL). Her corticosteroid therapy was reinitiated and her tacrolimus dose was adjusted based on variable blood trough concentrations. After intensive monitoring and management of her tacrolimus dosages, her tacrolimus blood trough level decreased to 10 ng/mL. This decrease in tacrolimus blood trough level to therapeutic range correlated with resolution of her symptoms, hyperkalemia and normalization of her renal allograft function. There was no further sequela to her renal allograft.

T.N. Weingarten MD (✉) • W.T. Nicholson MD, PharmD, MSc
Department of Anesthesiology, Mayo Clinic, Rochester, MN, USA
e-mail: Weingarten.toby@mayo.edu

C.M. Formea PharmD, BCPS
Pharmacy Research, Mayo Clinic, College of Medicine, Rochester, MN, USA

C. Marcucci et al. (eds.), *A Case Approach to Perioperative Drug-Drug Interactions*, DOI 10.1007/978-1-4614-7495-1_158

Discussion

This is an example of reversal of induction.

Tacrolimus is a commonly used immunosuppressant drug used to prevent allograft rejection in transplanted organ recipients. It has complex pharmacokinetics and considerable patient variability is observed.[1] Tacrolimus undergoes hepatic metabolism by cytochrome P450 (CYP) 3A enzymes which include CYP3A4 and CYP3A5.[2] Tacrolimus is also a substrate of P-glycoprotein (MDR1, multidrug resistance protein1) which transports it across cell membranes and affects tacrolimus absorption in the intestines and biliary excretion.[3] Polymorphisms for both CYP3A5 and P-glycoprotein exist, although the influence of polymorphic the CYP3A5 gene is greater than that of P-glycoprotein on tacrolimus metabolism.[4,5] Based on these polymorphic genes, patients may metabolize tacrolimus slower or faster and demonstrate lower or higher tacrolimus requirements, respectively.[5]

Drugs that induce or suppress CYP3A and/or P-glycoprotein influence tacrolimus plasma concentration. Interactions between corticosteroids and tacrolimus in renal transplant patients have been observed. Corticosteroids induce CYP3A isoenzymes[6] and P-glycoproteins[7] decreasing tacrolimus bioavailability. Increased tacrolimus dose requirements have been observed in renal transplant patients that use corticosteroids.[8,9] Conversely, tacrolimus blood trough levels have been shown to increase when corticosteroids are discontinued.[10] These effects are more pronounced in patients that have genetic polymorphisms that result in slower metabolism of tacrolimus.[5] Tacrolimus is a narrow therapeutic index drug and symptoms and signs of toxicity include (but are not limited to) hypertension, worsening renal allograft function, hyperkalemia, and mental status changes. Therefore, it is important for clinicians to closely monitor tacrolimus blood trough levels when corticosteroid dosages are being adjusted.

In this case, by self-discontinuing prednisone, the patient inadvertently reversed the induction of CYP3A and P-glycoprotein, which resulted in slower drug metabolism of tacrolimus. The tacrolimus blood trough level increased to a supratherapeutic level, and she developed signs and symptoms of tacrolimus drug toxicity.

Take-Home Points

- Tacrolimus has complex pharmacokinetics and undergoes hepatic metabolism by CYP3A isoenzymes and is also a substrate of P-glycoprotein that influences its uptake in the intestines.

- Genetic polymorphisms exist that may increase or decrease metabolism and clearance of tacrolimus.

- Tacrolimus is a narrow therapeutic index drug.

- Corticosteroids induce CYP3A4, CYP3A5, and P-glycoprotein, which results in increased metabolism of tacrolimus and increased tacrolimus dose requirements.

- When corticosteroids are discontinued, the induction of these proteins is reversed, hepatic metabolism rate decreases, and tacrolimus drug requirements are decreased.

Summary

Interaction: pharmacokinetic
Substrate: tacrolimus
Enzyme/transporter: CYP3A family including CYP3A4 and CYP3A5; P-glycoprotein
Inducer: prednisone
Clinical effect: decreased metabolism of tacrolimus by a reversal of induction leading to tacrolimus toxicity

References

1. Chen JS, Li LS, Cheng DR, et al. Effect of CYP3A5 genotype on renal allograft recipients treated with tacrolimus. Transplant Proc. 2009;41:1557–61.
2. Sattler M, Guengerich FP, Yun CH, et al. Cytochrome P-450 3A enzymes are responsible for biotransformation of FK506 and rapamycin in man and rat. Drug Metab Dispos. 1992;20:753–61.
3. Saeki T, Ueda K, Tanigawara Y, et al. Human P-glycoprotein transports cyclosporin A and FK506. J Biol Chem. 1993;268:6077–80.
4. Renders L, Frisman M, Ufer M, et al. CYP3A5 genotype markedly influences the pharmacokinetics of tacrolimus and sirolimus in kidney transplant recipients. Clin Pharmacol Ther. 2007;81:228–34.
5. Stratta P, Quaglia M, Cena T, et al. The interactions of age, sex, body mass index, genetics, and steroid weight-based doses on tacrolimus dosing requirement after adult kidney transplantation. Eur J Clin Pharmacol. 2012;68(5):671–80.
6. McCune JS, Hawke RL, LeCluyse EL, et al. *In vivo* and *in vitro* induction of human cytochrome P4503A4 by dexamethasone. Clin Pharmacol Ther. 2000;68:356–66.
7. Demeule M, Jodoin J, Beaulieu E, et al. Dexamethasone modulation of multidrug transporters in normal tissues. FEBS Lett. 1999;442:208–14.
8. Anglicheau D, Flamant M, Schlageter MH, et al. Pharmacokinetic interaction between corticosteroids and tacrolimus after renal transplantation. Nephrol Dial Transplant Off Publ Eur Dial Transpl Assoc Eur Ren Assoc. 2003;18:2409–14.

9. Hesselink DA, Ngyuen H, Wabbijn M, et al. Tacrolimus dose requirement in renal transplant recipients is significantly higher when used in combination with corticosteroids. Br J Clin Pharmacol. 2003;56:327–30.
10. van Duijnhoven EM, Boots JM, Christiaans MH, et al. Increase in tacrolimus trough levels after steroid withdrawal. Transpl Int Off J Eur Soc Organ Transplant. 2003;16:721–5.

The Fall Guy (I)

159

Fatal Forty DDI: tamoxifen, metoclopramide, CYP2D6

Catherine Marcucci MD and Neil B. Sandson MD

Abstract

This case discusses the interaction of tamoxifen and metoclopramide. Tamoxifen is a cytochrome P450 2D6 prodrug and metoclopramide is a 2D6 inhibitor.

Case

A 62-year-old woman was admitted to the postanesthesia care unit (PACU) after a hysterectomy under general anesthesia. As the epidural was being dosed for postoperative analgesia, the PACU resident received report from the operating room team. The patient had a history of obesity, food-related gastroesophageal reflux, and breast cancer 3 years earlier (stable on an oral tamoxifen dosage of 20 mg/d). Preinduction, she had received "GI premeds" of metoclopramide 10 mg IV and ranitidine 50 mg IV. The epidural placement, intubation, and extubation were without difficulty.

Anticipating an uneventful PACU course before transfer to the floor, the anesthesia resident went off to eat lunch in the staff lounge. Thirty minutes later, he heard loud voices coming from around the corner in the PACU. His phone rang a few seconds later. The patient's husband was at the bedside, asking to speak with an anesthesiologist immediately. Apparently, the patient's son was starting a pharmacy technician program in the fall and he had just spoken with his father by cell phone. What followed

C. Marcucci MD (✉)
Anesthesia Services Department, Philadelphia Veterans Affairs Medical Center, Philadelphia, PA, USA
e-mail: sandson.marcucci@comcast.net

N.B. Sandson MD
Department of Psychiatry, University of Maryland Medical System, Baltimore, MD, USA

Department of Psychiatry, VA Maryland Health Care System, Baltimore, MD, USA

C. Marcucci et al. (eds.), *A Case Approach to Perioperative Drug-Drug Interactions*, DOI 10.1007/978-1-4614-7495-1_159

was a brief and very difficult exchange with the agitated husband, starting with "Why did my wife get Reglan® when it says right in her record that she's taking tamoxifen for her breast cancer?" and ending with "This is on Wikipedia, don't you people know *anything*?" The unfortunate resident realized that the patient's family was aware of a drug–drug interaction (DDI) that he was not. He managed to stammer that he would check with the pharmacist and get back to them. So as not to be caught again without adequate information to give to the patients, he also decided to study perioperative DDIs during the whole of his upcoming vacation in 3 weeks.

Discussion

This is an example of an inhibitor added briefly to a prodrug substrate.

Tamoxifen is actually a prodrug, (ie, its prime antiestrogenic effects depend on an intact metabolic pathway for the formation of one or more metabolites that then achieve the desired pharmacologic effect). One of the major metabolites of tamoxifen is N-desmethyltamoxifen, which is further converted to 4-hydroxy-n-desmethytamoxifen (endoxifen) by cytochrome P450 (CYP) 2D6. Endoxifen is the physiologically relevant metabolic byproduct of tamoxifen, as it has much more potent antiestrogenic properties than tamoxifen itself.

Metoclopramide is a moderate inhibitor of CYP2D6. Both pharmacokinetic and clinical effects of 2D6 inhibition on tamoxifen metabolism and efficacy have been reported. Early P450 investigators showed that inhibitors of 2D6 impair the conversion to the more active compound.[1–3] Subsequent studies reported that impaired conversion of tamoxifen to endoxifen by either exogenous inhibition of 2D6 (or by a 2D6 genotype that codes for less active forms of the enzyme) can result in poorer clinical outcomes, such as decreased time to breast cancer recurrence.[4]

After checking with the pharmacy department, the anesthesiologist was able to give the patient and her family some reassuring information. Serum levels of tamoxifen and its metabolites show a biphasic pattern. The first peak is within hours and there is a second peak several days later—the overall serum half-life from a single dose is estimated to be as long as 5 to 7 days. Also, because the patient had been on tamoxifen for several years, she was almost certainly at steady-state serum concentrations. Inhibition of the cytochrome P450 enzymes (including CYP2D6) generally takes several days of continued administration. In this situation, a single dose of a metabolic inhibitor of a steady-state drug with a long half life would have little if any effect on serum drug levels.

This case also highlights another important issue—namely, that patients and their families are often surprisingly conversant on the drugs they take. There is a wealth of quite specific and detailed information on the Internet—it is a trivial matter to obtain the package insert on just about any drug. In fact, Wikipedia does indeed address the pharmacokinetics of tamoxifen in some detail, but without the qualifying information above.[5] In this case, the anesthesia resident found that a partially informed patient can be as challenging to deal with as a misinformed patient.

Take-Home Points

- Phase I (oxidative) metabolism via the cytochrome P450 system is necessary not only for elimination of active compounds from the body, but also for the conversion of prodrugs, such as tamoxifen, into their more active metabolites.
- Inhibition of the P450 enzymes takes on the order of several days, a single dose in most cases does not produce clinically relevant effects in drug levels.
- Families and patients are increasingly knowledgeable about the drugs they take and hence potential DDIs. For some reason, the editors have found that patients and families get particularly upset about DDIs, perhaps because they are adverse events that are easily traced to one or a few missteps in prescribing. Thus, it may seem to the families that they could have been easily avoided.
- Just as this resident planned with his study course, mastery of perioperative DDIs can be greatly facilitated by placing them in clinical context.

Summary

Interaction: pharmacokinetic
Substrate: tamoxifen
Enzyme: CYP2D6
Inhibitor: metoclopramide
Clinical effects: potential DDI caught in time, but a very upset family!

References

1. Borges S, Desta Z, Li L, et al. Quantitative effect of CYP2D6 genotype and inhibitors on tamoxifen metabolism: implication for optimization of breast cancer treatment. Clin Pharmacol Ther. 2006;80:61–74.
2. Jin Y, Desta Z, Stearns V, et al. CYP2D6 genotype, antidepressant use, and tamoxifen metabolism during adjuvant breast cancer treatment. J Natl Cancer Inst. 2005;97:30–9.

3. Stearns V, Johnson MD, Rae JM, et al. Active tamoxifen metabolite plasma concentrations after coadministration of tamoxifen and the selective serotonin reuptake inhibitor paroxetine. J Natl Cancer Inst. 2003;95:1758–64.
4. Goetz MP, Knox SK, Suman VJ, et al. The impact of cytochrome P450 2D6 metabolism in women receiving adjuvant tamoxifen. Breast Cancer Res Treat. 2007;101:113–21.
5. Tamoxifen. Wikipedia. 2012. http://en.wikipedia.org/wiki/Tamoxifen. Last accessed 4 May 2012.

The Fall Guy (2)

160

Fatal Forty DDI: tamoxifen, diphenhydramine, CYP2D6

Catherine Marcucci MD and Neil B. Sandson MD

Abstract
This case discusses the interaction of tamoxifen and diphenhydramine. Tamoxifen is a cytochrome P450 2D6 prodrug substrate and diphenhydramine is a 2D6 inhibitor.

Case

The patient in the previous case (**The Fall Guy**) had a moderately prolonged postoperative hospital course due to nausea and difficulty tolerating oral intake. She also had pain management issues, necessitating continuation of her epidural patient-controlled analgesia (PCA) device for 5 days postoperatively. On the night of surgery (a Friday) she reported good pain relief, but was greatly bothered by pruritis and insomnia. The patient asked for "something to help me sleep and something for the itching." A standing diphenhydramine (Benadryl®) dosage (25 mg intravenously every 6 hours) was added to the PCA template orders. On Monday, the anesthesia resident in the preceding case was called to a meeting in the office of the chief of anesthesia services, chiefly to answer the question of why he had not "passed along" the tamoxifen drug–drug interaction (DDI) information to the pain and surgical services. It seems that there had been something of a repeat confrontation with the patient's family, this time over the administration of 10 doses of diphenhydramine over the weekend. The house officer covering the surgical service was unaware of the previous encounter in the postanesthesia care unit and disavowed *a priori* knowledge of the drug–drug

C. Marcucci MD (✉)
Anesthesia Services Department, Philadelphia Veterans Affairs Medical Center, Philadelphia, PA, USA
e-mail: sandson.marcucci@comcast.net

N.B. Sandson MD
Department of Psychiatry, University of Maryland Medical System, Baltimore, MD, USA

Department of Psychiatry, VA Maryland Health Care System, Baltimore, MD, USA

C. Marcucci et al. (eds.), *A Case Approach to Perioperative Drug-Drug Interactions*, DOI 10.1007/978-1-4614-7495-1_160

interaction (DDI) issues. The husband and son had contacted both the patient advocate and the risk management office and were hinting darkly at legal action.

Discussion

This is an example of an inhibitor added to a prodrug substrate.

Because diphenhydramine is a high-affinity substrate of cytochrome P450 (CYP) 2D6, it acts as a relatively potent competitive inhibitor of that enzyme.[1] As stated in the preceding case, the formation of endoxifen, the most physiologically active anti-estrogenic form of tamoxifen, depends on several metabolic steps, including one that is catalyzed by 2D6.

This time, it was a bit more difficult for the anesthesia department to provide reassuring words to the family. Insofar as the patient received diphenhydramine as a standing medication over a number of days, some reduction in the magnitude of this conversion likely occurred. Ultimately, the anesthesia providers (including the pain specialists) and the oncology service spent a considerable amount of time with the family. They acknowledged a real impairment in conversion of tamoxifen to the active metabolite, but were ultimately able to reassure the family that the relatively brief and reversible lapse in tamoxifen therapy would not meaningfully impact on her overall breast cancer prognosis.

The very shaken anesthesia resident never missed another tamoxifen or prodrug drug interaction for the rest of his career.

Take-Home Points

- Meaningful inhibition of a cytochrome P450-mediated metabolic pathway can occur in a matter of days.
- Adding or subtracting a standing medication to a regimen in the perioperative period (as opposed to administration of a single dose) requires a different level of surveillance for DDIs.
- The occurrence of a DDI should be communicated to other perioperative care providers.
- When tamoxifen is in the medication regimen, always look for the presence of CYP2D6 inhibitors (eg, paroxetine, fluoxetine, bupropion, etc.) And remember, there are no 2D6 inducers.

Summary

Interaction: pharmacokinetic
Substrate: tamoxifen
Inhibitor: diphenhydramine
Clinical effects: inhibition of CYP2D6-mediated conversion of tamoxifen to active metabolites without likely meaningful change in cancer prognosis

Reference

1. Akutsu T, Kobayashi K, Sakurada K, et al. Identification of human cytochrome p450 isozymes involved in diphenhydramine N-demethylation. Drug Metab Dispos. 2007;35(1):72–8.

161 The Topic of the Day

Fatal Forty DDI: cimetidine, lidocaine, CYP1A2, CYP3A4

Catherine Marcucci MD

Abstract
This case discusses two pharmacokinetic interactions between lidocaine and cimetidine (metabolic and distribution) resulting in lidocaine toxicity.

Case

A 58-year-old mill worker presented to the operating room for a cholecystectomy. He had a history of obesity and gastroesophageal reflux disease (GERD). Two years earlier he had been in an industrial accident at the mill. His back and torso were protected by his fire-retardant clothing, but he had suffered significant and debilitating burns on his neck and face and had had a long inpatient hospitalization requiring tracheostomy. He was managed at a comprehensive burn center for debilitating post-burn skin conditions including intermittent but severe pruritis. His medication panel was remarkable only for an occasional sleep aid and cimetidine, which was prescribed to treat his GERD and as an off-label therapy for his burn pruritis.

Because of very poor ability to open his mouth and his other airway issues, an awake fiberoptic intubation was planned. He had suffered terribly with previous attempts at awake intubation and the anesthesia team promised that they would "topicalize" him thoroughly. The attending told the senior resident on the airway rotation to take the patient into the room, start a lidocaine nebulizer, and to begin to dilate his nares with nasal trumpets lubricated with lidocaine jelly, while he started his other room. He was detained longer than he expected and was just leaving his second room when he heard the overhead stat call to the urology room. A nurse hurried by him with the backup airway cart saying, "Here's your next grand rounds. The patient's seizing and I think the resident's about to have a seizure, too."

C. Marcucci MD
Anesthesia Services Department, Philadelphia Veterans Affairs Medical Center, Philadelphia, PA, USA
e-mail: sandson.marcucci@comcast.net

C. Marcucci et al. (eds.), *A Case Approach to Perioperative Drug-Drug Interactions*, DOI 10.1007/978-1-4614-7495-1_161

Discussion

This is an example of a pharmacokinetic interaction involving a substrate added to an inhibitor. There is also a pharmacokinetic interaction involving distribution.

Cimetidine was the first H_2 receptor antagonist approved by the Food and Drug Administration (FDA) for use in inhibition of gastric acid secretion. It was in wide use for many years, and was in fact one of the first billion-dollar "blockbuster" drugs. Recently, its use has been somewhat supplanted by other H_2 antagonists such as ranitidine and famotidine. However, it is still actively marketed in the US and is currently used off-label and being studied for a number of conditions. These include dermatological conditions, chronic pain conditions, and interstitial cystitis.[1] Cimetidine is a known cytochrome P450 (CYP) paninhibitor, including inhibition of CYP isozymes 1A2, 3A4, 2C9, 2C19, 2D6, and 2E19.[2,3] Cimetidine is also known to decrease hepatic perfusion.[4]

Lidocaine is a known CYP 1A2 and 3A4 substrate.[5–7] The plasma levels of lidocaine will reliably be raised by both CYP1A2 and CYP3A4 inhibitors, although the contribution is greater from 1A2 inhibition.[8] It has been used for many years as a topical anesthetic for the oral mucosa. Although there is known to be significant plasma absorption of topical lidocaine anesthesia to the airway, usually toxic serum levels are not reached in healthy individuals. However, seizures have been reported with as little as 300 mg of lidocaine administered for bronchoscopy in a chronically debilitated patient with congestive heart failure and cardiomyopathy. It is certainly likely that this patient, although he was not of small stature, could have received a considerably higher lidocaine dose, considering the administration of nebulized lidocaine and lidocaine jelly to his nares and oropharynx.

This patient suffered from a well-recognized drug–drug interaction (DDI) between cimetidine and lidocaine.[9] Two pharmacokinetic mechanisms were at work. First, there was a metabolic DDI involving the administration of lidocaine in the presence of strong inhibitor, thereby raising serum lidocaine levels into the toxic range. Second, the effect of decreased blood flow to the liver with relative higher distribution of lidocaine in the plasma served as a compounding pharmacokinetic DDI.

Take-Home Points

- Cimetidine is an older drug that is still in use and may be finding new off-label use.
- Cimetidine is a paninhibitor of multiple enzymes including CYP1A2 and CYP3A4. It also decreases hepatic blood flow.

- Lidocaine is a CYP1A2 and CYP3A4 substrate.
- Lidocaine toxicity is possible at much lower than normal doses in patients with comprised hepatic blood flow due to disease states or drugs.

Summary

Interaction 1: pharmacokinetic (metabolic)
Substrate: lidocaine
Enzyme: CYP1A2 and CYP3A4
Inhibitor: cimetidine
Clinical effect: lidocaine toxicity manifesting as seizures

Interaction 2: pharmacokinetic (distribution)
Substrates: lidocaine
Inhibitor: cimetidine
Mechanism: decreased hepatic blood flow and effective increased distribution to plasma leading to greater bioavailability of lidocaine
Clinical effect: increased incidence of lidocaine toxicity

References

1. Scheinfeld N. Cimetidine: a review of the recent developments and reports in cutaneous medicine. Dermatol Online J. 2003;9(2):4.
2. Martínez C, Albet C, Agúndez JA, et al. Comparative *in vitro* and *in vivo* inhibition of cytochrome P450 CYP1A2, CYP2D6, and CYP3A by H2-receptor antagonists. Clin Pharmacol Ther. 1999;65(4):369–76.
3. Nation RL, Evans AM, Milne RW. Pharmacokinetic drug interactions with phenytoin (Part I). Clin Pharmacokinet. 1990;18(1):37–60.
4. Feely J, Wilkinson GR, Wood AJ. Reduction of liver blood flow and propranolol metabolism by cimetidine. N Engl J Med. 1981;304(12):692–5.
5. Wang JS, Backman JT, Taavitsainen P, et al. Involvement of CYP1A2 and CYP3A4 in lidocaine N-deethylation and 3-hydroxylation in humans. Drug Metab Dispos. 2000;28(8): 959–65.
6. Wang B, Zhou SF. Synthetic and natural compounds that interact with human cytochrome P450 1A2 and implications in drug development. Curr Med Chem. 2009;16(31):4066–218.
7. Olkkola KT, Isohanni MH, Hamunen K, et al. The effect of erythromycin and fluvoxamine on the pharmacokinetics of intravenous lidocaine. Anesth Analg. 2005;100(5):1352–6.
8. Naguib M, Magboul MM, Samarkandi AH, et al. Adverse effects and drug interactions associated with local and regional anaesthesia. Drug Saf. 1998;18(4):221–50.
9. Knapp AB, Maguire W, Keren G, et al. The cimetidine-lidocaine interaction. Ann Intern Med. 1983;98(2):174–7.

Bounce Back

162

Ondansetron, CYP2D6 ultra-rapid metabolism

Erica D. Wittwer MD, PhD,
Wayne T. Nicholson MD, PharmD, MSc,
and Juraj Sprung MD, PhD

Abstract
This case discusses a drug–gene interaction involving ondansetron. Ondansetron is a cytochrome P450 2D6 substrate. The patient depicted in this clinical scenario is a 2D6 ultrarapid metabolizer.

Case

An otherwise healthy 29-year-old woman came to the operating room for a vaginal hysterectomy for a large uterine leiomyoma. The patient had undergone a tonsillectomy at age 14 years with no complications and had no allergies. Her only medication was an oral contraceptive. The patient underwent an uncomplicated intravenous induction and inhalational general anesthesia. There were no intraoperative complications and the patient was extubated in the operating room. The patient received ketorolac and granisetron at the end of the procedure and was discharged to home late in the afternoon.

That night, the patient was seen in the emergency department due to severe nausea and vomiting. She received intravenous fluids, ondansetron hydrochloride, and droperidol, which improved her symptoms, and was discharged to home with a prescription for ondansetron tablets. Late the next day, the patient contacted her surgeon because of severe nausea and vomiting. She had been unable to tolerate any food or drink since leaving the emergency department and could not keep her oral contraception down, despite taking the ondansetron tablets as prescribed. She was admitted to the hospital for treatment with intravenous fluids and antiemetics. She received

E.D. Wittwer MD, PhD (✉) • W.T. Nicholson MD, PharmD, MSc • J. Sprung MD, PhD
Department of Anesthesiology, Mayo Clinic, Rochester, MN, USA
e-mail: Wittwer.erica@mayo.edu

C. Marcucci et al. (eds.), *A Case Approach to Perioperative Drug-Drug Interactions*, DOI 10.1007/978-1-4614-7495-1_162

a dose of intravenous ondansetron, which did not improve her symptoms. The anesthesiologists were asked to see the patient and noted that she received granisetron in the operating room and initially had done well after surgery. The patient was administered a dose of granisetron and her symptoms improved; she then was given a dose of droperidol, with complete resolution of her symptoms. She received a subsequent dose of granisetron the following day and stayed in the hospital until late that day, when she and the surgical team were confident that her symptoms would not recur and she was tolerating food. The patient was seen in the clinic 1 day later to follow up on her condition, and she was doing well.

Discussion

This is an example of a drug–gene interaction.

More specifically, this is an example of ultra-extensive drug metabolism (of ondansetron) leading to ineffective therapy.

Ondansetron is a selective 5-hydroxytryptamine (5-HT) type 3 receptor antagonist commonly used to prevent or treat nausea and vomiting in various circumstances, including chemotherapy-induced or postoperative nausea and vomiting. The cytochrome P450 (CYP) 2D6 isozyme is the primary enzyme responsible for metabolism of ondansetron, with other CYP isozymes (eg, 1A1, 1A2, 3A) also contributing to its metabolism.[1,2] Genotypic variation in the CYP2D6 isozyme can cause an individual to metabolize certain medications poorly, extensively, or ultrarapidly. Because of the existence of numerous pathways for ondansetron metabolism, it had been thought that 2D6 genotype variation would not impact the drug's effect. However, studies have shown an increased risk of vomiting for patients with ultrarapid metabolism who receive ondansetron compared with patients without the ultrarapid metabolism genotype.[3,4]

In general, persons who metabolize medications poorly at the CYP2D6 isozyme may not have significantly impaired total clearance of drugs because of the alternative metabolic pathways. However, genotypic variation leading to ultra-rapid metabolism is due to duplicate (total of 3, 5, 7, 9, 11, or 13) copies of the CYP2D6 allele and increased metabolic ability. When the active form of a drug is the *parent drug*, persons with ultrarapid metabolism have a risk for treatment failure due to rapid clearance of the drug; when the active form of a drug is the *metabolite*, those with ultra-rapid metabolism are at risk for increased drug effect or adverse effects, or both, due to "ultraextensive" metabolism. In the case of ondansetron and some other 5-HT type 3 receptor antagonists, individuals with ultra-rapid metabolism may not respond to antiemetic therapy because of greater-than-expected clearance of the drug, thereby decreasing its effectiveness.

To prevent treating patients who have ultra-rapid metabolism with functionally inadequate (although in this case "standard") doses of ondansetron, patients at high risk for nausea and vomiting could undergo genetic testing to determine their genotype. It has been estimated that 50 patients would need to have genotype tests to prevent one treatment failure due to the ultrarapid metabolism genotype for CYP2D6.[4] The cost-effectiveness of treating patients on the basis of genotype is not known. An alternative to genotyping and creating a personalized treatment and dosing regimen is use of a 5-hydroxytryptamine type 3 receptor antagonist not metabolized with the CYP2D6 isozyme, such as granisetron, which is metabolized through the CYP3A4 isozyme.[5] The patient in the present example had relief from her nausea and vomiting when she received granisetron to achieve the antiemetic effect, because it was not metabolized by the same enzyme as ondansetron.

Take-Home Points

- Ondansetron, a commonly used antiemetic, is metabolized by the CYP2D6 isozyme, which has genetic variability. Persons with duplicate copies of the CYP2D6 allele metabolize ondansetron ultrarapidly and may have reduced effectiveness from standard dosages.
- Consider the possibility of CYP2D6 ultrarapid metabolism when you are having great difficulty controlling perioperative nausea and vomiting!
- The choice of which drug to use in a class of medications may be impacted by the route of metabolism of the drugs in that class. Use of granisetron may reduce treatment failure because it is metabolized by an alternative route compared with ondansetron.
- Genetic evaluation could lead to more effective treatment or prevention of nausea and vomiting, but the cost-effectiveness of such a strategy is unknown.

Summary

Interaction: pharmacokinetic (drug–gene)
Substrate: ondansetron
Enzyme: CYP2D6
Clinical effect: decreased antiemetic efficacy

References

1. Fischer V, Vickers AE, Heitz F, et al. The polymorphic cytochrome P-4502D6 is involved in the metabolism of both 5-hydroxytryptamine antagonists, tropisetron and ondansetron. Drug Metab Dispos. 1994;22:269–74.
2. Dixon CM, Colthup PV, Serabjit-Singh CJ. Multiple forms of cytochrome P450 are involved in the metabolism of ondansetron in humans. Drug Metab Dispos. 1995;23:1225–30.
3. Candiotti KA, Birnbach DJ, Lubarsky DA, et al. The impact of pharmacogenomics on postoperative nausea and vomiting: do CYP2D6 allele copy number and polymorphisms affect the success or failure of ondansetron prophylaxis? Anesthesiology. 2005;102:543–9.
4. Kaiser R, Sezer O, Papies A, et al. Patient-tailored antiemetic treatment with 5-hydroxytryptamine type 3 receptor antagonists according to cytochrome P-450 2D6 genotypes. J Clin Oncol. 2002;20:2805–11.
5. Janicki PK. Cytochrome P450 2D6 metabolism and 5-hydroxytryptamine type 3 receptor antagonists for postoperative nausea and vomiting. Med Sci Monit. 2005;11:RA322–8.

163 Call the Cath Lab!

Fatal Forty DDI: omeprazole, clopidogrel, CYP2C19

Anna Dubovoy MD and Erin B. Payne MD

Abstract
This case discusses the pharmacokinetic interaction between clopidogrel and omeprazole, possibly resulting in loss of antiplatelet efficacy. Clopidogrel is a cytochrome P450 2C19 prodrug. Omeprazole inhibits conversion of clopidogrel to the active metabolite.

Case

Mr. M. was a 65-year-old man with a history of coronary artery disease, type 2 diabetes, renal insufficiency, and gastroesophageal reflux disease, who presented to the Emergency Room with possible acute appendicitis versus small bowel obstruction. Unfortunately, he also had severe substernal chest pain that radiated to the left jaw. Three months ago, Mr. M. underwent drug-eluting stent placement in the right coronary artery (RCA). Today, his electrocardiogram performed in the emergency room showed ST elevation in leads II, III and aVF. His heart rate was 55 beats per minute, blood pressure was 110/78 mm Hg, and respiratory rate was 14 breaths per minute. His medications included aspirin, clopidogrel, metoprolol, amlodipine, and omeprazole. His laboratory values were significant for creatinine 1.8 mg/dL, potassium 4.8 meq/L, and troponin 1.85 ng/ml. Given his symptoms, electrocardiogram changes and elevated troponin, Mr. M. was taken to the cardiac catheterization laboratory for diagnostic catheterization. Catheterization revealed in-stent thrombosis of RCA stent and angioplasty was performed. Mr. M. was admitted to the intensive

A. Dubovoy MD (✉)
Department of Anesthesiology, University of Michigan Hospital Center, Ann Arbor, MI, USA
e-mail: aodnopoz@med.umich.edu

E.B. Payne MD
Preoperative Assessment Clinic, University of Michigan Health System, Plymouth, MI, USA

C. Marcucci et al. (eds.), *A Case Approach to Perioperative Drug-Drug Interactions*, DOI 10.1007/978-1-4614-7495-1_163

care unit for observation of his abdominal pain and restarted on his home regimen of clopidogrel and aspirin for drug-eluting stent, however his omeprazole was changed to ranitidine.

Discussion

Clopidogrel is a prodrug that undergoes a two-step metabolic activation by multiple hepatic cytochrome P450 isoenzymes including cytochrome P450 (CYP) enzymes 3A4 and 2C19.[1,2] The active metabolite of clopidogrel works through the platelet $P2Y_{12}$ receptor to irreversibly inhibit adenosine-diphosphate (APD)–induced platelet aggregation. Variable patient response to clopidogrel has been attributed to variable expression of cytochrome genes, $P2Y_{12}$ receptor polymorphism, and multiple interactions with other classes of medications.[3] It has also been shown *in vitro* that proton pump inhibitors (PPI) decrease the antiplatelet activity of clopidogrel.[4]

Proton pump inhibitors (PPIs) including, but not limited to omeprazole, esomeprazole, and lansoprazole are metabolized by the hepatic CYP2C19 isoenzyme.[2] In patients taking a 2C19-metabolized PPI, there is attenuation of 2C19 metabolic activity for the activation of clopidogrel. Currently, this interaction remains a controversial topic in the literature since more patients are placed on dual antiplatelet therapy with clopidogrel and aspirin, according to the most recent American College of Cardiology/American Heart Association (ACC/AHA) guidelines and increasing number of those patients are on a PPI, according to American College of Cardiology Foundation/American College of Gastroenterology/American Heart Association (ACCF/ACG/AHA) 2008 expert consensus.[5,6]

A meta-analysis of studies published before October 2010 noted that small randomized control trials of clopidogrel with PPI therapy versus clopidogrel alone failed to identify a difference in the rate of cardiovascular events. However, the observational studies showed a strong attenuation of antiplatelet function of clopidogrel by PPI with approximately 50% increased risk for major adverse events (MACE), stroke, and hospital readmission.[7] In a 2011 retrospective analysis of BASKET study data, Burkard et al. evaluated 801 patients on clopidogrel, 109 (14%) of whom also received a PPI.[2] Patients receiving a combination of clopidogrel/PPI therapy had higher rates of MACE (30.3% vs. 20.8%, $P=.027$) and myocardial infarction (14.7% vs. 7.4%, $P=0.01$).[2] In another recent study of 1270 Japanese patients on clopidogrel, 331 patients (26%) were also taking a PPI. This study failed to show any negative PPI–clopidogrel drug interaction.[8]

Concerned with the current controversy in literature about PPI attenuation of clopidogrel antiplatelet action by PPIs, the Federal Drug Administration and the European Medicines Agency issued a warning regarding the interaction of clopidogrel with omeprazole and other PPIs, respectively. Given a growing patient population that is prescribed both clopidogrel and PPI, if patients are at high risk for gastrointestinal bleeding, a PPI therapy is still recommended. However, if patients do not have acid-peptic symptoms and/or they are at low risk for gastrointestinal bleeding, PPI therapy may be discontinued or an acid-suppressive regimen intensity may be decreased.[9]

Take-Home Points

- Clopidogrel is a prodrug that is activated primarily by multiple hepatic enzymes, including CYP2C19.
- PPIs are metabolized by CYP2C19.
- PPIs attenuate clopidogrel antiplatelet actions *in vitro*, however *in vivo* studies show variable results. Most observational studies show an increased rate of MACE in patients on combined clopidogrel–PPI therapy.
- A large, randomized controlled study of clopidogrel alone and clopidogrel–PPI combination needs to be performed to better analyze the interaction. However, national drug safety organizations have issued warnings about potential interaction of clopidogrel with omeprazole.
- This case is an example of a patient who was on dual antiplatelet therapy for a drug-eluting stent in the coronary artery. This patient was also prescribed omeprazole, a PPI, which potentially attenuates clopidogrel antiplatelet action. Therefore, his in-stent thrombosis could be potentially attributed to this interaction. Replacing this patient's omeprazole with ranitidine may potentially increase the number of active clopidogrel metabolites.

Summary

Interaction: pharmacokinetic
Substrate: clopidogrel
Enzyme: CYP2C19
Inhibitor: omeprazole
Clinical effect: loss of antiplatelet efficacy

References

1. Hall R, Mazer CD. Antiplatelet drugs: a review of their pharmacology and management in the perioperative period. Anesth Anal. 2011;112(2):292–318.
2. Burkard T, Kaiser CA, et al. Combined clopidogrel and proton pump inhibitor therapy is associated with higher cardiovascular event rates after percutaneous coronary intervention: a report from the BASKET trial. J Inter Med. 2012;(3):257–63.

3. Bates ER, Lau WC, Angiolillo DJ. Clopidogrel-drug interactions. J Am Coll Cardiol. 2011; 57:1251–63.
4. Siller-Matula J, Spiel A, et al. Effects of pantoprazole and esomeprazole on platelet inhibition by clopidogrel. Am Heart J. 2009;157:148.e1–5.
5. King 3rd SB, Smith SJ, Hirshfield JJ, et al. 2007 Focused update of the ACC/AHA/SCAI 2005 guideline update for percutaneous coronary intervention: a report of the American College of Cardiology/American Heart Association task force on practice guidelines: 2007 writing group to review new evidence and update the ACC/AHA/SCAI 2005 guideline update for percutaneous coronary intervention, writing on behalf of the 2005 writing committee. Circulation. 2008;117:261–95.
6. Bhatt D, Scheiman J, Abraham N, et al. ACCF/ACG/AHA 2008 expert consensus document on reducing the gastrointestinal risks of antiplatelet therapy and NSAID use: a report of the American College of Cardiology Foundation Task Force on Clinical Expert Consensus Documents. J Am Coll Cardiol. 2008;52:1502–17.
7. Chen M, Wei JF, et al. A meta-analysis of impact of proton pump inhibitors on antiplatelet effect of clopidogrel. Cardiovasc Ther. 2012;30(5):e227–33.
8. Chitose T, Hokimoto S, et al. Clinical outcomes following coronary stenting in Japanese patients treated with and without proton pump inhibitor. Circ J. 2012;76(1):71–8.
9. Madanick R. Proton pump inhibitor side effects and drug interactions: much ado about nothing? Cleve Clin J Med. 2011;78(1):39–49.

The Imatinib Inquiry: A Theoretical Case (for Now)

164

Imatinib, metoprolol, midazolam, fentanyl, CYP3A4

Stephen J. Gleich MD, Erica D. Wittwer MD, PhD, Juraj Sprung MD, PhD, and Nicole Henwood MD

Abstract
This case discusses a possible interaction between imatinib and anesthetic drugs. Many anesthetic drugs are cytochrome P450 3A4 substrates. Imatinib is a 3A4 inhibitor. The interaction is mechanistically possible and perhaps even likely, but has not yet been reported.

Case

A 73-year-old woman was admitted to the hospital to undergo a diagnostic knee arthroscopy for chronic knee arthritis. She had a history of chronic myelogenous leukemia (CML) that was in remission for 2 years and was currently being treated with imatinib (Gleevec®). She was very concerned about information she found on Internet relating to the interaction of imatinib and anesthetic agents. The anesthesia resident quickly checked a popular online drug information program, but did not

Editor's Note: Many of the example cases in the present book are prepared based on current drug–drug interaction information. New information should always be incorporated before making any clinical decisions. It is the responsibility of the individual practitioners to review the newest drug information to ensure proper therapy. This chapter was composed based on present knowledge regarding imatinib, and reflects absence of current reports of clinically significant interaction with midazolam and propofol.

S.J. Gleich MD (✉) • E.D. Wittwer MD, PhD • J. Sprung MD, PhD
Department of Anesthesiology, Mayo Clinic, Rochester, MN, USA
e-mail: Gleich.stephen@mayo.edu

N. Henwood MD
West Chester Anesthesia Associates, West Chester, PA, USA

C. Marcucci et al. (eds.), *A Case Approach to Perioperative Drug-Drug Interactions*, DOI 10.1007/978-1-4614-7495-1_164

find any reported drug–drug interactions (DDI) between imatinib and the standard anesthesia medications. However, he discovered that imatinib is primarily metabolized by cytochrome P450 isoenzyme 3A4 (CYP3A4) and may competitively inhibit the metabolism of other drugs that are substrates for the same pathway. He further recalled that midazolam is also primarily metabolized by CYP3A4, inviting the possibility of a DDI. He postulated that coadministration of imatinib with midazolam could reduce midazolam clearance.

The resident discussed this finding with his attending and together, they recommended a spinal anesthetic. The resident brought the patient to the operating room to proceed with the planned surgery. Just as the incision was about to be made, the patient became increasingly anxious and indicated she couldn't tolerate the procedure without some sedation. The anesthetic level induced by spinal anesthesia was rechecked and found to be appropriate. Additional intravenous sedation was given with standard doses of midazolam and propofol. Subsequently, the patient tolerated the procedure well and awoke at the end of the procedure without prolonged sedation. In the recovery room, the patient was comfortable and had an uneventful recovery (*personal communication, Nicole Henwood, MD, 2009*).

Discussion

This is an example of a theoretical drug interaction, with (as yet) no reported clinically significant interactions.

The tyrosine kinase inhibitor, imatinib, has tremendously improved the treatment and prognosis of CML. Imatinib's mechanism of action includes inhibition of the tyrosine kinase Bcr-Abl, which is a fusion oncoprotein that results from the translocation t(9;22) and is associated with the Philadelphia chromosome. Imatinib is metabolized primarily by CYP3A4, with its metabolites eliminated through biliary excretion.[1]

Imatinib may competitively inhibit the metabolism of drugs that are CYP3A4 substrates, including midazolam. Consequently, midazolam levels may be increased with an associated enhanced pharmacodynamic effect when administered concurrently with imatinib.[1] Despite this theoretical DDI, there are no reported clinically significant interactions with imatinib and midazolam.

A clinically relevant DDI exists between the intravenous anesthetic propofol and midazolam with a similar mechanism as the *theoretical* imatinib interactions. Propofol has been shown to decrease the clearance of midazolam *via* competitive inhibition of CYP3A4, producing a synergistic hypnotic effect.[2] Yet, propofol and midazolam are routinely administered together safely by experienced anesthesia providers. Further, propofol's inhibition of CYP3A4 could potentially increase plasma imatinib levels. However, when imatinib is at steady-state levels (taken for

2 months or more), the potent CYP3A4 inhibitor, ritonavir, did not change imatinib plasma levels, indicating that alternate elimination pathways may exist.[3] This would also suggest that short term administration of propofol to a patient on chronic imatinib therapy would have a minimal DDI.

Imatinib affects the clearance of other commonly used (nonanesthetic) drugs that also utilize the CYP3A4 metabolic pathway. For example, simvastatin, calcium channel blockers (verapamil and diltiazem), amiodarone, and quinidine may have significantly decreased clearance when administered to patients on imatinib. Due to imatinib's extensive metabolism by 3A4, strong inhibitors of 3A4 including ketoconazole, voriconazole, levothyroxine, and amiodarone, should be utilized with caution to avoid causing supratherapeutic imatinib levels. Imatinib also inhibits the hepatic glucuronidation of acetaminophen, leading to hepatotoxicity. As a result, the use of acetaminophen should be limited in patients on imatinib therapy.[1]

Finally, although the main metabolic pathway of imatinib is via CYP3A4, CYP2D6 also plays a small role. Metoprolol is a selective β_1 adrenoceptor antagonist and is metabolized via 2D6. Concurrent administration of imatinib and metoprolol have demonstrated small to moderate increases in metoprolol plasma levels.[4] Although the pharmacodynamic effects were not reported, perhaps this is why our patient only required a low dose of metoprolol for adequate blood pressure control.

In summary, the 73-year-old patient with CML on chronic imatinib therapy in this scenario was an informed patient who dutifully researched her medications and encountered information on DDIs with imatinib on the Internet. Despite the *theoretical* DDIs with imatinib and commonly used anesthetics, no clinically significant interactions have been reported to date. Significant DDIs with imatinib and many drugs not commonly used in anesthesia practice are known and these interactions should be reviewed for any patient on imatinib therapy.

Take-Home Points

- Patients, especially those who are more informed and proactive, may encounter information that they discover on the Internet or through other sources that may not have clinical relevance or may be incorrect.
- Imatinib, despite several theoretical interactions with anesthetic agents, can and should be continued throughout the perioperative period to maintain therapeutic levels.
- Imatinib does interact to a clinically significant degree with several common nonanesthetic medications and imatinib use should prompt a thorough review of concurrently used medication for potential interactions.

Summary

Interaction: theoretical pharmacokinetic interaction
Substrates: anesthetic drugs such as midazolam and propofol
Enzyme: CYP3A4
Inhibitor: imatinib (theoretical)
Significant clinical effect: none reported to date

References

1. Haouala A, Widmer N, Duchosal MA, et al. Drug interactions with the tyrosine kinase inhibitors imatinib, dasatinib, and nilotinib. Blood. 2011;117(8):e75–87.
2. Hamaoka N, Oda Y, Hase I, et al. Propofol decreases the clearance of midazolam by inhibiting CYP3A4: an in vivo and in vitro study. Clin Pharmacol Ther. 1999;66(2):110–7.
3. van Erp NP, Gelderblom H, Karlsson MO, et al. Influence of CYP3A4 inhibition on the steady-state pharmacokinetics of imatinib. Clin Cancer Res. 2007;13(24):7394–400.
4. Wang Y, Zhou L, Dutreix C, et al. Effects of imatinib (Glivec) on the pharmacokinetics of metoprolol, a CYP2D6 substrate, in Chinese patients with chronic myelogenous leukaemia. Br J Clin Pharmacol. 2008;65(6):885–92.

A HAART-breaking Tale

165

Metformin, tenofovir

Dean Laochamroonvorapongse MD
and Kirk Lalwani MD, FRCA, MCR

Abstract
This case discusses the synergistic pharmacodynamic interaction between metformin and tenofovir, resulting in lactic acidosis and renal failure.

Case

A 40-year-old man presented to the Emergency Department with a 2-day history of vomiting, severe abdominal pain, and lethargy. He had a history of non-insulin-dependent diabetes mellitus (NIDDM) with microalbuminuria and has been taking metformin (1000 mg BID) for the past five years. The patient's family was extremely distraught and stated that he looked "completely healthy" when they saw him the previous month and that he was always meticulous about his diet and exercise regimen. The patient was noted to be dehydrated and tachycardic with extreme right lower quadrant tenderness and guarding. His fingerstick glucose reading was 100 mg/dL. The laboratory values showed a white blood cell count of 20,000/μL with a left shift, sodium 140 mEq/L, potassium 5.2 mEq/L, chloride 94 mEq/L, bicarbonate 16 mEq/L, anion gap of 30, BUN 50 mg/dL, and creatinine 2.5 mg/dL. An arterial blood gas was drawn on room air and showed a metabolic acidosis with a serum lactate of 15 mmol/L. An intravenous infusion of normal saline was started and a Foley catheter was inserted, which revealed scant amounts of tea-colored urine. The patient was taken to the preoperative holding area for an emergent appendectomy.

The attending anesthesiologist arrived and found an ill-appearing and tearful patient. He confessed that he was recently diagnosed with human immunodeficiency virus (HIV) and started on a highly active antiretroviral therapy (HAART) regimen

D. Laochamroonvorapongse MD (✉) • K. Lalwani MD, FRCA, MCR
Department of Anesthesiology and Perioperative Medicine,
Oregon Health and Science University, Portland, OR, USA
e-mail: laochamr@ohsu.edu

C. Marcucci et al. (eds.), *A Case Approach to Perioperative Drug-Drug Interactions*, DOI 10.1007/978-1-4614-7495-1_165

including tenofovir at a city health clinic (not his primary care provider). He was also very concerned about being upsetting his family and even being "disowned." The anesthesiologist reassured the patient as he was being wheeled into the operating room him and called his intensive care unit (ICU) colleague to tell her to expect a sicker-than-normal acute appendicitis patient. Postoperatively, the patient required six sessions of continuous veno-venous hemofiltration and his serum lactate and urine output normalized on the third postoperative day. He was eventually discharged home off his HAART regimen and instructed to tell his primary care provider about his new HIV diagnosis during their follow-up appointment.

Discussion

This is an example of a synergistic pharmacodynamic drug effect.

The biguanide metformin (Glucophage®) is the most commonly prescribed oral antidiabetic agent, with over 42 million prescriptions written in 2005.[1] It works by inhibiting hepatic glycogenesis, increasing muscle and fat tissue sensitivity to insulin, and reducing gastrointestinal absorption of glucose. Metformin has become a first-line treatment for NIDDM due to its lack of hypoglycemic effect and favorable effects on lipid profile.[2] Metformin-associated lactic acidosis (MALA) has been described in several clinical settings but the pathophysiology is not completely understood, with impaired hepatic clearance of lactate considered the predominant mechanism. Elderly patients and those with renal insufficiency are often cited to be at the highest risk. However, a recent Cochrane Database review of 176 studies found no evidence supporting a link between metformin and lactic acidosis, even in patients with renal insufficiency or medical comorbidities.[3]

Tenofovir (Viread®) is a nucleotide analog approved for treatment of HIV and works by blocking RNA-dependent DNA synthesis by reverse transcriptase. It also has some affinity for mitochondrial DNA polymerase, which may lead to mitochondrial toxicity and associated lactic acidosis, nephrotoxicity, hepatic steatosis, peripheral neuropathy, and pancreatitis.[4]

Lactic acidosis can be divided into two broad categories: those associated with impairment in systemic tissue oxygenation (type A) and those resulting from a deregulation in cell metabolism (type B). Causes of type A lactic acidosis include hypoxemia and tissue hypoperfusion resulting from hypovolemia, sepsis, and heart failure. Causes of type B lactic acidosis such as toxins, hepatic failure, and thiamine deficiency are frequently overlooked. There have been at least three case reports of lactic acidosis and acute renal failure after concomitant treatment with metformin and tenofovir.[5–7] The interaction between metformin and tenofovir is complex and poorly understood, but likely involves the synergistic effect of metformin and tenofovir-induced mitochondrial toxicity, markedly impairing hepatic clearance of lactate. It is important to note that these patients may have chronic renal insufficiency, leading to decreased elimination of both drugs. Furthermore, all the usual causes of tissue hypoperfusion may lead to renal and hepatic dysfunction, setting the patient up for this dangerous interaction. Treatment once the diagnosis is confirmed usually involves discontinuation of both drugs and renal replacement therapy in order to clear the lactate, metformin, and tenofovir.

Take-Home Points

- This case emphasizes the importance of taking a thorough history utilizing open-ended questions from the patient in a private setting. Some patients may also be reluctant to provide accurate information about sensitive (a potentially stigmatizing diagnosis such as HIV) or embarrassing issues when other persons are present.
- Work hard to familiarize yourself and stay current with the drug cocktails (such as HAART) that are commonly used by the patients you treat—not just the "initials" of the cocktails, but the individual drugs included in the regimens.
- Both metformin and tenofovir have been independently linked to the development of lactic acidosis, but the concomitant administration of both agents may cause marked impairment of hepatic lactate clearance.
- Keep this interaction in mind when a previously stable patient on one of these drugs has the other added to his or her medication regimen and develops nonspecific symptoms such as abdominal pain, nausea,vomiting, muscle weakness, and dyspnea.

Summary

Interaction: pharmacodynamic
Substrates: metformin and tenofovir
Sites of action/enzyme: unknown, possible mitochondria
Clinical effect: lactic acidosis and renal failure

References

1. Perrone J, Phillips C, Gaieski D. Occult metformin toxicity in three patients with profound lactic acidosis. J Emerg Med. 2011;40(3):271–5.
2. Fisman EZ, Tenenbaum A. A cardiologic approach to non-insulin antidiabetic pharmacotherapy in patients with heart disease. Cardiovasc Diabetol. 2009;8:38.

3. Salpeter S, et al. Risk of fatal and nonfatal lactic acidosis with metformin use in type 2 diabetes mellitus. Cochrane Database Syst Rev. 2004;(3):CD002967.
4. Patel V, Hedayati SS. Lactic acidosis in an HIV-infected patient receiving highly active antiretroviral therapy. Nat Clin Pract Nephrol. 2006;2(2):109–14.
5. Aperis G, et al. Lactic acidosis after concomitant treatment with metformin and tenofovir in a patient with HIV infection. J Ren Care. 2011;37(1):25–9.
6. Dupont C, Meier F, Loupy A. Acute renal failure and tenofovir: two new cases. Antivir Ther. 2003;8(Suppl 1), abstract 694.
7. Kazazis C. A case of lactic acidosis (LA) after administration of tenofovir and metformin in a diabetic patient with recently diagnosed HIV infection. J Ren Care. 2011;37(3):174.

Drug–Drug Interactions Involving Neuropsychiatric Drugs

XV

Introduction 166

Neil B. Sandson MD

Abstract
This section introduces drug–drug interactions involving neuropsychiatric medications.

Although clinically significant drug–drug interactions (DDIs) can occur with drugs from any functional drug class, the history of this topic has been closely linked to the neuropsychiatric drugs. One of the most infamous DDIs in American medical history occurred in the "Libby Zion" case, in which an interaction between phenelzine and meperidine was implicated in this young woman's death. While this case served as a clarion call around the issue of resident work hours, it also highlighted the seriousness of monoamine oxidase inhibitor (MAOI) drug interactions. In the early 1990s, the advent of selective serotonin reuptake inhibitors (SSRIs) was soon followed by an appreciation of potentially grave selective serotonin reuptake inhibitor-tricyclic antidepressant (SSRI-TCA) interactions. As a result, in the ensuing years, a greater proportion of psychiatrists gained familiarity with this topic than any of the other broad medical specialties. This was and continues to be driven by very real practice-based, need-to-know considerations given that at least a dozen of the **Fatal Forty** drugs are neuropsychiatric drugs.

As the DDI evidence base expands with time, the details can be difficult to remember with exactness, but within the neuropsychiatric area, some reasonably reliable generalizations can be made. For instance, when antidepressants (except for TCAs) are involved in significant DDIs, they are probably acting as inhibitors, with fluoxetine (Prozac®) as our most ubiquitous pan-inhibitor. When an antipsychotic, valproate, lamotrigine, lithium, or TCAs are involved in a DDI, these drugs are probably the substrates or "victims." In contrast, many of our anticonvulsants, such as carbamazepine, oxcarbazepine, phenytoin, and phenobarbital, are enzymatic inducers, with all (except for oxcarbazepine) acting as pan-inducers.

N.B. Sandson MD
Department of Psychiatry, University of Maryland Medical System, Baltimore, MD, USA

Department of Psychiatry, VA Maryland Health Care System, Baltimore, MD, USA
e-mail: sandson.marcucci@comcast.net

C. Marcucci et al. (eds.), *A Case Approach to Perioperative Drug-Drug Interactions*, DOI 10.1007/978-1-4614-7495-1_166

Several of the "older" agents—such as TCAs, lithium, carbamazepine, phenytoin, and clozapine—have lower therapeutic indices, making them deadlier in overdose or if their levels are increased by coadministration of an inhibitor of their metabolism or some other pharmacokinetic mechanism. The broad appeal of many of the newer psychotropic agents derives from their higher therapeutic indices, although these newer agents are often either less effective, or have other liabilities.

In many ways, the story of modern neuropsychiatric drug development mirrors the evolution of the DDI narrative, but a consciousness of this topic has been there all along, on some level. One need only look at Sinemet® (levodopa + carbidopa) to see that. In the modern era, we have created Nuedexta® (quinidine + dextromethorphan) for the treatment of pseudobulbar affect (uncontrollable emotional lability) in amyotrophic lateral sclerosis, a virtually analogous development. The quinidine serves no therapeutic purpose except to prevent peripheral breakdown of dextromethorphan (which crosses the blood–brain barrier) into dextrorphan (which does not cross) by potently inhibiting the activity of cytochrome P450 (CYP) 2D6, so that effective concentrations of the parent drug can exist in the periphery long enough to be absorbed into the central nervous system.

Clearly, the sophistication with which DDIs are being utilized in drug development is growing. It behooves us to gain greater comfort and mastery of this topic, so we are not left behind the curve, using drugs when we don't understand how they work, or how other drugs might unexpectedly hinder or enhance their effects. It is a challenge, but a rewarding one, for both clinicians and their patients!

Phenytoin (I): Going Crazy! 167

Fatal Forty DDI: phenytoin, quetiapine, CYP3A4

Sara M. Skrlin MD and Ansgar M. Brambrink MD, PhD

Abstract
This case discusses a pharmacokinetic interaction between quetiapine and phenytoin resulting in breakthrough of psychotic symptoms. Quetiapine is a cytochrome P450 3A4 substrate and phenytoin is a 3A4 inducer.

Case

An anesthesia resident went to see a 32-year-old postoperative patient who had undergone an uneventful general anesthetic for the repair of a humerus fracture the previous day. Eleven days ago, the patient had been hit by a truck while walking his dog and he sustained multiple orthopedic injuries, a large subdural bleed, and a generalized tonic-clonic seizure. Phenytoin had been started at the time of evacuation of the subdural hematoma. He also had a preoperative history of schizophrenia, which had been well managed for the past 2 years on a stable dose of quetiapine (Seroquel®).

As the resident entered the patient's room, the patient was having a vivid conversation with someone in the air conditioning vent. The patient was anxious, agitated, diaphoretic, and complained of a headache. The orthopedic surgeon had ordered haloperidol to treat the hallucinations to no avail.

On the way to the neurointensive care unit (ICU) by way of the computed tomography (CT) scanner, the anesthesia resident wondered if the patient's quetiapine had been discontinued. When the patient's medication list showed that he had been maintained on his home dose of quetiapine , the resident placed a call to the ICU pharmacist who confirmed her suspicions. After a discussion with neurosurgery and psychiatry, the patient was continued on his quetiapine at the same dose and also

S.M. Skrlin MD (✉) • A.M. Brambrink MD, PhD
Department of Anesthesiology and Perioperative Medicine,
Oregon Health and Science University, Portland, OR, USA
e-mail: skrlins@ohsu.edu

C. Marcucci et al. (eds.), *A Case Approach to Perioperative Drug-Drug Interactions*, DOI 10.1007/978-1-4614-7495-1_167

started on levetiracetam (Keppra®). The phenytoin was discontinued. In order to effectively manage the patient's hallucinations, extra doses of quetiapine were ordered to effect for the next 24 hours. The CT scan revealed no signs of intracranial pathology and the patient recovered within a few hours. He was transferred back to the ward on the next day with normal cognition and neurologically intact.

Discussion

This is an example of an inducer added to a substrate.

Quetiapine is an atypical antipsychotic predominantly and extensively metabolized by cytochrome P450 (CYP) enzyme 3A4. The major metabolites are inactive. It is used for the treatment of schizophrenia, schizoaffective disorder, and bipolar disorder. Compared to traditional antipsychotics, it is associated with a reduced incidence of extrapyramidal symptoms. Quetiapine has also been used in lower dosages to treat insomnia or delirium in hospitalized patients and new evidence shows benefits in particular in the critically ill.

Phenytoin is an anticonvulsant and known to be a potent inducer of CYP3A4. It is a commonly used, effective anticonvulsant that is indicated for the control and prevention of generalized tonic-clonic and complex partial seizures. Status epilepticus and other acute seizures are often treated with phenytoin intravenously due to its fast onset. Dosage adjustments can be made reasonably well by monitoring serum phenytoin and albumin levels.

In this case, phenytoin treatment was initiated acutely in a patient who was well controlled with a stable dose of quetiapine for several years. Given the pharmacokinetics of the two drugs, it is highly likely that the induction of 3A4 by the newly added phenytoin resulted in an increased amount of enzyme available that is responsible for the clearance of quetiapine. This resulted in an accelerated metabolism and increased clearance of quetiapine, lowering plasma concentration and possibly decreasing its clinical effect.[1,2] Most inducing agents given in therapeutic doses produce their maximum effects on enzyme activity within 3 weeks.

This interpretation is supported by evidence from the literature: A small case series explored the pharmacokinetic impact of phenytoin by looking at quetiapine administration alone or in combination with phenytoin in 17 men with diagnosed schizophrenia, schizoaffective disorder, or bipolar disorder. They found that the concomitant administration of phenytoin and quetiapine resulted in a fivefold increase in the clearance of quetiapine and the mean steady-state area under the concentration-time curve was reduced to 19% of its value prior to phenytoin administration. Trough concentrations of phenytoin were minimally affected.[3]

Symptoms associated with quetiapine withdrawal, including nausea, dizziness, headache, diaphoresis, and agitation have also been reported.[3,4] In patients receiving quetiapine and phenytoin, a fivefold increase in quetiapine dosage would be necessary to compensate for the accelerated metabolism of quetiapine, which is not practical clinically. A better choice would be to choose a different anticonvulsant or antipsychotic medication. Alternative noninducer anticonvulsants are levetiracetam and sodium valproate.[2,5] Levetiracetam is not extensively metabolized in humans and is not dependent on, nor does it have an impact on, the cytochrome P450 enzymes. Protein binding is less than 10%. It is not associated with clinically significant pharmacokinetic interactions with other drugs, including other anti-epileptic drugs. Renal clearance is the major route of elimination and dose adjustments may be required in patients with renal failure. Extra doses of quetiapine may be given to clinical effect until the phenytoin has been cleared.

Care must also be taken with use of other CYP3A4 inducers such as carbamazepine, barbiturates, rifampin, and glucocorticoids, which may also lower the effectiveness of quetiapine. On the other hand, CYP3A inhibitors like ketoconazole, itraconazole, fluconazole, and erythromycin can cause an increase in the plasma quetiapine concentration by inhibiting its clearance.[6]

Take-Home Points

- Patients treated concomitantly with quetiapine and phenytoin may need to be switched to an alternative anticonvulsant medication to control psychiatric symptoms due to the induction of CYP3A4 enzyme and subsequent increased clearance of quetiapine. An alternative noninducer anticonvulsant is levetiracetam.

- Quetiapine can be used very effectively for the treatment of delirium in hospitalized patients. If quetiapine is being used on an as needed basis, such as for ICU delirium, the healthcare provider should be aware that dose adjustments may be required to achieve therapeutic goals in patients who concomitantly receive drugs that induce or inhibit the P450 3A pathway. As a general rule, the doses used for delirium tend to be lower than those used in schizophrenia.

- Enzymatic induction with ensuing effects on drug metabolism and drug levels may take 3 weeks for maximal changes to be seen. Health care providers need to keep this in mind when multiple specialties are contributing to a patient's care and prescribing medications during the hospital stay so as not to miss a drug–drug interaction.

Summary

Interaction: pharmacokinetic
Substrate: quetiapine
Enzyme: CYP3A4
Inducer: phenytoin
Clinical effects: increased psychotic signs and symptoms

References

1. Besag FMC, Berry D. Interactions between antiepileptic and antipsychotic drugs. Drug Saf. 2006;29:95–118.
2. DeVane CL, Nemenoff CB. Clinical pharmacokinetics of quetiapine. An atypical antipsychotic. Clin Pharmacokinet. 2001;40:507–22.
3. Wong YW, Yeh C, Thyrum PT. The effects of concomitant phenytoin administration on the steady-state pharmacokinetics of quetiapine. J Clin Psychopharmacol. 2001;21:89–93.
4. Thurstone CC, Alahi P. A possible case of quetiapine withdrawal syndrome. J Clin Psychiatry. 2000;61:602–3.
5. Keppra XR® [package insert]. Smyrna: UCB, Inc: 2009.
6. Quetiapine [package insert]. Wilmington: AstraZeneca Pharmaceuticals: 2009.

Phenytoin (II): The Wrong Drug for the Schizophrenic 168

Fatal Forty DDI: phenytoin, quetiapine, CYP3A4

Melisa N. Weingarten RN, MS, Juraj Sprung MD, PhD, and Toby N. Weingarten MD

Abstract
This case discusses the pharmacokinetic interaction between quetiapine and phenytoin, resulting in acute psychosis in a postoperative patient. Quetiapine is a cytochrome P40 3A4 substrate and phenytoin is a 3A4 inducer.

Case

At 3 AM, a call for the rapid response team was made by a nurse caring for a 45-year-old, 80 kg man on the orthopedic surgical ward because the patient was causing behavioral disturbances including yelling and throwing objects at the health care staff. The man had a long history of schizophrenia and had been living in a group home. His schizophrenia had been moderately controlled with oral quetiapine fumarate (400 mg daily). He had been hospitalized for a week for injuries sustained from falling from a tree that included a compound femur fracture, a cranial subdural hematoma, and an apparent seizure in the field. He had undergone emergent craniotomy via burr hole for evacuation of the hematoma and open reduction and internal fixation of his femur. Intraoperatively fosphenytoin (1600 mg) was administered intravenously (IV) for seizure prophylaxis. Postoperatively he had no obvious neurological deficits and was started on oral phenytoin sodium (300 mg daily).

M.N. Weingarten RN, MS (✉)
Patient Education, Mayo Clinic, Rochester, MN, USA
e-mail: Weingarten.melisa@mayo.edu

J. Sprung MD, PhD • T.N. Weingarten MD
Department of Anesthesiology, Mayo Clinic, Rochester, MN, USA

C. Marcucci et al. (eds.), *A Case Approach to Perioperative Drug-Drug Interactions*, DOI 10.1007/978-1-4614-7495-1_168

The resident on the rapid response team administered intravenous haloperidol decanoate to the patient for sedation. In the morning, a psychiatric consultation was obtained. Oral levetiracetam was substituted for phenytoin while the oral quetiapine fumarate was continued. The patient remained seizure free and had no more behavioral disturbances.

Discussion

This is an example of an inducer added to a substrate.

More specifically this is an example of decreased efficacy of quetiapine due to enhanced metabolism secondary to induction of the cytochrome P450 (CYP) 3A4 isoenzyme caused by coadministration of phenytoin.

Quetiapine is an atypical dibenzothiazepine antipsychotic that is frequently used to treat the symptoms of schizophrenia as it has a more desirable side-effect profile including less extrapyramidal symptoms than traditional antipsychotics.[1] Quetiapine fumarate is inactivated primarily by hepatic metabolism by the 3A4 isoenzyme into the pharmacologically inactive quetiapine sulfoxide and N- and O-desalkylquetiapine.[2,3] Phenytoin is a potent inducer of the CYP3A4 isoenzyme which can increase the plasma clearance of quetiapine by fivefold.[4] The increased clearance results in a substantial decline in plasma levels of quetiapine (Fig. 168.1). In this case, the coadministration of phenytoin to a schizophrenic patient on a stable dose of quetiapine resulted in a return of psychotic symptoms. However, the stress of the hospital environment may have also have been a contributing factor to his clinical decline. Levetiracetam does not induce the cytochrome P450 3A4 enzyme and does not interfere with clearance of quetiapine.

Take-Home Points

- Quetiapine fumarate is primarily cleared via hepatic metabolism by CYP3A4.
- Inducers of CYP3A4, such as phenytoin, can increase the clearance of quetiapine resulting in a loss of clinical effect.
- When anticonvulsant therapy is required in a patient on quetiapine, an antiepileptic that does not induce the cytochrome P450 system (and more specifically CYP3A4) better choice.

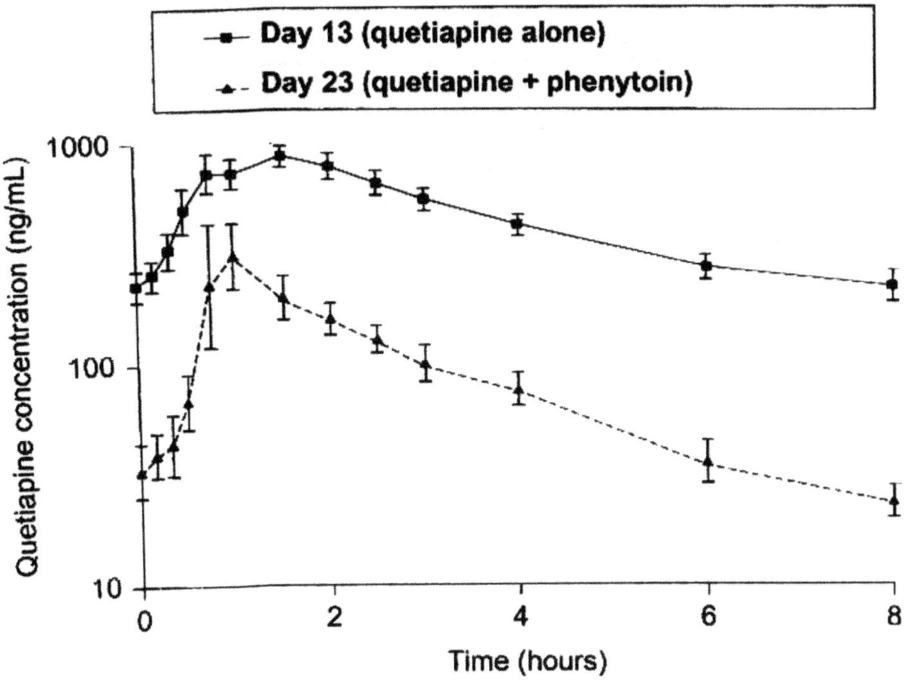

Fig. 168.1 Mean (SE) plasma concentration-versus-time profiles for morning doses of quetiapine (250 mg TID) without coadministration of phenytoin (solid line) verses quetiapine (250 mg TID) with coadministration of phenytoin (100 mg TID) (dotted line) [Wong YW, Yeh C, Thyrum PT. The effects of concomitant phenytoin administration on the steady-state pharmacokinetics of quetiapine. J Clin Psychopharmacol. 2001;21:89-93. With permission from Wolter Kluwers Health.]

Summary

Interaction: pharmacokinetic
Substrate: quetiapine
Enzyme: CYP3A4
Inducer: phenytoin
Clinical effects: acute psychosis

References

1. Small JG, Hirsch SR, Arvanitis LA, et al. Quetiapine in patients with schizophrenia. A high- and low-dose double-blind comparison with placebo. Seroquel Study Group. Arch Gen Psychiatry. 1997;54:549–57.

2. DeVane CL, Nemeroff CB. Clinical pharmacokinetics of quetiapine: an atypical antipsychotic. Clin Pharmacokinet. 2001;40:509–22.
3. Grimm SW, Richtand NM, Winter HR, et al. Effects of cytochrome P450 3A modulators ketoconazole and carbamazepine on quetiapine pharmacokinetics. Br J Clin Pharmacol. 2006;61:58–69.
4. Wong YW, Yeh C, Thyrum PT. The effects of concomitant phenytoin administration on the steady-state pharmacokinetics of quetiapine. J Clin Psychopharmacol. 2001;21:89–93.

Dizzy and Depressed

169

Fatal Forty DDI: nefazodone, carbamazepine, CYP3A4

William A. Shakespeare MD and Juraj Sprung MD, PhD

Abstract
This case discusses the pharmacokinetic interaction between carbamazepine and nefazodone leading to supratherapeutic carbamazepine levels. Carbamazepine is a cytochrome P450 3A4 substrate and nefazodone is a 3A4 inhibitor.

Case

A 54-year-old, morbidly obese woman with a history of bipolar disorder and dysfunctional uterine bleeding presented to the operating room for a total abdominal hysterectomy. Her bipolar disorder was well controlled with carbamazepine (500 mg BID). She had required three blood transfusions in the past because of uterine bleeding. The patient underwent general endotracheal anesthesia, and the operative course was unremarkable. Unfortunately, the patient suffered a wound infection that required a long postoperative inpatient hospitalization.

The psychiatry service was consulted during the first postoperative due to the patient's persistent and severe dysphoria. Therapy with nefazodone (200 mg daily) was started. As the postoperative course progressed, the house staff became concerned that the patient's depression was becoming a vegetative depression as she was increasingly somnolent, reluctant to get out of bed, and difficult to understand due to slow, slurred speech. The perceptive surgical chief resident also confirmed alteration in depth perception on physical examination. When a serum chemistry panel showed no abnormalities the computed tomographic scan of the head showed no acute evidence of pathology, the resident ordered a serum carbamazepine level. The level was found to be 17 mcg/mL (therapeutic level, 4–12 mcg/mL). The

W.A. Shakespeare MD (✉) • J. Sprung MD, PhD
Department of Anesthesiology, Mayo Clinic, Rochester, MN, USA
e-mail: washakespeare@gmail.edu

C. Marcucci et al. (eds.), *A Case Approach to Perioperative Drug-Drug Interactions*, DOI 10.1007/978-1-4614-7495-1_169

psychiatry and surgical pharmacy services were consulted and the nefazodone was discontinued and a selective serotonin reuptake inhibitor (sertraline) was started. Over the next 2 days, carbamazepine values decreased to reference levels, and the somnolence, visual changes, and ataxia resolved.

Discussion

This is an example of a complex pharmacokinetic interaction involving both an inhibitor added to a substrate and a substrate added to an inducer.

Nefazodone is an antidepressant that acts as a potent 5-hydroxytryptamine-2 (5-HT) antagonist, a moderate inhibitor of neuronal reuptake of 5-HT, and a mild inhibitor of norepinephrine uptake. Carbamazepine is an anticonvulsant agent that has been used for epilepsy treatment, as an analgesic for trigeminal neuralgia, and as a mood stabilizer for bipolar disorders.[1] It is metabolized in the liver by cytochrome P450 (CYP) 3A4 and it is known to induce multiple hepatic CYP enzymes. The concentration of carbamazepine-10,11-epoxide, a main and active metabolite generated through the 3A4 pathway, may reach up to 50% of the concentration of the parent compound. Nefazodone is metabolized by and is a potent inhibitor of 3A4.

The coadministration of an agent that is both a substrate and inducer of CYP3A4 (carbamazepine) and an agent that is both a substrate and inhibitor of CYP3A4 (nefazodone) leads to unpredictable concentrations of both agents. Two contrasting interactions are reported in the medical literature.[2,3] The induction of CYP3A4 by carbamazepine may lead to more rapid metabolism of nefazodone and cause an inability to maintain therapeutic levels of the antidepressant. Clinically, this effect is subtle; it appears as an inability to achieve mood improvement and could be interpreted as a therapeutic failure of nefazodone.

In contrast, a more clinically apparent reaction occurs when the inhibition of CYP3A4 by nefazodone slows the metabolism of carbamazepine, resulting in an increase in the concentration of carbamazepine, and producing toxic symptoms. Symptoms of carbamazepine toxicity include depression of the central nervous system, headache, ataxia, and diplopia. Thus, although the unpredictable pharmacokinetics may lead to two contrasting outcomes; an increase in the levels of carbamazepine produces new neurologic symptoms and is the most acutely concerning interaction. In two cases documenting toxicity from the accumulation of carbamazepine, the symptoms resolved after the carbamazepine dose was decreased or the nefazodone therapy was discontinued.[2]

A study to evaluate the effect of the coadministration of carbamazepine and nefazodone on serum levels of each drug found that both drugs may be used safely for healthy persons when medication levels are tightly controlled, monitoring is frequent, and dosing is low.[3] However, clinically meaningful doses were not evaluated in the study, and with many alternative antidepressant therapies available, the combination of nefazodone and carbamazepine is not advisable.

Take-Home Points

- Nefazodone inhibits CYP3A4 and carbamazepine induces CYP3A4.
- Coadministration of these two agents leads to unpredictable serum levels of both drugs.
- Nefazodone may slow the metabolism of carbamazepine, which can lead to development of supratherapeutic or even toxic levels of carbamazepine (depression of the central nervous system, headache, ataxia, and diplopia) even when the dosages of both nefazodone and carbamazepine are in the normal range.
- Carbamazepine may increase the metabolism of nefazodone, making the achievement of therapeutic nefazodone levels difficult.
- Coadministration of nefazodone and carbamazepine is not recommended.

Summary

Interaction: pharmacokinetic (complex)
Substrates: carbamazepine and nefazodone
Enzyme: CYP3A4
Inducer: carbamazepine
Inhibitor: nefazodone
Clinical effect: carbamazepine toxicity

References

1. Kerr BM, Thummel KE, Wurden CJ, et al. Human liver carbamazepine metabolism: role of CYP3A4 and CYP2C8 in 10,11-epoxide formation. Biochem Pharmacol. 1994;47:1969–79.
2. Ashton AK, Wolin RE. Nefazodone-induced carbamazepine toxicity. Am J Psychiatry. 1996;153:733.
3. Laroudie C, Salazar DE, Cosson JP, et al. Carbamazepine-nefazodone interaction in healthy subjects. J Clin Psychopharmacol. 2000;20:46–53.

The Funeral Is on Monday

170

Fatal Forty DDI: phenytoin, valproic acid, CYP2C9

Elizabeth Macri MD, Ansgar M. Brambrink MD, PhD, and Neil B. Sandson MD

Abstract
This case discusses a complex pharmacokinetic interaction between phenytoin and valproic acid involving both metabolism and distribution.

Case

A 30-year-old woman was admitted to the intensive care unit (ICU) with apparent "cryptogenic" fulminant liver failure in the hopes that she would be a candidate for orthotopic liver transplant in the ensuing days. The diligent ICU fellow and pharmacist carefully reviewed her history to ascertain the cause of the liver failure.

She was known to have a history of complex partial seizures with secondary generalization. She had been compliant with her phenytoin therapy (300 mg daily) and her liver function tests were normal. However, she continued to have seizures with episodes of status epilepticus. Her neurologic status had deteriorated and she starting having ataxia and mental disturbances. This was felt to be compounded by anoxic complications of status epilepticus. She was started on divalproex sodium (750 mg daily). Three weeks after starting valproic acid, she had another episode of status epilepticus. At that

Editor's Note: Normal serum phenytoin levels: total = 10-20 mcg/mL, free = 1-2 mcg/mL; normal serum valproic acid levels: total = 50-100 mcg/mL, free = 5-10 mcg/mL.

E. Macri MD (✉)
Department of Neurology, Presbyterian Medical Group, Albuquerque, NM, USA
e-mail: elizabethmacri@yahoo.com

A.M. Brambrink MD, PhD
Department of Anesthesiology and Perioperative Medicine, Oregon Health and Science University, Portland, OR, USA

N.B. Sandson MD
Department of Psychiatry, University of Maryland Medical System, VA Maryland Health Care System, Baltimore, MD, USA

C. Marcucci et al. (eds.), *A Case Approach to Perioperative Drug-Drug Interactions*, DOI 10.1007/978-1-4614-7495-1_170

time, her valproic acid level was within normal limits at 55 mcg/mg. Because her liver function tests remained normal, the divalproex dosage was increased to 1250 mg daily. One month later on reevaluation, she was unable to stand, had developed new choreoathetoid movements, diaphragmatic myoclonus, and difficulty speaking. The valproic acid level at that time was 59 mcg/mL and the phenytoin level was 17.1 mcg/mL. Her divalproex dosage was then increased again to 1750 mg daily.

The ICU staff obtained immediate labs and discovered that her phenytoin level was 18.4 mcg/mL, and her valproic acid level was 63 mcg/mL, with unbound phenytoin and divalproex fractions of approximately 40%. Both drugs were immediately discontinued. Unfortunately, she did not survive the acute liver failure or receive a donor liver, and she died approximately 12 weeks after initiation of valproic acid therapy. Autopsy demonstrated extensive hepatic cell necrosis not consistent with viral hepatitis. Brain autopsy was consistent with multiple system atrophy as well as diffuse gliosis.

Discussion

This is a complex pharmacokinetic interaction involving both metabolism and distribution.

Valproic acid is an antiepileptic drug that moderately inhibits CYP2C9 and displaces phenytoin from serum protein binding sites.[1–3] This can cause an unpredictable change in free and total phenytoin concentrations.[4] The free concentration can increase initially due to displacement which exposes additional free phenytoin to hepatic metabolism.[2–5] Total phenytoin concentrations can be decreased by 20% to 50% due to this additional free phenytoin metabolism. The nonlinear kinetics of phenytoin and inhibition of 2C9 by valproate can increase total phenytoin concentrations and lead to significantly sustained free phenytoin concentrations.[4,5] This interaction can lead to increased risk of phenytoin toxicity or decreased seizure control.[6–12]

Phenytoin is an antiepileptic drug that is a CYP2C9 inducer, for which valproic acid is a substrate, leading to decreased serum levels of valproic acid by an average of 50%.[10] Phenytoin may increase the production of a hepatotoxic metabolite of valproic acid – 2 propyl-4-pentenoic acid.[12,13] Metabolism of phenytoin follows first-order kinetics at lower dosages and zero-order kinetics at higher dosages. Any other drug or change in liver function or albumin level that alters the amount of drug metabolized by the liver can therefore lead to unpredictable drug levels.[14,15]

This case serves to illustrate that liver function tests must be checked routinely when on these medications and when dosages are increased. In this case, the patient's total phenytoin concentration went down to subtherapeutic levels when valproate therapy was initiated, then went to supratherapeutic levels when her valproate dose was increased seven weeks later. However, it is most likely that free phenytoin concentrations increased significantly almost immediately after the addition of valproate, despite the decrease in the total concentration. The increased free phenytoin concentration likely led to increased metabolism of valproate, producing a real decrease in valproate concentrations and thus prompting an increase in the valproate dosage to achieve therapeutic total levels. Ultimately, the patient succumbed to liver failure likely due to the hepatotoxic effect of valproate metabolites.

Given the complex and potentially unpredictable nature of the interaction of these two drugs, combining them should be avoided if possible. There are newer antiepileptic medications that do not undergo hepatic metabolism that would be preferred in patients already on one of these two drugs. If indeed a patient requires both phenytoin and valproate, close monitoring of the liver function tests is paramount. For such cases the recommendation is testing prior to initiation of therapy, with every dose increase, and every 3 months the patients receive the two drugs.[11]

The free phenytoin level is a better indicator of antiepileptic efficacy than the total serum level in patients that receive drugs, in this case valproate, that may displace phenytoin from serum protein-binding sites.

Not available in this case were the patient's free valproate concentration nor the serum albumin levels. When a drug is extensively plasma protein bound, addition of another protein-bound drug can cause the total drug level to appear subtherapeutic when in fact the free, unbound level may be therapeutic or even supratherapeutic. Both phenytoin and valproate are extensively protein-bound and only the free drug is therapeutically active.[5,8–10] In this case, free concentrations of both should have been measured. Since both drugs are bound to serum albumin, fluctuations in serum albumin levels can lead to the appearance of decreased total drug concentrations with an increase in free drug concentrations. A significant change in serum albumin levels, such as that seen following severe illness or injury, should prompt free drug level checks.

Phenytoin can cause hepatic toxicity that manifests as an increase in liver enzyme levels.[6,11,13] This typically occurs within the first 6 weeks of drug initiation and is an idiosyncratic reaction. It may be accompanied by fever, rash and eosinophilia. In the case above, the patient had been on phenytoin for 2 ½ years with normal liver function tests and her liver failure was not due to phenytoin alone. Elevations of ALT to less than three times the upper limit of normal are generally tolerated and tend to decrease over time. Elevations above three times the upper limit of normal should prompt discontinuation of the drug.

Liver function tests should be measured prior to initiation of valproate therapy and during therapy.[12–15] New-onset confusion should prompt testing of serum ammonia levels. Most liver function elevations occur during the first 6 months of therapy. Elevated serum ammonia levels with normal ALT have been demonstrated on valproic acid. The most severe form of hepatotoxicity, liver cell necrosis, may occur within 2 to 3 months of initiation of therapy.[12] Platelet and coagulation levels should be measured before and during therapy and prior to surgery. An elevated of ALT to greater than three times normal range is an indication to discontinue the new drug. In contrast to phenytoin hypersensitivity-type hepatotoxicity, valproate-related hepatotoxicity typically presents with fatigue, nausea and vomiting. Preliminary studies have demonstrated increased survival with carnitine treatment in those with significant valproate-induced hepatotoxicity.[12,13]

In summary, phenytoin toxicity can present with ataxia, confusion, nystagmus, choreoathetoid movements, and dysarthria. Valproate toxicity can present as ataxia, confusion, and dysarthria. The above case presented 7 weeks after initiation of valproate therapy with symptoms most consistent with phenytoin toxicity. Confusing the clinical picture was her concomitant diagnosis of multisystem atrophy, which could explain the diaphragmatic myoclonus. The patient died secondary to liver failure caused by increasing dosages of valproate, which were prescribed to bolster the anticonvulsant efficacy of phenytoin, but that decision was never revisited and the two anticonvulsants were not monitored appropriately.

Take-Home Points

- Phenytoin is a cytochrome P450 pan-inducer (except for 1A2). Any drug metabolized via CYP2C9 may be subtherapeutic at standard doses when taken concomitantly.
- Valproic acid is a CYP2C9 inhibitor. Any drug metabolized via CYP2C9 may be supratherapeutic at standard doses when taken concomitantly.
- Valproic acid and phenytoin are both highly protein-bound drugs. Measurement of free drugs concentrations is a more accurate measure of likely therapeutic and/or toxic effects than total drug levels when a patient is on both agents.
- Because phenytoin and valproate are both highly bound to plasma proteins, when these drugs are coadministered, any significant change in albumin levels should prompt rechecking free concentrations of both drugs.
- Valproic acid is associated with liver toxicity. Prior to initiation of valproic acid treatment, liver function tests should be checked and repeated after initiation and after dosage increase. Elevation of ALT beyond three times upper limit of normal should prompt drug discontinuation.

Summary

Interaction 1: pharmacokinetic (metabolism)
Substrate: valproate
Enzyme: assorted UGTs
Inducer: phenytoin
Clinical effect: subtherapeutic valproate levels leading to breakthrough seizures

Interaction 2: pharmacokinetic (metabolism)
Substrate: phenytoin
Enzyme: CYP2C9
Inhibitor: valproate
Clinical effect: phenytoin toxicity

Interaction 3: pharmacokinetic (distribution)
Substrates: phenytoin and valproate
Mechanism/site of action: mutual displacement from plasma protein binding sites
Clinical effect: phenytoin toxicity (in synergy with metabolic inhibition of DDI 2 above)

References

1. Yap KY, Chui WK, Chan A. Drug interactions between chemotherapeutic regimens and antiepileptics. Clin Ther. 2008;30:1385–407.
2. Mamiya K, Yukawa E, Matsumoto T, et al. Synergistic effect of valproate co-administration and hypoalbuminemia on the serum-free phenytoin concentration in patients with severe motor and intellectual disabilities. Clin Neuropharmacol. 2002;25:230–1.
3. Johnson GJ, Kilpatrick CJ, Bury RW, et al. Unbound phenytoin plasma concentrations in patients co-medicated with sodium valproate–the predictive value of plasma albumin concentration. Br J Clin Pharmacol. 1989;27:843–9.
4. Tsanaclis LM, Allen J, Perucca E, et al. Effect of valproate on free plasma phenytoin concentrations. Br J Clin Pharmacol. 1984;18:17–20.
5. Dahlqvist R, Borgå O, Rane A, et al. Decreased plasma protein binding of phenytoin in patients on valproic acid. Br J Clin Pharmacol. 1979;8:547–52.
6. Palm R, Silseth C, Alvan G. Phenytoin intoxication as the first symptom of fatal liver damage induced by sodium valproate. Br J Clin Pharmacol. 1984;17:597–9.
7. Levy RH, Koch KM. Drug interactions with valproic acid. Drugs. 1982;24:543–56.
8. Monks A, Richens A. Effect of single doses of sodium valproate on serum phenytoin levels and protein binding in epileptic patients. Clin Pharmacol Ther. 1980;27:89–95.
9. Perucca E, Hebdige S, Frigo GM, et al. Interaction between phenytoin and valproic acid: plasma protein binding and metabolic effects. Clin Pharmacol Ther. 1980;28:779–89.
10. Suzuki Y, Nagai T, Mano T, et al. Interaction between valproate formulation and phenytoin concentrations. Eur J Clin Pharmacol. 1995;48:61–3.
11. von Winckelmann SL, Spriet I, Willems L. Therapeutic drug monitoring of phenytoin in critically ill patients. Pharmacotherapy. 2008;28:1391–400.
12. Nau H, Loscher W. Valproic acid and metabolites. Pharmacological and toxicological studies. Epilepsia. 1984;25 suppl 1:S14–22.
13. Björnsson E. Hepatotoxicity associated with antiepileptic drugs. Acta Neurol Scand. 2008;118:281–90.
14. Product Information: Depakote® Tablets, divalproex sodium delayed-release tablets. North Chicago: Abbott Laboratories; 2002.
15. Product Information: Depakene® Valproic acid. North Chicago: Abbott Laboratories; 1998.

This Antacid Is Making Me Sick! 171

Fatal Forty DDI: phenytoin, cimetidine, CYP2C9, CYP2C19

Arun Subramanian MBBS, Toby N. Weingarten MD, and Juraj Sprung MD, PhD

Abstract
This case discusses a pharmacokinetic interaction between cimetidine and phenytoin. Phenytoin is a cytochrome P450 2C9 and 2C19 substrate and cimetidine is a cytochrome P450 2C9 and 2C19 inhibitor. Coadministration results in phenytoin toxicity.

Case

A 56-year-old, 65 kg man presented to the preoperative clinic for evaluation prior to elective hernia repair. He was unsteady on his feet but made it to the examination room where he was dizzy and vomited when attempting to get on the examination table. He reported that he had a history of epilepsy treated with extended-release oral phenytoin (300 mg daily) and gastroesophageal reflux disease (GERD) which had been treated with extended-release pantoprazole (40 mg daily) until 2 weeks prior. The patient had run out of his pantoprazole 2 weeks prior and had not gotten the prescription refilled. Instead, he had purchased an over-the-counter medication for heartburn and had been taking it in the morning and at night. He complained that instead of decreasing his bothersome GERD, he had lately been experiencing worse symptoms.

The patient was noted to be tachycardic and somewhat hypotensive. When the knowledgeable nurse practitioner also ascertained that had nystagmus, tremor, and hyperreflexia, the patient and his spouse were sent to the Emergency Department.

A. Subramanian MBBS (✉) • T.N. Weingarten MD • J. Sprung MD, PhD
Department of Anesthesiology, Mayo Clinic, Rochester, MN, USA
e-mail: Subramanian.arun@mayo.edu

C. Marcucci et al. (eds.), *A Case Approach to Perioperative Drug-Drug Interactions*, DOI 10.1007/978-1-4614-7495-1_171

A call was placed to the patient's daughter at home to check on the "heartburn medicine," which proved to be cimetidine. Routine laboratory values were within reference ranges, but his phenytoin level was elevated at 35 mcg/mL (reference therapeutic range, 10-20 mcg/mL) and a diagnosis of phenytoin toxicity was made. The cimetidine was immediately stopped, and the phenytoin dose was decreased temporarily. The patient's plasma phenytoin levels decreased to the therapeutic range and his symptoms resolved during the next few days. He underwent an uneventful anesthetic and surgery 2 weeks later.

Discussion

This is an example of an inhibitor added to a substrate.

Phenytoin is an anticonvulsant agent that inhibits the spread of cortical seizure activity. It acts by binding to neuronal sodium ion channels in a frequency-dependent manner, decreasing transmembrane sodium ion flux and thus stabilizing neuronal cell membranes. Phenytoin has a narrow therapeutic index (total phenytoin plasma concentration range, 10-20 mcg/mL). It is extensively metabolized in the liver through the cytochrome P450 (CYP) system, with approximately 80% metabolized by CYP2C9 and 20% by CYP2C19.[1] Phenytoin metabolism also displays saturable kinetics.[1] When the CYP system is not saturated, the metabolism of phenytoin displays first-order kinetics. When the CYP system is saturated, its metabolism kinetics displays zero-order kinetics, thus appreciably increasing its plasma concentration half-life.

Phenytoin toxicity can manifest in a number of different ways. Acute toxicity results in cerebellar and vestibular symptoms and cardiac dysrhythmias, and chronic toxicity can lead to a paradoxical increase in seizures, megaloblastic anemia, hirsutism, gingival hyperplasia, gastrointestinal symptoms, and lymphoid hyperplasia. Occasionally, such serious adverse effects as agranulocytosis, leukopenia, pancytopenia, thrombocytopenia, and toxic epidermal necrolysis can occur.[2]

Cimetidine is a histamine receptor subtype 2 (H_2) antagonist. It decreases gastric secretions and increases gastric pH by inhibiting the effects of histamine in gastric parietal cells. Also, it is an inhibitor of the CYP enzymes 2C9, 2C19, 2D6, and 3A4.[1] Inhibition of these CYP isozymes by cimetidine is known to inhibit the half-life of numerous drugs, including the half-life of phenytoin through inhibition of 2C9 and 2C19. Administration of cimetidine has been shown to decrease the plasma clearance of phenytoin by 16% to 59%.[3,4] The increase in plasma concentration of phenytoin after treatment with cimetidine normalizes after cimetidine use is discontinued.[4]

In the present patient, cimetidine use resulted in inhibition of CYP2C9 and CYP2C19 and, subsequently, an increase of phenytoin plasma levels, leading to signs of phenytoin toxicity.

Take-Home Points

- Phenytoin works by blocking voltage-gated sodium channels in a frequency-dependent manner.
- Its elimination displays nonlinear kinetics, being first-order at low plasma concentrations and zero-order at greater concentrations.
- The common adverse effects of phenytoin toxicity are nystagmus, dysarthria, ataxia, and confusion.
- Medications that inhibit the CYP system, such as cimetidine, can increase the plasma concentration of phenytoin, sometimes to toxic levels.

Summary

Interaction: pharmacokinetic (metabolism)
Substrate: phenytoin
Enzymes: CYP2C9 and CYP2C19
Inhibitor: cimetidine
Clinical effect: phenytoin toxicity

References

1. Patsalos PN, Froscher W, Pisani F, et al. The importance of drug interactions in epilepsy therapy. Epilepsia. 2002;43:365–85.
2. Porter RJ, Meldrum BS. Antiseizure drugs. In: Katzung BG, Masters SB, Trevor AJ, editors. Basic & clinical pharmacology. 11th ed. New York: McGraw-Hill Medical; 2009. p. 399–422.
3. Sambol NC, Upton RA, Chremos AN, et al. A comparison of the influence of famotidine and cimetidine on phenytoin elimination and hepatic blood flow. Br J Clin Pharmacol. 1989;27:83–7.
4. Neuvonen PJ, Tokola RA, Kaste M. Cimetidine-phenytoin interaction: effect on serum phenytoin concentration and antipyrine test. Eur J Clin Pharmacol. 1981;21:215–20.

Young at Heart

172

Fatal Forty DDI: pimozide, nefazodone, CYP3A4

Catherine Marcucci MD

Abstract
This case discusses the pharmacokinetic interaction between pimozide and nefazodone, resulting in QTc prolongation. Pimozide is cytochrome P450 3A4 substrate and nefazodone is a 3A4 inhibitor.

Case

One Sunday evening, the anesthesia resident on the remote anesthesia rotation called her attending, mentioning that a case had been added onto Monday's schedule. The patient was a 27-year-old male veteran with renal calculi, who was coming over from the small, affiliated Veterans Affairs (VA) hospital, as that facility lacked a modern lithotripsy machine. The resident had managed to contact the preoperative evaluation clinic at the VA hospital and was told that he had "pretty bad posttraumatic stress disorder (PTSD) from the battle of Fallujah" but since returning from active duty was managing to hold down a part-time job as a pit-crew member at the local speedway. He was absent the traditional cardiovascular risk factors, such as hypertension and diabetes, seen in older patients. Happily, he did not smoke. When the anesthesia resident asked the referring VA internist about the preoperative laboratory values and echocardiogram (ECG), she was told "they are not necessary in a sedation case for an active 23-year-old without risk factors who does heavy lifting at his job."

In the preoperative area, she encountered an extremely restless and nervous-appearing young man, who was intermittently drumming his fingers on the bed rail. The resident inquired if it was due to nerves and was told, "No, it keeps pace

C. Marcucci MD
Anesthesia Services Department, Philadelphia Veterans Affairs Medical Center, Philadelphia, PA, USA
e-mail: sandson.marcucci@comcast.net

C. Marcucci et al. (eds.), *A Case Approach to Perioperative Drug-Drug Interactions*, DOI 10.1007/978-1-4614-7495-1_172

with my heart." While the nurse went to get the ECG machine, the resident looked at the preoperative evaluation note the patient had brought with him. What had been lumped together as "pretty bad PTSD" in the verbal report was in actuality a documented history of schizoaffective disorder, along with the onset 3 weeks ago of dysphoria, anergy, and insomnia. The final assessment by the VA primary care practitioner noted "multiple psych meds, no cardiac risks factors, may undergo the procedure without further testing." On further questioning, the patient gave his medication regimen as a longstanding dosage of pimozide (Orap®, 6 mg/day) and with the recent addition (in the past 2 weeks) of nefazodone, which had been titrated to 400 mg/day at the small VA satellite clinic where he obtained his psychiatric care and medications. His 12-lead ECG showed a sinus tachycardia of 98 bpm with a QTc interval of 535 msec. The resident remembered that this was a case very similar to one she had just read about and a quick check online confirmed her suspicions. She informed her attending of her findings and the case was postponed.

Discussion

This is an example of an inhibitor (nefazodone) added to a substrate (pimozide)

The pimozide/nefazodone drug pair is a very dangerous combination. The editors feel that there are few, if any, clinical situations that warrant exposing patients to this level of drug–drug interaction (DDI) risk. Regrettably, perioperative clinicians may still see these drugs being used concurrently—this scenario is based on a real case from the files of one of the consulting editors.[1]

Pimozide is a potent typical antipsychotic medication with a severe side-effect profile. Even when used as monotherapy, it may be associated with life-threatening QTc prolongation and arrhythmias as well as akathisia, tardive dyskinesia, neuroleptic malignant syndrome, and lowered seizure threshold. In the United States, it is used on-label only for the treatment of debilitating Tourette's symptoms, but off-label for the treatment of psychotic symptoms such as auditory hallucinations and paranoid delusions. Additionally, pimozide is a cytochrome P450 (CYP) 3A4 substrate.[2,3]

Nefazodone is an antidepressant that was added to this patient's drug list in order to address the vegetative symptoms of depression (anhedonia, insomnia, etc.). It is a strong competitive inhibitor of 3A4.[4] Nefazodone will reliably increase the blood level of pimozide, resulting in a toxic state that can readily manifest as exaggeration or new onset of akathisia and QTc prolongation.[5,6] Discontinuation of the nefazodone and substitution with an antidepressant that does not inhibit 3A4, such as escitalopram or bupropion, would be expected to lower pimozide blood levels (via withdrawal of inhibition) within a week or so. The patient should then be re-evaluated, especially with respect to the ECG abnormalities, before proceeding with anesthesia for an elective surgery.

Take-Home Points

- It is incumbent on perioperative clinicians to recognize risk factors (such as potentially dangerous DDIs) that may not have been accounted for in the large epidemiological studies used in the development of practice guidelines. Remember that guidelines are just that—guidelines.

- You will find that is not unusual for primary care notes or preoperative "clearance" notes to fail to note psychiatric DDIs. More than one primary care practitioner has found it overwhelming to completely master the basic clinical pharmacology of the dozens of antipsychotics, antidepressants, sedatives, and mood stabilizers in use, much less tease out the potential DDIs. As such, psychopharmacologic agents unwittingly tend to be lumped together as "the psych meds," accompanied by a sincere hope that they are not causing too much mischief with each other. Of course, in actuality there is as much variation in the pharmacologic actions and metabolic pathways in this pharmacopeia as there is for the "anesthesia meds."

- Spend some time learning the DDIs that, while hopefully rare, are the most dangerous. ***If it can be at all be helped***, do not take a potentially pimozide-toxic patient to the OR.

Summary

Interaction: pharmacokinetic
Substrate: pimozide
Enzyme: CYP3A4
Inhibitor: nefazodone
Clinical effect: QTc prolongation

References

1. Neil B, Sandson M. Drug-drug interaction primer: a compendium of case vignettes for the practicing clinician. Washington, DC: American Psychiatric Press, Inc.; 2007. p. 27–8.
2. Desta Z, Kerbusch T, Soukhova N, et al. Identification and characterization of human cytochrome P450 isoforms interacting with pimozide. J Pharmacol Exp Ther. 1998;285:428–37.
3. Desta Z, Kerbusch T, Flockhart DA. Effect of clarithromycin on the pharmacokinetics and pharmacodynamics of pimozide in healthy poor and extensive metabolizers of cytochrome P450 2D6 (CYP2D6). Clin Pharmacol Ther. 1999;65:10–20.
4. von Moltke LL, Greenblatt DJ, Harmatz JS, et al. Triazolam biotransformation by human liver microsomes in vitro: effects of metabolic inhibitors and clinical confirmation of a predicted interaction with ketoconazole. J Pharmacol Exp Ther. 1996;276:370–9.
5. Dresser GK, Spence JD, Bailey DG. Pharmacokinetic-pharmacodynamic consequences and clinical relevance of cytochrome P450 3A4 inhibition. Clin Pharmacokinet. 2000;38:41–57.
6. Gate Pharmaceuticals: Orap (pimozide) (package insert). Sellersville: Gate Pharmaceuticals; 1999.

Shiver Yes, Die No

Selegiline patch, meperidine, serotonin syndrome

173

Ahmed F. Zaky MD, MPH and Michael J. Bishop MD

Abstract
This case discusses the interaction between an unsuspected source of selegiline in a transdermal patch and meperidine, resulting in serotonin syndrome.

Case

A 53-year-old female veteran with comorbidities of hypertension and type 2 diabetes mellitus arrived for a laparoscopic cholecystectomy. Three years previously she had developed severe depression when her only son was killed in Afghanistan and was started on the tricyclic antidepressant amitriptyline, which she did not tolerate after a period of 3 months. She was then started on 6 mg daily of Emsam® (a selegiline patch) as an alternative. The patient understood that the patch delivered the monoamine oxidase inhibitor (MAOI) selegiline via a transdermal route and that she was to report to the Emergency Room if she developed headaches, severe elevation in blood pressure, or visual changes. The patient was also given clear instructions to avoid sympathomimetic decongestants. She did not smoke, drink, or use illicit drugs.

The patient's anesthetic was uneventful except for some episodes of hypotension after induction of general anesthesia. In the recovery room, the patient started to shiver. The postanesthesia care unit (PACU) nurse asked the resident to write "something for shivering." The diligent resident checked the anesthesia chart to

A.F. Zaky MD, MPH (✉)
Department of Anesthesiology and Pain Medicine, VA Puget Sound Health Care Center/
University of Washington, Seattle, WA, USA
e-mail: drazaky@yahoo.com

M.J. Bishop MD
Department of Anesthesiology, University of Washington School of Medicine,
Seattle, WA, USA

C. Marcucci et al. (eds.), *A Case Approach to Perioperative Drug-Drug Interactions*, DOI 10.1007/978-1-4614-7495-1_173

make sure the patient was not on tranylcypromine (Parnate®) or phenelzine (Nardil®). The chilly patient was also asked if she had ever been told to avoid aged cheese and wine and replied truthfully that she had not. Reassured, the resident then wrote for meperidine (25 mg) for shivering and the PACU nurse concurred stating, "Oh, that works the best."

Five minutes later, the patient started to complain of headaches, became tachycardic, hypertensive, hyperthermic, and diaphoretic. A few minutes later, the patient experienced difficulty in breathing and was noticed to have a rigid chest, interfering with respiration A cardiac arrest protocol was initiated. An anesthesiologist rushed to the patient, administered propofol (200 mg), a nondepolarizing muscle relaxant (rocuronium 50 mg), secured the airway, and initiated mechanical ventilation. A wide-bore intravenous line was started and a bolus of 1L of normal saline was given. Sodium nitroprusside was started and the patient was transferred to the surgical intensive care unit (ICU). The ICU team placed a nasogastric tube and began active cooling using iced saline. A full neurologic exam was performed after neuromuscular function returned and revealed right lower extremity clonus.

The results of an electrocardiogram, brain computed tomography scan, serum electrolytes, renal and liver function tests were all normal. A diagnosis of serotonin syndrome was made and the patient was given cyproheptadine (4 mg/8h) via the nasogastric route. The patient was weaned from mechanical ventilation and extubated within 24 hours. Vital signs returned to baseline and the patient was weaned from antihypertensives within 72 hours. The patient was discharged home 2 days later.

Discussion

This is an example of a pharmacodynamic drug interaction.

Selegiline is a newer MAOI of which clinicians should take special note. It is an effective anti-depressant and in the lowest patch dose (6 mg) does not require dietary restrictions. This fact and the availability of the drug in a patch formulation are often considered favorably when prescribing to patients and have even led to a modest increase in the use of MAOIs to treat depression. However, at all doses, selegiline will interact pharmacodynamically in drug–drug interactions (DDIs) much as the "traditional" MAOIs do.

The combination of a MAOI and meperidine can be fatal. The vignette above describes "serotonin toxicity," originally described by Oates in 1995.[1] This is an excitatory phenomenon characterized by mental, autonomic, and neuromuscular changes due to intrasynaptic accumulation of serotonin in the brainstem and spinal cord.[2] Selegiline inhibits serotonin metabolism presynaptically while meperidine blocks the reuptake of serotonin in nerve terminals.[3] The diagnosis of serotonin toxicity is based on the Hunter Serotonin Toxicity Criteria with clonus, hyperreflexia, and hyperkinesia being the most specific signs.[4] The most commonly confused neurotoxic syndrome is the neuroleptic malignant syndrome. The latter syndrome, however, is characterized by an insidious onset, bradykinesia, and extrapyramidal manifestations.[5] Selegiline patches, especially in the lowest dosage (6 mg/day), do not appear to put the patient at risk for tyramine-induced hypertensive crises from dietary causes. However, they do place the patient at risk for a central serotonin syndrome when combined with serotonergically active agents (such as meperidine), as well as hypertensive crises when combined with sympathomimetic agents.

Treatment of serotonin toxicity centers on discontinuation of the offending drug and immediate stabilization of airway, breathing and circulation. Muscle relaxants and sedatives can be used to secure the airway. Active and passive cooling should be provided to treat hyperthermia. After the initial period of stabilization, detoxification and antidotes should be provided. Activated charcoal can be given, if the incriminated drug was ingested in the preceding hour. Cyproheptadine, available only in an oral form, can be given orally to moderately severe cases. Chlorpromazine can be given intravenously in severe cases, however the accompanying hypotension necessitates volume preloading.[6]

Patients with serotonin toxicity should be intensively monitored for the first 6 to 12 hours. Symptoms will usually subside within 24 hours of discontinuing the offending agent.

Take-Home Messages

- Even transdermal medications can have drug interactions.
- Selegiline is an MAOI that does not require dietary restrictions, however, it interacts with meperidine, much as tranylcypromine and phenelzine do. Remember, if you give the drug, you are responsible for the drug–drug interaction—stay vigilant!
- Serotonin toxicity should be considered for any patient who is receiving a MAOI.
- Clonus, hyperreflexia and hyperkinesis are the most specific signs of serotonin toxicity.

Summary

Interaction: pharmacodynamic
Substrates: selegiline and meperidine
Mechanism/site of action: inhibition of serotonin metabolism by selegiline and blockage of serotonin reuptake by meperidine
Clinical effects: serotonin toxicity including clonus, hyperreflexia, and hyperkinesis

References

1. Oates JA, Sjoerdsma A. Neurologic effects of tryptophan in patients receiving a monamine oxidase inhibitor. Neurology. 1960;10:1076–8.
2. Gillman PK. The serotonin syndrome and its treatment. J Psychopharmacol. 1999;13:100–9.
3. Isbister GK, Buckley NK, Whyte IM. Serotonin toxicity: a practical approach to diagnosis and treatment. Med J Aust. 2007;187:361–5.
4. Dunkley EJ, Isbister GK, Sibritt D, et al. The Hunter Serotonin Toxicity Criteria: simple and accurate diagnostic decision rules for serotonin toxicity. Q J Med. 2003;96:635–42.
5. Gillman PK. Serotonin syndrome: history and risk. Fundam Clin Pharmacol. 1998;12:482–91.
6. Chan BS, Graudins A, Whyte IM, et al. Serotonin syndrome from drug interactions. Med J Aust. 1998;169:523–5.

Clip and Dip 174

Fatal Forty DDI: carbamazepine, felodipine, CYP3A4

David W. Barbara MD, Randall Flick MD,
and Juraj Sprung MD, PhD

Abstract
This case discusses the pharmacokinetic interaction between felodipine, carbamazepine, and phenytoin, resulting in decreased antihypertensive efficacy. Felodipine is a cytochrome P450 3A4 substrate and carbamazepine and phenytoin are 3A4 inducers.

Case

A 72-year-old man who was the owner of a dog-grooming salon presented for removal of a 2-cm supratentorial mass. His past medical history was notable for hypertension, controlled with oral felodipine (10 mg/d), and mild asthma, for which he used an albuterol inhaler once a month. Three months before his scheduled surgery, the patient began to have partial complex seizures, and the cerebral mass was discovered. He had been adamant about postponing the surgery until after the peak of dog-grooming season. Carbamazepine therapy was started to control his seizures until he consented to surgery.

The patient's medical record showed that preoperative blood pressure readings had been 125/84 mm Hg. On his arrival at the hospital on the day of surgery, his blood pressure was 189/112 mm Hg. The patient denied new medication changes, noncompliance, or other changes in his medical history. The decision was made to proceed with the surgery. The patient's blood pressure was 184/111 mm Hg on his arrival in the operating room. The surgeon requested a controlled hypotensive technique for this patient. After tracheal intubation, anesthesia was maintained with isoflurane and fentanyl citrate. Adequate control of the blood pressure required both

D.W. Barbara MD (✉) • R. Flick MD • J. Sprung MD, PhD
Department of Anesthesiology, Mayo Clinic, Rochester, MN, USA
e-mail: barbara.david@mayo.edu

C. Marcucci et al. (eds.), *A Case Approach to Perioperative Drug-Drug Interactions*, DOI 10.1007/978-1-4614-7495-1_174

labetalol hydrochloride and sodium nitroprusside. The operation was uneventful, the patient was extubated at the end of the surgery, and he was found to be neurologically intact.

Discussion

This is an example of an inducer added to a substrate.

Felodipine, a second-generation dihydropyridine calcium channel blocker, is an orally administered arterial vasodilator with minimal direct effects on heart rate or cardiac contractility. It inhibits calcium influx through L-type calcium channels in the myocardium and vascular smooth muscle and exerts a greater affinity for vascular calcium channels than cardiac calcium channels, making it an attractive antihypertensive. Common adverse effects are due to excessive peripheral vasodilation and may include hypotension, cutaneous flushing, dizziness, headache, and syncope. Felodipine is known to also secondarily increase heart rate through indirect activation of the sympathetic nervous system, which can result in reflex tachycardia and palpitations. It undergoes extensive phase I metabolism in the liver through cytochrome P450 (CYP) 3A4.[1]

Carbamazepine is an antiepileptic whose mechanism of action involves the blockade of sodium channels. This blockade causes inhibition of the generation and propagation of repetitive action potentials, resulting in a highly effective drug for the treatment of partial seizures. It also is used to treat tonic-clinic seizures and trigeminal neuralgia. Carbamazepine is a potent inducer of CYP3A4, which can decrease the plasma levels and effects of drugs that undergo Phase I metabolism through this common enzymatic pathway.

Phenytoin sodium, another effective antiepileptic for the treatment of partial and tonic-clonic seizures, exerts its therapeutic effect by binding to voltage-gated sodium channels in their inactive states. This binding results in a prolonged recovery rate for the ion channel and a reduction in the spread of abnormal action potentials from epileptogenic foci. Similar to carbamazepine, phenytoin induces hepatic CYP3A4, resulting in decreased serum levels of drugs metabolized by this isozyme.

Capewell et al. matched 10 patients taking antiepileptic therapy (carbamazepine monotherapy [n=4], phenytoin monotherapy [n=2], carbamazepine and phenytoin together [n=3], and phenobarbitone monotherapy [n=1]) with 12 control patients not taking regular medications.[2] Each group received felodipine for 4 days, and felodipine levels were measured on day 5. The epileptic patients had a mean maximum felodipine concentration that was only 18% that of the control patients (Fig. 174.1), and their mean area under curve for concentration versus time was only 6.6% that of the control patients. Additionally, 83% of the control patients had vasodilatory

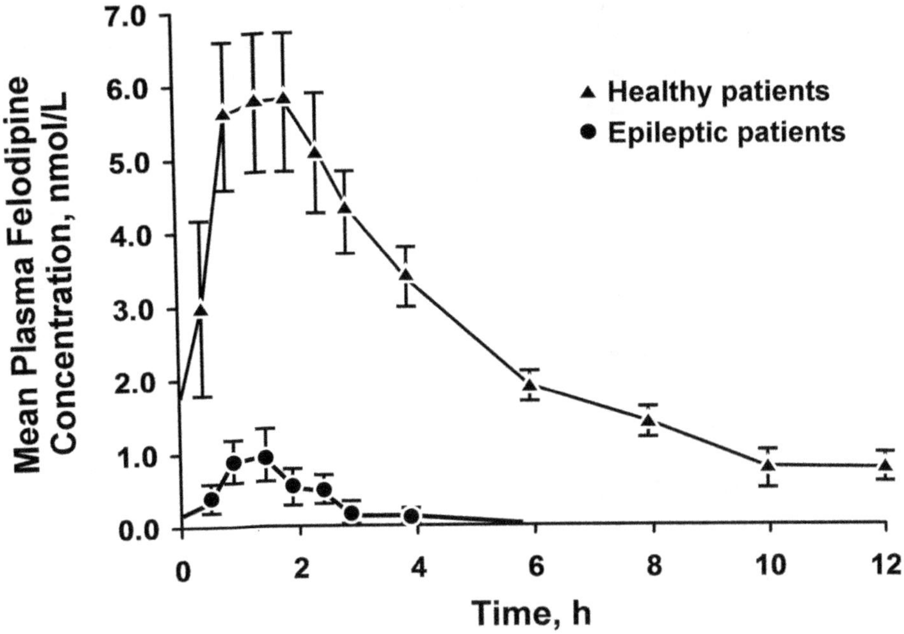

Fig. 174.1 Felodipine concentrations of healthy study participants and of treated epileptic patients. Error bars represent standard error of the mean [Adapted from Capewell S, Freestone S, Critchley JA et al. Reduced felodipine bioavailability in patients taking anticonvulsants. Lancet. 1988;2:480–482. With permission from Elsevier]

adverse effects, but no patient taking antiepileptic therapy had any of these adverse effects. By administering and measuring concentrations of antipyrine, an indicator of CYP3A4 induction, on day 6, the investigators noted significant correlations between the half-life of antipyrine, the felodipine maximum concentration, and the area under the curve, indicating that felodipine levels had been reduced because of an increase in metabolism of the drug through the cytochrome P450 system.

There is evidence that phenytoin and carbamazepine can affect concentrations of other calcium channel blockers. Tartara et al. examined 8 patients taking CYP-inducing anticonvulsive therapy (carbamazepine, phenobarbitone sodium, or phenytoin, either alone or in combination), eight patients taking CYP-inhibiting anticonvulsive therapy (sodium valproate monotherapy), and eight drug-free control patients.[3] Nimodipine was administered as a single dose, and blood levels were measured. The area under the curve of patients receiving CYP-inducing therapy was seven times less than that of control patients. The area under the curve of patients receiving CYP-inhibiting therapy was 50% greater than that of control patients. Other sources have noted similar reductions in calcium channel blockers, such as verapamil hydrochloride, with CYP3A4 inhibitors, such as phenytoin.[4]

In patients who are starting or continuing therapy with carbamazepine or phenytoin, an increased dose of felodipine may be necessary to ensure adequate plasma concentrations of the drug to achieve the desired therapeutic effect.

Take-Home Points

- Felodipine is a dihydropyridine calcium channel blocker that acts chiefly as a peripheral vasodilator.
- The hepatic CYP3A4 isozyme extensively metabolizes felodipine.
- Carbamazepine and phenytoin are potent inducers of CYP3A4.
- Antiepileptic therapy with phenytoin or carbamazepine, or their combination, can reduce plasma concentrations of felodipine drastically.
- In patients who are starting or continuing therapy with carbamazepine or phenytoin, increased doses of felodipine may be necessary because of the increased metabolism of felodipine with CYP3A4 induction.

Summary

Interaction: pharmacokinetic
Substrate: felodipine
Enzyme: CYP3A4
Inducer: carbamazepine, phenytoin
Clinical Effect: decreased antihypertensive efficacy

References

1. Todd PA, Faulds D. Felodipine: a review of the pharmacology and therapeutic use of the extended release formulation in cardiovascular disorders. Drugs. 1992;44:251–77.
2. Capewell S, Freestone S, Critchley JA, et al. Reduced felodipine bioavailability in patients taking anticonvulsants. Lancet. 1988;2:480–2.
3. Tartara A, Galimberti CA, Manni R, et al. Differential effects of valproic acid and enzyme-inducing anticonvulsants on nimodipine pharmacokinetics in epileptic patients. Br J Clin Pharmacol. 1991;32:335–40.
4. Woodcock BG, Kirsten R, Nelson K, et al. A reduction in verapamil concentrations with phenytoin. N Engl J Med. 1991;325:1179.

Blue Fog

175

Citalopram, methylene blue, serotonin syndrome

Toby N. Weingarten MD,
Wayne T. Nicholson MD, PharmD, MSc,
and Juraj Sprung MD, PhD

Abstract
This case discusses a pharmacodynamic interaction between citalopram and methylene blue, resulting in serotonin syndrome. Citalopram is a selective serotonin reuptake inhibitor and methylene blue is a reversible monoamine oxidase inhibitor.

Case

A 60 kg, 30-year-old woman underwent laparoscopic excision of endometriosis under general anesthesia. She had a history of depression which was treated with the serotonin reuptake inhibitor (SSRI) citalopram (40 mg daily). One hour into the procedure, a large endometrial tumor was found to be adherent to the left ureter. The surgeon was concerned about intraoperative damage to the ureter and requested administration of 100 mg IV of methylene blue (methylthioninium chloride) to facilitate visualization of extraluminal urine. At the end of the operation, the patient opened her eyes spontaneously, but not to command. Because her movements were interpreted as somewhat purposeful (reaching for the endotracheal tube), her trachea was extubated.

In the recovery room, she was confused, agitated, tachycardic, hypertensive, diaphoretic, and febrile with tympanic membrane temperature measured at 38.2°C. Her pupils were dilated. In addition to altered mental state, her neurologic examination was notable for muscle rigidity, hyperreflexia, and clonus. She was

T.N. Weingarten MD (✉) • W.T. Nicholson MD, PharmD, MSc • J. Sprung MD, PhD
Department of Anesthesiology, Mayo Clinic, Rochester, MN, USA
e-mail: Weingarten.toby@mayo.edu

C. Marcucci et al. (eds.), *A Case Approach to Perioperative Drug-Drug Interactions*, DOI 10.1007/978-1-4614-7495-1_175

reintubated and transferred to the intensive care unit where a diagnosis of serotonin toxicity (serotonin syndrome) was made. Her sensorium cleared after 8 hours and she was extubated. She was observed overnight and was discharged home the next day.

Discussion

This is an example of a pharmacodynamic interaction.

Serotonin (5-hydroxytryptamine, 5-HT) is a widely distributed monoamine neurotransmitter in the gastrointestinal tract, platelets and central nervous system (CNS). Serotonin has an important role in modulating brain function by interacting with a variety of pre- and postsynaptic receptors. Its role is implicated in several psychiatric disorders, and thus is an important target for many psychiatric drugs. The central effects of serotonin following release by nerve terminals are terminated by specific presynaptic reuptake system which clears serotonin from the synaptic cleft back into the nerve terminal. Inhibition of serotonin reuptake by SSRI drugs (citalopram, fluoxetine, and sertraline) potentiates the effect of serotonin at the postsynaptic receptors. After reuptake, serotonin is stored in the nerve terminal vesicles. However, any free serotonin in the neuronal cytoplasm is metabolized primarily by monoamine oxidase type A (MAO-A) isoenzyme into 5-hydroxyindoleacetaldehyde which undergoes further metabolism by aldehyde dehydrogenase into 5-hydroxyindoleacetic acid (5-HIAA). Inhibition of the MAO-A isoenzyme results in increased levels of serotonin in the nerve terminal which leads to hyperstimulation of postsynaptic 5-HT-1A and 5-HT-2A serotonin receptors, and may result in development of serotonin syndrome.[1]

Serotonin syndrome is a potentially fatal disorder characterized by mental status changes, autonomic hyperactivity, and neuromuscular abnormalities.[1] In this patient the syndrome was manifested by agitation, confusion, hypertension and tachycardia, muscle rigidity, hyperreflexia and clonus. This disorder can mimic the hypermetabolism observed in malignant hyperthermia. Treatment includes removal of the offending agents as well as supportive measures including control of hemodynamic instability, protection of the airway, and sedation with benzodiazepines.[2] Additionally a serotonin antagonist, cyproheptadine, may be considered, however this drug is available only in an oral formulation.

Methylene blue is used in several clinical situations including treatment of methemoglobinemia, cardiotomy-related vasoplegia, and to facilitate diagnosis of traumatic disruption of the urinary system during surgery. It has recently been recognized that methylene blue is a potent reversible inhibitor of MAO-A.[5] There have been several recent reports of patients developing the serotonin syndrome following intravenous administration of methylene blue in patients that are chronically

Drugs associated with the serotonin syndrome

Selective serotonin-reuptake inhibitors: sertraline, fluoxetine, fluvoxamine, paroxetine, and citalopram
Antidepressant drugs: trazodone, nefazodone, buspirone, clomipramine, and venlafaxine
Monoamine oxidase inhibitors: phenelzine, moclobemide, clorgiline, and isocarboxazid
Anticonvulsants: valproate
Analgesics: meperidine, fentanyl, tramadol, and pentazocine
Antiemetic agents: ondansetron, granisetron, and metoclopramide
Antimigraine drugs: sumatriptan
Bariatric medications: sibutramine
Antibiotics: linezolide (a monoamine oxidase inhibitor) and ritonavir (through inhibition of cytochrome P-450 enzyme isoform 3A4)
Over-the-counter cough and cold remedies: dextromethorphan
Drugs of abuse: methylenedioxymethamphetamine (MDMA, or "ecstasy"), lysergic acid diethylamide (LSD), 5-methoxydiisopropyltryptamine ("foxy methoxy"), Syrian rue (contains harmine and harmaline, both monoamine oxidase inhibitors)
Dietary supplements and herbal products: tryptophan, *Hypericum perforatum* (St. John's wort), Panax ginseng (ginseng)
Other: lithium

Drug interactions associated with severe serotonin syndrome

Zoloft, Prozac, Sarafem, Luvox, Paxil, Celexa, Desyrel, Serzone, Buspar, Anafranil, Effexor, Nardil, Manerix, Marplan, Depakote, Demerol, Duragesic, Sublimaze, Ultram, Talwin, Zofran, Kytril, Reglan, Imitrex, Meridia, Redux, Pondimin, Zyvox, Norvir, Parnate, Tofranil, Remeron

Phenelzine and meperidine
Tranylcypromine and imipramine
Phenelzine and selective serotonin-reuptake inhibitors
Paroxetine and buspirone
Linezolide and citalopram
Moclobemide and selective serotonin-reuptake inhibitors
Tramadol, venlafaxine, and mirtazapine

Fig. 175.1 Drugs and drug interactions associated with the serotonin syndrome [Reprinted from Boyer EW, Shannon M. The serotonin syndrome. N Engl J Med. 2005;352:1112–20. With permission from Massachusetts Medical Society]

administered serotonergic antidepressants (see Fig. 175.1 for drugs associated with serotonin syndrome and potential drug interactions associated with serotonin syndrome).[3,4] Most of the serotonin toxicity cases occurred when methylene blue dosages were between 5 and 10 mg/kg.[6] Currently, it is recommended that intravenous methylene blue dosages be limited to 1 to 2 mg/kg, as was the dose used in our patient.[4] However, a case of serotonin toxicity has been reported in a patient treated chronically with paroxetine who received only 1 mg/kg of intravenous methylene blue.[6] Currently, methylene blue is not a US FDA-approved drug, thus precise information regarding its use is lacking and it is unknown if doses lower than 1 mg/kg pose risk.[7] The manufacturers product information for 1% methylene blue instructs that SSRI must be ceased prior to treatment.[8] Considering that some SSRI agents have long half-lives (fluoxetine 4–6 days), serotonin toxicity may be noted for a long time after discontinuation.[3] Therefore, the use of methylene blue in patients taking medications with serotonergic action should be avoided or used only when the benefit clearly outweighs the risk.

Take-Home Points

- Serotonin syndrome is a potentially fatal condition caused by excessive accumulation of serotonin at postsynaptic receptors.
- Methylene blue is a potent reversible MAO-A inhibitor (blocks metabolism of free serotonin) which if used in combination with SSSI (antidepressants citalopram, etc.) may result in substantial increase in central serotonergic activity and serotonin syndrome.
- Some SSRI medications have long half-lives and the risk for serotonin syndrome (interaction with medications) may persist beyond the immediate discontinuation of SSRI agent.

Summary

Interaction: pharmacodynamic
Substrates: methylene blue and citalopram
Sites of action/enzyme: serotonin reuptake transporter and monoamine oxidase
Clinical effect: serotonin syndrome

References

1. Boyer EW, Shannon M. The serotonin syndrome. N Engl J Med. 2005;352:1112–20.
2. Gillman PK. The serotonin syndrome and its treatment. J Psychopharmacol. 1999;13:100–9.
3. Ng BK, Cameron AJ. The role of methylene blue in serotonin syndrome: a systematic review. Psychosomatics. 2010;51:194–200.
4. Methylthioninium chloride (methylene blue): update on CNS toxicity with serotonergic drugs. Drug Safety Update. 2009;2:3.

5. Ramsay RR, Dunford C, Gillman PK. Methylene blue and serotonin toxicity: inhibition of monoamine oxidase A (MAO A) confirms a theoretical prediction. Br J Pharmacol. 2007;152: 946–51.
6. Schwiebert C, Irving C, Gillman PK. Small doses of methylene blue, previously considered safe, can precipitate serotonin toxicity. Anaesthesia. 2009;64:924.
7. FDA Drug Safety Communication: updated information about the drug interaction between methylene blue (methylthioninium chloride) and serotonergic psychiatric medications. http://www.fda.gov/Drugs/DrugSafety/ucm276119.htm. Last accessed 12 Dec 2011.
8. Product information: Methylene Blue Injection USP 1 % American Regent Inc. Rev. 3/11

Confiscated Contraceptives

176

Fatal Forty DDI: lamotrigine, ethinyl estradiol, UGT1A4

Erica D. Wittwer MD, PhD, Juraj Sprung MD, PhD, and Wayne T. Nicholson MD, PharmD, MSc

Abstract
This case discusses a pharmacokinetic interaction between lamotrigine and ethinyl estradiol, resulting in seizures.

Case

One night in July, an intensive care unit (ICU) fellow received a phone call from the hospital's transfer access line. The patient was an 18-year-old woman with a history of seizures, who had been stably maintained on lamotrigine (200 mg/d). She had apparently had a seizure and fallen while on a ski trip with her new boyfriend at a local ski resort and had suffered an open femur fracture that had required an open reduction and internal fixation under general anesthesia at the initial hospital. After waking postoperatively and initially doing well, she began to experience an increased frequency of seizures. When her parents arrived in town, they stated that she had been on a number of different antiepileptic medications before her seizure disorder was controlled with lamotrigine. They reported that she had approximately one or two seizures per year on the medication. After a negative head computed tomography (CT) scan, the physician at the local hospital had increased the dose of lamotrigine to 400 mg/day in order to treat her increased seizure frequency. She was transferred to allow her to be monitored in a neuro-ICU.

Shortly after arrival, she suffered another seizure and she was kept in the ICU for monitoring. She was transferred to a regular nursing floor on postoperative day 4, after 2 days in the ICU, and she remained seizure free. On postoperative day 8, the

E.D. Wittwer MD, PhD (✉) • J. Sprung MD, PhD • W.T. Nicholson MD, PharmD, MSc
Department of Anesthesiology, Mayo Clinic, Rochester, MN, USA
e-mail: Wittwer.erica@mayo.edu

C. Marcucci et al. (eds.), *A Case Approach to Perioperative Drug-Drug Interactions*, DOI 10.1007/978-1-4614-7495-1_176

patient was transferred from the ICU to the regular nursing floor and plans were made for discharge the following morning.

That evening an urgent call was made to the ICU fellow requesting that she be seen. On arrival to her room, he found her very anxious and reporting dizziness, blurred vision, and a headache. Acetaminophen and ibuprofen had been administered without effect. Due to her abrupt symptom onset she was sent for a repeat head CT scan and then was transferred back to the ICU.

The patient's mother was called to inform her of the change in her daughter's status and she came into the hospital to be with her. The ICU fellow and nurse went over the patient's symptom onset and course in extreme detail as well as all medications she had taken since leaving the ICU. When the fellow left the room, the patient's mother informed him that she had discovered oral contraceptive pills in her daughter's purse. She was upset by the discovery and had taken the pills away. She asked if her daughter had been receiving the medication in the hospital, but the fellow stated that she had not been given the medication while in the hospital.

As part of the workup for her symptoms, a lamotrigine level was drawn and found to be elevated. After consultation with the critical care pharmacist, her dose was decreased back to her original 200 mg/day and her symptoms improved quickly. She admitted that she started taking the oral contraceptive pills one month previously without her parent's or primary doctor's knowledge. After being educated on the interaction between oral contraceptive pills and lamotrigine, she was discharged from the hospital in good condition two days later.

Discussion

This is an example of an inducer added to a substrate causing decreased serum substrate levels. This was followed by compensatory dosage increase of the substrate, and then discontinuation of the inducer.

Lamotrigine is an antiepileptic medication that is also used to treat other conditions such as bipolar disorder. It is metabolized via glucuronidation and excreted primarily in the urine. Lamotrigine has the ability to induce its own metabolism and lamotrigine pharmacokinetics can be affected by medication coadministration. Specifically, it has been demonstrated that lamotrigine serum concentrations are decreased when oral contraceptives are taken concomitantly. Wegner et al. compared the pharmacokinetics of lamotrigine between young women who were taking oral contraceptives and women who were non-users.[1] Clearance of lamotrigine was 126 L per 24 hours in subjects taking oral contraceptives compared to 49 L per 24 hours in non-users.[1] Lamotrigine is metabolized via UDP-glucuronosyltransferase 1A4 (UGT1A4), while estradiol, a steroid hormone, is metabolized via multiple pathways including UGT1A1. Interestingly, it appears that the steroid hormone

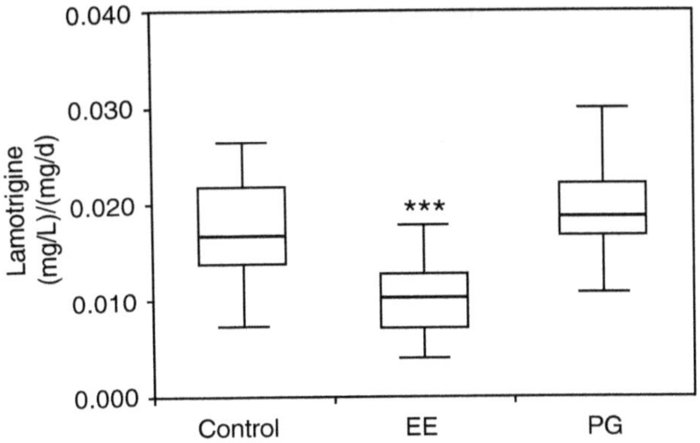

Fig. 176.1 Ethinyl estradiol (EE)-based contraceptives, but not progestogen (PG)-based contraceptives reduce lamotrigine serum concentrations. Box plot showing the median (*horizontal line*), interquartile range (*lower and upper edge of the box*), and total range of the serum lamotrigine concentration-to-dose ratio of the three groups of female patients of childbearing age. Group 1 used no hormonal contraception (**control**), Group 2 used an EE contraceptive, and Group 3 PG only contraceptives. Control vs. either EE or PG group $P = .003$ [Reprinted from Reimers A, Helde G, Brodtkorb E. Ethinyl estradiol, not progestogens, reduces lamotrigine serum concentrations. Epilepsia. 2005;46(9):1414–7. with permission from John Wiley & Sons, Inc]

effects UGT1A4, possibly by upregulation,[2] resulting in the increased clearance of lamotrigine.[3,4] It has also been demonstrated that the changes in lamotrigine metabolism are relatively rapid. Cessation of an oral estradiol administration for a little as 1 week leads to an 84% increase in the serum lamotrigine concentration.[5] Therefore, adverse events may potentially be observed within the 7-day period between the 21-day treatment cycle of a estradiol contraceptive regimen.[5] In contrast, progesterone based contraceptives do not decrease serum levels of lamotrigine (Fig. 176.1).[6] When our patient started taking oral contraceptives, her lamotrigine serum concentration decreased, resulting in seizures. After she was hospitalized, the oral contraceptives were not administered and her lamotrigine dose was simultaneously increased. This led to an increase in the lamotrigine serum concentration, resulting in lamotrigine-associated adverse effects including anxiety, blurred vision, dizziness, and headaches.

Take-Home Points

- Lamotrigine is an antiepileptic. When oral contraceptives containing ethinyl estradiol are taken in conjunction with lamotrigine, plasma concentrations of lamotrigine decrease and seizures may occur.

- Progesterone-only oral contraceptives do not decrease lamotrigine plasma concentrations.

- Lamotrigine concentrations increase rapidly when oral contraceptives are discontinued.

Summary

Interaction: pharmacokinetic
Substrate: lamotrigine
Inducer: ethinyl estradiol
Enzyme: UGT1A4
Clinical effect: breakthrough seizures

References

1. Wegner I, Edelbrock PM, Bulk S, et al. Lamotrigine kinetics within the menstrual cycle, after menopause, and with oral contraceptives. Neurology. 2009;73(17):1388–93.
2. Chen H, Yang K, Choi S, et al. Up-regulation of UDP-glucuronosyltransferase (UGT) 1A4 by 17beta-estradiol: a potential mechanism of increased lamotrigine elimination in pregnancy. Drug Metab Dispos. 2009;37(9):1841–7.
3. Johannessen SI, Landmark CJ. Antiepileptic drug interactions – principles and clinical implications. Curr Neuropharmacol. 2010;8(3):254–67.
4. Gaffield ME, Culwell KR, Lee CR. The use of hormonal contraception among women taking anticonvulsant therapy. Contraception. 2011;83(1):16–29.
5. Christensen J, Petrenaite V, Atterman J, et al. Oral contraceptives induce lamotrigine metabolism: evidence from a double blind, placebo-controlled trial. Epilepsia. 2007;48(3):484–9.
6. Reimers A, Helde G, Brodtkorb E. Ethinyl estradiol, not progestogens, reduces lamotrigine serum concentrations. Epilepsia. 2005;46(9):1414–7.

Gotta Love Derm

Fatal Forty DDI: lamotrigine, valproic acid, UGT1A4

177

Jonathan Anson MD and Richard C. Month MD

Abstract
This case discusses a pharmacokinetic interaction between lamotrigine and divalproex, sodium resulting in Stevens-Johnson syndrome.

Case

A 61-year-old woman was posted for the operating room (OR) late one early January night for repair of an open radial fracture after falling off the drop-down ladder to the attic while putting away the Christmas decorations. The patient's daughter was worried about the surgery as her mother had been lethargic and a little confused with flu-like symptoms. She had also seemed dehydrated over the past 2 days, and had dry, cracked, ulcerated lips. However, the repair of the open fracture could not be postponed.

The patient had a history of bipolar I disorder, well-controlled hypertension, thyroid cancer status post-thyroidectomy with neck radiation, and asymptomatic carotid artery stenosis. Carotid Doppler studies 1 year previously had revealed 60% stenosis of the right internal carotid artery. Surgical history was also notable for cervical fusion 8 years ago. Her medications included lamotrigine (200 mg daily), hydrochlorothiazide (12.5 mg daily), lisinopril (10 mg daily), and

J. Anson MD (✉)
Department of Anesthesiology, Penn State Milton S. Hershey Medical Center, Hershey, PA, USA
e-mail: janson@hmc.psu.edu

R.C. Month MD
Department of Anesthesiology and Critical Care, University of Pennsylvania Health System, Philadelphia, PA, USA

C. Marcucci et al. (eds.), *A Case Approach to Perioperative Drug-Drug Interactions*, DOI 10.1007/978-1-4614-7495-1_177

divalproex sodium (trade name Depakote®, 250 mg BID), which was started by her psychiatrist 1 week earlier, as she had had persistent mood lability over the extended holiday season. On exam, the patient appeared confused but was not in acute distress. Her temperature was 100.8°C. and she was mildly tachycardic.

After the uneventful surgical repair, the patient did not arouse sufficiently to be extubated. She arrived intubated and sedated in the intensive care unit around 3:30 AM and the anesthesia resident met the ICU fellow at the bedside to take signout from the OR team. They were going over the medical record performing an examination of the patient's head and neck and discussing whether they should consult with neurology due to concern for transient ischemic attack or cerebrovascular accident secondary to carotid stenosis, when the anesthesia fellow noticed the patient's ulcerated lips and said, "Call dermatology now!"

The dermatologist doing ICU consults that month was contacted without delay. He was in the habit of swimming laps every morning at 5 AM but agreed to come straight to the hospital instead. He rapidly made the diagnosis of early Stevens-Johnson syndrome and requested that a lamotrigine level be sent immediately. The level later was found to be 5.2 mcg/mL. A review of previous labs showed a baseline lamotrigine level of 2.4 mcg/mL. The ICU clinical pharmacist was consulted and the patient's lamotrigine and divalproex were discontinued. Over the next few days, her flu-like symptoms and her oral ulcers subsided. A psychiatrist was consulted and she was started on quetiapine as a new mood stabilizer. The patient was ultimately discharged to home.

Discussion

This is an example an inhibitor added to a substrate.

Lamotrigine is a phenyltriazine anticonvulsant compound that is approved for use in the US for treatment of seizures and bipolar I disorder. It has a specific on-label application for severe seizure disorders in children characterized by atonic seizures or "drop attacks." It is used off-label for the treatment of a variety of neuropsychiatric conditions including bipolar II disorder, neuropathic pain, neuropathy, trigeminal neuralgia, cluster and migraine headaches, and posttraumatic stress disorder. Lamotrigine has a serum half-life of about 13 hours and is metabolized in the liver by phase II glucuronidation by way of the uridine 5′-diphosphate glucuronyltransferase (UGT) 1A4 enzyme.[1] The major metabolite (76%) is the inactive 2-N-glucuronide conjugate and the drug is primarily cleared through the kidney (94%).[2] Divalproex is an inhibitor of UGT1A4.[3] Thus, by inhibiting UGT1A4, divalproex is able to significantly inhibit the metabolism of Lamotrigine.[4] Coadministration of lamotrigine and divalproex will consistently and reliably raise serum lamotrigine levels.

Lamotrigine is chemically unrelated to other anticonvulsant drugs and is associated with a number of side effects. It is not primarily metabolized by the cytochrome P450 system and is generally considered to be involved in fewer drug–drug interactions than other anticonvulsant medications. Paradoxically, however, it is associated with Stevens-Johnson syndrome (SJS), a rare but clinically significant and possibly fatal syndrome in which there is full thickness epidermal necrosis and separation from the dermis. The coadministration of lamotrigine and sodium divalproex is well-recognized as an additional risk factor for the development of both benign rashes as well as SJS.[5–8] Other medications associated with SJS are the sulfonamide antibiotics, penicillin, barbiturates, NSAIDS, and phenytoin.

SJS is considered to be a true dermatological emergency on the spectrum of toxic epidermal necrolysis and is highlighted with a black box warning in lamotrigine prescribing information.[2] It is seen more often in women than men and is often preceded by flu-like symptoms including fever and sore throat. Early dermatological signs involve a red or purplish rash or blisters, especially in the mouth or on the lips, anal, or genital regions presentation. Any and all suspected inciting agents should be immediately discontinued. The balance of treatment is supportive, including transfer to a burn center if necessary.

Take-Home Points

- Lamotrigine is an anticonvulsant drug used in a wide range of on-label and off-label neuropsychiatric conditions. It is metabolized by UGT1A4.
- Lamotrigine, even as monotherapy, is associated with the Stevens-Johnson syndrome, a threatening dermatological emergency that can be fatal.
- Sodium divalproex (valproic acid) is a UGT1A4 inhibitor.
- Drug–drug interactions between lamotrigine and valproic acid are known to represent an increased risk for Stevens-Johnson syndrome.

Summary

Interaction: pharmacokinetic
Substrate: lamotrigine
Enzyme: UGT1A4
Inhibitor: divalproex sodium
Clinical effects: early Stevens-Johnson syndrome

References

1. Hiller A, Nguyen N, Strassburg C, et al. Retigabine N-glucuronidation and its potential role in enterohepatic circulation. Drug Metab Dispos. 1999;27:605–12.
2. GlaxoSmithKline: Lamictal (package insert). Available http://dailymed.nlm.nih.gov/dailymed/about.cfm. Accessed 14 Mar 2010.
3. Hachad H, Ragueneau-Majlessi I, Levy RH. New antiepileptic drugs: review on drug interactions. Ther Drug Monit. 2002;24:91–103.
4. Bottiger Y, Svensson JO, Stahle L. Lamotrigine drug interactions in a TDM material. Ther Drug Monit. 1999;21:171–4.
5. Ertam I, Sezgin AO, Unal I. A case with Stevens Johnson syndrome triggered by combination of clobazam, lamotrigine, and valproic acid treatment. Int J Dermatol. 2009;48(1):98–9.
6. Kocak S, Girisgin SA, Gul M, et al. Stevens-Johnson syndrome due to concomitant use of lamotrigine and valproic acid. Am J Clin Dermatol. 2007;8(2):107–11.
7. Famularo G, De Simone C, Minisola G. Stevens-Johnson syndrome associated with single high dose of lamotrigine in a patient taking valproate. Dermatol Online J. 2005;11(1):25.
8. Yalçin B, Karaduman A. Stevens-Johnson syndrome associated with concomitant use of lamotrigine and valproic acid. J Am Acad Dermatol. 2000;43(5 Pt 2):898–9.

Desperate for a Drink

178

Fatal Forty DDI: amitriptyline, CYP2D6 poor metabolizer

Erica D. Wittwer MD, PhD, Juraj Sprung MD, PhD, and Wayne T. Nicholson MD, PharmD, MSc

Abstract
This case discusses a drug–gene interaction involving the poor metabolism of amitriptyline by the cytochrome P450 2D6 enzyme pathway, leading to toxicity.

Case

A 33-year-old woman was scheduled for an exploratory laparoscopy to determine the cause of her chronic pelvic and lower abdominal pain. She had been seen for preoperative evaluation by her primary care physician. She had a history of anxiety and depression and had recently been started on amitriptyline because treatment with citalopram and then fluoxetine had failed. She had no other medical issues. Her preoperative laboratory results were within reference limits and an electrocardiogram (ECG) showed normal sinus rhythm and a heart rate of 80 beats per minute.

In the preoperative area, the patient appeared mildly somnolent but reported that, other than her prescribed medication, she had not had anything to eat or drink since the night before. She reported severe thirst and asked whether she could have a drink of water. She was noted to be tachycardic, with a flushed face and dilated pupils, and she reported blurred vision. The resident discussed the case with the attending anesthesiologist because the patient's status appeared changed since the recent preoperative visit. A new 12-lead ECG was done and showed tachycardia of 125 beats per minute, a prolonged QRS (0.12 sec), and a prolonged QTc interval (0.55 sec). When the anesthesia team reviewed the ECG findings, the resident

E.D. Wittwer MD, PhD (✉) • J. Sprung MD, PhD • W.T. Nicholson MD, PharmD, MSc
Department of Anesthesiology, Mayo Clinic, Rochester, MN, USA
e-mail: Wittwer.erica@mayo.edu

C. Marcucci et al. (eds.), *A Case Approach to Perioperative Drug-Drug Interactions*, DOI 10.1007/978-1-4614-7495-1_178

informed the consultant that the only recent change the patient could identify was starting amitriptyline therapy for depression.

The laparoscopy was cancelled and the patient was admitted for cardiac monitoring, which was continued for 12 hours until ECG findings normalized. Amitriptyline therapy was discontinued. The patient was instructed to follow up with her primary care physician regarding alternative treatments for depression.

Discussion

This is an example of a drug–gene interaction.

More specifically, this is an example of a pharmacogenomic problem of poor metabolism of amitriptyline by the cytochrome P450 (CYP) 2D6 enzyme pathway, leading to toxicity.

Amitriptyline is a tricyclic antidepressant that is both hydroxylated and demethylated by CYP2D6, and also demethylated by the cytochrome P450 enzymes 1A2, 2C19, and 3A4 to nortriptyline. Nortriptyline is subsequently further metabolized by the 2D6 enzyme to 10-OH-nortriptyline. Nortriptyline is an active metabolite; however, 10-OH- nortriptyline is an inactive one. All of these enzymes have the potential to impact amitriptyline toxicity, but only *CYP2D6* genotypic variation resulting in the poor metabolism phenotype has been found to correlate with increased adverse effects.[1] The *CYP2C19* mutation, for instance, resulted in decreased metabolism of amitriptyline to nortriptyline but did not correlate with increased adverse effects.[1,2] Persons with the *CYP2D6* mutation have decreased ability to metabolize 2D6 substrates, such as amitriptyline and nortriptyline. There are ethnic population differences in the prevalence of such poor metabolizer status. For example, only 1% of persons of Asian descent poorly metabolize CYP2D6 substrates, compared with 7% of Caucasians.[3]

Amitriptyline toxicity presents primarily with adverse anticholinergic effects: sinus tachycardia, dry mouth, dilated pupils (blurred vision), flushing, and urinary retention. Ataxia, nystagmus, drowsiness, respiratory depression, acidosis, hypotension, seizures, and coma can occur. ECG changes include prolonged QRS and prolonged QTc interval, and may progress to ventricular tachycardia.[4] Inhibitors of CYP2D6 may worsen toxicity of amitriptyline in persons with otherwise normal metabolism, depending on the clinical situation. Many antipsychotic agents and antidepressants, including some of the selective serotonin reuptake inhibitors (SSRIs), are clinically significant 2D6 inhibitors. In addition, other commonly used medications also inhibit CYP2D6, including cimetidine, metoclopramide, and promethazine.[5–7] In fact, one risk factor for elevated or toxic levels of tricyclic antidepressants is the concurrent use of the SSRIs paroxetine hydrochloride or fluoxetine.[4,8] Additionally, because of the long half-life of fluoxetine, this inhibition may continue for several days or weeks after drug discontinuation. Other risk factors include female sex and an increasing tricyclic antidepressant dose.[4]

Take-Home Points

- Persons who have poor CYP2D6 metabolism have an increased risk for amitriptyline toxicity.
- Ethnic differences among persons with poor CYP2D6 metabolism include an increased frequency of poor metabolism in white persons compared with persons of Asian descent.
- Amitriptyline toxicity may involve anticholinergic symptoms; cardiac toxicity, including QRS prolongation, prolonged QTc interval, and ventricular tachycardia; seizures; hypotension; and coma.
- Patients at highest risk for amitriptyline toxicity may be those with poor CYP2D6 metabolism whose dose was increased recently, who started SSRI therapy, or who received a CYP2D6 inhibitor, such as cimetidine or metoclopramide hydrochloride.

Summary

Interaction: pharmacogenomic (drug–gene)
Substrate: amitriptyline
Enzyme: CYP2D6 ("poor metabolizer" genetic variant)
Clinical effect: amitriptyline toxicity including prolonged QRS and prolonged QTc interval

References

1. Steimer W, Zopf K, von Amelunxen S, et al. Amitriptyline or not, that is the question: pharmacogenetic testing of CYP2D6 and CYP2C19 identifies patients with low or high risk for side effects in amitriptyline therapy. Clin Chem. 2005;51(2):376–85. Epub 2004 Dec 8.
2. Shimoda K, Someya T, Yokono A, et al. The impact of CYP2C19 and CYP2D6 genotypes on metabolism of amitriptyline in Japanese psychiatric patients. J Clin Psychopharmacol. 2002;22(4):371–8.
3. Poolsup N, Li Wan Po A, Knight TL. Pharmacogenetics and psychopharmacotherapy. J Clin Pharm Ther. 2000;25(3):197–220.
4. Billups SJ, Delate T, Dugan D. Evaluation of risk factors for elevated tricyclic antidepressant plasma concentrations. Pharmacoepidemiol Drug Saf. 2009;18(3):253–7.

5. Martinez C, Albet C, Agundez JA, et al. Comparative in vitro and in vivo inhibition of cytochrome P450 CYP1A2, CYP2D6, and CYP3A by H2-receptor antagonists. Clin Pharmacol Ther. 1999;65(4):369–76.
6. Desta Z, Wu GM, Morocho AM, et al. The gastroprokinetic and antiemetic drug metoclopramide is a substrate and inhibitor of cytochrome P450 2D6. Drug Metab Dispos. 2002;30(3):336–43.
7. He N, Zhang WQ, Shockley D, et al. Inhibitory effects of H1-antihistamines on CYP2D6- and CYP2C9-mediated drug metabolic reactions in human liver microsomes. Eur J Clin Pharmacol. 2002;57(12):847–51.
8. Downs JM, Downs AD, Rosenthal TL, et al. Increased plasma tricyclic antidepressant concentrations in two patients concurrently treated with fluoxetine. J Clin Psychiatry. 1989;50(6):226–7.

Drug–Drug Interactions Involving QT-Prolonging DDIs

XVI

179 Introduction

Matthew DeCaro MD, FACC, FACP

Abstract
This section introduces drug–drug interactions resulting in prolongation of the QT interval and torsades de pointes.

Prolongation of the QT interval can occur in a variety of settings including genetic predisposition, fluid and electrolyte abnormalities, presence of structural heart disease, and from the use of a variety of cardiovascular and non-cardiovascular pharmacologic agents. The final common pathway in the vast majority of situations is inhibition of the I_{Kr} rectifying potassium current mediated by the potassium channel which is encoded by HERG (human ether-a-go-go–related gene). It is easily diagnosed from a 12-lead electrocardiogram (ECG). The ECG parameter most commonly used is the corrected QT (QTc) based on Bazett's formula: $QTc = QT / \sqrt{(RR\ interval)}$. The problem is that a marked prolongation is associated with a life-threatening arrhythmia: polymorphic ventricular tachycardia (PMVT). When PMVT occurs in the setting of QT prolongation, it is called torsades de pointes (TdP).

Mild prolongation of this interval is relatively common, and not particularly dangerous. Marked prolongation, often with a QTc > 500, entails a much higher risk for TdP, although there is by no means a linear relationship between QT prolongation and the risk of TdP. QT dispersion — the difference in duration between the lead with the longest QT minus the lead with the shortest on the 12-lead ECG — appears to play a significant role as well. This may explain why the drug with perhaps the greatest lengthening of the QT, amiodarone, has a relatively rare incidence of TdP. This agent prolongs the QT significantly in all leads to a similar extent, such that the QT dispersion is low.

Other "electrical" properties of the heart can modify the likelihood of development of TdP with QT prolongation. Since transmembrane ion flux is integrally related to

M. DeCaro MD, FACC, FACP
Coronary Care Unit, Thomas Jefferson University Hospital, Jefferson Medical College, Philadelphia, PA, USA
e-mail: Matthew.DeCaro@jefferson.edu

C. Marcucci et al. (eds.), *A Case Approach to Perioperative Drug-Drug Interactions*, DOI 10.1007/978-1-4614-7495-1_179

depolarization and repolarization of myocardial cells, absolute concentrations of the various minerals responsible for modulation of the transmembrane potential such as potassium, magnesium, calcium, and sodium play a role in susceptibility to this arrhythmia. Heart rate can also play a significant role. Bradyarrhythmias are common in the time frame immediately prior to the development of TdP and appear to play a mechanistic role, particularly in acquired, often drug-induced, prolongation of the QT.

Sick hearts, often with macroscopic (post-myocardial infarction) and microscopic (cardiomyopathic) scarring are more likely to support arrhythmias of any type, including TdP. Congenital or genetic abnormalities of the sodium and potassium channel have been found to be very important, particularly the various genetic long QT syndromes (LQTS), of which there are several varieties. Long QT syndromes 1, 2, and 3 are the most common. Although the prevalence of these mutations is low in the general population, the incidence of TdP in their presence is significant. In addition, there are a number of drugs that have an effect on the QT, many due to less well-defined mutations in the HERG complex. These have been postulated to lower the "repolarization reserve", making them more susceptible to other QT prolonging events.

Unfortunately for the practitioner, the frequency of acquired LQTS, usually due to drugs, is significant. There are several classes of drugs with the ability to prolong the QT and this problem is compounded by the fact that there are many more drugs that interact with these agents to increase their blood levels, and thereby potentiate the likelihood of an adverse arrhythmic event. The level of complexity introduced by this cascade of interactions is daunting to pharmacologists whose careers are devoted to the study of this process. To the average physician, it is a morass.

The solution is not simple, but a systematic approach is possible and mandatory, considering the impact on patient outcomes. Luckily, the number of drug classes that directly affect the QT is manageable. Of course, antiarrhythmic drugs whose therapeutic effects hinge on manipulation of ion channels, fit the bill and comprise a good percentage of the culprit events. Other drug classes include non-sedating antihistamines, macrolide antibiotics, psychotropic medications, and gastric motility agents, in addition to many miscellaneous drugs with a high propensity, such as methadone. Cases within this book chapter illustrate some common potential problems with these types of agents. A comprehensive list of offending agents compiled by the University of Arizona Center for Education and Research on Therapeutics can be found at the website http://www.qtdrugs.org.

The next step involves a systematic analysis for the drugs that impact the metabolism of these agents. There are several ways to accomplish this. The most elementary as well as an often nonspecific and nonsensitive method is to utilize the functionality on the electronic health record that alerts one to the presence of potential adverse interactions. Additionally, many institutions have access to proprietary programs such as MICROMEDEX® that can assist in identifying these types of interactions. Practitioners can also use one of the freely available smartphone or web applications. However, as is discussed elsewhere in this book, all such drug–drug interaction (DDI) programs, while better than nothing, have their significant limitations. The best option would be to use this book (in general) and this section (in particular) as a way of gaining the kind of mastery of this material that would obviate the need for relying exclusively on these DDI programs or make checking the commercially available DDI software a matter of double-checking as opposed to a first-line defense against these morbid clinical events.

The key to success is a heightened awareness of the problem and its impact. This requires a review of all medications and over-the-counter preparations used by the patient at the first preoperative contact. If one of these agents is identified, the clinical context needs to be considered. What is the QTc interval? What overall risk does an arrhythmia pose to the patient? When these factors have been considered the patient's record needs to be labeled in a clear fashion to indicate the patient's at-risk status to all intraoperative and postoperative caregivers. In addition, those patients with higher risk of arrhythmias due to preexisting cardiac conditions should be identified. These individuals may require a higher level of cardiac monitoring, with particular attention to assessment of the QT interval. In addition, modifiable risk factors such as myocardial ischemia, heart failure, and electrolyte abnormalities, especially hypokalemia, need to be identified and promptly treated.

No system is perfect, but careful attention to details is usually rewarded with fewer untoward, preventable arrhythmic events.

Delusion at Heart

180

Fatal Forty DDI: thioridazine, ondanestron, QT-prolongation

Arun Subramanian MBBS, Toby N. Weingarten MD, and Juraj Sprung MD, PhD

Abstract
This case discusses the interaction of ondansetron and thioridazine resulting in synergistic prolongation of QTc interval.

Case

A 25-year-old woman with a history of schizophrenia presented to the emergency department reporting severe abdominal pain because "I have an alien baby in my belly." Her past medical history was notable for severe schizophrenia that was diagnosed at age 20 years. Her psychiatrist had prescribed trials of numerous antipsychotics that had no therapeutic benefit and eventually had resorted to treatment with a stable dose of thioridazine hydrochloride. With this therapy she was able to reside in a group home facility. An ultrasonographic scan of the patient's abdomen failed to show a pregnancy but did show torsion of the left ovary.

The patient underwent laparoscopic ovarian cystectomy, however, she had severe nausea and vomiting in the postanesthesia care unit. A dose of ondansetron was administered by the anesthesiology resident. When the attending anesthesiologist was doing the signout, he suddenly remembered the the risk for QTc prolongation due to interaction between ondansetron and thioridazine. Sure enough, an urgent electrocardiogram (ECG) showed that the QTc was prolonged at 495 msec. Her psychiatry records included an ECG obtained while she was on a stable dose of thioridazine documented a QTc of 450 msec. No further ondansetron therapy was given to the patient. She was admitted to the hospital, where her cardiac rhythm was

A. Subramanian MBBS (✉) • T.N. Weingarten MD • J. Sprung MD, PhD
Department of Anesthesiology, Mayo Clinic, Rochester, MN, USA
e-mail: Subramanian.arun@mayo.edu

C. Marcucci et al. (eds.), *A Case Approach to Perioperative Drug-Drug Interactions*, DOI 10.1007/978-1-4614-7495-1_180

monitored continuously because of her increased risk for torsades de pointes (TdP). The patient also had serial ECGs over the next 24 hours that documented a decrease in her QTc. Her cardiac monitoring was discontinued the following day after her QTc returned to baseline. The consulting psychiatrist elected to continue thioridazine, but recommended that other medications with the potential to prolong the QTc be avoided. The patient was dismissed to her group home the next day after an uneventful hospital stay.

Discussion

This is an example of a synergistic pharmacodynamic interaction.

More specifically, this demonstrates the effects of two QT segment prolonging drugs (ondansetron and thioridazine) on the cardiac conduction system causing synergistic prolongation of QTc interval.

Ondansetron is an antiemetic agent commonly used to treat chemotherapy-induced and radiation-induced, as well as anesthesia-induced, nausea and vomiting. It works by selectively inhibiting the 5-hydroxytryptamine subtype 3 (5-HT_3) receptor (Fig. 180.1). 5-HT_3 receptors are found in both the central nervous system (in the area postrema) and the peripheral nervous system (especially on vagus nerve terminals). Stimulation of these receptors leads to nausea and vomiting.

Ondansetron blocks the central and peripheral 5-HT_3 receptors, thus exerting its therapeutic effects. One of the notable adverse effects of ondansetron—and of all the 5-HT_3–receptor blockers—is a small, dose-dependent increase in QTc, especially when used in its intravenous form.[1] Surprisingly, one study showed that this QT prolongation is comparable between ondansetron and droperidol, a drug that received a black box warning for excessive prolongation of QT associated with TdP.[2] Despite this effect on QTc, it has been concluded that in the absence of other diseases or medications affecting QTc, the effects of ondansetron alone on QTc are probably not clinically significant.[1]

Thioridazine is a piperidine phenothiazine antipsychotic agent used for both initial and maintenance treatments of refractory schizophrenia. It exerts its therapeutic effects by blocking dopamine type 2 receptors in the central nervous system. Thioridazine also displays potassium channel, calcium channel, and β-adrenoceptor blocking properties at therapeutic doses, a feature responsible for its cardiac adverse effects.[3–5]

The major cardiac adverse effect of concern with thioridazine use is TdP, which can frequently present with sudden death. In fact, of all antipsychotic medications, thioridazine poses the highest risk for TdP.[6] This is why thioridazine generally is

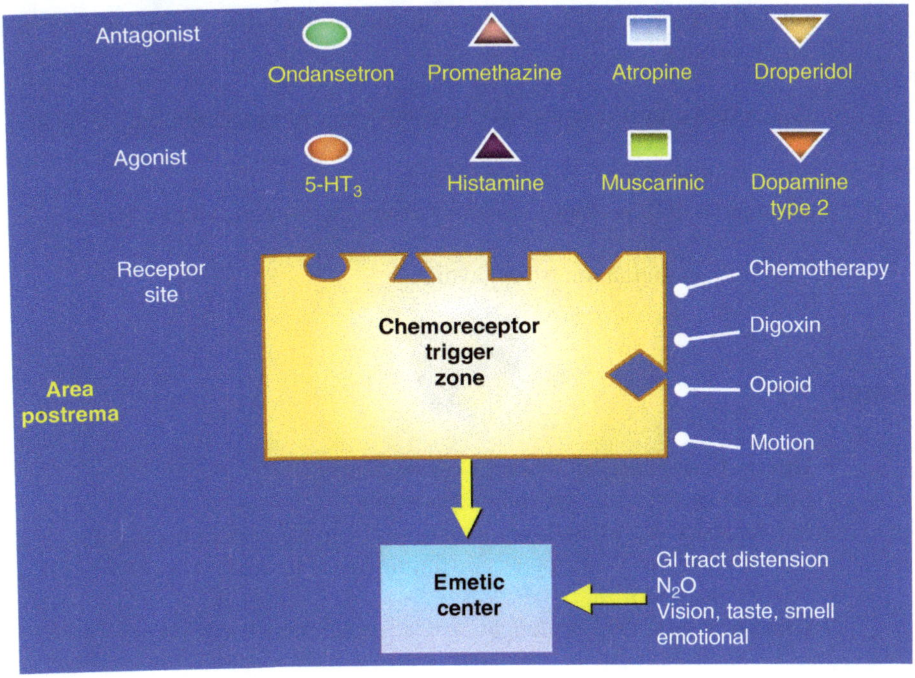

Fig. 180.1 Chemoreceptor trigger zone and the main agonists and antagonists involved with nausea and vomiting. 5-HT_3 indicates 5-hydroxytryptamine subtype 3; GI, gastrointestinal

reserved for schizophrenia that is recalcitrant to other medications, as was the case for the present patient. QTc prolongation is seen frequently in patients who subsequently have TdP and is used clinically as a marker for risk for TdP.[7]

The understanding of the interaction between ondansetron and thioridazine is based on the clinical observation that the increase in QTc can be synergistic when drugs that can prolong the QTc by different mechanisms are administered in combination. Therefore, though there is no direct clinical evidence of TdP from the combination of these two drugs, it is recommended that the combination be avoided.

Take-Home Points

- Thioridazine, an antipsychotic, works through blocking the dopamine type 2 receptor. It also blocks potassium channels, calcium channels, and the β-adrenoceptor.
- One of the important adverse effects of thioridazine use is QTc prolongation.

- Ondansetron is a 5-HT_3–receptor blocker used in the treatment of nausea and vomiting.
- Ondansetron prolongs the QTc slightly when administered intravenously.
- The combination of intravenous ondansetron and thioridazine can lead to substantial QTc prolongation and thereby increase the risk of TdP.
- This drug combination is best avoided.

Summary

Interaction: pharmacodynamic (synergism)
Substrates: thioridazine and ondansetron
Mechanism/site of action: potassium channels, calcium channels, and β-adrenergic receptors (thioridazine) and 5-HT_3–receptor (ondansetron)
Clinical effect: QTc prolongation can lead to torsades de pointes

References

1. Navari RM, Koeller JM. Electrocardiographic and cardiovascular effects of the 5-hydroxytryptamine3 receptor antagonists. Ann Pharmacother. 2003;37:1276–86.
2. Charbit B, Albaladejo P, Funck-Brentano C, et al. Prolongation of QTc interval after postoperative nausea and vomiting treatment by droperidol or ondansetron. Anesthesiology. 2005;102:1094–100.
3. Drolet B, Vincent F, Rail J, et al. Thioridazine lengthens repolarization of cardiac ventricular myocytes by blocking the delayed rectifier potassium current. J Pharmacol Exp Ther. 1999;288:1261–8.
4. Gould RJ, Murphy KM, Reynolds IJ, et al. Calcium channel blockade: possible explanation for thioridazine's peripheral side effects. Am J Psychiatry. 1984;141:352–7.
5. Albrecht CA. Proarrhythmia with non-antiarrhythmics: a review. Cardiology. 2004;102:122–39.
6. Glassman AH, Bigger Jr JT. Antipsychotic drugs: prolonged QTc interval, torsade de pointes, and sudden death. Am J Psychiatry. 2001;158:1774–82.
7. Gupta A, Lawrence AT, Krishnan K, et al. Current concepts in the mechanisms and management of drug-induced QT prolongation and torsade de pointes. Am Heart J. 2007;153:891–9.

At Long Last

181

Fatal Forty DDI: ziprasidone, moxifloxacin, CYP3A4, CYP2D6, QT-prolongation

Kristen B. McCullough PharmD, BCPS, BCOP
and Wayne T. Nicholson MD, PharmD, MSc

Abstract
This case discusses two separate drug–drug interactions. There is a pharmacokinetic interaction between fluoxetine and cyclobenzaprine and a pharmacodynamic interaction with droperidol. The drug interactions are compounded by an electrolyte imbalance, resulting in prolongation of the QTc.

Case

A 62-year-old, 70 kg man required a laparoscopic abdominal hernia repair. He had a history major depressive disorder that was well controlled with fluoxetine (40 mg daily). The patient also suffered from back spasms, which were managed on cyclobenzaprine (10 mg as needed), up to three doses per day. At his preoperative evaluation, he reported some anxiety about receiving general anesthesia which had resulted in nausea and vomiting many years ago during a tonsillectomy. His laboratory values were normal, with the exception of his potassium value, which was slightly low (3.3 mEq/L). The electrocardiogram (ECG) On reading the ECG, showed a heart rate of 82 beats per minute, QRS duration of 110 msec, and QTc interval of 465 msec.

The patient received a total intravenous anesthesia (TIVA) technique with propofol and fentanyl and the surgical repair was uneventful. In the postoperative care unit the patient complained of nausea and was given a dose of droperidol 0.625 mg for

K.B. McCullough PharmD, BCPS, BCOP (✉)
Department of Pharmacy Services, Mayo Clinic, Rochester, MN, USA
e-mail: mccullough.kristen@mayo.edu

W.T. Nicholson MD, PharmD, MSc
Department of Anesthesiology, Mayo Clinic, Rochester, MN, USA

C. Marcucci et al. (eds.), *A Case Approach to Perioperative Drug-Drug Interactions*, DOI 10.1007/978-1-4614-7495-1_181

symptom relief. He subsequently developed a brief period of polymorphic ventricular tachycardia, review of the recorded strip demonstrated torsades de pointes with a QTc interval of 560 msec. Notably his potassium was 3.0 mEq/L. He was admitted to the intensive care unit (ICU), where he was treated with magnesium sulfate and electrolyte repletion with potassium chloride. The ICU pharmacist recommended immediate discontinuation of the cyclobenzaprine. Over the next day, electrolytes were further repleted and his QTc interval normalized to 430 msec. A full cardiac work up was within normal limits and the patient was advised to discontinue cyclobenzaprine therapy on a permanent basis.

Discussion

This is an example of an inhibitor (fluoxetine) administered in a standing medication panel with a substrate (cyclobenzaprine). It is also an example of a pharmacodynamic interaction between multiple drugs with the potential for QT prolongation and an electrolyte imbalance.

The QT interval represents the duration of time between onset of ventricular depolarization (Q wave) and repolarization (T wave), as visualized on an electrocardiogram. This interval is shortened as heart rate increases, thus equations are used to calculate a corrected interval (QTc)[1]. A normal QTc for men is less than 430 msec; for women, it is less than 450 msec. Various formulas exist for QT interval correction, including the Bazett formula, which is commonly used. The main concern of a prolonged QT interval is the risk of polymorphic ventricular tachycardia or torsades de pointes, which can be fatal.

Most drugs that cause QT interval prolongation do so through targeting the rapid potassium current component of the delayed potassium rectifier channel (I_{Kr}).[2] The I_{Kr} is responsible for potassium efflux out of the cell and the subsequent return of resting membrane potential.[3] When this flow is impeded, which happens with some drug therapy, release of potassium is delayed and the cells remain depolarized for an extended duration of time, resulting in QT interval prolongation. Hypokalemia causes a paradoxical reduction in I_{Kr} through various proposed mechanisms, including enhanced inactivation.[4] Even a modest reduction in serum potassium concentration, such as a decrease to between 2.8 to 3.5 mEq/L, can lead to QT intervals of 660 msec.[5]

In this case, the mechanism of QT interval prolongation may be explained in part by pharmacokinetics. Fluoxetine is a strong inhibitor of cytochrome P450 (CYP) 2D6. In addition fluoxetine's primary metabolite, norfluoxetine, has a moderate inhibitory effect on CYP3A4.[6] Cyclobenzaprine, a structural derivative of tricyclic antidepressants is primarily metabolized by CYP3A4 and CYP1A2 with CYP2D6 being a minor metabolic pathway.[7] Therefore, the norfluoxetine metabolite likely has the greatest effect on reducing cyclobenzaprine clearance.

In addition, the mechanism of QT interval prolongation may also be explained in part by pharmacodynamics. Postoperative nausea and vomiting is often managed with agents that have the potential of prolonging QT. These include serotonin antagonists, phenothiazines, or butyrophenones such as droperidol. In the case of droperidol, the manufacturer highlights the QT_c interval prolongation in a "Black Box Warning". Here, use is contraindicated for a QT_c greater than 450 msec for females and 440 msec for males. This would also include patients with congenital long QT syndrome.[8] Relative safety of low dose of droperidol within the practice of anesthesiology has been demonstrated in both clinical and epidemiological studies.[9,10] Therefore, clinical decisions for use of antiemetic drugs with QT prolonging effects should be taken into consideration along with other patient risk factors. To assist practitioners, many institutions have instituted their own administration guidelines to ensure the safe use of these agents.

The proposed mechanism of QT interval prolongation in this case example is multifactorial. Tricyclic antidepressants and butyrophenone antipsychotics (such as amitriptyline and haloperidol, respectively) have been involved in QT prolongation and torsades de pointes.[11] In addition a case report similar to the example case, has previously documented the additive effects of droperidol in patients utilizing fluoxetine and cyclobenzaprine.[12] This case resulted in torsades de pointes which progressed to ventricular fibrillation. This patient was successfully resuscitated and two days following discontinuing the cyclobenzaprine the QT was normal. Many medications from several classes can result in QT prolongation (Table 181.1). Because

Table 181.1 Examples of Commonly Used Medications that Cause QT Prolongation

Class	Examples	
Antiarrhythmics	Amiodarone (Cordarone) Disopyramide (Norpace) Dofetilide (Tikosyn) Ibutilide (Corvert)	Procainamide (Pronestyl) Quinidine (Quinaglute) Sotalol (Betapace)
Antipsychotics	Chlorpromazine (Thorazine) Clozapine (Clozaril) Haloperidol (Haldol)	Quetiapine (Seroquel) Risperidone (Risperdal) Thioridazine (Mellaril)
Antibiotics	Azithromycin (Zithromax) Ciprofloxacin (Cipro) Clarithromycin (Biaxin) Erythromycin (Erythrocin) Fluconazole (Diflucan) Gatifloxacin (Tequin) Itraconazole (Sporanox)	Ketoconazole (Nizoral) Levofloxacin (Levaquin) Moxifloxacin (Avelox) Ofloxacin (Floxin) Sparfloxacin (Zagam) Telithromycin (Ketek) Trimethoprim-Sulfa (Bactrim)
Antidepressants	Amitriptyline (Elavil) Citalopram (Celexa) Desipramine (Pertofrane) Doxepin (Sinequan) Fluoxetine (Prozac)	Imipramine (Norfranil) Nortriptyline (Pamelor) Paroxetine (Paxil) Sertraline (Zoloft) Venlafaxine (Effexor)
Antiemetics	Ondansetron (Zofran)	Prochlorperazine (Compazine)

[Adapted from Ayad RF, Assar MD, Simpson L, Garner JB, Schussler JM. Causes and management of drug-induced long QT syndrome. Proc (Bayl Univ Med Cent). 2010 Jul;23(3):250–5. With permission from BUMC Proceedings]

this type of adverse effect could be additive, it is imperative that health care providers be knowledgeable about the classes of medication which have a large propensity for QT interval prolongation.

Take-Home Points

- The QT interval represents the point between ventricular depolarization and subsequent repolarization. This activity is dependent on heart rate and, therefore, is mathematically adjusted for this factor. The adjusted interval, QTc, has different normal values for men and women.
- QT interval prolongation occurs through impedance of potassium ion flow via the I_{Kr}. This flow is responsible for repolarization of the membrane potential.
- Hypokalemia also results in a paradoxical reduction in the I_{Kr} potassium ion flow, and its effects on QT intervals have been documented.
- Numerous drugs are known to create QT interval prolongation, and combinations of these medications, as well as electrolyte imbalances, can increase the likelihood of QT interval prolongation occurrence.
- Prompt recognition of the medications that are in these categories and subsequent avoidance of them or close monitoring when they are administered can prevent QT interval prolongation and the likelihood of its worsening to torsades de pointes, which can be fatal.

Summary

Interactions: pharmacokinetic and pharmacodynamic
Substrate (pharmacokinetic): cyclobenzaprine
Enzyme: CYP3A4 and CYP2D6
Inhibitor: fluoxetine
Substrates (pharmacodynamic): droperidol, fluoxetine, cyclobenzaprine, and hypokalemia
Mechanism/site of action: slowing of potassium current through potassium channels in cardiac cells
Clinical effect: QTc prolongation with an increased risk for ventricular dysrhythmias and torsades de pointes

References

1. Haddad PM, Anderson IM. Antipsychotic-related QTc prolongation, torsade de pointes and sudden death. Drugs. 2002;62:1649–71.
2. Roden DM, Viswanathan PC. Genetics of acquired long QT syndrome. J Clin Invest. 2005;115:2025–32.
3. De Ponti F, Poluzzi E, Montanaro N. QT-interval prolongation by non-cardiac drugs: lessons to be learned from recent experience. Eur J Clin Pharmacol. 2000;56:1–18.
4. Kannankeril PJ, Roden DM. Drug-induced long QT and torsade de pointes: recent advances. Curr Opin Cardiol. 2007;22:39–43.
5. Curry P, Fitchett D, Stubbs W, et al. Ventricular arrhythmias and hypokalaemia. Lancet. 1976;2:231–3.
6. Hemeryck A, Belpaire FM. Selective serotonin reuptake inhibitors and cytochrome P-450 mediated drug-drug interactions: an update. Curr Drug Metab. 2002;3(1):13–37.
7. Wang RW, Liu L, Cheng H. Identification of human liver cytochrome P450 isoforms involved in the in vitro metabolism of cyclobenzaprine. Drug Metab Dispos. 1996;24(7):786–91.
8. Inapsine [package insert]. Decateur: Taylor Pharmaceuticals; 2006.
9. White PF, Song D, Abrao J, et al. Effect of low-dose droperidol on the QT interval during and after general anesthesia: a placebo-controlled study. Anesthesiology. 2005;102(6):1101–5.
10. Nuttall GA, Eckerman KM, Jacob KA, et al. Does low-dose droperidol administration increase the risk of drug-induced QT prolongation and torsade de pointes in the general surgical population? Anesthesiology. 2007;107(4):531–6.
11. Ayad RF, Assar MD, Simpson L, Garner JB, Schussler JM. Causes and management of drug-induced long QT syndrome. Proc (Bayl Univ Med Cent). 2010;23(3):250–5.
12. Michaelets EL, Smith LK, Van Tassel ED. Torsade de pointes resulting from the addition of droperidol to an existing cytochrome P450 drug interaction. Ann Pharmacother. 1998;32:761–5.

Metha-don't!

182

Fatal Forty DDI: methadone, amitriptyline, levofloxacin, CYP2D6, QT-prolongation

Bryan C. Hoelzer MD, Juraj Sprung MD, PhD, and Wayne T. Nicholson MD, PharmD, MSc

Abstract
This case discusses pharmacokinetic and pharmacodynamic drugs interactions between methadone, amitriptyline, and moxifloxacin leading to QT prolongation.

Case

A 48-year-old, 73 kg woman underwent radical hysterectomy for cervical carcinoma. She had poorly controlled postoperative pain which required hydromorphone patient-controlled analgesia. Subsequently, her treatment was successfully transitioned to an oral pain regimen. At her 3-month follow-up, the patient reported severe life-altering right-groin and inner-thigh pain, which she attributed to her postoperative course of radiation therapy and chemotherapy with cisplatin. She described the pain as and a shooting and burning sensation, rating it as 5 of 10 on a visual analog scale at baseline, with exacerbations reaching 10 of 10. The workup showed right obturator neuropathy.

Multimodal pain management therapy was started and included neuropathic and opioid pain medications. The patient found that she had reasonable quality of life and amelioration of her pain symptoms on a regimen of gabapentin (900 mg TID), amitriptyline to help with the neuropathic pain, as well as her sleep pattern (75 mg each night), and methadone (30 mg TID).

Several months later, the patient had a purulent, productive cough with fevers and felt "lightheaded." She was prescribed moxifloxacin (400 mg daily) for 10 days by

B.C. Hoelzer MD (✉) • J. Sprung MD, PhD • W.T. Nicholson MD, PharmD, MSc
Department of Anesthesiology, Mayo Clinic, Rochester, MN, USA
e-mail: hoelzer.bryan@mayo.edu

C. Marcucci et al. (eds.), *A Case Approach to Perioperative Drug-Drug Interactions*, DOI 10.1007/978-1-4614-7495-1_182

an urgent care center. Approximately 4 days after starting the antibiotic, she had a syncopal episode at her hospital volunteer job and was admitted to the intensive care unit after her electrocardiogram (ECG) showed normal sinus rhythm and a QTc interval of 650 msec. Moxifloxacin therapy was discontinued, and the patient was retained in the hospital for cardiac monitoring because of suspicion of intermittent torsades de pointes dysrhythmia.

Discussion

This is an example of a mixed pharmacodynamic and pharmacokinetic interaction producing cardiac toxicity due to QT interval prolongation.

The present case represents a clinical situation leading to prolongation of the QT interval. The patient already was taking two medications (methadone and amitriptyline) known to prolong the QT interval when a third medication with the same potential, moxifloxacin, was added.[1–3] Moxifloxacin is associated with the greatest risk for QTc-interval prolongation of all of the currently available fluoroquinolones.[4] However, all fluoroquinolones prolong the QT interval, and caution has to be used when they are taken with methadone simultaneously.[1]

Methadone is a synthetic opioid with unique pharmacokinetic and pharmacodynamic profiles that separate it from other opioid agonists. Methadone's action as both an *N*-methyl-D-aspartate antagonist and a μ-receptor agonist and its low cost have resulted in its increased use for treating chronic pain. Methadone causes a dose-dependent prolongation of the QT interval, which has been reported to result in torsades de pointes (a potentially fatal arrhythmia).[5] This is illustrated in the following figures: Figure 182.1A shows an example of an ECG from the patient taking methadone, with long QT interval and QTc and Fig. 182.1B shows an ECG rhythm strip of torsades de pointes caused by QT interval prolongation due to methadone. Recent reports have showed a sharp increase in methadone-related deaths.[6] Some of these deaths could have been avoided with better understanding of methadone's interaction with other medications known to prolong the QT interval.

The medications that have been shown in case reports and clinical studies to prolong the QT interval include several antiarrhythmics, antibiotics including levofloxacin, ciprofloxacin, moxifloxacin (see below), gemifloxacin, oxofloxacin, sparfloxacin, pentamidine, trimethoprim, azithromycin, clarithromycin, and erythromycin, antiemetics including droperidol and ondansetron, and antidepressants including amitriptyline, nortriptyline, desipramine, trimipramine, doxepin, sertraline, citalopram and fluoxetine. Drug-induced QT-interval prolongation and torsades de pointes frequently occur through inhibition of the rapidly activating component of the delayed rectifier potassium current.[7,8] The increased QT interval caused by medications can be worse when other contributing factors are present, such as structural conduction abnormalities or bradycardia.[7]

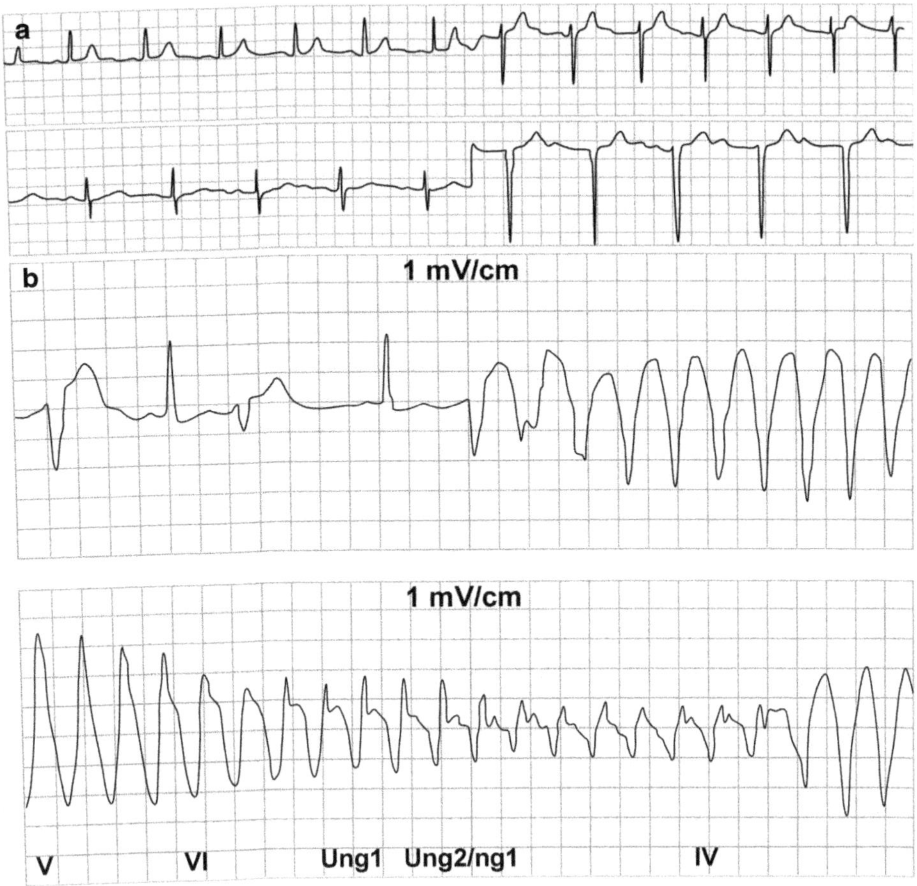

Fig. 182.1 **A**, Electrocardiogram showing QT interval prolongation due to methadone therapy. **B**, Electrocardiogram rhythm strip showing sustained torsades de pointes of a patient taking methadone [Adapted from Sticherling C, Schaer BA, Amman P et al. Methadone-induced torsades de pointes tachycardias. Swiss Med Wkly. 2005;135:282–285. With permission from EMH Swiss Medical Publishers Ltd]

Methadone is primarily metabolized by the cytochrome P450 (CYP) system—specifically, CYP3A4 and, to a lesser extent, CYP2D6 and CYP1A2.[9] Additionally, CYP2B6 is also considered to have a secondary role, although one recent study suggested a more significant role for 2B6 in methadone metabolism and disposition.[10] The biotransformation of methadone is not entirely predictable, since there is an up to 17-fold interindividual variation of methadone blood concentration for a given dosage, this may be explained in a large part by interindividual variability of CYP enzymes.[11] As dose-related effects of methadone on QT prolongation are seen, the inherent pharmacokinetics of this agent may contribute to the toxicity.[12]

Amitriptyline is a tricyclic antidepressant (TCA) that is metabolized by a number of CYP enzymes—it is hydroxylated by 2D6 and demethylated by 2C19, 1A2, and 3A4 to nortriptyline. Nortriptyline is also subsequently hydroxylated by 2D6. Drugs that inhibit these enzymes have the potential to produce amitriptyline toxicity; however, so far it has been shown that only inhibition of amitriptyline's metabolism by 2D6 is correlated with increased adverse effects.[13] Because methadone is a moderate inhibitor of 2D6, it has the potential of decreasing amitriptyline metabolism and subsequent clearance.[14] In the case of the TCA desipramine, concomitant use of methadone and desipramine have been shown to increase desipramine serum concentrations.[15]

Patients who simultaneously take methadone and amitriptyline have to be monitored closely for ECG signs of toxicity. Recent recommendations advise an ECG, to assess QTc, at the start of therapy with either methadone or amitriptyline and a second ECG at 30 days after initiating therapy. In addition, an ECG should be considered when escalating the methadone dose or when adding another medication that can prolong the QT interval.[16] The present patient did not receive an ECG until after symptoms developed, but she should have received at least four—at the initiation of methadone, 30 days later, annually, and before starting moxifloxacin therapy.

Take-Home Points

- Methadone is a synthetic opioid agonist that also functions as an *N*-methyl-D-aspartate antagonist. Because of its potential efficacy against neuropathic pain and its relatively low cost, prescriptions of methadone have increased. Concurrently, there has been an increase in methadone-related deaths.
- Methadone causes a dose-dependent prolongation in the QT interval that is associated with malignant dysrhythmias (eg, torsades de pointes).
- It is recommended that a baseline ECG be obtained before a patient starts methadone therapy. A follow-up ECG should be obtained at 30 days and annually.
- The QT interval should be reassessed before and after an escalation in methadone dose.
- The QT interval should be reassessed when a new medication is added to a patient's treatment regimen that is known to be associated with prolongation of QT interval.

- The QT interval should be reassessed when a potential for pharmacokinetic drug–drug interaction may alter the serum concentrations of an arrhythmogenic drug.

Summary

Interaction 1: pharmacodynamic
Substrates: methadone, amitriptyline, and moxifloxacin
Mechanism/site of action: inhibition of the rapidly activating component of the delayed rectifier potassium current
Clinical effects and ECG effects: prolonged QTc and increased risk for torsades de pointes

Interaction 2: pharmacokinetic
Substrate: amitriptyline
Enzyme: CYP2D6
Inhibitor: methadone
Clinical and ECG effects: amitriptyline toxicity including prolonged QTc

References

1. Weschules DJ, Bain KT, Richeimer S. Actual and potential drug interactions associated with methadone. Pain Med. 2008;9:315–44.
2. Krantz MJ, Lewkowiez L, Hays H. Torsade de pointes associated with very-high-dose methadone. Ann Intern Med. 2002;137:501–4.
3. Badshah A, Janjua M, Younas F, et al. Moxifloxacin-induced QT prolongation and torsades: an uncommon effect of a common drug. Am J Med Sci. 2009;338:164–6.
4. Li EC, Esterly JS, Pohl S, Scott SD, McBride BF. Drug-induced QT-interval prolongation: considerations for clinicians. Pharmacotherapy. 2010;30(7):684–701.
5. Fanoe S, Hvidt C, Ege P, et al. Syncope and QT prolongation among patients treated with methadone for heroin dependence in the city of Copenhagen. Heart. 2007;93:1051–5.
6. Hall AJ, Logan JE, Toblin RL. Patterns of abuse among unintentional pharmaceutical overdose fatalities. JAMA. 2008;300:2613–20.
7. Roden DM. Drug-induced prolongation of the QT interval. N Engl J Med. 2004;350:1013–22.
8. QT Drug Lists by Risk Groups. Arizona Cert. 2012. http://www.azcert.org/medical-pros/drug-lists/drug-lists.cfm. Last Accessed on 27 July 2012.
9. Ferrari A, Coccia CP, Bertolini A, et al. Methadone: metabolism, pharmacokinetics and interactions. Pharmacol Res. 2004;50:551–9.
10. Totah RA, Sheffels P, Roberts T, et al. Role of CYP2B6 in stereoselective human methadone metabolism. Anesthesiology. 2008;108:363–74.
11. Eap CB, Buclin T, Baumann P. Interindividual variability of the clinical pharmacokinetics of methadone: implications for the treatment of opioid dependence. Clin Pharmacokinet. 2002;41(14):1153–93.

12. Krantz MJ, Kutinsky IB, Robertson AD, Mehler PS, et al. Dose-related effects of methadone on QT prolongation in a series of patients with torsade de pointes. Pharmacotherapy. 2003;23(6):802–5.
13. Steimer W, Zopf K, von Amelunxen S, et al. Amitriptyline or not, that is the question: pharmacogenetic testing of CYP2D6 and CYP2C19 identifies patients with low or high risk for side effects in amitriptyline therapy. Clin Chem. 2005;51:376–85.
14. Wu D, Otton SV, Sproule BA, et al. Inhibition of human cytochrome P450 2D6 (CYP2D6) by methadone. Br J Clin Pharmacol. 1993;35(1):30–4.
15. Maany I, Dhopesh V, Arndt IO, Burke W, Woody G, O'Brien CP. Increase in desipramine serum levels associated with methadone treatment. Am J Psychiatry. 1989;146:1611–3.
16. Krantz MJ, Martin J, Stimmel B, et al. QTc interval screening in methadone treatment. Ann Intern Med. 2009;150:387–95.

Flash Fire

183

Fatal Forty DDI: amiodarone, haloperidol, CYP1A2, CYP3A4, CYP2D6; QT-prolongation

Michael P. Hutchens MD, Catherine Marcucci MD, and Neil B. Sandson MD

Abstract
This case discusses a mixed synergistic pharmacodynamic and pharmacokinetic interaction involving haloperidol and amiodarone. The pharmacodynamic interaction between these drugs resulted in QTc prolongation and torsades de pointes. In addition, haloperidol is a substrate of cytochrome P450 enzymes 1A2, 2D6, and 3A4. Amiodarone is an meaningful inhibitor of these enzymes.

Case

A 63-year-old Vietnam veteran underwent successful hand-reattachment surgery after partially severing his right hand in a motorcycle accident. He had a long smoking history, diabetes, a remote diagnosis of bipolar disease type I, and a poor psychosocial history due to severe posttraumatic stress disorder (PTSD) as a result of surviving a helicopter crash during his combat tour. His admission electrocardiogram (ECG) showed at QTc of 444 msec. On the first postoperative day, he

M.P. Hutchens MD (✉)
Department of Anesthesiology and Perioperative Medicine,
Oregon Health and Science University, Portland, OR, USA
e-mail: hutchenm@ohsu.edu

C. Marcucci MD
Anesthesia Services Department, Philadelphia Veterans Affairs Medical Center,
Philadelphia, PA, USA

N.B. Sandson MD
Department of Psychiatry, University of Maryland Medical System, Baltimore, MD, USA

Department of Psychiatry, Baltimore VA Medical Center, VA Maryland Health Care System,
Baltimore, MD, USA

C. Marcucci et al. (eds.), *A Case Approach to Perioperative Drug-Drug Interactions*, DOI 10.1007/978-1-4614-7495-1_183

began complaining of chest pain. A repeat ECG showed a narrow complex tachycardia and ST depressions in lateral leads. Metoprolol (15 mg) was given intravenously (IV) over 20 minutes which did not resolve the tachycardia but caused a significant drop in blood pressure. Amiodarone (150 mg) was then given IV over 30 minutes and an amiodarone infusion was initiated at 1 mg/min. Ten minutes later, the patient converted to sinus rhythm with improvement in his blood pressure.

On the second postoperative day, the patient began to suffer hallucinations of being burned in a fire. He ripped out his IV, and was combative with staff. The intensive care unit (ICU) nurse yelled for help, stating, "I think he's having a flashback." He was restrained and successfully sedated with haloperidol (10 mg IM), and his IV replaced. During the episode a brief run of supraventricular tachycardia (SVT) occurred. Because of continued paranoid ideation, disorientation, and staff safety concerns, the patient was placed on a standing haloperidol dose (2 mg IV q8h). Daily ECGs were ordered to follow the QTc. The amiodarone infusion was continued at 0.5 mg/min. to treat the recurrent SVT.

At 6 AM on the third postoperative day, the ECG was done by the night-shift nurse prior to going home. It showed sinus bradycardia at 55 beats per minute with a QTc of 575 msec, but unfortunately no report was given to the day-shift staff. At 7:30 AM. the intensivist rounded on the patient and noted the prolonged QTc. He discontinued the haloperidol, and, after discussion with the consultation-liaison (C-L) psychiatrist, ordered fluphenazine (5 mg IM q6h PRN agitation) instead.

At 7:50 AM, as the intensivist was walking over to the step-down unit, the telemetry alarm sounded. The patient was unresponsive and the rhythm on the monitor was torsades de pointes. The advanced cardiopulmonary resuscitation protocol was initiated and magnesium sulfate (2 g IV) was given without effect. Defibrillation was transiently effective. A transvenous pacer was placed and the patient was successfully paced with continued recovery of spontaneous circulation. He remained intubated on a short-term propofol infusion for sedation. Anticipating the patient's extubation, the ICU physician also asked the C-L psychiatry fellow to come to afternoon rounds to discuss the use of sedation and antipsychotics for treatment of behavioral dyscontrol in the ICU setting in general and for patients on amiodarone specifically.

Discussion

This is an example of a mixed pharmacodynamic and pharmacokinetic interaction. The pharmacodynamic interaction involves the synergism of two arrhythmogenic drugs. In addition, this is an example of an inhibitor (amiodarone) added to a substrate (haloperidol).

This interaction was caused by the synergistic activity of two potentially arrhythmogenic agents: haloperidol and amiodarone. Haloperidol is prone to produce QT prolongation.[1,4] Thus, it is relatively contraindicated to coadminister it with a Class III antiarrhythmic agent, such as amiodarone. The combination of these agents produced a much greater degree of QT prolongation than would have occurred with either agent alone, which led to the episode of torsades.

In addition to this pharmacodynamic synergy, there is also a significant pharmacokinetic interaction between these agents. While much of haloperidol's metabolism is catalyzed by Phase II enzymes, a large component is also handled by several cytochrome P450 (CYP) enzymes, specifically CYP1A2, CYP2D6, and CYP3A4. Amiodarone is a meaningful inhibitor of the activity of all of these enzymes, thus producing greater haloperidol level than would have been typically expected at the administered dosages. This pharmacokinetic drug–drug interaction (DDI) made a dangerous outcome even more likely than would have been anticipated from the mere fact of combining two arrhythmogenic agents.

Torsades de pointes (TdP) is initiated by R-on-T in the setting of prolonged QTc. As the heart rate slows and the QTc lengthens, the probability that an early afterdepolarization (EAD) of the ventricle will occur while normal conduction pathways are refractory, increases. Patients with heightened sympathetic tone (in this case induced by agitated paranoid delirium) are more likely to have EADs and hence have increased risk of TdP if the QTc becomes prolonged. Most treatments for conventional ventricular tachycardia prolong the QT interval and are therefore not effective for torsades. The standard treatment is magnesium sulfate, which suppresses EADs.[5] If the underlying rhythm is slow, atropine, β-agonists, or overdrive pacing may be helpful in shortening the QT, although beta agonists are considered contraindicated in patients with congenital prolonged QT.[2, 3]

Although there is no ideal pharmacologic choice for the management of ICU delirium in the presence of amiodarone, fluphenazine is often recommended by the knowledgeable C-L consultant, as it is another high-potency typical antipsychotic. It provides all of the advantages of haloperidol in terms of reliably sedating with minimal changes in blood pressure and minimal anticholinergic effects. However, haloperidol is a butyrophenone antipsychotic, and all butyrophenones have been implicated as having a "definite association" with significant QT prolongation and subsequent development of TdP. In contrast, fluphenazine is a phenothiazine, and in that class, only thioridazine and its metabolite mesoridazine have been similarly implicated.[6] Thus, it is essentially a less arrhythmogenic alternative to haloperidol.

As a final note, the careful ICU provider will remember that it has now been well established that lorazepam and other benzodiazepines are generally contraindicated in the management of delirium, as they are among the worst offenders in worsening and prolonging delirium.[7, 8]

Take-Home Points

- This is an acute-on-chronic scenario. The patient was suffering acute ICU delirium with psychotic features. The specific content of his hallucinations was informed by his prior traumatic experiences.
- Although haloperidol has for many years been a mainstay of treatment for the hospitalized patient with acute behavioral dyscontrol, it is a poor choice for patients on amiodarone or for whom cardiac arrhythmias are a pressing concern.
- Haloperidol has been described as causing QT prolongation and increasing the risk for TdP in a variety of doses and clinical situations.
- The QT prolonging effect of haloperidol is pronounced when administered with a class III arrhythmogenic agent such as amiodarone—this is a classic synergistic pharmacodynamic interaction.
- Haloperidol also undergoes metabolism to a significant degree by CYP1A2, CYP2D6, and CYP3A4.
- Amiodarone is a meaningful inhibitor of CYP1A2, CYP2D6, and CYP3A4.
- The combination of haloperidol and amiodarone poses a special risk for patients, especially those with heightened sympathetic tone.
- When an ICU patient on amiodarone requires treatment for acute psychotic symptoms and behavioral dyscontrol in the context of ICU delirium, consider the use of other drugs, such as the antipsychotic fluphenazine, that have less association of QT prolongation and/or TdP.

Summary

Interaction 1: pharmacodynamic
Substrates (pharmacodynamic): amiodarone and haloperidol
Mechanism: synergistic QTc prolongation and arrhythmogenicity
Clinical effect: torsades de pointes

Interaction 2: pharmacokinetic
Substrate (pharmacokinetic): haloperidol
Enzymes: CYP1A2, CYP2D6, and CYP3A4
Inhibitor: amiodarone
Clinical effect: decreased metabolism of drug associated with QTc prolongation leading to increased and prolonged risk for torsades de pointes

References

1. Di Salvo TG, O'Gara PT. Torsade de pointes caused by high-dose intravenous haloperidol in cardiac patients. Clin Cardiol. 1995;18:285–90.
2. Hassaballa HA, Balk RA. Torsade de pointes associated with the administration of intravenous haloperidol:a review of the literature and practical guidelines for use. Expert Opin Drug Saf. 2003;2:543–7.
3. Hassaballa HA, Balk RA. Torsade de pointes associated with the administration of intravenous haloperidol. Am J Ther. 2003;10:58–60.
4. Jackson T, Ditmanson L, Phibbs B. Torsade de pointes and low-dose oral haloperidol. Arch Intern Med. 1997;157:2013–5.
5. O'Brien JM, Rockwood RP, Suh KI. Haloperidol-induced torsade de pointes. Ann Pharmacother. 1999;33:1046–50.
6. Crouch MA, Limon L, Cassano AT. Drug-related QT interval prolongation: drugs associated with QT prolongation. Medscape Today News. www.Medscape.com. Last accessed 11 Apr 2012.
7. Jones SF, Pisani MA. ICU delirium: an update. Curr Opin Crit Care. 2012;18(2):146–51.
8. Trompeo AC, Vidi Y, Locane MD, et al. Sleep disturbances in the critically ill patients: role of delirium and sedative agents. Minerva Anesthesiol. 2011;77(6):604–12.

I Am Dizzy When I Stand Up

184

Fatal Forty DDI: thioridazine, propranolol, CYP2D6, QT prolongation

Tasha L. Welch MD, Toby N. Weingarten MD, and Juraj Sprung MD, PhD

Abstract
This case discusses a pharmacokinetic interaction between thioridazine and propranolol leading to QTc prolongation. Thioridazine is a cytochrome P450 2D6 substrate. Propranolol is a 2D6 inhibitor.

Case

A 75-year-old man presented for an anesthesia preoperative evaluation before his cystectomy for bladder cancer. He had a history of heavy smoking, and a diagnosis of hypertension made 4 months earlier when he presented to a community health clinic with blood in his urine. He was taking oral propranolol (80 mg TID). He had a history of schizophrenia that presented while he was teenager and had undergone trials of numerous antipsychotic medications and a long-term internment in a state-run psychiatric hospital. He had been relatively stable over the past 20 years with a standing oral thioridazine dose (200 mg BID) and he was able to reside in a community-based group home.

During the preoperative visit, the patient reported that since taking propranolol, he felt lightheaded on standing and sometimes needed to sit or lie down for relief. His vital signs showed mild bradycardia, and normotension while seated. He was markedly hypotensive but when standing, although with no corresponding increase in

T.L. Welch MD (✉)
Department of Anesthesiology, Mayo Clinic College of Medicine, Rochester, MN, USA
e-mail: welch.tasha@mayo.edu

T.N. Weingarten MD • J. Sprung MD, PhD
Department of Anesthesiology, Mayo Clinic, Rochester, MN, USA

C. Marcucci et al. (eds.), *A Case Approach to Perioperative Drug-Drug Interactions*, DOI 10.1007/978-1-4614-7495-1_184

heart rate. Routine laboratory values were unremarkable, however an electrocardiogram showed mild sinus bradycardia with normal QRS and T waves and a prolonged QTc interval of 580 msec. He was admitted to the cardiac care unit for monitoring. His evening and morning doses of thioridazine were held and lisinopril was substituted for propranolol for hypertension control. A repeated electrocardiogram on the following day showed normal sinus rhythm and a shortened QTc interval of 450 msec. Because of the severe nature of his schizophrenia, it was elected to restart his thioridazine therapy; a repeated electrocardiogram on the following day showed that the QTc interval stayed normal.

Discussion

This is an example of an inhibitor added to a substrate.

Thioridazine is a phenothiazine neuroleptic (postsynaptic dopamine D_2 receptor antagonist) used for treatment of symptoms of schizophrenia, psychotic depression, and schizoaffective psychosis. It has several important adverse effects. They include anticholinergic, H1 antagonism, and α_1-adrenergic receptor antagonism, as well as cardiac repolarization abnormalities (eg, potential to prolong the QTc interval and thus cause severe life-threatening dysrhythmias, such as torsades de pointes).[1] The cardiac adverse effects of thioridazine are believed to be caused by blockade of the delayed inward rectifier potassium channels.[2] Because of these serious adverse effects, thioridazine is used infrequently in Western countries compared with the newer antipsychotic drugs, but it still is used as a second-line agent or for patients for whom discontinuation is not possible. Also, it continues to be used in the developing world.

Thioridazine is metabolized to the pharmacologically active metabolites mesoridazine and sulforidazine through several cytochrome P450 (CYP) pathways.[3] The cytochrome enzymes 1A2 and 3A4 are the main enzymes responsible for its 5-sulfoxidation and *N*-demethylation (34% and 52%, respectively); CYP2D6 is the primary enzyme that catalyzes the mono-2-sulfoxidation and di-2-sulfoxidation of thioridazine in the human liver (49% and 64%, respectively). CYP2C19 contributes to a minor degree to the *N*-demethylation of thioridazine.[4]

Propranolol is a lipid-soluble β-adrenergic receptor antagonist that was added to the patient's regimen as an antihypertensive. A nonselective β-blocker, propranolol reduces chronotropic, inotropic, and vasodilator responses to β-adrenergic stimulation by competing for available binding sites that stimulate the β-adrenergic receptors. Propranolol is a substrate and a moderate inhibitor of CYP2D6. It also has mild to moderate inhibiting activity against CYP1A2.[5,6]

Concurrent administration of thioridazine and propranolol can result in inhibited metabolism of thioridazine, leading to a three- to five fold increase in plasma levels of thioridazine.[7] Propranolol induces dose-related elevations in thioridazine plasma levels.[8] This interaction can have several serious cardiac consequences. First, thioridazine effects on the cardiac conduction system are dose related, and for this patient probably were reflected in the prolonged QTc interval on the electrocardiogram. This known interaction has made the simultaneous use of thioridazine and propranolol contraindicated. Second, other medications that inhibit the metabolism of thioridazine, such as cimetidine and many antidepressants, are similarly contraindicated. Third, thioridazine should not be used simultaneously with drugs that prolong the QT interval (some antiarrhythmics and most antipsychotics) or for patients who already have a prolonged (≥500 msec) QTc interval. Thioridazine should be withdrawn or its dose reduced to achieve a QTc interval of less than 500 msec. In the present case, the patient was at risk for serious, life-threatening cardiac arrhythmia. With discontinuation of propranolol therapy, his electrocardiogram results returned to normal and he was able to resume his thioridazine therapy.

The cause of hypotension in this patient was also related to interactions between propranolol and thioridazine. The inhibition of thioridazine metabolism and the subsequent increased plasma concentration resulted in an increase in α_1-adrenergic receptor antagonism and contributed to the patient's orthostatic hypotension. The β-adrenergic antagonism of propranolol blunted the reflex tachycardiac response that should have accompanied the orthostatic hypotension, thus potentiating the patient's symptoms. The use of lisinopril as the antihypertensive for this patient is a better choice than propranolol because it does not interfere with thioridazine metabolism.

Take-Home Points

- Thioridazine is metabolized through the CYP2D6 pathway.
- Propranolol is a moderate inhibitor of CYP2D6.
- Concurrent administration of thioridazine and propranolol can result in a three- to five fold increase of thioridazine concentration in patients taking large doses of thioridazine.
- Signs and symptoms of thioridazine toxicity may not be seen even with thioridazine levels in the toxic range. However, potential adverse effects are so severe (ie, hypotension, prolonged QTc interval, and torsades de pointes) that the combined use of thioridazine and propranolol is contraindicated.
- Lisinopril would have been a better choice for this patient.

Summary

Interaction: pharmacokinetic
Substrate: thioridazine
Enzymes: CYP2D6 and CYP1A2
Inhibitors: propranolol
Clinical effects: QT prolongation, hypotension

References

1. Kelly HG, Fay JE, Laverty SG. Thioridazine hydrochloride (Mellaril): its effect on the electrocardiogram and a report of two fatalities with electrocardiographic abnormalities. Can Med Assoc J. 1963;89:546–54.
2. Drolet B, Vincent F, Rail J, et al. Thioridazine lengthens repolarization of cardiac ventricular myocytes by blocking the delayed rectifier potassium current. J Pharmacol Exp Ther. 1999;288:1261–8.
3. Murray M. Role of CYP pharmacogenetics and drug-drug interactions in the efficacy and safety of atypical and other antipsychotic agents. J Pharm Pharmacol. 2006;58:871–85.
4. Wojcikowski J, Maurel P, Daniel WA. Characterization of human cytochrome p450 enzymes involved in the metabolism of the piperidine-type phenothiazine neuroleptic thioridazine. Drug Metab Dispos. 2006;34:471–6.
5. Rowland K, Yeo WW, Ellis SW, et al. Inhibition of CYP2D6 activity by treatment with propranolol and the role of 4-hydroxy propranolol. Br J Clin Pharmacol. 1994;38:9–14.
6. Gillam EM, Reilly PE. Phenacetin O-deethylation by human liver microsomes: kinetics and propranolol inhibition. Xenobiotica. 1988;18:95–104.
7. Silver JM, Yudofsky SC, Kogan M, et al. Elevation of thioridazine plasma levels by propranolol. Am J Psychiatry. 1986;143:1290–2.
8. Greendyke RM, Kanter DR. Plasma propranolol levels and their effect on plasma thioridazine and haloperidol concentrations. J Clin Psychopharmacol. 1987;7:178–82.

Drug–Drug Interactions Involving Foods and Nutrition

XVII

185 Introduction

Kevin W. Cleveland PharmD and David G. Metro MD

Abstract
This section introduces drug interactions involving food.

Perioperative health care providers have the goal of providing patients with the safest possible perioperative care. During patient preoperative evaluation, factors such as the patient's medical, surgical, and anesthetic history; current medications; and allergies are gathered to ensure that the patient's care is optimized while minimizing any risk during surgery and post-surgery. However, one of the most overlooked areas of a patient's history is the evaluation of their diet and the potential effects of diet on their medications. To confound our ability to evaluate the potential drug–food interactions in our patients, the medical literature has limited and conflicting information to guide clinicians in identifying true dietary risks to pharmacotherapy, with the possible exception of drug interactions with grapefruit and tyramine containing-foods are well documented and known to most health care providers.

Drug–food interactions are of clinical importance because 1) food can decrease the response of the medication, 2) food can cause acute or chronic drug toxicity, and 3) medications can interfere with the nutritional status of the patient. All of these can dramatically affect the patient's care by potentially prolonging treatment or hospitalization.

To help mitigate or avoid potential drug–food interactions, the individual characteristics of medications and diets need to be considered and evaluated. An understanding of the physical and chemical properties of a drug, such as the stereochemistry,

K.W. Cleveland PharmD (✉)
Idaho Drug Information Service, Idaho State University College of Pharmacy,
Pocatello, ID, USA
e-mail: kevin@pharmacy.isu.edu

D.G. Metro MD
Department of Anesthesiology, University of Pittsburgh School of Medicine,
Pittsburgh, PA, USA

C. Marcucci et al. (eds.), *A Case Approach to Perioperative Drug-Drug Interactions*, DOI 10.1007/978-1-4614-7495-1_185

molecular weight, solubility, pKa/pH, is essential in determining if a drug will interact with food. Likewise, dietary macronutrient effects on medications need to be recognized. Increased dietary fat can enhance the absorption and availability of lipophilic medications and supplements but a decreased dietary fat intake can lead to poor absorption. Diets high in fiber can bind to medication in the gastrointestinal tract thus limiting the medications bioavailability. Protein in the diet can have variable effects on the availability, actions, and absorption of medications. High protein diets can decrease the availability of medications by directly competing with medications for absorption sites, increasing protein binding of medications in the blood, and up regulating hepatic enzymes thus increasing hepatic clearance of medications. Lastly, medication interactions with dietary carbohydrates are highly variable and generally considered not significant.

To further our understanding, drug–food interactions can largely be divided into two categories—pharmacological interactions and nutritional interactions. Pharmacological food interactions can be further subdivided into either pharmacokinetic or pharmacodynamic interactions. Pharmacokinetic drug–food interactions happen when the food affects the absorption, distribution, metabolism, or elimination of the medication, which can lead to an increase or decrease in drug response. Of these, the most important drug–food interaction is the one that affects medication absorption. Absorption of a drug can be affected by either direct chemical interactions (ie, chelation), changes in gastrointestinal environment, or changes in gastrointestinal motility. Conversely, food interactions that affect metabolism, distribution, or elimination are not as common but can impact the patient's pharmacotherapy. For example, the most notable interaction is grapefruit inhibition of the ability of the cytochrome P450 (CYP) 3A4 to metabolize medications thus increasing drug availability and risk for adverse effects.

Pharmacodynamic drug–food interactions are ones that affect the pharmacologic action of a medication and are generally not as common. However, the significant pharmacodynamic interaction between vitamin K and warfarin is well documented. Lastly, nutritional interactions are the result of a medication interfering with the nutritional status of patient. These can either manifest as altered food intake, nutrient malabsorption, or electrolyte imbalances.

Because health care providers have a solemn duty to ensure patient's safety while under their care, it is important that they know, identify, and minimize potential risks for the patient. Although information on drug–food interactions is limited, there are consistent concepts that can guide a clinician to minimize these potential interactions in our patients. This section will explore how different aspects of the patient's diets can interact with their pharmacotherapy and how to identify and manage potential food–drug interactions in the perioperative setting.

High Fat Diet (I): No Juice For The Ketotic Kid

186

Ketosis, carbohydrates, seizures

Denise M. Hall Burton MD, Miya Asato MD, and Charles Boucek MD

Abstract
This case discusses the food–drug interactions encountered with children on a ketogenic diet.

Case

An 8-year-old boy presented for extensive dental restoration due multiple deep painful dental caries and extraction of two primary teeth under general anesthesia. His past medical history was significant for refractory epilepsy with frequent breakthrough seizures despite a regimen of phenytoin, phenobarbital, and valproic acid. He also had been on a ketogenic diet (KGD) for the past 15 months, which was effective in decreasing the frequency of his seizures and allowed him to attend school and participate in other activities. The general anesthetic proceeded without incident or apparent complication. Before leaving the surgical center he was given sweetened fruit juice to drink to demonstrate that postoperative nausea would not lead to dehydration at home. Shortly after consuming this he had a seizure.

D.M. Hall Burton MD (✉)
Department of Anesthesiology, Children's Hospital of Pittsburgh, University of Pittsburgh Medical Center, Pittsburgh, PA, USA
e-mail: hallburtondm@upmc.edu

M. Asato MD
Division of Child Neurology, Department of Pediatrics and Psychiatry, Children's Hospital of Pittsburgh, Pittsburgh, PA, USA

C. Boucek MD
Department of Anesthesiology, University of Pittsburgh Medical Center, Pittsburgh, PA, USA

C. Marcucci et al. (eds.), *A Case Approach to Perioperative Drug-Drug Interactions*, DOI 10.1007/978-1-4614-7495-1_186

Discussion

This is an example of a food–drug pharmacodynamic interaction at the end-organ level. It is also a possible interaction at the neurotransmitter level.

This case highlights the importance of maintaining perioperative dietary homeostasis in children on dietary therapies for epilepsy. The KGD is a strictly controlled alternate therapy for epilepsy and should be considered in anesthesia care planning and management.

The KGD is a carefully prescribed high-fat, low-carbohydrate, and low protein dietary regimen that has been used since the 1920s as an effective therapy for epilepsy, primarily in children. Most tissues, including the brain, preferentially utilize carbohydrate as an energy source but can switch to metabolizing fat when carbohydrates are scarce. During starvation, ketosis induces changes of brain function including suppression of seizures. Metabolism of this diet results in the formation of ß-hydroxybutyrate (structurally similar to GABA), acetoacetate, and acetone, collectively referred to as "ketone bodies." These compounds may have direct anticonvulsant or anti-epileptogenic effects. The KGD may also change the expression of excitatory and inhibitory neurotransmitters but the exact mechanism of action has not been completely elucidated despite the long history of the diet's use for seizure control.[1–5]

Important medical considerations in patients on the KGD undergoing anesthesia include common laboratory findings in these patients including metabolic acidosis, hyponatremia, hypocalcemia, hypoalbuminemia, and alteration in liver and pancreatic enzymes. Children commonly have low serum glucoses but tolerate lower serum levels with chronic adaptation to the diet. All intravenous or orally administered fluids or medication should be free of glucose and other sugar forms. Blood products can also contain glucose products. The sudden addition of excess carbohydrate in the case example in the form of sweetened juice can switch cerebral metabolism back to glucose dependence with increase in seizure activity.[6–8]

Resources available to the medical team prior to surgery include the consulting specialized dietician who typically works closely with patients and families, the consulting neurology team who can assist with medication plans for seizure prevention and occurrence, and the family who is often the most knowledgeable about their child's medical needs and need for certain precautions. Measures should be taken to ensure effective communication with nursing and pharmacy staff to provide safe care to children on the KGD.

Take-Home Points

- Severe carbohydrate restriction with ketosis may improve seizure control.
- The exact neurotransmitter mechanism for the efficacy in seizure control is not known.
- The sudden addition of carbohydrate can precipitate seizures in a patient using the ketogenic diet (KGD) for seizure control.
- Postoperative patients who are on a ketogenic diet should not be given popsicles or juice of any kind.

Summary

Interaction: pharmacodynamic
Substrates: high-fat ketogenic diet and acute administration of high-carbohydrate foodstuffs
Mechanism/site of action: seizure suppression resulting from induction of ketosis by high-fat diet is offset by acute administration of carbohydrates with increase in seizure potential
Clinical effect: acute onset of seizures

References

1. Huffman J, Kossoff EH. State of the ketogenic diet(s) in epilepsy. Curr Neurol Neurosci Rep. 2006;6:332–40.
2. Kossoff EH. More fat and fewer seizures: dietary therapies for epilepsy. Lancet Neurol. 2004;3:415–20.
3. Lefevre F, Aronson N. Ketogenic diet for the treatment of refractory epilepsy in children: a systematic review of efficacy. Pediatrics. 2000;105:e46.
4. Nordli D. The ketogenic diet: uses and abuses. Neurology. 2002;58(12 Supplement 7):S21–4.
5. Sinha S, Kossoff EH. The ketogenic diet. Neurologist. 2005;11(3):161–70.
6. Ichikawa J, Nishiyama K, Ozaki K, et al. Anesthetic management of a pediatric patient on a ketogenic diet. J Anesth. 2006;20:135–7.
7. McNeely JK. Perioperative management of a paediatric patient on a ketogenic diet. Paediatr Anaesth. 2000;10:103–6.
8. Valencia I, Pfeifer H, Thiele E. General anesthesia and the ketogenic diet. Epilepsia. 2002;43(5):525–9.

Protein Huffing and Puffing 187

Fatal Forty DDI: theophylline, dietary protein, CYP1A2

Brian C. Bane MD
and James Gordon Cain MD, MBA, FAAP

Abstract
This case discusses a pharmacokinetic interaction between theophylline and high dietary protein levels.

Case

Upon entering the preoperative area, the anesthesiologist noticed that her patient appeared anxious and had labored breathing. The patient was a moderately obese 26-year-old scheduled for an esophagogastroduodenoscopy to evaluate gastroesophageal reflux symptoms. The patient's husband explained that, "She has been wheezing for a few days, but walking in from the parking garage this morning really set her off." She had a distant history of poorly controlled asthma due to noncompliance with inhaled bronchodilators. She had enjoyed much better control after starting on oral theophylline 3 years earlier, but over the past week had needed to use her albuterol inhaler multiple times per day. The patient's room air SaO_2 was noted to be 92%. She was particularly exasperated because she had expected improvement in her breathing after a 5-kg weight loss over the previous 2 weeks while on a high-protein diet.

Because of the patient's asthma exacerbation, her procedure was canceled. She received an albuterol nebulizer and demonstrated mild improvement. Upon further examination of the patient's records, the anesthesiologist noted that previous theophylline levels had been consistently in the low therapeutic range, between

B.C. Bane MD (✉)
Anesthesia Element, RAF Lakenheath, Suffolk, UK
e-mail: bcbane@hotmail.com

J.G. Cain MD, MBA, FAAP
Department of Anesthesiology, Children's Hospital of Pittsburgh of UPMC, Pittsburgh, PA, USA

C. Marcucci et al. (eds.), *A Case Approach to Perioperative Drug-Drug Interactions*, DOI 10.1007/978-1-4614-7495-1_187

10 and 11 mcg/mL. A new theophylline level was obtained, which was subtherapeutic at 6 mcg/mL. The patient was started on oral steroids and admitted for overnight observation. A pulmonologist was consulted who suggested that the low theophylline level may have been associated with the recent change to a high-protein diet.

Discussion

This is an example of an inducer added to a substrate.

More specifically, this is an example of a macronutrient (high-protein diet) altering the metabolism of theophylline.

Dietary habits are rarely addressed when obtaining a patient's medical history. Nonetheless, the content of a patient's diet has been demonstrated to affect the bioavailability and metabolism of certain drugs.

A high-protein diet may affect the bioavailability and metabolism of drugs via decreased absorption, increased protein binding, increased hepatic metabolism, and/or increased renal clearance.[1] Drugs that have been shown to be affected by a high-protein diet include theophylline, warfarin, and propranolol.[2,3,6,7]

In this case, a patient in the preoperative holding area was noted to have signs and symptoms of an asthma exacerbation, despite her asthma having been well controlled on theophylline maintenance therapy until several days prior to the scheduled procedure. Upon further questioning, it was discovered that 2 weeks before the date of surgery, the patient had initiated a high-protein, low-carbohydrate diet in order to lose weight before her procedure under general anesthesia.

Several controlled studies have shown that theophylline clearance is increased in patients on a high-protein diet.[2,3] Theophylline is a known substrate of cytochrome P450 (CYP) 1A2.[9] Cimetidine is a pan-inhibitor.[10,11] Kennedy et al. performed a series of dietary manipulations of subjects on theophylline and found that a high-protein diet was able to partially offset cimetidine's inhibitory effects on theophylline metabolism and the subsequent rise in theophylline levels, that is, a high-protein diet was acting as a specific CYP1A2-mediated inducer of theophylline metabolism.[8] In comparison, high-carbohydrate diets do not affect theophylline levels in the blood.[2,3]

Theophylline is rarely used as a first-line agent for the treatment of asthma; however, it may still be utilized in patients who have failed inhaled bronchodilator therapy.[4] The therapeutic range of theophylline is narrow. It is conceivable that increased hepatic metabolism due to a high-protein diet may make a patient's theophylline blood level subtherapeutic.

High dietary protein has also been reported to affect clinical levels of warfarin. Case reports have shown decreased international normalized ratio (INR) and the need for dose escalation in patients acutely increasing their protein intake. If patients discontinue their high-protein diet, the INR begins to rise and the medication dosage must be reduced to maintain an INR within a therapeutic range.[5,6]

Although a high-protein diet has only been shown to affect the bioavailability and metabolism of a handful of medications, differences in dietary macronutrients may help explain the interpatient differences in drug response seen with a wide range of medications.

Take-Home Points

- Many patients are on a weight loss diet at the time of surgery. Beyond a patient's time since last oral intake, specific information about diet is rarely elicited, although certain dietary components may interact with medications.
- The metabolism of theophylline may be altered by dietary macronutrients. This could predispose patients to an asthma exacerbation.
- Warfarin is another example of a drug with decreased clinical effects when combined with a high-protein diet. Patients who have an unexplained decrease in INR should have a history of changes in dietary protein elicited.
- Differences in dietary protein intake between patients may play a role in wide interpatient variability in drug and dose responses.

Summary

Interaction: pharmacokinetic
Substrate: theophylline
Enzyme: CYP1A2
Inducer: high levels of dietary protein
Clinical effects: subtherapeutic theophylline levels leading to exacerbation of asthma

References

1. Anderson KE. Influences of diet and nutrition on clinical pharmacokinetics. Clin Pharmacokinet. 1988;14(6):325–46.
2. Kappas A, Anderson KE, Conney AH, et al. Influence of dietary protein and carbohydrate on antipyrine and theophylline metabolism in man. Clin Pharmacol Ther. 1976;20(6):643–53.
3. Juan D, Worwag EM, Schoeller DA, et al. Effects of dietary protein on theophylline pharmacokinetics and caffeine and aminopyrine breath tests. Clin Pharmacol Ther. 1986;40(2): 187–94.
4. Weinberger M, Hendeles L. Theophylline in asthma. N Engl J Med. 1996;334(21):1380–8.
5. Hornsby LB, Hester EK, Donaldson AR. Potential interaction between warfarin and high dietary protein intake. Pharmacotherapy. 2008;28(4):536–9.
6. Beatty SJ, Mehta BH, Rodis JL. Decreased warfarin effect after initiation of high-protein, low-carbohydrate diets. Ann Pharmacother. 2005;39(4):744–7.
7. Fagan TC, Walle T, Oexmann MJ, et al. Increased clearance of propranolol and theophylline by high-protein compared with high-carbohydrate diet. Clin Pharmacol Ther. 1987; 41(4):402–6.
8. Anderson KE, McCleery RB, Vesell ES, et al. Diet and cimetidine induce comparable changes in theophylline metabolism in normal subjects. Hepatology. 1991;13(5):941–6.
9. Zhang ZY, Kiminsky LS. Chararacterization of human cytochromes P450 involved in theophylline 8-hydroxylation. Biochem Pharmacol. 1995;50:205–11.
10. Martinez C, Albet C, Agundez JA, et al. Comparative in vitro and in vivo inhibition of cytochrome P450 CYP1A2, CYP2D6, and CYP3A by H2-receptor antagonists. Clin Pharmacol Ther. 1999;65:369–76.
11. Nation RL, Evans AM, Milne RW. Pharmacokinetic drug interactions with phenytoin, part I. Clin Pharmacokinet. 1990;18:37–60.

Salty Sam

188

High-salt diet, nitroprusside

Robert Scott Lang MD and Li Meng MD, MPH

Abstract
This case reviews the physiology of dietary salt and discusses the possible exaggerated effects of sodium nitroprusside in patients with high salt ingestion.

Case

Samuel S. Saltinstall was a mildly obese 57-year-old who presented for emergent laparotomy for an enlarging subcapsular hematoma of his liver. Mr. Saltinstall had apparently fallen at home and impacted a sharp table corner. He delayed seeking medical care, insisting that he was just clumsy and often fell and bruised himself. Sam stated he was much more upset about his recent marital separation and his weight gain since being a bachelor and living on "salami slammers" and beef jerky. After prompting from his son, he did finally admit to a history of bipolar disease, which was well controlled with lithium. He also admitted that he had been on other medications but he was unsure of the names, stating his recently departed wife had always taken care of his prescriptions. The patient's son also indicated that his father suffered from a bleeding disorder. The son did not know the name of his condition, but reported that his father bruised easily and had significant blood loss during a previous surgery.

R.S. Lang MD (✉)
Department of Anesthesiology, University of Pittsburgh Medical Center, Pittsburgh, PA, USA
e-mail: langrs@upmc.edu

L. Meng MD, MPH
Department of Anesthesiology, University of Pittsburgh School of Medicine,
Pittsburgh, PA, USA

C. Marcucci et al. (eds.), *A Case Approach to Perioperative Drug-Drug Interactions*, DOI 10.1007/978-1-4614-7495-1_188

The patient underwent an uncomplicated induction of anesthesia and central line placement. During the surgery, there was substantial blood loss. The surgery team asked if sodium nitroprusside could be used to induce hypotension in an effort to decrease the amount of blood loss.

Discussion

This is an example of a pharmacodynamic interaction of unknown mechanism.

Sodium chloride is ubiquitous, and has long been a part of our diets. It is used as an intravenous solution regularly throughout hospitals and other health care facilities. Dietary sodium intake can be classified into low, normal, and high with many ranges of milligrams per day reported in the literature. A majority of the US population ingests much more sodium chloride daily than is required for homeostasis, with little thought to its effects on the body. There is still debate and conjecture on the physiologic effects caused by changes in dietary sodium. It has widely been preached that a high-sodium diet causes hypertension and that lowering intake has favorable effects on hemodynamics. Understanding salt's relationship with our body is an important step in elucidating these changes and in managing patients like the one in the case.

Sodium is an essential electrolyte in our body; helping to regulate fluid balance, continuing the action potential of nervous conduction, and playing an important role in cardiac contraction. The control of sodium is regulated in the body by several hormones. The key factors in this regulation include the natriuretic peptides as well as the renin-angiotensin-aldosterone system. The peptides include atrial natriuretic peptic (ANP), brain natriuretic peptide, and C-type. The amount of sodium in the body is dependent on intake, the actions of these hormones, and modifying factors such as the stress of surgery.

In trying to understand how a high-salt diet affects an anesthetic, one needs to understand the effects it has on the body. It would be unlikely for the patient in this case to suffer the effects of hypernatremia. Rather, more chronic changes in his body's chemistry should be considered. A diet high in sodium chloride has been implicated in hypertension, increased risk for stroke, increased cardiovascular mortality, left ventricular hypertrophy, insulin resistance, nephrolithiasis, as well as changes in renin, aldosterone, catecholamines, cholesterols, and triglycerides.[1–3] In addition to these alterations, vascular regulation may be disrupted due to a high-salt diet. Some research has indicated the possibility that a high salt diet is associated with altered vascular control in salt-sensitive hypertensive individuals, as well as having an effect on vascular regulation in normotensive subjects.[4] Data suggest that normotensive individuals on a high-salt diet may have impaired regulation of tissue perfusion due to oxidative stresses.[5] Other studies have indicated that a high-salt diet enhances GABA receptor-mediated responses in the brain, which can affect arterial pressure.[6] Furthermore, a high-salt diet may affect the metabolism of vasoactive intestinal peptide, which has numerous consequences to the gastrointestinal system such as smooth muscle relaxation of the lower esophageal sphincter and the stomach.[7]

The most prominent and widely discussed effect of a high-salt diet is hypertension.[8] Hypertension can have a complex etiology, with various factors all potentially playing a role.[9] Sodium and water retention are the end points of this pathophysiology. Any patient may have chronic hypertension when he or she presents to the operating room. Anesthesiologists will need to use hypotensive agents with care, as they would with any chronic hypertensive. Fluid volume status needs to be assessed to adequately treat these patients. Increased sodium intake can cause fluid retention. Anesthesiologists must be careful when correcting blood pressure through medications such as hydralazine, nitroglycerin, and nitroprusside,

Sodium nitroprusside is a potent vasodilator that acts on the smooth muscles, which cause both arterial and venous dilation. Researchers have studied the effects of nitroprusside on the human forearm. The study suggested that a salt loading prior to nitroprusside injection intra-arterially enhanced the vasodilatory effects.[10] In Mr. Saltinstall's case, as presented above, the patient might have had an increased reaction to the nitroprusside suggested by the surgery team. This may be explained by previous studies in animal models demonstrating increased sensitivity to nitric oxide during a high-salt diet. There needs to be further research in this area before generalized guidelines can be made. If these results are consistent, the prepared anesthesiologist should consider either adjusting the dose or slowly titrating nitroprusside intraoperatively when the patient has recently had a high-salt intake.

A diet high in sodium has also been linked to interactions with other medications. A well-known interaction is that of dietary salt and lithium. Lithium is used mainly for bipolar disorders as well as some forms of schizophrenia. Steady-state blood levels of lithium have been shown to significantly rise and fall with consistent alterations of sodium intake. The physicians taking care of the patient in this case may see a change in his normally well-controlled condition. A high-salt diet has been reported to decrease the lithium level in the blood; whereas a low-salt diet can cause the level to rise. As the body adjusts to a low-salt diet, the kidneys try to retain sodium. Monovalent cations like lithium are "mistaken" for sodium and are retained as well, causing an increase in plasma lithium levels. Conversely, as the body adjusts to a high-salt diet, the kidneys will excrete sodium and concomitantly excrete lithium and other monovalent cations.

Dietary sodium has also been linked to changes in function of the cytochrome P450 (CYP) enzyme system in animals.[11,12] The exact physiologic relationships of the liver, intestinal, and renal P450 enzyme systems with a high-salt diet in humans have not yet been elucidated, although the early work is interesting. For example, a recent study suggested an association between CYP2C9 polymorphism and activation of the renin-angiotensin-aldosterone system in normotensive men.[13]

Take-Home Points

- A high-sodium diet is common in the United States population and can have significant physiologic effects on the body both chronically and acutely during surgery.

- Sodium is regulated in the body by several hormones such as antidiuretic hormone and the renin-angiotensin-aldosterone system. The function of these hormones can be altered by stressful states such as surgery and anesthesia.

- Certain drugs such as nitroprusside and lithium may have altered effects due to a high-salt diet or an abrupt change in diet.

- Changes on the P450 cytochrome system in humans due to a high-salt diet are not yet fully identified.

- Careful titration of medications and a quick investigation into patients' habits can help avoid problematic events during the course of anesthesia.

Summary

Interaction: pharmacodynamic
Substrates: dietary salt and sodium nitroprusside
Mechanism/site of action: unknown, increased sensitivity to nitric oxide during a high-salt diet shown in animals
Clinical effects: possible exaggerated hypotensive effects

References

1. Ferrari AU, Mark AL. Sensitization of aortic baroreceptors by high salt diet in dahl salt-resistant rats. Hypertension. 1987;10:55–60.
2. Hu G, Qiao Q, Tuomilehto J. Nonhypertensive cardiac effects of a high salt diet. Curr Hypertens Rep. 2002;4:13–7.
3. Jürgens G, Graudal NA. Effects of low sodium diet versus high sodium diet on blood pressure, renin, aldosterone, catecholamines, cholesterols, and triglycerides. Cochrane Database Syst Rev. 2004;(1):CD004022. doi:10.1002/14651858.CD004022.pub2.

4. Wang J, Roman RJ, Falck JR, et al. Effects of high-salt diet on CYP450-4A ω-hydroxylase expression and actibve tone in mesenteric resistance arteries. Am J Physiol Heart Circ Physiol. 2005;288:H1557–65.
5. Zhu J, Huang T, Lombard H. Effect of high-salt diet on vascular relaxation and oxidative stress in mesenteric resistance arteries. J Vasc Res. 2007;44:382–90.
6. Masubuchi Y, Tsukamoto K, Isogai O, et al. Effect of a high-salt diet on γ-aminobutyric acid-mediated responses in the nucleus tractus solitarius of Sprague-Dawley rats. Brain Res Bull. 2004;64:221–6.
7. Davis RE, Shelley S, Macdonald GJ, et al. The effects of a high sodium diet on the metabolism and secretion of vasoactive intestinal peptide in the rabbit. J Physiol. 1992;451:17–23.
8. Bazilinski N. Salt, diet and health: Neptune's poisoned chalice: the origins of high blood pressure. JAMA. 1999;282(2):196–7.
9. Ortiz P, Stoos BA, Hong NJ, et al. High-salt diet increases sensitivity to NO and eNOS expression but not NO production in THALs. Hypertension. 2003;41(part 2):682–7.
10. Stein CM, Nelson R, Brown M, et al. Dietary sodium intake modulates vasodilation mediated by nitroprusside but not by methacholine in the human forearm. Hypertension. 1995;25:1220–3.
11. Lui J, Callahan SM, Brunner LJ. Effect of sodium alterations of hepatic cytochrome P450 3A2 and 2C11 and renal function in rats. Drug Dev Ind Pharm. 2003;29(7):767–75.
12. Vences-Melja A, Caballero-Ortega H, Dorada-Gonzalez V, et al. Cytochrome P450 expression in rat gastric epithelium with intestinal metaplasia induced by high dietary NaCl level. Environ Toxicol Pharmacol. 2005;20(1):57–64.
13. Bolbrinker J, Beige J, Huber M, et al. Role of CYP2C9 genetic variants for salt sensitivity and the regulation of then rennin-angiotensin-aldosterone system in normotensive men. J Hypertens. 2011;29(1):56–61.

A Peak Potassium Problem 189

Salt substitute, spironolactone, lisinopril

Justin McCray MD and Steven L. Orebaugh MD

Abstract
This case discusses a pharmacokinetic drug–drug interaction (excretion) between a high-potassium salt substitute, spironolactone, and lisinopril.

Case

A 67-year-old man presented for inguinal hernia repair. He had a history of chronic hypertension, mild congestive heart failure, and mild, chronic renal insufficiency with a glomerular filtrate rate 40% of normal. He had good functional status except for occasional shortness of breath and lower extremity edema. He had had two previous surgeries without anesthetic complications. His medications included metoprolol (25 mg BID), lisinopril (40 mg daily), furosemide (40 mg BID), spironolactone (50 mg daily), and aspirin (81 mg daily). His vital signs were acceptable and preoperative laboratory values showed a potassium of 4.4 mEq/L, BUN 16 mg/dL, and creatinine 1.2 mg/dL. An electrocardiogram (ECG) showed normal sinus rhythm. An echocardiogram 6 months ago showed no wall motion abnormalities and an ejection fraction of 45%.

Five minutes after an uneventful induction, peaked T-waves were noted on the ECG monitor, which progressed to include a prolonged PR interval, decreased P-wave amplitude, and widened QRS. The patient had a brief run of ventricular tachycardia, which resolved spontaneously. Hyperkalemia was suspected. An arterial blood gas (ABG) revealed a potassium of 6.8 mEq/L. Calcium gluconate, sodium bicarbonate, and insulin were administered along with furosemide (40 mg). The case was cancelled and he was admitted to the intensive care unit. He was treated for ongoing

J. McCray MD (✉)
Department of Anesthesiology, University of Pittsburgh Medical Center, Pittsburgh, PA, USA

S.L. Orebaugh MD
Department of Anesthesiology and Critical Care, University of Pittsburgh School of Medicine, Pittsburgh, PA, USA
e-mail: orebaughsl@anes.upmc.edu

C. Marcucci et al. (eds.), *A Case Approach to Perioperative Drug-Drug Interactions*, DOI 10.1007/978-1-4614-7495-1_189

moderate hyperkalemia with furosemide and sodium polystyrene sulfonate (Kayexalate®) per rectum and extubated later that evening.

Upon questioning the patient denied any recent medication changes. However, he did admit to recently using potassium-containing salt substitutes, which he began two weeks ago after his primary care physician recommended decreasing his sodium intake.

Discussion

This is an example of a pharmacokinetic food–drug interaction.

Hyperkalemia (serum potassium > 5.5 mEq/L) rarely occurs in normal individuals because of the capacity to renally excrete excess potassium.[1] The patient discussed in this hypothetical case was at risk for several reasons. He had a history of mild renal insufficiency with a decreased glomerular filtration rate (GFR) that, coupled with hypovolemia from fasting for surgery, can further decrease his GFR.[2]

In addition, the patient was taking spironolactone, an aldosterone antagonist, and lisinopril, an angiotensin-converting enzyme inhibitor (ACEI) that acts to impair production of aldosterone. Both of these drugs can raise potassium levels. However, despite his medications and renal status, the patient had been normokalemic until recently. In patients with renal insufficiency, increased dietary intake of potassium can alter potassium levels.[2] Salt substitutes, such as those that this patient had been ingesting, allow decreased sodium intake and improved control of hypertension by substitution of potassium chloride for sodium chloride. Indeed, most commercially available salt substitutes contain approximately two-thirds KCl and one-third NaCl.[3] Using a salt substitute in conjunction with his medications and renal insufficiency, his baseline potassium was elevated. With an elevated potassium that was not apparent the morning of surgery it is not surprising that receiving succinylcholine would produce symptomatic hyperkalemia.[1]

The prevalence of salt substitute use is not known, but may be increasing. One large multicenter randomized control trial conducted in China and published in the *Journal of Hypertension* in 2007 showed a statistically significant mean reduction of systolic blood pressure of 3.4 mm Hg when 100% NaCl dietary supplementation was switched to one containing 65% NaCl, 25% KCl, and 10% magnesium sulfate.[4] The reduction in systolic blood pressure was also shown to increase over time with a maximum net reduction of 5.4 mm Hg after 1 year. Given the prevalence of hypertension worldwide, it follows that dietary salt supplements are an inexpensive method that can contribute to maintaining normal blood pressure. However, certain patient populations are at risk for developing hyperkalemia. There are case reports in the literature of patients developing life-threatening hyperkalemia when using salt substitutes if they are in chronic renal failure or if taking an ACEI.[3,5] In the case of salt substitute use with an ACEI, the hyperkalemia was initially attributed to ACEI use alone until further history was elicited from the patients.

Take-Home Points

- Potassium-containing salt substitutes used in conjunction with medications known to raise serum potassium levels can potentially lead to symptomatic hyperkalemia, especially in patients with impaired ability to excrete potassium.
- Salt substitutes are available in any supermarket and there are no regulations governing their purchase. At least one such salt substitute, Lo-Salt, contains a warning that states that people who are taking medications for diabetes, heart disorders, or kidney disorders should consult their physician before using.[6] However, as the product is available without regulation many customers may be unaware of the potential dangers of using them.
- A dietary history to exclude the use of salt substitutes should be considered in patients taking drugs known to cause increased serum potassium levels, and in patients with impaired renal function for any reason.

Summary

Interaction: pharmacokinetic (excretion)
Substrate: potassium-containing salt substitute
Inhibitors (of excretion): spironolactone, and lisinopril
Mechanism/site of action: increased potassium intake combined with decreased renal excretion of potassium
Clinical effects: cardiac arrhythmias

References

1. Morgan GE, Mikhail MS, Murray MJ. Clinical anesthesiology. 3rd ed. McGraw Hill Professional: New York; 2005.
2. Barash PG, Cullen BF, Stoelting RK. Clinical anesthesia. 6th ed. Wolters Kluwer/Lippincott Williams & Wilkins: Philadelphia; 2006.
3. Doorenbos CJ, Vermeij CG. Danger of salt substitutes that contain potassium in patients with renal failure. BMJ. 2003;326(7379):35–6.
4. Li N, Neal B, Yangfeng W, et al. Salt substitution: a low-cost strategy for blood pressure control among rural Chinese. A randomized controlled trial. J Hypertens. 2007;10:2011–8.
5. Ray KK, Dorman S, Watson RDS. Severe hyperkalemia due to concomitant use of salt substitutes and ACE inhibitors in hypertension. A potentially life threatening interaction. J Hum Hypertens. 1999;13:717–20.
6. LoSalt. 2009. http://www.losalt.com. Last Accessed 25 Sept 2012.

Awake?

190

Vitamin C, general anesthetics

Nicole Scouras MD and David G. Metro MD

Abstract

This case discusses a hypothetical interaction between vitamin C and general anesthetics leading to increased incidence of intraoperative awareness

Case

A healthy but very nervous 28-year-old man presented to the Perioperative Anesthesia Clinic and expressed significant concern over the possibility of intraoperative awareness during his upcoming shoulder surgery under general anesthesia. While in college, he had seen the movie *Awake*. Since then, although he recognized that the movie "was just Hollywood" he had been concerned that something like this would happen to him. While searching the Internet he found websites devoted to an interaction between increased awareness under general anesthesia and vitamin C supplementation. He had been taking 1000 mg of vitamin C daily and was very concerned that he would be awake during surgery.

N. Scouras, MD (✉)
Department of Anesthesiology, University of Pittsburgh Medical Center, Pittsburgh, PA, USA

D.G. Metro, MD
Department of Anesthesiology, University of Pittsburgh School of Medicine, Pittsburgh, PA, USA

C. Marcucci et al. (eds.), *A Case Approach to Perioperative Drug-Drug Interactions*, DOI 10.1007/978-1-4614-7495-1_190

Discussion

This is an example of a hypothetical food–drug interaction, supported at this time only by personal anecdotal reports in the non–peer-reviewed literature and media.

Vitamin C, also known as ascorbic acid, is an essential micronutrient that cannot be synthesized by humans and, therefore, must be obtained from the diet. It is found in vegetables and fruits, particularly citrus fruits. Besides being used to prevent or treat the common cold, vitamin C may be of benefit in preventing cardiovascular disease, cancer, and cataracts.[1] Vitamin C also has an important use as a treatment of methemoglobinemia and also has been considered for use as a prevention of methemoglobinemia when using prilocaine.[2]

Awareness is usually defined as a patient remembering an event that occurred during general anesthesia. The true prevalence is not fully understood, however, it has been reported to occur in between one and two cases per thousand.[3,4]

Dr. Allan Spreen, a nutrition expert, on a Health Sciences Institute e-Alert entitled "C-saw," stated "Before surgery I deliberately suggest [tapering vitamin C] to people, as high-dose C is very detoxifying and many times I've had patients tell me that their anesthesiologist was surprised at how much medication was required to knock them out. This happened to a friend of mine and my sister-in-law, both of whom tapered before a subsequent surgical procedure."[5]

Although there is a vast medical literature on the biology and pharmacology of ascorbic acid (vitamin C), there are few reports of clinically significant drug–food or drug–drug interactions. Those studies that have been done have looked at the occurrence of drug interactions between ascorbic acid and oral contraceptives, finding either no significant pharmacologic or clinical effects or increased serum concentrations of the hormonal constituents.[6]

No clinical trials have been done to support the claim that vitamin C increases a person's anesthetic requirement, but the Pennsylvania Patient Safety Advisory on Anesthesia Awareness included that "a high level of vitamin C may interfere with anesthetic effect."[7]

Take-Home Points

- Vitamin C is used for the prevention of the common cold, cardiovascular disease, cancer, cataracts, and methemoglobinemia.

- There are anecdotal reports suggesting that people who take high doses of Vitamin C supplementation may require a greater depth of anesthesia in order to prevent intraoperative awareness but no retrospective or prospective trials have been conducted.

- The entertainment world has capitalized on this as yet unsupported association and it may be a concern for some patients undergoing anesthesia.

- If vitamin C is administered preoperatively, there should be increased vigilance by the anesthesia providers for potential signs of intraoperative awareness and these steps can be discussed with the patient.

- It is important to inquire about and document all medications that a patient is taking. Although, vitamin C supplementation may seem benign, it may have implications for anesthetic management.

- Just as knowledge and awareness of real and possible drug interactions is increasing in the medical community, it is increasing in the cohort of health care consumers, although it may be less reliable. Be prepared for this and be prepared to answers questions!

Summary

Interaction: hypothetical
Substrates: vitamin C and general anesthetics
Mechanisms: unreported
Clinical effect (claimed): increased incidence of anesthetic awareness

References

1. Enstrom JE. Vitamin C, in prospective epidemiological studies. In: Packer L, Fuchs J, editors. Vitamin C in health and disease. New York: Marcel Dekker Inc; 1997. p. 381–98.
2. Korthgen A. Methemoglobinemia due to prilocaine after plexus anesthesia. Reduction by prophylactic administration of ascorbic acid? Anaesthesist. 2003;52:1020–6.
3. Ghoneim MM. Awareness during anesthesia. Anesthesiology. 2000;92:597–602.
4. Sebel PS, Bowdle RA, Ghoneim MM, et al. The incidence of awareness during anesthesia: a multicenter United States study. Anesth Analg. 2004;99:833–9.
5. Health Sciences Institute. Vitamin dosages vs vitamin absorption: C-saw. Health Sciences Institute e-Alert [online] May 2003 [accessed 2 May 2009]. Available from Internet: http://hsionline.com/2003/05/28/. Last accessed 28 Nov 2012.
6. Back DJ, Breckenridge AM, MacIver M. Interaction of ethinyloestradiol with ascorbic acid in man. Br Med J. 1981;281:1516.
7. Pennsylvania Patient Safety Reporting System. Anesthesia Awareness. Patient Safety Advisory [online] 2005. Available from Internet: http://www.psa.state.pa.us/psa/lib/psa/advisories/v2n3september2005/vol_2-3-sept-05-article_i-anesthesia_awareness.pdf. Accessed 2 May 2009.

Tropical Punch Packing a Real Knockout

191

Fatal Forty DDI: grapefruit juice, midazolam, CYP3A4

Brian Blasiole MD, PhD and Shawn T. Beaman MD

Abstract
This case discusses the interaction of midazolam and grapefruit juice. Midazolam is a cytochrome P450 3A4 substrate. Grapefruit juice is an irreversible and cumulative inhibitor of intestinal 3A4.

Case

An anesthesiologist was posted for an elective right inguinal herniorrhaphy for a 14-year-old boy. As she greeted the patient and his family, she noted the patient was large for his age, rocking back and forth, and avoided eye contact. His mother confirmed that he had been diagnosed with an autism spectrum disorder and other developmental delays, but was otherwise healthy and had no prior surgeries.

The patient took no medications and had no known drug allergies. His last oral intake was the previous evening when he drank a large glass of grapefruit juice per his nightly routine. He weighed 116 kg. Finally, the mother was concerned because the patient experienced significant difficulties and could be very aggressive when uncomfortable or forced from his routine. She asked if he could be given something "like a clear juice" to help keep him calm as he loved flavored drinks and fruit juices of all kinds. The anesthesiologist ordered midazolam syrup (20 mg) to be administered by mouth 15 minutes before going to the operating room.

B. Blasiole MD, PhD (✉)
Department of Anesthesiology, Children's Hospital of Pittsburgh of UPMC, Pittsburgh, PA, USA
e-mail: blasioleb@upmc.edu

S.T. Beaman MD
Department of Anesthesiology, University of Pittsburgh School of Medicine, Pittsburgh, PA, USA

C. Marcucci et al. (eds.), *A Case Approach to Perioperative Drug-Drug Interactions*, DOI 10.1007/978-1-4614-7495-1_191

Twenty minutes later, the overhead paging system announced an emergency in the preoperative area. Upon arriving, the anesthesiologist found the patient apneic and being ventilated by bag-valve mask. The upset mother reported that shortly after drinking the preoperative midazolam cocktail, the child stopped rocking in his chair, became unconscious, and slumped to the ground.

Discussion

This is an example of a substrate added to an inhibitor.

This case illustrates a grapefruit juice–drug interaction. The child in this scenario became apneic after a relatively low dose of oral midazolam for his weight, due to an increased plasma concentration of midazolam caused by grapefruit juice inhibition of presystemic drug metabolism. Grapefruit juice selectively and irreversibly inhibits intestinal cytochrome P450 (CYP) 3A4, resulting in increased bioavailability of orally administered drugs metabolized by CYP3A4, such as midazolam.[1] This interaction was first discovered in 1989 when concomitant ingestion of grapefruit juice and the dihydropyridine calcium channel antagonist felodipine caused excessive hypotension.[2] The effect of grapefruit juice on CYP3A4 activity is immediate, causes decreased levels of 3A4 by 47% within 4 hours of juice ingestion, and is still detected at 24 hours.[3] Consuming grapefruit juice in large amounts or in concentrated form causes a cumulative effect on CYP activity. Grapefruit juice irreversibly inhibits 3A4 via increased enzyme degradation and by reduced mRNA translation, requiring *de novo* synthesis of CYP 3A4 for full recovery of metabolic function.[4] The components of grapefruit juice thought to be responsible for CYP 3A4 enzyme inhibition have yet to be elucidated, however the furanocoumarin, 6′,7′-dihydroxybergamottin, is currently the main focus of attention.[5]

Grapefruit juice is consumed by 21% of US households. Its popularity is enhanced among the health conscious by medical evidence suggesting grapefruit juice reduces atherosclerosis and inhibits breast cancer cell formation.[6,7] The clinically important grapefruit juice–drug interactions that have been studied include the dihydropyridines, terfenadine, saquinavir, cyclosporine, midazolam, triazolam, and verapamil. The interactions with midazolam and triazolam are of particular importance since benzodiazepines cause dose-dependent respiratory depression. Studies in healthy human volunteers who drank just 8 ounces of grapefruit juice 1 hour prior to oral midazolam administration showed 1.5-fold increase in plasma levels and significantly reduced clearance levels of the drug.[8] Similar results have also been observed with triazolam, however, alprazolam is unaffected by grapefruit juice due to high baseline bioavailability. These data strongly suggest that caution is warranted when administering oral midazolam and triazolam to patients who consume grapefruit juice.

Take-Home Points

- Grapefruit juice inhibits intestinal more than hepatic CYP3A4; therefore, the grapefruit juice–drug interaction predominantly increases the plasma levels of orally, as opposed to parenterally, administered drugs.

- The effect of grapefruit juice on enteric CYP3A4 is unique and does not pertain to other juices, including orange juice or pomegranate juice.

- If there is a possibility of an interaction with grapefruit juice, oral midazolam and triazolam should be avoided or the dose decreased by 50%.

Summary

Interaction: pharmacokinetic
Substrate: midazolam
Enzyme: CYP3A4
Inhibitor: grapefruit juice
Clinical effect: increased sedation

References

1. Bailey DG, Spence JD, Munoz C, et al. Interaction of citrus juices with felodipine and nifedipine. Lancet. 1991;337:268–9.
2. Bailey DG, Spence JD, Edgar B, et al. Ethanol enhances the hemodynamic effect of felopdipine. Clin Invest Med. 1989;12:357–62.
3. Lundahl J, Regardh CG, Edgar B, et al. Effects of grapefruit juice ingestion-pharmacokinetics and haemodynamics of intravenously and orally administered felopdipine in healthy men. Eur J Clin Pharmacol. 1995;52:139–45.
4. Lown KS, Baily DG, Fontana RJ, et al. Grapefruit juice increases felodipine oral availability in humans by decreasing intestinal CYP 3A protein expression. J Clin Invest. 1997;99:2545–53.
5. Paine MF, Criss AB, Watkins PB. Two major grapefruit juice components differ in time to onset of intestinal CYP3A4 inhibition. J Pharmacol Exp Ther. 2005;312:1151–60.
6. Cerda JJ, Normann SJ, Sullivan MP, et al. Inhibition of atherosclerosis by dietary pectin in microswine with sustained hypercholesterolemia. Circulation. 1994;89:1247–53.
7. So FV, Guthrie N, Chambers AF, et al. Inhibition of human cancer cell proliferation and delay of mammary cell tumorogenesis by flavonoids and citrus juices. Nutr Cancer. 1996;26:167–81.
8. Farkas D, Oleson LE, Zhao Y, Harmatz JS, Zinny MA, Court MH, Greenblatt DJ. Pomegranate juice does not impair clearance of oral or intravenous midazolam, a probe for cytochrome P450-3A activity: comparison with grapefruit juice. J Clin Pharmacol. 2007;47:286–94.

When the Fire Won't Go Out

192

Pomegranate juice, sildenafil, CYP3A4

Thomas P. Pontinen MD and Randal O. Dull MD, PhD

Abstract

This case discusses the pharmacokinetic interaction between pomegranate juice and sildenafil, resulting in priapism. Sildenafil is a cytochrome P450 3A4 substrate and pomegranate juice is a 3A4 inhibitor.

Case

The Urology chief resident called the operating room desk to schedule surgical intervention for a case of priapism and asked if anyone from the Anesthesiology on-call team was available to pre-op the patient and consult for pain control. The junior Anesthesiology on-call resident was dispatched to the ED (no pun intended) and found a 56-year-old man in significant distress having experienced an erection that began 7 hours ago. A thorough history and physical was done and was significant for hypertension, hypercholesterolemia, and erectile dysfunction. The patient was an occasional cigar smoker. His medications included lisinipril, atorvastatin, and sildenafil, the later taken "as needed." He stated that he had no known drug allergies. Further questions about NPO status led to the patient revealing that he drank approximately a liter of pomegranate juice every day because he was told in his "men's group" that that particular juice can help with erectile dysfunction.

The Anesthesiology resident had majored in food science in college and was married to a lady who was just finishing her PharmD program and so was keenly aware

T.P. Pontinen MD (✉)
Department of Anesthesiology, University of Illinois Hospital and Health Sciences System, Chicago, IL, USA
e-mail: tompontinen@gmail.com

R.O. Dull MD, PhD
Department of Anesthesiology, University of Illinois at Chicago, Chicago, IL, USA

C. Marcucci et al. (eds.), *A Case Approach to Perioperative Drug-Drug Interactions*, DOI 10.1007/978-1-4614-7495-1_192

of the association between nutritional supplements and commonly prescribed medications. He alerted the patient and the Urology resident to the biologically activate compounds in pomegranate juice and grapefruit juice.

Discussion

This is an example of a substrate added to an inhibitor.

Sildenafil is phosphodiesterase type-5 inhibitor that is used for treatment of erectile dysfunction and pulmonary hypertension. There are numerous drug–drug interactions (DDIs) with sildenafil, notably nitrates, α-blockers, and ß-blockers, which may all cause severe hypotension. Sildenafil is metabolized by cytochrome P450 (CYP) 3A4 (80%) and CYP2C9 (20%); in addition to known DDIs, patients are advised to avoid grapefruit juice when taking sildenafil.

Pomegranate juice has high concentrations of antioxidants and has been recommend as part of a heart-healthy diet and as a nutritional treatment of erectile dysfunction. However, like grapefruit juice, pomegranate juice has been reported to inhibit CYP enzymes based on laboratory studies. In our patient in this scenario, regular ingestion of pomegranate juice with concurrent administration of sildenafil likely resulted in inhibition of CYP3A4 which in turn resulted in elevated plasma levels of sildenafil. This then resulted in increased risk for side effects including priapism. Case reports of priapism associated with both grape fruit juice and pomegranate juice have been reported.[1]

Take-Home Points

- A thorough preanesthesia history and physical must include questions regarding the patient's nutritional habits and consumption of vitamins, herbs, and other supplements that may possess biologically active compounds.
- Both pomegranate juice and grapefruit juice are inhibitors of CYP3A4 and possible other members of the CYP family.[2]
- Sildenafil is metabolized by two members of the CYP family, CYP3A4 and CYP2C9. The astute practitioner must develop an awareness for CYP-mediated DDIs and know where to expediently locate information regarding perioperative implications.[3]

Summary

Interaction: pharmacokinetic
Substrate: sildenafil
Enzyme: CYP3A4
Inhibitor: pomegranate juice
Clinical effects: priapism

References

1. Senthilkumaran S, Balamurugan N, Suresh P, et al. Priapism, pomegranate juice and sildenafil; is there a connection? Urol Ann. 2012;4(2):108–10.
2. Nagata M, Hidaka M, Sekiya H, et al. Effects of pomegranate juice on human cytochrome P450 2C9 and tolbutamide pharmacokinetics in rats. Drug Metab Dispos. 2007;35:302–5.
3. Sildenafil. PubMed Health; 2010. http://www.ncbi.nlm.nih.gov/pubmedhealth/PMH0001046/. Last accessed 25 Sept 2012.

Peppermint Patty 193

Fatal Forty DDI: peppermint, felodipine, CYP3A4

Ryan D. Ball MD and Karen Boretsky MD

Abstract
This case discusses a pharmacokinetic interaction between felodipine and peppermint. Felodipine is a cytochrome P450 3A4 substrate and peppermint is a 3A4 inhibitor.

Case

Mrs. Patricia Patterson was a generally healthy, 78-year-old women with long-standing essential hypertension and irritable bowel syndrome (IBS). She was scheduled for an outpatient colonoscopy and, because of a recent Emergency Department (ED) visit, her gastroenterologist requested that she be seen by a nurse practitioner in the preoperative clinic at the local hospital and that her colonoscopy be done there instead of at a free-standing center.

The preoperative nurse practitioner had a bit of a story to untangle about the recent ED visit when trying to decide if further workup was necessary. Patty gave a history of being transported to the ED with low blood pressure and a "faint pulse." She reported that she had been admitted to the "observation unit" for a day and a half, but could give no other details about her hospitalization. However, she was able to give more detail about her preceding medical history. Her only prescription medication was felodipine for control of her hypertension. And although her IBS was mild, she occasionally used over-the-counter-medications when her symptoms worsened. Over time, Patty found that peppermint oil capsules were most effective in reducing IBS symptoms, and the fact that peppermint oil is an herbal remedy increased her confidence in its safety.

Just prior to the ED visit, Patty had been experiencing increased IBS-related symptoms with worsened pain. She had tried to schedule an appointment with her family

R.D. Ball MD (✉) • K. Boretsky MD
Department of Anesthesiology, University of Pittsburgh Medical Center, Pittsburgh, PA, USA
e-mail: ballrd@upmc.edu

C. Marcucci et al. (eds.), *A Case Approach to Perioperative Drug-Drug Interactions*, DOI 10.1007/978-1-4614-7495-1_193

physician, but was unable to get an appointment for several weeks, While awaiting the appointment, Patricia increased her intake of peppermint oil to try to improve her symptoms. On a particularly painful morning, she planned to spend the day with her grandchildren and used much more peppermint oil than usual. Later that day, Patty was preparing lunch and fainted. She lost consciousness only briefly and was brought immediately to the ED by her neighbors for further evaluation. Fortunately, our astute preoperative nurse practitioner immediately recognized the likely cause of the syncopal episode and further unnecessary workup was avoided.

Discussion

This is an example of an inhibitor added to a substrate.

Patty's hypotension-induced syncopal episode was due to an increased plasma concentration of felodipine resulting from an inhibition of felodipine metabolism by peppermint. Peppermint oil and its primary constituent menthol are moderately potent, reversible inhibitors of the cytochrome P450 (CYP) 3A4, the primary enzyme responsible for the metabolism of felodipine. In one study, the administration of oral peppermint oil (600 mg) versus placebo (water) increased felodipine concentrations by a mean of 140%.[1] Levels of cyclosporine and simvastatin may also be increased by concurrent use of peppermint.[2] Conversely, menthol has been reported to increase the clearance of warfarin, leading to decreased International Normalized Ratios.[3,8]

Peppermint is one of the oldest used medicinal herbs. Today, peppermint is used for many different reasons, and it is commercially sold in several forms. Peppermint oil capsules are used for dyspepsia and as an antispasmodic and have been shown to provide relief from the symptoms related to IBS in both children and adults.[4,5] Peppermint oil is also sold diluted in a topical preparation and has shown promising results in the treatment of pain related to postherapeutic neuralgia.[6] Using over-the-counter peppermint oil capsules in excess, such as in the case above, can lead to high doses of peppermint ingestion and potentially to inhibition of the CYP3A4 enzyme.

Aside from its drug interactions, peppermint also has clinically significant side effects. Some people have been shown to be allergic to peppermint oil, with rash being most commonly associated, and these folks would be ill advised to use the capsule or topical form. Although peppermint oil has been used in the treatment of dyspepsia, it also causes relaxation of the lower esophageal sphincter and can actually make heartburn and acid reflux worse in some instances.[7]

Take-Home Points

- Medicinal use of peppermint oil should be avoided in combination with drugs that are metabolized by the CYP3A4 enzyme.
- Over-the-counter medications are not devoid of side effects and/or drug interactions, and should be discussed with a physician to determine safety.

Summary

Interaction: pharmacokinetic
Substrate: felodipine
Enzyme: CYP3A4
Inhibitor: peppermint
Clinical effect: increased antihypertensive effect

References

1. Dresser GK, Wacher V, Wong S, et al. Evaluation of peppermint oil and ascorbyl palmitate as inhibitors of cytochrome P4503A4 activity *in vitro* and *in vivo*. Clin Pharmacol Ther. 2002;72(3):247–55.
2. Wacher VJ, Wong S, Wong HT. Peppermint oil enhances cyclosporine oral bioavailability in rats: comparison with D-alpha-tocopheryl poly(ethylene glycol 1000) succinate (TPGS) and ketoconazole. J Pharm Sci. 2002;91(1):77–90.
3. Kassebaum PJ, Shaw DL, Tomich DJ. Possible warfarin interaction with menthol cough drops. Ann Pharmacother. 2005;39:365–7.
4. Cappello G, Spezzaferro M, Grossi L, et al. Peppermint oil (Mintoil) in the treatment of irritable bowel syndrome: a prospective double blind placebo-controlled randomized trial. Dig Liver Dis. 2007;39(6):530–6.
5. Kline RM, Kline JJ, Di Palma J, et al. Enteric-coated, pH-dependent peppermint oil capsules for the treatment of irritable bowel syndrome in children. J Pediatr. 2001;138:125–8.
6. Davies SJ, Harding LM, Baranowski AP. A novel treatment of postherpetic neuralgia using peppermint oil. Clin J Pain. 2002;18(3):200–2.
7. Charrois TL, Hrudey J, Gardiner P, et al. Peppermint oil. Pediatr Rev. 2006;27:49–51.
8. Coderre K, Faria C, Dyer E. Probable warfarin interaction with menthol cough drops. Pharmacotherapy. 2010;30(1):110.

From Bleeding Gums to Green Thumbs: A True Story

194

Fatal Forty DDI: warfarin, green vegetables

Audra M. Webber MD and Patricia L. Dalby MD

Abstract
This case discusses the pharmacodynamic interaction between leafy green vegetables and warfarin, resulting in loss of anticoagulant effect.

Case

A 60-year-old anesthesiologist was on call for his practice and completed a tiring overnight shift. Early the next morning he began to experience palpitations and felt some chest discomfort. His first instinct was to brush it off and head home, however, the anesthesiologist coming on call convinced him to go to the emergency department for evaluation. As soon as the electrocardiogram (ECG) leads were placed, it was apparent he was experiencing intermittent atrial fibrillation, as well as short periods of supraventricular tachycardia. He was also significantly hypertensive. He elected for medical therapy - flecainide, atenolol, and lisinopril, as well as warfarin for primary prevention of stroke with the goal of an International Normalized Ratio (INR) around 3.0.

Shortly after this regimen was initiated, the patient was scheduled for knee arthroscopy and mentioned at his preoperative appointment that his gums were bleeding

A.M. Webber MD (✉)
Department of Anesthesiology, Kosair Children's Hospital, Louisville, KY, USA
e-mail: audra.webber@gmail.com

P.L. Dalby MD
Department of Anesthesiology, Magee-Womens Hospital, University of Pittsburgh School of Medicine, Pittsburgh, PA, USA

C. Marcucci et al. (eds.), *A Case Approach to Perioperative Drug-Drug Interactions*, DOI 10.1007/978-1-4614-7495-1_194

when he brushed his teeth. His INR was found to be elevated at 6.7, and his warfarin frequency was decreased to every other day. In the meantime, the physician had embarked on a healthier lifestyle, including significant changes in exercise habits and nutrition. When next evaluated, his INR had dropped to 0.9, even though the patient was utterly compliant with his warfarin regimen. None of his current medications were known to interact significantly with warfarin, so his cardiologist made inquiries about other recent changes the physician had made. The physician related his recent increase in aerobic exercise – 1/2 hour daily 4 days a week, and then mentioned his turnaround in dietary habits. He had increased his intake of whole grains, fruits, and especially leafy green vegetables. He had even started gardening, and had been cooking his way through a bumper crop of kale.

Discussion

This is an example of a pharmacodynamic interaction.

Warfarin is one of the most widely prescribed anticoagulant medications. Patients are placed on warfarin therapy for a variety of reasons, often for atrial fibrillation, cardiac valve replacement, or deep vein thromboses. Response to therapy is notoriously variable, and derangements in INR can have a number of unwanted side effects. Studies have shown that at any one time point only 50% to 60% of patients on warfarin therapy are within their therapeutic range.[2,5] Inhibition of the drug's activity can lead to subtherapeutic INR and increased likelihood of clotting and thromboemboli. Potentiation of warfarin can lead to a supratherapeutic INR and side effects of excessive anticoagulation like bleeding gums, hematomas, and gastrointestinal or intracranial bleeds.

Warfarin works by interfering with with vitamin K-dependent coagulation factors, specifically by inhibiting vitamin K epoxide reductase such that the resultant vitamin KH2 is not available as a substrate for carboxylation of coagulation factors II, VII, IX, and X, rendering them functionally inactive.[5] Patient response to warfarin can be influenced by individual genetic components, interactions with coadministered medications, and dietary vitamin K intake.[4] Vitamin K from plants, specifically the phylloquinone which is available as vitamin K1, can bypass the warfarin sensitive pathway and be reduced to vitamin KH2 without VK epoxide reductase.[1,3,5] Obviously this effect varies as diet varies, which is one of the reasons INR is so difficult to keep in the therapeutic range. A diet low in dietary vitamin K, for example in cases of malnutrition or patients with poor fat-soluble vitamin absorption (such as gastric bypass patients), can potentiate the activity of warfarin. Conversely, a diet rich in leafy greens (which have the highest phylloquinone content of all vegetables), or one that includes vitamin supplementation, can inhibit the action of warfarin. As in the above case, it is often when patients embark on a healthier lifestyle regimen that their vitamin K intake changes significantly from baseline. It is

Table 194.1 Vitamin K Content of Common Foods

300–600 mcg/serving	70–100 mcg/serving	>10 mcg/serving	10 mcg/serving
Kale	Brussels sprouts	Sauerkraut/Cabbage	Olive oil
Collard greens	Broccoli	Peas	Potatoes
Spinach	Asparagus	Lettuce	Carrots
Turnip or beet greens		Canola oil	
Rapini		Artichokes	
		Pasta sauce	
		Tomato paste	
		Peppers	
		Salsa	

[Based on data from Refs. [2, 6]]

those patients with poor baseline vitamin K status that are most susceptible to large changes in INR with relatively small changes in vitamin K intake, especially with regard to vitamin supplements.[6]

Which foods contribute most to dietary vitamin K content varies with food habits, some of which may be influenced by culture. The vitamin K content of common foods in shown in Table 194.1. The US Recommended Daily Allowance of vitamin K for men is 120 mcg/daily and for women is 90 mcg /daily. A recent Brazilian study showed that kidney beans and soy oil were the most significant contributors to dietary vitamin K in a Brazilian population.[2] This is notable because as kidney beans have relatively small amounts of phylloquinones, but are eaten in such quantity that they make a significant contribution to the total. Although it is commonly thought that leafy green vegetables are the primary source of vitamin K in the American diet, tomato products such as pasta sauce and salsa can be consumed in sufficient quantity to contribute significantly, even though they are relatively low in phylloquinone. Cooking foods in oil also aids vitamin K absorption as it is a fat-soluble vitamin. The cooking oil itself can also contribute to dietary phylloquinone content.

Take-Home Points

- Diet has a significant impact on INR, often more so than medications and over and above any variation in response attributable to genetic variation.
- Leafy greens such a broccoli, kale, and rapini have the highest levels of phylloquinones, but cooked tomatoes, which are more common in the American diet, can also contribute a significant amount of vitamin K.
- Diet changes daily, but patients are often on a regimented warfarin dosing schedule. The goal is not to have patients omit these healthy foods from

their diet entirely, but to regularly consume the same amount of phylloquinone-rich foods. This requires patient education regarding the vitamin K content of foods common in the particular patient's diet. Additionally, any addition of vitamin supplementation or sweeping revamps of dietary intake should be accompanied by more frequent monitoring of INR.

- For patients undergoing surgery, an INR should be obtained within 1 day of the scheduled procedure. A 2-week-old INR is not necessarily reflective of the patient's current state of anticoagulation as their diet may have changed significantly in the weeks leading up to surgery.
- If warfarin therapy is being held or modified in the week preceding an elective surgery, patients should be counseled not to make any changes in their diet or to start or stop vitamin supplementation.
- Anticoagulation therapy with warfarin can result in quite erratic patient blood levels of the drug that is affected by many factors. Clinicians should look carefully for signs of supratherapeutic or subtherapeutic levels of anticoagulation.

Summary

Interaction: pharmacodynamic
Substrates: warfarin and leafy green vegetables
Site of action: vitamin K-associated coagulation cascade
Clinical effect: loss of warfarin efficacy

References

1. Ansell J, Hirsh J, Hylek E, et al. Pharmacology and management of the vitamin K antagonists: American college of chest physicians evidence-based clinical practice guidelines (8th edition). Chest. 2008;133(6 Suppl):160S–98.
2. Custodio das Dores SM, Booth SL, Martini LA, et al. Relationship between diet and anticoagulant response to warfarin: a factor analysis. Eur J Nutr. 2007;46(3):147–54.
3. Damon M, Zhang N, Haytowitz D, et al. Phylloquinone (vitamin K1) content of vegetables. J Food Comp Anal. 2005;18:751–8.
4. Greenblatt DJ, von Moltke LL. Interaction of warfarin with drugs, natural substances, and foods. J Clin Pharmacol. 2005;45(2):127–32.
5. Hirsh J, Fuster V, Ansell J, et al. American Heart Association, American College of Cardiology Foundation. American heart Association/American college of cardiology foundation guide to warfarin therapy. Circulation. 2003;107(12):1692–711.
6. Johnson MA. Influence of vitamin K on anticoagulant therapy depends on vitamin K status and the source and chemical forms of vitamin K. Nutr Rev. 2005;63(3):91–7.

Delicious but Malicious

195

Licorice, spironolactone, hypokalemia

Eric Fox BA and Kirk Lalwani MD, FRCA, MCR

Abstract
This case discusses the synergistic pharmacodynamic interaction between the mineralocorticoid activity of licorice, and the diuretic effects of hydrochlorothiazide, each contributing to the development of hypokalemia.

Case

One December evening, a 57-year-old man was seen in the Emergency Department (ED) with concerns about his heart "racing" and having a hard time catching his breath. He collapsed in the triage area and was immediately rushed to a bay by the ED staff. He was found to be in ventricular fibrillation, and successfully treated with cardiopulmonary resuscitation and defibrillation. A 12-lead electrocardiogram (ECG) showed significant ST segment depression, but his cardiac enzymes were normal, and the ST depression had resolved on a repeat ECG. Serum potassium was dramatically low at 1.9 mmol/L but other laboratory values were normal. The patient was transferred to the intensive care unit (ICU) for monitoring and administration of intravenous (IV) potassium chloride.

On initial workup, the ICU doctor obtained the history that patient was generally healthy, but had been on a low dose of hydrochlorothiazide to manage mild hypertension. A careful history revealed that the patient had a 24-year-old son, who had recently graduated from college and been hired to do marketing for a famous licorice company in California. In addition to supplying his son with gainful employment and fulfilling work, the company also liberally supplied their employees with confectionery products from the company's lineup. The son had just recently started

E. Fox BA (✉)
College of Medicine, Oregon Health and Science University, Portland, OR, USA
e-mail: foxe@ohsu.ed

K. Lalwani MD, FRCA, MCR
Department of Anesthesiology & Perioperative Medicine,
Oregon Health and Science University, Portland, OR, USA

C. Marcucci et al. (eds.), *A Case Approach to Perioperative Drug-Drug Interactions*, DOI 10.1007/978-1-4614-7495-1_195

shipping his dad a 4-pound mega-tub of black licorice every week or two. The patient's wife occasionally helped out, but the patient happily shouldered the burden of consuming the licorice before the next tub arrived. The intensivist, who also harbored a love of licorice (especially at the movies), faintly recalled hearing of a woman who had survived cardiac arrest secondary to eating heroic quantities of licorice (4.5 pounds per week).[1] Following correction of his hypokalemia and detailed discussions about the dangers of excessive licorice consumption, the patient was discharged without further incident.

Discussion

This is an example of a synergistic pharmacodynamic interaction.

Licorice has seen liberal use for centuries as a food sweetener and natural remedy for ailments such as peptic ulcers, indigestion, cough, bronchitis, and sore throats.[2] However, excess licorice consumption can result in symptoms of mineralocorticoid excess, such as hypokalemia, metabolic alkalosis, sodium retention, hypertension, and suppression of the renin-angiotensin-aldosterone system.[3] Licorice contains glycyrrhizic acid (GZA), which imparts both the sweet flavor and pharmacodynamic properties of licorice.[4] GZA is hydrolyzed in the intestines into glycyrrhetic acid (GTA) and other active metabolites, which are potent inhibitors of 11-β-hydroxysteroid dehydrogenase (11β-OHSD).[3,4]

Mineralocorticoids such as aldosterone act in the kidney to promote potassium and hydrogen ion secretion as well as sodium bicarbonate reabsorption. The mineralocorticoid receptors also have a high affinity for glucocorticoids such as cortisol, which are generally present at much higher plasma concentrations than aldosterone. These circulating glucocorticoids are prevented from exerting effects at the renal mineralocorticoid receptors by the presence of tissue localized 11β-OHSD, which converts cortisol to its inactive form, cortisone, but has no effect on aldosterone. When 11β-OHSD is inhibited by GTA and other GZA metabolites, the body's endogenous cortisol is not deactivated in the kidneys and is permitted to act on the mineralocorticoid receptors, producing the observed symptoms of apparent mineralocorticoid excess.[3]

The patient in this case suffered from a tachydysrhythmia followed by ventricular fibrillation due to dramatic hypokalemia brought about by his recent boost in licorice consumption. His tendency to lose potassium from his kidneys as a result of licorice's mineralocorticoid activity was further exacerbated by his concurrent use of a thiazide diuretic. Hypokalemia is a well-known side effect of thiazide diuretics, which increase delivery of sodium ions to the collecting duct and drive the secretion of potassium ions through the Na/K exchanger. Concurrent use of a thiazide diuretic and large quantities of licorice overwhelmed the body's ability to regulate potassium balance, resulting in the dramatic presentation of hypokalemia observed above.

It should be noted that although various cardiac dysrhythmias have been observed due to excess licorice consumption, ventricular fibrillation is relatively rare.[1,5] Hypokalemia secondary to excess licorice consumption responds to treatment with spironolactone, a mineralocorticoid receptor antagonist, and is reversible upon discontinuation of the patient's licorice habit.[5]

Take-Home Points

- This case emphasizes the overwhelming importance of a thorough history. Without the full story, seemingly superfluous details (such as the consumption of pounds of licorice per week) might escape the clinician, setting the patient up for misdiagnosis, relapse, or unnecessary investigations.
- Licorice is found in a surprising array of products, including the obvious confectionaries and teas, but also some less obvious products such as liquors (absinthe, ouzo, pastis, Belgian beers, etc.), herbal cough syrups, throat lozenges, gum, chewing tobacco, and as a stiffening agent in pills.[3]
- While the mineralocorticoid effects of licorice have been well established, the connection may be difficult to ascertain in acute presentations of mineralocorticoid excess.
- Given the prevalence of licorice containing products, the morbidity associated with accidental excess consumption could be substantial.[3]

Summary

Interaction: pharmacodynamic
Substrates: licorice and hydrochlorothiazide
Site of action: nephron
Clinical effect: hypokalemia

References

1. Gerritsen KG, Meulenbelt J, Spiering W, et al. An unusual cause of ventricular fibrillation. Lancet. 2009;373:1144.

2. Isbrucker RA, Burdock GA. Risk and safety assessment on the consumption of licorice root (Glycyrrhiza sp.), its extract and powder as a food ingredient, with emphasis on the pharmacology and toxicology of glycyrrhizin. Regul Toxicol Pharmacol. 2006;46:167–92.
3. Olukoga A, Donaldson D. Liquorice and its health implications. J R Soc Promot Health. 2000;120:83–9.
4. Ploeger B, Mensinga T, Sips A, et al. A population physiologically based pharmacokinetic/pharmacodynamic model for the inhibition of 11-beta-hydroxysteroid dehydrogenase activity by glycyrrhetic acid. Toxicol Appl Pharmacol. 2001;170:46–55.
5. Quinkler M, Stewart PM. Hypertension and the cortisol-cortisone shuttle. J Clin Endocrinol Metab. 2003;88:2384–92.

I Just Can't Lick This Problem

196

Fatal Forty DDI: licorice, electrolytes, digoxin

Koshy M. Mathai MD, Michael P. Hutchens MD, and Robert G. Krohner MD

Abstract

This case discusses a complex pharmacodynamic interaction between digoxin and natural licorice, resulting in digoxin toxicity.

Case

A 55-year-old man with a history of hypertension, atrial fibrillation, congestive heart failure, and a distant knee arthroscopy presented for elective laparoscopic cholecystectomy. His medication list included digoxin. The anesthesiologist noted the patient appeared diaphoretic and lethargic. When asked about his last oral intake, the patient said he had been nauseated and vomited several times since eating a whole bag of his favorite natural licorice candy – a staple part of his diet – which he had nervously binged on the afternoon before surgery. Having recently read about the effects of natural licorice, the anesthesiologist ordered an electrocardiogram (EKG), which demonstrated frequent premature ventricular contractions and a 10 beat run of ventricular tachycardia. The anesthesiologist cancelled the elective surgery and obtained an emergent cardiology consult, which resulted in an admission to the medical intensive care unit and treatment for digoxin toxicity.

K.M. Mathai MD (✉)
Division of Pain Management, Department of Neurosurgery, West Virginia University, Morgantown, WV, USA
e-mail: KMMATHAI@hsc.wvu.edu

M.P. Hutchens MD
Department of Anesthesiology & Perioperative Medicine, Oregon Health & Science University, Portland, OR, USA

R.G. Krohner MD
Department of Anesthesiology, Magee-Womens Hospital of UPMC, University of Pittsburgh School of Medicine, Pittsburgh, PA, USA

C. Marcucci et al. (eds.), *A Case Approach to Perioperative Drug-Drug Interactions*, DOI 10.1007/978-1-4614-7495-1_196

Discussion

This is an example a complex pharmacodynamic interaction

Glycyrrhiza is a genus classified into more than 20 species, all of which have been known as licorice and long used as flavoring and natural medicine.[1] The popular herb is found across the world and is native to central and southwestern Asia and the Mediterranean, in both temperate and subtropical regions.[2] It has been used across cultures; there is documented use by the Assyrians, Egyptians, Chinese, Indians, Greeks, and Romans for respiratory tract infections and symptoms of hepatitis.[2] In fact, it has been used within the past 60 years as an anti-hepatitis agent.[3]

There are several active components of the licorice herb: triterpene saponins, flavonoids, isoflavonoids, and chalcones. Glycyrrhizic acid (GLA) or glycyrrhizin is the main biologically active compound.[1] Glycyrrhizic acid is approximately 50 times sweeter than sugar.[1]

GLA competitively binds the enzyme 11-ß-dehydrogenase, which forms together with 11-oxoreductase to make the enzyme complex 11ß-HSD. It is this complex that is responsible for the interconversion of cortisol and cortisone. The binding of 11-ß-dehydrogenase by GLA results in the inhibition of oxidation of cortisol. Mineralocorticoid receptors in the distal nephron are thus activated by cortisol; the previous enzyme complex no longer protects it. The consequence is a state of apparent mineralocorticoid excess in which there is suppressed renin and aldosterone production secondary to sodium retention and volume expansion.[4] This syndrome is known as pseudohyperaldosteronism. Clinically, it is marked by hypertension, hypokalemia, and metabolic alkalosis.[5] Digoxin acts via inhibition of the sodium-potassium ATPase, resulting in higher intracellular sodium concentrations and lower intracellular potassium concentration. Patients suffer symptoms of toxicity (nausea, anorexia, lethargy, and a wide variety of dysrhythmias) at lower serum digoxin levels when the serum potassium level is subnormal.[6]

Metabolism of oral glycyrrhizin is initiated by ß-D-glucuronidase supplied by intestinal bacteria. This transforms the herbal component into its active form, GLA. If administered by IV, it is metabolized by liver lysosomal ß-D-glucuronidase to 3-mono-glycuronidase, which is then excreted into the bile and intestine, where ultimately, bacteria metabolize it further into GLA. The active metabolite then undergoes enterohepatic recirculation versus fecal excretion.[5] Enterohepatic circulation may prolong metabolic effects. Furthermore, even though the body may be rid of the drug within a few days, existing electrolyte abnormalities and hypertension from chronic use may take weeks to resolve after discontinuation.[5]

Although little evidence supports therapy with GLA, it is present in many products. As a flavoring agent, it has been used in chewing gum, chocolate, candy, cigarettes/snuff, and as a mask for bitter aloe/quinine. It has been used in toothpastes, mouth rinses, and cosmetics.[5,7] In addition GLA has been used as treatment for adrenal insufficiency, aphthous ulcers, dermatitis, Crohn's disease, croup, gastrointestinal ulceration, herpes simplex virus, and viral hepatitis. It has even been shown to reduce the thickness of subcutaneous thigh fat.[8]

The potential interaction between licorice and digoxin resulting in toxicity is highlighted here. Generally, the use of GLA is cautioned or contraindicated in four groups:[9]

- patients on warfarin, NSAID, and antiplatelet agents, because GLA can have anti-platelet effects.
- patients on nitrofurantoin, as GLA can lead to increased excretion of the drug.
- patients taking antihypertensives, diuretics, digoxin, laxatives, steroids, or hormone replacement therapy because electrolyte imbalances can be made evident.
- women who are pregnant because the effects on fetal growth are not well-delineated.

Take-Home Points

- Recommendations for safe dosing of GLA are in dispute. The US FDA states that current evidence does not support a definitive recommendation regarding safe levels of GLA consumption, and to date, there is no evidence that glycyrrhizin at currently consumed levels is teratogenic or mutagenic.[9,10]
- The amount of GLA in many products, and thus, the amount consumed by a patient, is unpredictable. Laboratory analysis may not be available. A good history and physical, including a thorough review of systems, will be what tips the clinician off to major abnormalities, including the possibility of life-threatening dysrhythmias.
- If GLA use is identified, and abnormal potassium/volume status is recognized, discontinuation of GLA for 2 weeks will generally result in adequate clearance and normalization of the electrolyte/volume status.
- As a general rule, a dietary history and a history of herbal compound/supplement can only be useful additions to the patient interview.

Summary

Interaction: pharmacodynamic (complex)
Substrates: digoxin and natural licorice
Sites of action: multisystem
Clinical effect: digoxin toxicity

References

1. Asi MN, Hosseinzadeh H. Review of pharmacological effects of Glycyrrhiza sp. and its bioactive compounds. Phytother Res. 2008;22:709–24.
2. Fiore C, Eisenhut M, Krausse R, et al. Antiviral effects of Glycyrriza species. Phytother Res. 2008;22:141–8.
3. Shibata S. A drug over the millennia: pharmacognosy, chemistry, and pharmacology of licorice. J Pharm Soc Jpn. 2000;120(10):849–62.
4. van Gelderen CE, Bijlsma JA, van Dokkum W, et al. Glycyrrhizic acid: the assessment of a no effect level. Hum Exp Toxicol. 2000;19(8):434–9.
5. Don BR, Lo JC. Endocrine hypertension. In: Gardner DG, Shoback D, editors. Greenspan's basic and clinical endocrinology. 8th ed. New York: McGraw-Hill Medical; 2007.
6. Sundar S, Burma DP, Vaish SK. Digoxin toxicity and electrolytes: a correlative study. Acta Cardiol. 1983;38:115–23.
7. Andersen FA. Final report on the safety assessment of glycyrrhetinic acid, potassium glycyrrhetinate, disodium succinoyl glycyrrhetinate, glyceryl glycyrrhetinate, glycyrrhetinyl stearate, stearyl glycyrrhetinate, glycyrrhizic acid, ammonium glycyrrhizate, dipotassium glycyrrhizate, disodium glycyrrhizate, trisodium glycyrrhizate, methyl glycyrrhizate, and potassium glycyrrhizinate. Int J Toxicol. 2007;26 Suppl 2:79–112.
8. Armanini D, Nacamulli D, Francini-Pesenti F, et al. Glycyrrhetinic acid, the active principle of licorice, can reduce the thickness of subcutaneous thigh fat through topical application. Steroids. 2005;70(8):538–42.
9. Lexi-Comp 1978–2009. Licorice (Glycyrrhiza glabra): Natural drug information. In: Basow DS, editor. UpToDate, Waltham: UpToDate; 2009.
10. Eisenbrand G. Glycyrrhizin: opinion of the Senate Commission on Food Safety (SKLM) of the German Research Foundation (DFG)-(shortened version). Mol Nutr Food Res. 2006; 50:1087–8.
10. Isbruckera RA, Burdock GA. Risk and safety assessment on the consumption of Licorice root (Glycyrrhiza sp.), its extract and powder as a food ingredient, with emphasis on the pharmacology and toxicology of glycyrrhizin. Regul Toxicol Pharmacol. 2006;46(3):167–92.

Sommelier's Surprise

197

Tyramine-rich foods, MAOI drugs, monoamine oxidase

Charles Lin MD and Joseph F. Talarico DO

Abstract
This case discusses a food–drug interaction the monoamine oxidase inhibitor tranylcypromine and tyramine, resulting in hypertensive emergency.

Case

A 64-year-old woman arrived in the trauma bay after suffering a fracture of the humerus when her scooter hit a tree. The patient was scheduled for an emergent external fixation of the humerus and the anesthesiologist was called to do her preoperative evaluation. The patient stated that she was returning home from a wine and cheese party when her scooter hit a wet patch on the road. Her vital signs included heart rate of 110 beats per minute and blood pressure of 240/110 mm Hg, although she stated that her blood pressure was normally well controlled with lisinopril. She complained of a headache that preceded the accident, but was getting worse. Review of the radiologic imaging obtained in the emergency room showed a normal computed tomography (CT) of the head without hemorrhage. An electrocardiogram (ECG) showed sinus tachycardia but no ST-wave changes. Her only medications were lisinopril and tranylcypromine (Parnate®) for depression. Despite multiple doses of fentanyl for pain control, the patient remained hypertensive. Her hypertension responded well to labetalol and decreased to 140/90 mm Hg after 10 minutes. The surgeons were impatiently waiting for the anesthesiologist's decision to bring the patient back to the operating room.

C. Lin MD (✉)
Department of Anesthesiology, University of Pittsburgh Medical Center, Pittsburgh, PA, USA
e-mail: linc4@upmc.edu

J.F. Talarico DO
Department of Anesthesiology, UPMC Presbyterian, University of Pittsburgh Medical Center, Pittsburgh, PA, USA

C. Marcucci et al. (eds.), *A Case Approach to Perioperative Drug-Drug Interactions*, DOI 10.1007/978-1-4614-7495-1_197

Discussion

This an example of a pharmacodynamic interaction.

Monoamine oxidase inhibitors and concomitant consumption of tyramine-rich foods should always be considered in the differential diagnosis of hypertensive crisis during the perioperative period.

Hypertensive crises or emergencies are defined as systolic blood pressure greater than 180 mm Hg or diastolic blood pressures greater than 110 mm Hg with associated end-organ damage such as cerebral hemorrhage, altered level of consciousness, retinopathy, angina, myocardial infarction, or renal failure.[1] The distinct difference between a hypertensive crisis from a hypertensive urgency is the absence of end-organ damage, not the degree of blood pressure elevation.[1] The patient in this clinical vignette manifests symptoms suggestive of a hypertensive urgency, because there are no focal neurological findings, and the CT revealed no abnormalities. The management of hypertensive crises and urgencies primarily involve controlling the blood pressure to mitigate end-organ damage, as opposed to lowering the blood pressure to normal levels. In fact, lowering the blood pressure should be controlled to avoid precipitous decrease which may result in cardiac or neurological complications. With the exception of acute aortic dissection, the goal in the use of intravenous anti-hypertensive therapies is to reduce the diastolic blood pressure by 10% to 15% or to 110 mm Hg within 30 to 60 minutes.[1] Appropriate anti-hypertensive medications include esmolol, phentolamine, nitroglycerin, and nitroprusside because they share qualities of rapid onset and short duration that permit titration. Alternatively, rapid onset agents with longer duration of action, such as labetalol or hydralazine, can be used when carefully titrated to avoid a precipitous decrease in blood pressure.

In trauma patients such as the one described, there are many causes for hypertension, the most common including pain or preexisting hypertension. One often overlooked cause is drug–drug or food–drug interactions, in this case the concurrent consumption of tyramine-rich foods with monoamine oxidase inhibitors (MAOIs) such as tranylcypromine. Monoamine oxidase inhibitors treat the symptoms of depression by blocking the action of monoamine oxidase (MAO) enzymes that inhibit the metabolism of biogenic amines including tyramine, dopamine, norepinephrine, epinephrine, and serotonin. Monoamine oxidase exists as two subtypes: MAO-A and MAO-B. MAO-A inhibition in the brain produces the antidepressant effect, but it also potentiates the adverse hemodynamic effects associated with a tyramine-rich diet when it works in the periphery.[2] Selective MAO-B inhibition is used in the treatment of Parkinson's disease because one of its preferred substrates is dopamine. It also accounts for 80% of the total MAO activity in the basal ganglia.[2] Hypertensive crises or urgencies arise when monoamine oxidase inhibitors block the peripheral MAO-A enzymes from controlling tyramine levels in the blood during the consumption of tyramine-rich foods such as aged wine and cheese. Tyramine has 1/20th to 1/50th of the vasopressor potency of epinephrine, but treatment with

Table 197.1 Foods and Beverages with Possible Interaction with Monoamine Oxidase Inhibitors

Aged cheese	Aged and cured meat including: pepperoni, salami, mortadella		Banana Peel
Beer: bottled, canned or tapped	Fava and broad bean pods	Spoiled meat	Poultry and fish
Sauerkraut	Soy products	Wine: Red and white	Marmite yeast concentrate

[Based on data from Refs. [2, 5]]

MAOI therapy can increase the pressor response to tyramine by 30-fold.[3] In addition, tyramine causes the release of stored norepinephrine from peripheral adrenergic nerve terminals.[2] Tranylcypromine is the most common offending drug at doses of 20 to 50 mg daily; however, case reports of hypertensive crises caused by administration of phenelzine (Nardil®) and pargyline have also been published.[3]

Tyramine exists naturally in cheeses and is formed during bacterial protein degradation in meats; spoiled or preserved foods may contain large amounts of tyramine.[4] The following table provides a useful guide for dietary restrictions (Table 197.1).

Take-Home Points

- One commonly overlooked cause for hypertensive crises is the interaction between the patient's diet and monoamine oxidase inhibitors.
- Tyramine is a vasopressor compound found in many foods and several beverages.
- An intact monoamine oxidase system will metabolize tyramine to prevent significant end-organ catecholaminergic effects from tyramine.
- Administration of a monoamine oxidase inhibiting drug such as tranylcypromine, phenelzine, and pargyline will prevent the breakdown of tyramine. Thus, tyramine indigested in the diet acts as an exogenous catecholamine surge.
- Hypertensive crises and urgencies require immediate management to reduce the blood pressure by 10 to 15% with intravenous antihypertensive medications.
- To best care for our patients, it is important to elicit a thorough medical and medication history to ensure that pertinent albeit unlikely differential diagnoses are not missed.

- As a general rule, tyramine is found in foods that have been degraded or preserved including aged cheeses, wines, and meats.
- Tranylcypromine is the monoamine oxidase inhibitor most commonly reported to be involved in hypertensive crises and urgencies.

Summary

Interaction: pharmacodynamic
Substrates: tranylcypromine (MAOI) and tyramine
Mechanism/site of action: inhibition of the enzyme in the central nervous system leads to catecholamine surge at peripheral catecholamine receptors
Clinical effects: hypertensive urgency

References

1. Varon J, Marik PE. Diagnosis and management of hypertensive crises. Chest. 2000; 118:214–27.
2. Rapaport MH. Dietary restrictions and drug interactions with monoamine oxidase inhibitors: the state of the art. J Clin Psychiatry. 2007;68:42–6.
3. Brown C, Taniguchi G, Yip K. Monoamine oxidase inhibitor-tyramine interaction. J Clin Pharmacol. 1989;29:529–32.
4. Marcason W. What is the bottom line for dietary guideline when taking monoamine oxidase inhibitors? J Am Diet Assoc. 2005;105:163.
5. Gardner DM, Shulman KI, Walker SE, et al. The making of a user friendly MAOI diet. J Clin Psychiatry. 1996;57:99–104.

Dairy Carefully

198

Fatal Forty DDI: dairy, fluoroquinolone

Kristin Ondecko Ligda MD and Erin A. Sullivan MD

Abstract
This case discusses reduced bioavailability of a fluoroquinolone due to consumption of calcium-containing food (dairy products).

Case

A 56-year-old, unrestrained man was involved in a motor vehicle crash and was ejected from the vehicle. He was intubated at the scene and transferred by helicopter to a tertiary care center, where he was noted to have multiple musculoskeletal injuries including multiple rib fractures, left scapular fracture, a pelvic fracture, and a right femur fracture. Physical exam and imaging were negative for any additional injuries.

On post-trauma day 1, he underwent open reduction and internal fixation of his pelvic and femur fractures and had paravertebral nerve blocks placed for his rib fractures. The patient was extubated, started on aggressive pulmonary toilet, and had his diet advanced. Despite pulmonary toilet including incentive spirometry and pain control, the patient developed tachypnea with shallow breathing which he attributed to pain from his ribs and he remained in the intensive care unit (ICU). On post-trauma day 3, the patient developed a fever and productive cough and there was a concern for nosocomial versus community-acquired pneumonia. A sputum culture was obtained and he was started on empiric cefepime and vancomycin. He responded well to the empiric antibiotic therapy with improved respiratory function. On

K.O. Ligda MD (✉)
Department of Anesthesiology, UPMC Mercy Hospital, University of Pittsburgh Medical Center, Pittsburgh, PA, USA
e-mail: ondeckoligdakm@upmc.edu

E.A. Sullivan MD
Department of Anesthesiology, University of Pittsburgh Medical Center, Pittsburgh, PA, USA

C. Marcucci et al. (eds.), *A Case Approach to Perioperative Drug-Drug Interactions*, DOI 10.1007/978-1-4614-7495-1_198

post-trauma day 5, his sputum culture grew methicillin-susceptible *Staphylococcus aureus,* which was sensitive to levofloxacin. The antibiotic regimen was then changed to oral levofloxacin. The patient was transferred to the ward and continued his regular diet, including snacks of fortified cereal and milk, orange juice, and a few ice cream treats brought in by his wife. Three days later, the patient became tachypneic and febrile with cough again productive of purulent sputum.

Discussion

This is an example of a pharmacokinetic (malabsorption) interaction.

Dairy products contain calcium, a divalent cation that is stored in teeth and bones and is essential to health. Calcium functions as a cellular messenger and is intimately involved with muscle contraction. For the average adult, the recommended daily requirement for calcium, the most abundant mineral in our body, is 1000 mg.

Calcium interacts with drugs through chemical interactions. Chelation interactions between calcium and various drugs may decrease drug absorption. Fluoroquinolones are chelated by calcium, and this interaction may have resulted in the patient's decompensation.

In vitro studies have long supported the decreased availability of levofloxacin in the presence of calcium.[2] In recent studies in humans, levofloxacin and gatifloxacin have both been shown to have decreased bioavailability when consumed with calcium-fortified orange juice.[3,4] Whether this is directly related to a chelation reaction or related to intestinal absorption mechanisms in the presence of calcium-containing juice has yet to be determined.

Most of the package inserts for these antibiotics suggest that the patient take the fluoroquinolone at least 2 hours before or after consuming a calcium-containing supplement, antacid, or calcium-containing food. However, yogurt taken with moxifloxacin had little effect on drug absorption and pharmacokinetics in healthy volunteers and thus, no specific dairy-related recommendations are needed for this antibiotic agent.[5,6]

Tetracycline, and to a lesser extent, minocycline, are also less well absorbed after milk ingestion while phenytoin may exhibit decreased absorption in the presence of caseinate salts and calcium chloride.[7,8] Bisphosphonates (alendronate, risedronate, and ibandronate) have low bioavailability, and little drug is absorbed when given with any type of food or beverage other than water; this is especially problematic with dairy products. Levels of cefuroxime, a cephalosporin antibiotic, are decreased when taken with dairy products. Other cephalosporins do not appear to be affected.[1] In addition, methotrexate levels are decreased with the consumption of milk-rich foods.[3] As a general rule, administration of dairy products and/or calcium supplements should be separated from the interacting drug by at least 2 to 4 hours.

Given the popularity of calcium-fortified foods, this and similar studies suggest the need to include consumption of such products in evaluating bioequivalence and bioavailability. It is especially important that patients be monitored for decreased therapeutic effects of oral quinolones if these antibiotics are coadministered with oral calcium supplements.

Take-Home Points

- Dairy products, as well as calcium supplements and calcium-fortified foods, may cause impaired bioavailability of certain antibiotics such as some of the fluoroquinolones and tetracyclines.
- Decreased absorption and thus bioavailability is due to chelation between the functional groups and calcium.
- Moxifloxacin, a newer fluoroquinolone, does not appear to have altered pharmacokinetics when taken with dairy products.
- Other medications such as phenytoin may have decreased absorption when taken concomitantly with enteral nutrition.

Summary

Interaction: pharmacokinetic (malabsorption) secondary to chemical interaction (chelation)
Substrates: calcium, fluoroquinolones
Site of action: gut lumen
Clinical effect: decreased absorption leading to decreased bioavailability and drug efficacy

References

1. Bailey DG, Malcom J, Arnold O, et al. Grapefruit juice-drug interactions. Br J Clin Pharmacol. 2001;52(2):216–7.
2. Sultana N, Arayne MS, Sharif S. Levofloxacin interactions with essential and trace elements. Pak J Pharm Sci. 2004;17(2):67–76.
3. Wallace AW, Victory JM, Amsden GW. Lack of bioequivalence when levofloxacin and calcium-fortified orange juice are coadministered to healthy volunteers. J Clin Pharmacol. 2003;43(5):539–44.

4. Wallace AW, Victory JM, Amsden GW. Lack of bioequivalence of gatifloxacin when coadministered with calcium-fortified orange Juice in healthy volunteers. J Clin Pharmacol. 2003;43(1):92–6.
5. Stass H, Kubitza D. Effects of dairy products on the oral bioavailability of moxifloxacin, a novel 8-methoxyfluoroquinolone, in healthy volunteers. Clin Pharmacokinet. 2001;40(Supp 1):33–8.
6. Stass H, Wandel C. No significant interaction between moxifloxacin and calcium supplements in healthy volunteers. J Antimicrob Chemother. 1999;44(Suppl A):132.
7. Leyden JJ. Absorption of minocycline hydrochloride and tetracycline hydrochloride. Effect of food, milk and iron. J Am Acad Dermatol. 1985;12:308–12.
8. Smith OB, Longe RL, Altman RE, et al. Recovery of phenytoin from solutions of caseinate salts and calcium chloride. Am J Hosp Pharm. 1988;45(2):365–8.

Cold and Sick, Sick and Cold

199

Fiber, thyroxine replacement, malabsorption

A. Murat Kaynar MD, MPH and Nikhil K. Bhatnagar MD

Abstract

This case discusses a pharmacokinetic interaction between dietary fiber and oral thyroid replacement therapy resulting in decreased absorption and lack of efficacy of thyroid hormone replacement.

Case

It was 3 PM on a Friday afternoon when the anesthesiologist at a Level 1 trauma center was informed by the operating room desk that an open reduction/internal fixation had been scheduled in her room. She went to the preoperative holding area and found an obtunded, mildly obese 71-year-old women who had fallen at her nursing home and had fractured her right hip. Her son was with her and told the anesthesiologist that her mental status was pretty typical as she suffered from Alzheimer's dementia and had steady and significant cognitive decline in the past 6 months. The patient also had a history of hypertension, hypothyroidism, hypercholesterolemia, chronic constipation, coronary artery disease, and a myocardial infarction 10 years earlier. She had undergone a cholecystectomy and appendectomy 3 years earlier and a thyroidectomy 7 months earlier for thyroid cancer. The patient's medicines were significant for aspirin, simvastatin, metoprolol, levothyroxine, donepezil (Aricept®), colace, senna, and hydrochlorothiazide.

A.M. Kaynar MD, MPH (✉)
Departments of Critical Care Medicine and Anesthesiology,
University of Pittsburgh School of Medicine, Pittsburgh, PA, USA
e-mail: kaynarm@upmc.edu

N.K. Bhatnagar MD
Department of Anesthesiology, University of Pittsburgh Medical Center, Pittsburgh, PA, USA

C. Marcucci et al. (eds.), *A Case Approach to Perioperative Drug-Drug Interactions*, DOI 10.1007/978-1-4614-7495-1_199

On physical exam, the anesthesiologist noted puffiness in the patient's hands and face, swollen lips, thickened nose and nonpitting edema in her legs. Her vital signs were significant for a temperature of 34.8°C checked both orally and maxillary as well as a blood pressure of 90/70 mm Hg. The patient's labs were significant for a sodium of 123 millimoles/L and a glucose of 54 mg/dL.

At this point, the anesthesiologist asked the son whether his mother had been getting her thyroid replacement therapy. The son responded by saying that his mother got her levothyroxine (Synthroid®) every morning with her breakfast of a bran muffin and whole-wheat toast, which the nursing home served to prevent constipation. The anesthesiologist recommended that the case be postponed because the patient was suffering from myxedema coma secondary to inadequate thyroid hormone replacement. The patient was admitted to the intensive care unit (ICU) where she was given 100 mg of intravenous hydrocortisone. Laboratory studies were drawn including thyroid-stimulating hormone (TSH), tetraiodothyronine (T_4), triiodothyronine (T_3), cortisol, and adrenocorticotropic hormone (ACTH).

Discussion

This is an example of a pharmacokinetic interaction involving absorption or (more accurately) malabsorption.

More specifically, this is an example of how changes in fiber intake can decrease oral bioavailability of certain drugs.

Dietary fibers have many beneficial effects on the body.[1,2] Fiber promotes greater chewing and increases salivation, which protects the teeth. Soluble fiber, found in fruits, vegetables, rye, and oats, forms a gel-like compound in the stomach, which slows down gastric motility.[1–3] This results in early satiety and also prevents rapid fluctuations in blood sugar, which is particularly beneficial in diabetics. Insoluble fiber, found in cereal grains and vegetables, stimulates the intestinal mucosa and absorbs water and other waste products promoting better gastrointestinal health. Several studies demonstrate that high fiber diets, specifically the consumption of vegetables and fruits, lowers the risk for colorectal cancer.[1–4] Fiber in the gastrointestinal (GI) tract also binds dietary cholesterol, lowering low-density lipoprotein (LDL) cholesterol and reducing the risk for heart disease.

However, dramatic and rapid changes in amount and timing of fiber consumed can affect oral bioavailability of certain drugs like digoxin, levothyroxine, lithium, and statins.[5–8] In addition, the blood concentrations of certain electrolytes like magnesium, zinc, and calcium can also be affected by dramatic changes in fiber intake.[9–11] The mechanism of action is presumably that fiber in the GI tract binds these medications before they are absorbed into the blood stream, hence reducing the concentration of these medications to subtherapeutic levels. In studies of levothyroxine and digoxin, it was shown that blood concentrations of these drugs were not decreased if there was a time delay between consumption of a high-fiber meal and the taking of these medications.[7,8]

Synthroid should be taken in a fasting state preferably in the morning at least an hour before breakfast to prevent any dietary interactions.[12] In addition, several studies have shown that dietary fibers greatly affect the absorption of levothyroxine from the jejunum and terminal ileum so TSH and T_4 levels should be checked if there are any changes in timing and quantity of fiber consumption.[13] It should be noted that although dietary fiber will delay absorption of levothyroxine, synthetic fibers at doses found in over-the-counter supplements do not have a significant effect on levothyroxine absorption.[14]

In this clinical scenario, the increase in fiber as well as the simultaneous administration of a high fiber breakfast with levothyroxine resulted in inadequate absorption of the levothyroxine. Although myxedema coma is very uncommon because of the ease of checking TSH and T_4, older women with dementia are a special subset of patients that can be missed because the signs and symptoms of myxedema coma could be confused with natural aging in these patients.[15] Myxedema coma is an endocrine emergency with up to 40% mortality and all elective surgeries should be cancelled until the patient is medically managed.

Take-Home Points

- Often during perioperative evaluation, physicians fail to inquire about changes in diet. The reason is because changes in a diet are often subtle and the interactions with medications are overlooked. However, several foods interact with medications resulting in variations in concentrations of medications, for example levothyroxine and high-fiber diets.

- It is important for perioperative physicians to spend enough time with a patient the day of surgery in order to do a focused history and physical. This is often difficult with debilitated nursing home patients but the perioperative physician must remember that he or she is the last safety check for the patient before surgery and must therefore remain vigilant.

- High-fiber diets have several positive effects on the body and it is not wise to counsel patients to eliminate fiber from their diets before surgery. However, if a patient starts consuming significantly less or more fiber over a short period of time, it is important to enquire about their medications and make sure that there is time delay between meal times and when medications are taken. This is especially crucial for medications that have narrow therapeutic ranges and high toxicity profiles like levothyroxine and digoxin.

- Levothyroxine has many drug and food interactions and therefore should be taken in a fasting state.

- Myxedema coma is an endocrine emergency and surgery must be delayed until all the physiologic perturbations are corrected.

Summary

Interaction: pharmacokinetic (absorption)
Substrates: thyroxine
Site of action: intestinal mucosa
Inhibitor: dietary fiber
Clinical effects: decreased absorption and bioavailability of thyroxine with resulting hypothyroidism

References

1. Trock B, Lanza E, Greenwald P. Dietary fiber, vegetables, and colon cancer: critical review and meta-analyses of the epidemiologic evidence. J Natl Cancer Inst. 1980;82(8):650–61.
2. Ludwig DS, Pereira MA, Kroenke CH, et al. Dietary fiber, weight gain, and cardiovascular disease risk factors in young adults. JAMA. 1999;282:1539–46.
3. Anderson JW, Smith BM, Gustafson NJ. Health benefits and practical aspects of high-fiber diets. Am J Clin Nutr. 1994;59:1242S–7.
4. Nomura A, Wilkens LR, Murphy SP, et al. Association of vegetable, fruit, and grain intakes with colorectal cancer: the Multiethnic Cohort Study. Am J Clin Nutr. 2008;88:730–7.
5. Decker BC. Drug-nutrient interactions. In: Hendricks KM, Duggan C, editors. Manual of pediatric nutrition. 4th ed. Ontario: BC Decker; 2005.
6. Eussen SR, Rompelberg CJ, Andersson KE, et al. Simultaneous intake of oat bran and atorvastatin reduces their efficacy to lower lipid levels and atherosclerosis in LDLr–/– mice. Pharmacol Res. 2011;64(1):36–43.
7. Johnson BF, Rodin SM, Hoch K. The effect of dietary fiber on the bioavailability of digoxin in capsules. J Clin Pharmacol. 1987;27:487–90.
8. Bach-Huynk TG, Nayak JL, Soldin S, et al. Timing of levothyroxine administration affects serum thyrotropin concentrations. J Clin Endocrinol Metab. 2009;94(10):3905–12.
9. Wolf RL, Cauley JA, Baker CE, et al. Factors associated with calcium absorption efficiency in pre- and perimenopausal women. Am J Clin Nutr. 2000;72(2):466–71.
10. Lönnerdal B. Dietary factors influencing zinc absorption. J Nutr. 2000;130(5S Suppl):1378S–83.
11. Bohn T, Davidsson L, Walczyk T, et al. Phytic acid added to white-wheat bread inhibits fractional apparent magnesium absorption in humans. Am J Clin Nutr. 2004;79(3):418–23.
12. Liwanpo L, Hershman J. Conditions and drugs interfering with thyroxine absorption. Best Pract Res Clin Endocrinol Metab. 2009;23:781–92.
13. Liel Y, Harman-Boehm I, Shany S. Evidence for a clinically important adverse effect of fiber-enriched on the bioavailability of levothyroxine in adult hypothyroid patients. J Clin Endocrinol Metab. 1996;81:857–9.
14. Chiu AC, Sherman SI. Effects of pharmacologic fiber supplements on levothyroxine absorption. Thyroid. 1998;8:667–71.
15. Haupt M, Kurz A. Reversibility of dementia in hypothyroidism. J Neurol. 1993;240:333.

TPN (I): A Review and Two Interactions

200

TPN basics and complications

Lavinia Kolarcyzk MD and Patrick J. Forte MD

Abstract
This case discusses an interaction between ceftriaxone and total parenteral nutrition (TPN) minerals, resulting in line precipitation, and a pharmacodynamic interaction between TPN solution and a nondepolarizing neuromuscular blocking agent. Other implications of the use of TPN in the perioperative period are reviewed.

Case

A 57-year-old man with a history of hypertension and alcoholism who was 5 weeks status post-motor vehicle accident presented to the operating room (OR) for percutaneous gastrostomy tube placement. He had been slow to wean from mechanical ventilation and required long-term enteral access. He had been receiving total parenteral nutrition (TPN) through a peripherally inserted central catheter (PICC) for the past week. In the OR, the anesthesiologist decided to disconnect the patient's TPN infusion and to induce general anesthesia through the PICC line. The patient received vecuronium for neuromuscular blockade. The anesthesia team gave 1g of ceftriaxone per surgeon request and immediately noticed white crystals in the line. The anesthesia resident secured a peripheral intravenous (IV) line for the remainder of the case. At the end of the case, the patient was unable to be extubated. He appeared weak despite full reversal of neuromuscular blockade and was not following commands. Postoperative labs revealed serum phosphate of 500 mg/dL (low) and serum glucose of 24 mg/dL. After sign-out to the intensive care team, there was

L. Kolarcyzk MD (✉)
Department of Anesthesiology, University of North Carolina, Chapel Hill, NC, USA
e-mail: lkolarczyk@aims.unc.edu

P.J. Forte MD
Department of Anesthesiology, University of Pittsburgh Medical Center, Pittsburgh, PA, USA

C. Marcucci et al. (eds.), *A Case Approach to Perioperative Drug-Drug Interactions*, DOI 10.1007/978-1-4614-7495-1_200

considerable discussion as to the etiology of the patient's weakness and unresponsiveness.

Discussion

This is an example of a physicochemical drug interaction. There is also a pharmacodynamic interaction involving combined drug effects superimposed on metabolic derangements resulting in neuromuscular weakness.

The potential complications of TPN infusions include both catheter-related and metabolic complications. The most common of these complications are drug interactions with TPN infusions (eg, precipitation of many drugs with calcium in the TPN solution) and metabolic derangements (eg, hypophosphatemia, hypo, and hyperglycemia). The patient in the above case scenario likely was weak from hypophosphatemia and unresponsive from hypoglycemia. Hypophosphatemia is commonly seen in malnourished patients and can worsen during the initial "refeeding stage" of TPN infusion therapy. This is commonly referred to as "refeeding syndrome." Additionally, TPN infusions can contain large amounts of dextrose and/or insulin, which could be the etiology for hyperglycemia and hypoglycemia in the perioperative period. TPN is rightfully considered to be a feeding modality, but it is actually a cocktail of a number of drugs, all with potential actions and interactions in the perioperative period. It is imperative that the perioperative provider understand the issues surrounding TPN infusions and identify patients at greatest risk for these complications.

When enteral feeding is contraindicated (eg, ileus), TPN is used as a way to provide nutritional support until enteral feedings can be resumed. However, aggressive nutritional support of the malnourished patient may lead to refeeding syndrome. Patients at high risk for this include those patients with a body mass index <16, unintentional weight loss >15% in the past three to six months, little or no nutritional support for >10 days, history of alcohol use, chemotherapy, or diuretic use.[1]

Refeeding syndrome is defined as shifts in fluids and electrolytes that may occur in malnourished patients receiving either parenteral or enteral nutrition, with the most remarkable biochemical disturbance being severe hypophosphatemia.[2] The pathophysiology is believed to be due to the metabolic and hormonal changes that occur in the starvation state; conversion to the use of fat and protein for energy sources (instead of carbohydrates), increase in serum ketone bodies, and decreased gluconeogenesis. Minerals and cofactors such as potassium, phosphate, magnesium, and thiamine are depleted during the starvation state, but their serum levels may appear normal due to the intracellular contraction. When enteral or parental feedings are initiated, glycemia causes insulin secretion, which in turn stimulates glycogen, fat, and protein synthesis.[2] These metabolic processes require the key minerals and cofactors listed above, which leads to critically low levels of these already depleted minerals.

Standard TPN infusions contain a mixture of amino acids, dextrose, and electrolytes (including sodium, potassium, calcium, magnesium, and phosphorus). Additives include insulin, vitamins, and lipid emulsions. Any patient on TPN should be closely monitored throughout the perioperative period for metabolic abnormalities, with particular attention to serum glucose, phosphate, magnesium, and potassium.[3] For example, hypophosphatemia may present as respiratory muscle failure and/or myocardial dysfunction, as phosphate is a key mineral in synthesis of ATP, 2,3-diphosphoglycerate, and membrane phospholipids.[4]

Catheter-related issues with TPN infusions arise from the need for a dedicated central venous line for infusion. Central venous lines carry inherent risks for injury during placement, as well as risks for infection and thrombosis. Several issues and questions arise when the patient arrives in the OR with only a PICC line and a TPN infusion. For example, TPN infusions should not be administered through a peripheral line. TPN solution is often very concentrated (hyperosmolar), as to prevent volume overload in critically ill patients. Connecting concentrated TPN solution to a peripheral IV may lead to thrombophlebitis.[5]

It is also imperative that the clinician be aware and understand the incompatibility of many drugs with TPN solutions. The chemical stability of many antibiotics and other drugs is jeopardized when these medications are given in the same intravenous line with TPN. The components of TPN most likely to cause issues with drug–nutrient incompatibility include calcium, phosphorus, and magnesium. For example, ceftriaxone precipitates with the calcium in the TPN infusion. Other drugs that are deemed incompatible with TPN infusions include metronidazole, acyclovir, imipenem, sulfamethoxazole-trimethoprim, diazepam, phenytoin, and sodium bicarbonate[6] If there are no other intravenous access lines available, it is recommended that the TPN be briefly discontinued and the line flushed with 0.9% saline or D_5W before giving any of the above mentioned medications.[6]

Take-Home Points

- Standard TPN infusions contain a mixture of amino acids, dextrose, and electrolytes (including sodium, potassium, calcium, magnesium, and phosphorus). Additives include insulin, vitamins, and lipid emulsions.
- The anesthesiologist must be cognizant of these components of TPN infusions and the potential for the clinical consequences of metabolic derangements. In particular, careful attention must be made to serum phosphate and glucose levels in the perioperative period.

- TPN infusions require a dedicated central venous access line. These central lines can become infected and thrombosed.
- Certain medications commonly given in the perioperative period, including several antibiotics, are chemically incompatible with trace elements in TPN solutions and can cause catheter blockage and/or precipitation with TPN solutions.

Summary

Interaction 1: physicochemical
Substrates: trace minerals in TPN solution (calcium, phosphorus, and magnesium) and ceftriaxone
Mechanism: chemical precipitation
Clinical effects: formation of precipitate with line occlusion

Interaction 2: pharmacodynamic
Substrates: TPN solution and vecuronium
Mechanism: neuromuscular blockade in the face of TPN-induced hypophosphatemia
Clinical: prolonged clinical neuromuscular weakness

References

1. National Institute for Health and Clinical Excellence. Nutrition support in adults. Clinical guideline CG32. 2006. www.nice.org.uk. Last accessed 25 Sept 2012.
2. Mehanna HM, Moledina J, Travis J. Reefeeding syndrome: what it is, and how to prevent and treat it. BMJ. 2008;336:1495–8.
3. Schneider AGL, Biebuyck JF. Intraoperative management of patients receiving total parenteral nutrition. Clin Anaesthesiol. 1983;1:697.
4. Barash PG, Cullen BF, Stoelting RK. Clinical anesthesia. Philadelphia: Lippincott Williams & Wilkins; 2006. p. 194–202.
5. Gupta K, Chopra SC. Total parenteral nutrition. J Anaesthesiol Clin Pharmacol. 2008;24(2):137–46.
6. Shikora SA, Martindale RG, Schwaitzberg SB. Nutritional considerations in the intensive care unit: science, rationale, and practice. Dubuque: Kendall/Hunt Publishing Company; 2002. p. 154–5.

TPN (II): A Traumatic Case of Increased Metabolism 201

TPN, valproic acid

Erica D. Wittwer MD, PhD,
Wayne T. Nicholson MD, PharmD, MSc,
and Juraj Sprung MD, PhD

Abstract

This case discusses increased clearance of the antiepileptic drug valproic acid in patients with traumatic brain injury during administration of total parenteral nutrition, resulting in subtherapeutic valproic acid levels.

Case

Following a motor vehicle accident, a 66-year-old man was flown by air ambulance to a Level 1 trauma center. His injuries included a traumatic brain injury, depressed skull fracture, a penetrating wound to his abdomen, and multiple rib fractures. He had a history of hypertension, gastroesophageal reflux disease, and alcohol abuse. His medications included aspirin, atenolol, and omeprazole. He was intoxicated but initially responsive, however, his mental status deteriorated. He required emergent surgical intervention for subdural hematoma evacuation and repair of a ruptured small bowel. His abdomen was left open, and he was transported to the neurosurgical intensive care unit sedated and with his trachea intubated.

The patient was prescribed total parenteral nutrition (TPN) on postoperative day 2. On postoperative day 3, while he was still sedated, his nurse noted generalized muscle movement consistent with seizure activity which was confirmed by electroencephalograph (EEG). Intravenous lorazepam was administered with resolution of the seizure activity, and point sodium valproate prophylaxis was instituted. Sedation was maintained with a continuous fentanyl infusion and boluses of lorazepam. On postoperative days 5, 7, 9, and 11 he was brought to the operating room for

E.D. Wittwer MD, PhD (✉) • W.T. Nicholson MD, PharmD, MSc • J. Sprung MD, PhD
Department of Anesthesiology, Mayo Clinic, Rochester, MN, USA
e-mail: Wittwer.erica@mayo.edu

C. Marcucci et al. (eds.), *A Case Approach to Perioperative Drug-Drug Interactions*, DOI 10.1007/978-1-4614-7495-1_201

abdominal reexploration and lavage, and his abdomen was finally closed on postoperative day 13. Following abdominal closure his sedation was weaned, but shortly after he became responsive his seizure activity returned. A blood valproic acid level was found to be below the therapeutic level. The valproic acid dose was increased, and blood levels were checked daily for the following week and every 3 days thereafter with dose adjustments as needed to assure the level remained therapeutic.

He did well over the next several days, TPN was stopped, and he slowly resumed oral intake. Interestingly, it was noted that after TPN was discontinued his valproic acid dose needed to be reduced to maintain the level within the therapeutic range.

Discussion

This is an example of an alteration in pharmacokinetic drug handling.

Valproic acid and its derivatives are antiepileptic medications that are commonly used to treat a variety of seizure disorders as well as migraine, manic bipolar disorder, and posttraumatic epilepsy. As a simple fatty acid, metabolism is via oxidation and glucuronidation with very little drug excreted unchanged in the urine.

Since the initial successful use of TPN in 1968, it has become a commonly implemented technique for providing nutrition in patients unable to receive oral intake or enteral feedings. Although formulations of TPN vary, most include a combination of water, carbohydrates, amino acids, essential fatty acids, vitamins, and minerals. The formulation can be adjusted based on information obtained from laboratory values. Central venous access is required for TPN administration because of the concentrated nature of the solution and risk for peripheral vein thrombosis. However, although TPN is a valuable tool, it is not without risk. Complications of TPN include but are not limited to complications due to central venous access, hyper- or hypoglycemia, sepsis, liver dysfunction, electrolyte abnormalities, and cholecystitis.[1]

With administration of a solution that may alter liver function, albumin concentration, and plasma osmolality, it is not surprising that drug pharmacokinetics and pharmacodynamics are impacted via alterations in metabolism or protein binding. Little is known about interactions between TPN and drugs including valproic acid. Much of the evidence has come from case reports and anecdotes.[2] However, in a prospective study, Anderson and colleagues examined the variability in valproic acid pharmacokinetics after traumatic brain injury demonstrating an increased clearance of both total and unbound valproic acid in this population.[3] This study investigated factors affecting valproic acid clearance in patients with traumatic brain injury and found that clearance was increased on average more than 75% by 2 to 3 weeks post-injury, presumably due to the presence of increased blood levels

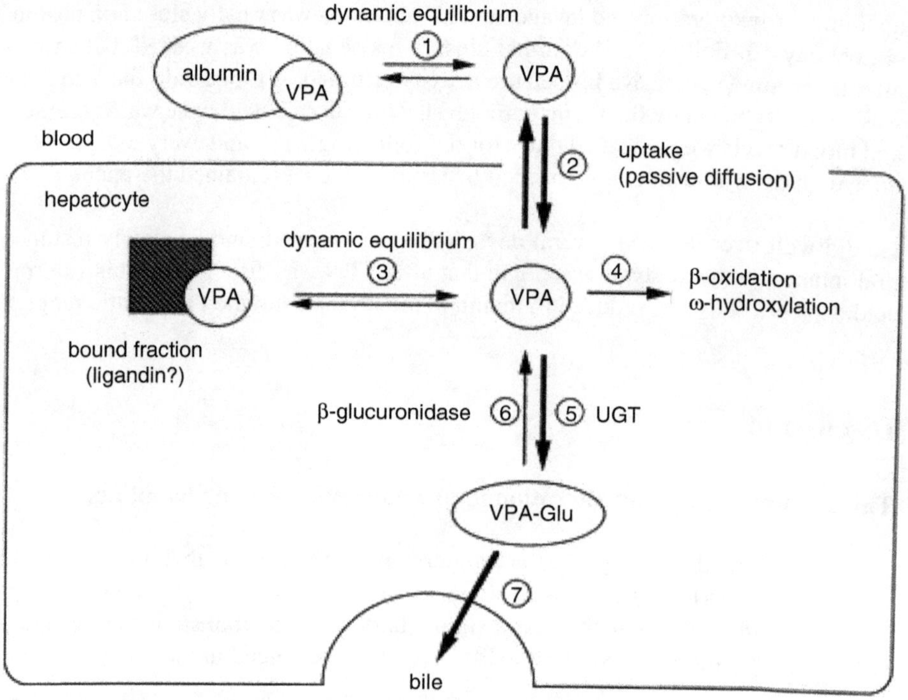

Fig. 201.1 Valproic acid (VPA) metabolism. Albumin decreases secondary to TPN or tube-feeding use. This decreases bound VPA to albumin. This subsequently increases free VPA. Increased hepatic metabolism *via* enzyme induction caused by traumatic brain injury or chronic ethanol use, results in increased VPA metabolism [Reprinted from Yamamura N, Imura K, Naganuma H et al. Panipenem, a carbapenem antibiotic, enhances the glucuronidation of intravenously administered valproic acid in rats. Drug Metab Dispos. 1999;27(6):724–30. With permission from American Society for Pharmacology and Experimental Therapeutics]

of proinflammatory mediators. While the severity of traumatic brain injury is associated *per se* with an increase in hepatic metabolism, increased total valproic acid clearance was also associated with decreased plasma albumin concentration, the presence of ethanol intoxication on admission, enteral feeding, and TPN. Increased unbound clearance (free valproic acid) is associated with older age, presence of ethanol on admission, increased severity of head injury, tube feeding, TPN, and if a postinjury neurosurgical procedure was performed.[3] Figure 201.1 illustrates the role of both plasma albumin and metabolism in valproic acid disposition.

Our 66-year-old patient in this scenario had decreased valproic acid serum concentrations due to increased clearance and required dose escalation to achieve seizure control. Because of the complexity of treatments for critically ill patients drug interactions could be considered inevitable. However, if we understand the nature of the interaction clinical decision making can be modified improving patient care.

Take-Home Points

- TPN is an important means of providing nutrition to patients in whom enteral feeding is not an option.
- Little is known about the effect of TPN on drug pharmacokinetics and pharmacodynamics.
- Valproic acid is a commonly used antiepileptic medication and it has been demonstrated that TPN use is associated with increased clearance in patients with traumatic brain injury.
- Using measurement of free valproic acid levels to guide dose adjustments may avoid complications due to low plasma level of the antiepileptic medication.

Summary

Interaction: pharmacokinetic
Substrates: TPN and valproate
Mechanism: unknown
Clinical effect: decrease in valproate levels

References

1. Total Parenteral Nutrition (TPN). The Merck Manual. 2009. http://www.merckmanuals.com/professional/sec01/ch003/ch003c.html. Last accessed 27 July 2012.
2. Salih MR, Bahari MB, Abd AY. Selected pharmacokinetic issues of the use of antiepileptic drugs and parenteral nutrition in critically ill patients. Nutr J. 2010;9:71.
3. Anderson GD, Temkin NR, Awan AB, et al. Effect of time, injury, age and ethanol on interpatient variability in valproic acid pharmacokinetics after traumatic brain injury. Clin Pharmacokinet. 2007;46:307–18.

Skin and Bones

202

Starvation, perioperative drugs

Mariam M. El-Baghdadi MD
and Ibtesam A. Hilmi MB, CHB, FRCA

Abstract
This case discusses the interplay of the physiologic derangements of starvation and the safe and appropriate administration of drugs in the perioperative period.

Case

A consultant anesthesiologist was paged to the emergency room. She arrived to find a 48-year-old cachectic homeless man in the trauma bay with an open right lower extremity wound and an obvious tibia and fibular fracture. When asked whether he had eaten within the past 12 hours, the patient disclosed that he had eaten nothing for the previous 3 days.

Discussion

This is a primer on the "interaction" between the physiologic derangements of starvation and the safe and appropriate administration of drugs in the perioperative period.

Patients with prolonged fasting states are malnourished. They are at risk for multi-organ system failure and subject to anesthetic complications if there is not adequate

M.M. El-Baghdadi MD (✉)
Department of Anesthesiology, University of Pittsburgh Medical Center, Pittsburgh, PA, USA
e-mail: melbaghdadi@yahoo.com

I.A. Hilmi MB, CHB, FRCA
Department of Anesthesiology, UPMC-Presbyterian Hospital, University of Pittsburgh Medical Center, Pittsburgh, PA, USA

C. Marcucci et al. (eds.), *A Case Approach to Perioperative Drug-Drug Interactions*, DOI 10.1007/978-1-4614-7495-1_202

adjustment for their prolonged fasting state. Prolonged fasting should be considered a possibility in patients who appear cachectic, are dysphagic, or have had recent weight loss. It is important to ask about prolonged fasting states as the condition may not reveal itself via physical appearance. Also, recognize that patients may opt to be in a prolonged fasting state due to religious conviction.

This homeless patient was in a prolonged fasting state. He had not eaten for 3 days, and was almost certainly malnourished prior to that, as suggested by his cachectic appearance. One of the most important initial considerations for our hypothetical malnourished patient was his volume status. Laboratory and physical findings that suggested this were low urine output, metabolic alkalosis if hypovolemia was mild, and lactic acidosis if hypovolemia was severe. Keep in mind that the serum creatinine, a product of muscle metabolism, can be low and misleading in the prolonged fasting state. Vasodilatory anesthetic induction agents and will have a profound effect in this patients like this who are significantly hypovolemic.

One of the major organs affected by prolonged fasting is the liver.[2] The liver is responsible for glucose homeostasis and synthesis of the proteins on which drug binding, coagulation, hydrolysis of ester linkages, and drug metabolism all depend. Laboratory findings can confirm the suspicion of malnutrition. Hepatocellular injury in patients with malnutrition results in an elevation in transaminases.[1] Case reports have described concentrations of alanine aminotransferase greater than 130 times the upper limit of normal. These abnormalities may be attributed to acute liver hypoperfusion from hypovolemia.[1]

If the liver is producing less protein, there will be fewer sites for drug binding; therefore, administered medications may be more effective than expected due to elevated levels of unbound agent. Because clearance of propofol exceeds hepatic blood flow, there is no impairment in clearance in liver disease but clearance can be slowed by low perfusion states. Etomidate hydrolysis occurs via hepatic microenzymes and plasma esterases. For decades, serum thiopental concentration has been known to parallel serum concentrations of albumin; higher free thiopental levels occur with lower levels of albumin.[6] Propofol at lower doses may therefore be the best induction choice in this malnourished patient.

Most providers would administer muscle relaxants during induction and maintenance of anesthesia in the case presented above. Remember, pseudocholinesterase is required for the hydrolysis of ester linkages in succinylcholine and local anesthetics with ester structures. Malnutrition has been established as a cause of acquired plasma cholinesterase deficiency. Unanticipated postoperative apnea following mivacurium administration in patients with previous uneventful exposure to both mivacurium and succinylcholine has resulted from acquired plasma cholinesterase deficiency.[5] Providers should keep this in mind and adjust doses accordingly.

Abnormalities in metabolic enzymes are common in outpatients with eating disorders combined with underweight status.[3] Additional abnormal laboratory findings may include prolonged prothrombin time and decreased platelet count. Providers may expect to see increased blood loss and potentially other complications such as pulmonary edema, acute renal failure, gastrointestinal bleeding, disseminated intravascular coagulation, and even death.[4]

Take-Home Points

- If there is a concern for malnutrition/prolonged fasting state, providers must recognize common abnormalities such as decreased plasma-binding proteins, decreased enzymes of metabolism, prolonged PT, and decreased platelet count.
- Patients in prolonged fasting states are hypovolemic and will have a more acute and exaggerated response to our vasodilatory anesthetics.
- Anesthesia providers must tailor the anesthetic; propofol may be the best induction choice as it exceeds hepatic blood flow and there is no impairment in clearance.
- Tailor induction and maintenance of pseudocholinesterase-dependent medications such as succinylcholine and ester local anesthetics. Providers will need to decrease dose as clearance is affected by acquired pseudocholinesterase deficiency in malnutrition.

Summary

Interaction: physiologic effects of starvation and perioperative drug administration

Effected mechanisms/sites of action: decreased plasma-protein binding, decreased plasma esterases, decreased hepatic microenzymes, acquired plasma cholinesterase deficiency

Clinical effects: various effects due to elevated unbound fractions of drugs, postoperative weakness, and apnea

References

1. Masayo T, Atsushi T, Motoe A, et al. Hepatocellular injuries observed in patients with an eating disorder prior to nutritional treatment. Intern Med. 2008;47:1447–50.
2. De Caprio C, Alfano A, Senatore I, et al. Severe acute liver damage in anorexia nervosa: two case reports. Nutrition. 2006;22:572–5.

3. Montagnese C, Scalfi L, Signorini A, et al. Cholinesterase and other serum liver enzymes in underweight outpatients with eating disorders. Int J Eat Disord. 2007;40(8):746–50.
4. Furuta S, Ozawa Y, Maejima K, et al. Anorexia nervosa with severe liver dysfunction and subsequent critical complications. Intern Med. 1999;38:575–9.
5. Niazi A, Leonard I, O'Kelly B. Prolonged neuromuscular blockade as a result of malnutrition induced pseudocholinesterase deficiency. J Clin Anesth. 2004;16:40–2.
6. Stoelting R. Pharmacology & physiology in anesthetic practice. Philadelphia: Lippincott Williams & Wilkins; 1999.

Enough to Make You Sick

203

Syrup of ipecac, general anesthesia

John Hache MD and Thomas M. Chalifoux MD

Abstract
This case discusses cardiomyopathy and muscle weakness secondary to syrup of ipecac abuse in a bulimic patient receiving general anesthesia.

Case

A 20-year-old college student presented to the operating room after breaking her ankle when she tripped on the library stairs during examination week. She was very anxious about missing her final exams. She denied any past medical history. Current medications included an oral contraceptive and occasional acetaminophen. She denied use of tobacco, alcohol, or illicit drugs. The physical examination was unremarkable. Emergency Department labs included a normal hemoglobin level and a negative drug screen.

General anesthesia was induced in the standard fashion and maintained with a volatile agent, supplemented with an opioid. During the case, mild hypotension responded to repeated fluid boluses. Frequent ectopic atrial and ventricular complexes were present on the electrocardiogram (ECG). Short runs of nonsustained ventricular tachycardia occurred throughout the case without causing hemodynamic instability. Near the end of the case, the oxygen saturation began to trend down despite measures to increase oxygen delivery and a small amount of pink frothy fluid was noted in the endotracheal tube. At completion of the surgery, sustained tetanus in response to peripheral nerve stimulation was demonstrated and neuromuscular blockade was antagonized. Despite being awake, the patient remained weak with

J. Hache MD (✉)
Department of Anesthesiology, University of Pittsburgh Medical Center, Pittsburgh, PA, USA
e-mail: johnhache@gmail.com

T.M. Chalifoux MD
Department of Anesthesiology, Magee-Womens Hospital Anesthesiology,
University of Pittsburgh School of Medicine, Pittsburgh, PA, USA

C. Marcucci et al. (eds.), *A Case Approach to Perioperative Drug-Drug Interactions*, DOI 10.1007/978-1-4614-7495-1_203

small spontaneous tidal volumes, weak handgrip, and inability to lift her head. She was taken to the intensive care unit with full mechanical ventilatory support. Further workup included a 12-lead ECG with low voltage QRS complexes and frequent ectopic ventricular and atrial complexes. An echocardiogram showed a poorly contracting left ventricle with an ejection fraction of 25% to 30%.

The cause of the cardiomyopathy remained elusive until the patient's condition improved and she was extubated several days later. She revealed that she had been "limiting her calories" by making herself vomit, especially after large meals. She often used syrup of ipecac, purchased in bulk over the Internet, to induce vomiting.

Discussion

This is an example of an "interaction" between the physiologic effects of chronic ingestion of syrup of ipecac, bulimia, and general anesthesia.

The prudent perioperative care provider is vigilant for cardiomyopathy, muscle weakness, and other physiologic derangements secondary to syrup of ipecac abuse in a bulimic patient receiving general anesthesia.

Syrup of ipecac was formerly recommended to induce vomiting after poisoning. The active ingredients are two alkaloids, cephaeline and emetine. Both act locally on the gastric mucosa and centrally act on the chemoreceptor trigger zone in the brainstem. Syrup of ipecac's efficacy in the treatment of poisoning has not been demonstrated however, and recently experts have recommended against its use.[1] Ipecac is available without a prescription and has been associated with abuse by patients with bulimia.

Chronic ingestion of syrup of ipecac can be toxic. The most serious manifestation can be cardiomyotoxicity, with death resulting from dysrhythmia or heart failure.[2,3] Skeletal muscles are also affected. Emetine-induced myopathy results from severe disruption of sarcomeres, inflammatory changes, and muscle fiber degeneration. With time, these changes may be reversible if syrup of ipecac use ends.[1,4] Metabolic derangements can also be present and contribute to cardiac morbidity. Loss of stomach acid establishes metabolic alkalosis and, often, compensatory depressed respiratory drive. Dehydration from vomiting, decreased oral intake, or possible diuretic abuse leads to increased serum aldosterone levels. The subsequent activation of the renin-aldosterone system and excessive potassium excretion by the kidneys establishes hypokalemia. Chronic hypokalemia may further damage the myocardium, in addition to the damage from chronic syrup of ipecac ingestion.[2,3] Patients with these metabolic derangements, combined with bradycardia and baseline preoperative hypotension, present significant challenges to safe anesthetic management.[4]

Ipecac use may be revealed on direct questioning, but if suspicion exists despite denial by the patient, laboratory assessment can confirm its use. Creatinine phosphokinase, lactate dehydrogenase, and transaminase levels may be increased and emetine can be detected in the urine and serum for several weeks after ingestion.[1]

Bulimic patients tend to be young women; however bulimia, can affect both men and older patients. Once identified, bulimic patients require careful preoperative evaluation and preparation. EKGs can provide valuable information. Common findings in the setting of syrup of ipecac abuse include atrioventricular block, ST- and T-wave changes, and findings consistent with hyponatremia. Electrolyte abnormalities may also contribute to prolonged QT interval and dysrhythmias such as wandering pacemaker, supraventricular tachycardia, and ventricular tachycardia. Hypokalemia can develop from repetitive vomiting or in patients suffering from volume depletion and dehydration.[4–6] A further consequence of profound electrolyte abnormalities is a reduction in the seizure threshold. In addition to routine electrolytes, calcium, magnesium, glucose, and phosphorus levels should be obtained.[7] If the patient complains of heart failure symptoms or admits to ipecac use, echocardiographic studies are indicated and elective cases should delayed if myocardial dysfunction or electrolyte abnormalities are discovered.

If significant preoperative cardiovascular involvement is suspected, invasive blood pressure monitoring may prove useful. In emergent or trauma cases, or if prolonged surgical time is expected, an arterial line will allow for blood gas and electrolyte monitoring in addition to close blood pressure monitoring.

For the anesthesiologist, examination of the oral cavity carries extra relevance in patients who self-induce vomiting. Identify and document damaged teeth. Protect at-risk teeth during laryngoscopy or instrumentation. Procedures that require instrumentation of the esophagus with probes, suction tubes, or scopes need to be done with extreme care and the risks and benefits should be weighed before placing these devices. Gastritis and reflux may not be uncovered on a routine review of symptoms, as these patients may not disclose complaints related to their disorder. The standard preoperative fasting guidelines may not ensure an empty stomach, as delayed gastric emptying, either from gastritis or from decreased metabolic rates seen in malnourished patients, may be present.[5] The combination of delayed gastric emptying and reflux places these patients at a significant risk for perioperative vomiting and aspiration of gastric contents. These problems become especially relevant during trauma or emergent cases. With decreased gastric emptying and an increased incidence of asymptomatic gastroesophageal reflux disease, a nonparticulate antacid such as sodium citrate may be useful. H_2-receptor antagonists may increase gastric pH. Promotility agents such as metoclopramide may improve gastric emptying.

Preoperative rehydration should be provided to hypovolemic patients, but should be performed cautiously in patients with cardiomyopathy. The optimization of electrolyte abnormalities should be initiated preoperatively, as these electrolyte abnormalities may prolong the effect of muscle relaxants and lead to dysrhythmias. In patients with either electrolyte abnormalities or a history of abusing syrup of ipecac, recovery from neuromuscular blockade should be carefully evaluated, with endotracheal extubation only attempted after full recovery has been demonstrated. Concern has been raised for the possibility of dysrhythmia associated with the antagonism of neuromuscular blockade, and the immediate availability of a defibrillator is warranted. Allowing these patients to spontaneously recover from paralytic agents without the use of reversal agents may be considered.[4,8]

Take-Home Points

- Muscle and cardiac damage can result from chronic syrup of ipecac abuse. The anesthetic implications will depend on the extent and severity of skeletal and cardiac muscle involvement. An ECG and an echocardiogram can provide vital information when managing these patients.

- Young healthy patients often require minimal preparation for anesthesia and surgery. However, bulimic patients, particularly those abusing syrup of ipecac or other agents, require more extensive preoperative evaluation. The identification of these patients may be difficult and physical exam findings may provide clues when assessing these patients.

- Fluid and electrolyte changes are commonly found with implications for increased sensitivity to neuromuscular blockade and cardiac dysrhythmias.

- Effects on the gastrointestinal system include decreased gastric emptying and esophageal pathology associated with self-induced vomiting. These patients cannot be assumed to have an empty stomach, even in cases where fasting time has been judged to be adequate. Preoperative preparation may include the use of nonparticulate antacids, H_2-receptor antagonists, and promotility agents. Esophageal pathology may result from repetitive vomiting, and the relative risks and merits of instrumenting the esophagus must be carefully considered.

Summary

Interaction: physiologic effects of syrup of ipecac use, bulimia, and general anesthesia

Effected mechanisms/sites of action: gastric mucosa, chemoreceptor zone in the brainstem, renin-aldosterone system

Clinical effects: neuromuscular weakness, exaggerated cardiodepressant effects of anesthetic agents, decreased seizure threshold

References

1. Silber TJ. Ipecac syrup abuse, morbidity, and mortality: isn't it time to repeal its over-the-counter status? J Adolesc Health. 2005;37:256–60.
2. Adler AG, Walinsky P, Krall RA, et al. Death resulting from ipecac syrup poisoning. JAMA. 1980;243:1927–8.
3. Dawson JA, Yager J. A case of abuse of syrup of ipecac resulting in death. J Am Coll Health. 1986;34:280–2.
4. Seller CA, Ravalia A. Anaesthetic implications of anorexia nervosa. Anaesthesia. 2003;58:437–43.
5. Yager J, Powers PS. Clinical manual of eating disorders. 1st ed. Washington, DC: American Psychiatric Pub; 2007.
6. Palla B, Litt IF. Medical complications of eating disorders in adolescents. Pediatrics. 1988;81:613–23.
7. Goldstein DJ. The management of eating disorders and obesity. 2nd ed. Totowa: Humana Press; 2005.
8. Arnold DE, Rose RJ, Stoddard P. Intraoperative cardiac dysrhythmias in a patient with bulimic anorexia nervosa. Anesthesiology. 1987;67:1003–5.

Determined and Desperate to Diet 204

Fatal Forty DDI: orlistat, warfarin

Lisa Chan MD and Kirk Lalwani MD, FRCA, MCR

Abstract
This case discusses the drug interactions between orlistat, vitamin K, and warfarin that lead to changes in coagulability.

Case

A sedentary, obese 39-year-old woman embarked on a drastic weight loss and exercise program prior to making an appointment to start treatment at an infertility clinic, as she had read that normalizing her weight would make an ensuing pregnancy safer and more likely to go to term. However, she was unable to even walk her bike up to the bike trail due to shortness of breath.

She reluctantly saw her primary care provider, who heard a loud murmur and sent her for a transthoracic echocardiogram (TTE). TTE showed a redundant mitral valve with severe regurgitation due to vegetations on the posterior leaflet. A workup for etiology came back negative, and she underwent a mechanical valve replacement of her mitral valve. Her surgery was uneventful as was her postoperative course.

The patient was started on warfarin and her International Normalized Ratio (INR) rose to therapeutic levels. Following treatment for a wound infection she was scheduled to be discharged on postoperative day 14, but that morning she was found coughing

L. Chan MD (✉)
Department of Pediatric Cardiac Anesthesiology,
Memorial Regional Hospital, Hollywood, FL, USA
e-mail: lisaychan@gmail.com

K. Lalwani MD, FRCA, MCR
Department of Anesthesiology & Perioperative Medicine,
Oregon Health and Science University, Portland, OR, USA

C. Marcucci et al. (eds.), *A Case Approach to Perioperative Drug-Drug Interactions*, DOI 10.1007/978-1-4614-7495-1_204

blood over the toilet. She confessed to purging, but only because she had not lost the weight in the hospital that she had hoped she would, despite secretly doubling, and tripling her usual dose. Once stabilized, she was transferred to inpatient cardiac rehabilitation under close observation by psychiatry, who discontinued her diet pills.

She was discharged from inpatient rehabilitation a few days later with her INR in the therapeutic range. However, the day after coming home, her mother found her confused, disoriented, and short of breath. In the emergency department, physical exam revealed a loud heart murmur, and an emergent TTE found a large clot on the mechanical valve. She was rushed to the OR and a decision was made to change out her clotted mechanical valve for a bioprosthetic one.[1] While on bypass, the anesthesiologist reviewed her chart more closely. An "event" note prior to her transfer mentioned she had used a diet pill called orlistat to help her purge. The anesthesiologist realized that orlistat prevented her from absorbing fat-soluble vitamins, which raised her INR quickly. At rehabilitation, her INR had begun to decrease rapidly despite aggressive warfarin dosing because she had stopped taking orlistat; the warfarin regimen was no longer adequate at the previous dosage, and despite increased dosing did not achieve sustained therapeutic levels in time to prevent thromboembolism.

Discussion

This is an example of a pharmacokinetic (absorption) drug–drug interaction.

Orlistat (trade name Alli® or Xenical® in the United States) is an FDA-approved over-the-counter drug to treat obesity. It is advertised as a diet supplement that is optimally used with a low-calorie diet for maximal weight-loss results. Orlistat prevents the breakdown of triglycerides in the gastrointestinal tract by inhibiting lipases, approximately 46% to 91% of pancreatic lipases and 51% to 81% of gastric lipases.[2] The breakdown products, monoglycerides and fatty acids, are what the body actually absorbs. When compared to those not taking orlistat, the mean maximum percentage of ingested fat excreted in the feces was 32% compared to 5%.[3] It is reported to have negligible systemic absorption.[4] Therefore, orlistat works by reducing the amount of dietary fat that the body is able to absorb from the gut.

Common side effects are steatorrhea, diarrhea, flatulence, and abdominal pain; other rare but serious effects that have been reported are pancreatitis, cholestatic hepatitis, and subacute liver failure. There seems to be no deleterious effect on the absorption of calcium, vitamin D, phosphorus, magnesium, iron, copper, or zinc balance. Studies have shown that while there are decreased levels of fat-soluble vitamins, the levels are usually still within normal limits.[5]

There are several means by which orlistat may interfere with other drugs. It can decrease the absorption of lipophilic drugs such as amiodarone, cyclosporine, thyroxine, and lamotrigine. Decreased absorption of fat-soluble vitamins leading to a raised INR in an elderly patient taking warfarin and orlistat has been reported.[6] Orlistat has also been suspected of binding directly to thyroxine in the gut, preventing its absorption. Lastly, it has been shown to augment the effects of antidiabetic drugs, leading to a risk for hypoglycemia.

Take-Home Points

- Orlistat is an over-the-counter dietary supplement that inhibits intestinal lipases from breaking down triglycerides for absorption.
- It may interfere with the absorption of fat-soluble vitamins resulting in potentiation of warfarin's anticoagulant effects as a result of reduction in absorption of vitamin K.
- Drug levels of the following should be monitored when coadministered with orlistat: warfarin, amiodarone, cyclosporin, lamotrigine, valproic acid, vigabatrin, gabapentin, and thyroxine.

Summary

Interaction: pharmacokinetic (absorption)
Substrate: warfarin
Mechanism/site of action: inhibition of intestinal lipases by Orlistat prevents absorption of fat-soluble vitamin K
Clinical effect: enhanced anticoagulant effect of warfarin

References

1. Masiello P, Mastrogiovanni G, Santoro G, et al. Early massive thrombosis of a mechanical mitral valve. Tex Heart Inst J. 1998;25:303–5.
2. Carriere F, Fenou C, Ransac S, et al. Inhibition of gastrointestinal lipolysis by orlistat during digestion of test meals in healthy volunteers. Am J Physiol Gastrointest Liver Physiol. 2001;28:G16–28.
3. Zhi J, Melia AT, Guerciolini R, et al. Retrospective population-based analysis of the dose-response (fecal fat excretion) relationship of orlistat in normal and obese volunteers. Clin Pharmacol Ther. 1994;56:82–5.
4. Zhi J, Melia AT, Funk C, et al. Metabolic profiles of minimally absorbed orlistat in obese/overweight volunteers. J Clin Pharmacol. 1996;36:1006–11.
5. Filippatos TD, Derdemezis CS, Gazi IF, et al. Orlistat-associated adverse effects and drug interactions. Drug Saf. 2008;31:53–65.
6. MacWalter RS, Fraser HW, Armstrong KM. Orlistat enhances warfarin effect. Ann Pharmacother. 2003;37(4):510–2.

XVIII

Drug–Drug Interactions Involving Spices and Supplements

Introduction

205

Kirk Lalwani MD, FRCA, MCR

Abstract
This section introduces drug–drug interactions involving spices and supplements.

"May they protect this man from the disease sent by the gods, the herbs whose father is the sky, whose mother is the earth, whose root is the ocean." *Hymn to all magic and medicinal plants: The Atharva Veda, circa 1200–900 B.C.E*

Plants are the basis of life as we know it. There are an estimated 380,000 species of plants, many of which have medicinal properties that are utilized in health care. Herbal medicine is a booming industry in many nations, with estimated 2007 herbal dietary supplement sales of $4.79 billion in the US alone.

There is a common misconception that these remedies are "natural", and therefore harmless. This may also be the reason that patients often do not voluntarily disclose their consumption of herbal supplements, unless questioned specifically about them. However, nothing is further from the truth regarding potential safety; published scientific literature describes numerous studies and case reports of interactions between a variety of herbal supplements and prescribed medications, with significant and sometimes fatal effects. These effects may occur as a result of induction or inhibition of cytochrome P450 enzymes, synergism or antagonism at receptor sites, alteration of bioavailability, or direct organ-specific toxicity. Some herbal supplements may have multiple effects via different mechanisms, some of which are poorly understood. For example, *Ginkgo biloba* is an inducer of cytochrome P450 (CYP) 2C19, which may lead to subtherapeutic levels of the antiepileptic drug phenytoin. It is also possibly an inducer of CYP2C9, producing decreases in tolbutamide levels and thus producing hyperglycemia. In patients on other antidiabetic drugs such as glyburide, it may cause a decrease in insulin levels, thus producing hyperglycemia through yet another mechanism. Finally, it can also cause serious

K. Lalwani MD, FRCA, MCR
Department of Anesthesiology & Perioperative Medicine,
Oregon Health and Science University, Portland, OR, USA
e-mail: lalwanik@ohsu.edu

C. Marcucci et al. (eds.), *A Case Approach to Perioperative Drug-Drug Interactions*, DOI 10.1007/978-1-4614-7495-1_205

bleeding in patients on anticoagulants as a result of its inhibition of platelet-activating factor, as well as by enhancing thrombolysis.

An additional difficulty is the popularity of herbal concoctions that may contain several different herbs in order to achieve a specific purpose, such as remedies for weight loss or depression. Confronted with these situations, practitioners should obtain details of each ingredient in order to prevent or diagnose potential interaction-related side effects.

This section explores some of the well-known herb drug interactions for which published clinical reports exist; it must be emphasized that Level I evidence for such interactions is rare. It is important to note that many additional potential interactions have been described based solely on *in vitro* studies; the absence of published clinical reports to support these interactions justify their exclusion from this book. On the other hand, the interactions highlighted in these chapters do not form a comprehensive list, but rather a selection of clinically relevant vignettes from which, it is hoped, the practitioner will acquire an awareness of the significance of these alternative remedies, and perhaps retain the more memorable or frequently encountered ones.

Caffeine Crash

206

Fatal Forty DDI: caffeine, ethinyl estradiol, ciprofloxacin, CYP1A2

Brian Gierl MD and Ryan Romeo MD

Abstract
This case discusses the pharmacokinetic interaction of caffeine, ethinyl estradiol, and ciprofloxacin, resulting in caffeine toxicity Caffeine is a cytochrome P450 1A2 substrate. Both ciprofloxacin and ethinyl estradiol inhibit 1A2. The physiologic effects of ingestion of high doses of caffeine are also reviewed.

Case

The patient was a 20-year-old female college student who was a restrained driver in a motor vehicle accident (MVA). She was belligerent and required intubation after being extracted from the vehicle. The patient vomited during the intubation. She had extensive knee swelling and deformity and was taken to the nearest trauma center for evaluation.

Her boyfriend reported that she had been up all night fretting and cramming for an oral examination. He also reported had a history of asthma, migraine headaches, and anaphylactic reaction to penicillin. Her medications included an oral contraceptive pill (OCP) and sumatriptan for migraine symptoms, which she had not taken recently as she had run out and did not have time to refill the prescription in the middle of finals week. He reluctantly reported that she had consumed four "no-dozing" maximum-strength tablets and three cans of "high-test" energy drinks in order to stay awake and review her notes. To stave off a headache, prior to the

B. Gierl MD (✉)
Department of Anesthesiology,
University of California San Diego, San Diego, CA, USA
e-mail: gierl.brian@gmail.com

R. Romeo MD
Department of Anesthesiology,
University of Pittsburgh School of Medicine, Pittsburgh, PA, USA

C. Marcucci et al. (eds.), *A Case Approach to Perioperative Drug-Drug Interactions*, DOI 10.1007/978-1-4614-7495-1_206

Table 206.1 Arterial Blood Gas

Species	Value
pH	7.10
P_aO_2 (mm Hg)	210
P_aCO_2 (mm Hg)	32
HCO_3^- (mEq)	18
Na+	139
K+	3.1
Hgb (g/dL)	11.2
HCT (%)	34
Lactate	7

examination, she took two ergotamine tartrate and caffeine (Cafergot®) tablets and repeated that dose midway through the examination. Her friend also reported that she "zoned out" and started shaking while she was driving, entering an intersection where another vehicle struck their vehicle on the driver's side.

The patient's left lower extremity was cyanotic and cold and she was taken to the operating room emergently for repair of her popliteal artery injury. Prior to incision, the anesthesiologist started ciprofloxacin as per the surgeon's request, due to the patient's penicillin allergy. The anesthesiologist also administered prophylactic albuterol down the patient's endotracheal tube for her asthma. After the infusion of 3 L of normal saline, she remained tachycardic and appeared flushed. He then checked an arterial blood gas that showed a metabolic acidosis. See Table 206.1.

The patient's blood pressure was stable with continued tachycardia and premature ventricular contractions, but after vascular repair the intraoperative angiogram showed continued poor flow to the lower limb. The anesthesiologist and surgeon decided to dose nicardipine for possible vasospasm and the vascular flow normalized shortly thereafter. Over the subsequent 24 to 48 hours, the patient's metabolic acidosis corrected and her potassium and lactate levels returned to baseline.

Discussion

This is an example of inhibitors added to a substrate.

This patient suffered from caffeine toxicity due to ingestion of several caffeine-containing over- the-counter (OTC) products as well as chronic oral contraceptive use that prolonged the half-life of the caffeine. Her caffeine ingestion combined with her sleep deprivation caused the seizure that led to the MVA. At the scene she demonstrated symptoms of caffeine intoxication, including tachycardia and dysphoria. Her popliteal artery injury required vascular surgery repair. Physical examination of a person who has ingested a large amount of caffeine may reveal agitation, restlessness, sweating, tachycardia, and a flushed face. Patients often complain of increased bowel motility and may present with aspiration.

Caffeine is naturally present in coffee, cola, tea, and cocoa. It is also the active component in guarana (also known as Brazilian cocoa or zoom) where it is present in concentrations of 3.6% to 5.8%. While the Food and Drug Administration limits the amount of caffeine in soft drinks to a maximum of 32.4 mg/6 oz, it does not regulate energy drinks, which may contain large amounts of caffeine. A single serving may provide up to 1000 mg of caffeine, which is the equivalent of 10 cups of coffee.[1]

Data are mixed regarding caffeine's impact on alertness. The US Army performed a series of studies to assess caffeine's impact on sleep-deprived individuals. After a period of sleep deprivation, caffeine increased vigilance without impacting recovery sleep, and improved psychomotor response speed and decreased subjective rating of sleepiness.[2] Some authors determined that caffeine only improved cognitive performance in subjects suffering from caffeine withdrawal, but others concluded that the benefit was a stimulant effect, independent of withdrawal.[3]

Caffeine increases seizure rates in persons susceptible to seizure and toxic doses of caffeine may cause seizures. A thorough analysis determined that the mechanism of methylxanthine-induced seizures may involve pyridoxine depletion as well as γ-aminobutyric acid (GABA) and adenosine inhibition. The anesthesiologist may employ caffeine clinically in patients undergoing electroconvulsive therapy (ECT) who do not achieve sufficient seizures despite maximal electrical stimulus.[4] Caffeine is the preferred methylxanthine because patients receiving theophylline to treat pulmonary disease have suffered status epilepticus during ECT. There was a trend to both a faster and higher rate of clinical response in patients treated with caffeine as an adjunct to ECT. Patients receiving caffeine before ECT have experienced cardiac dysrhythmias, anxiety, tremors and olfactory sensations.

Adenosine causes muscle vasodilation in areas of ischemia and by blocking this effect, caffeine may prevent vasodilation and is not recommended for patients undergoing vascular surgery.[5] For this patient, the high level of caffeine resulted in vasospasm that required treatment with a calcium channel blocker.

The prophylactic ciprofloxacin prolonged the symptom of tachycardia by inhibiting caffeine degradation. Like other methylxanthines, the liver metabolizes the majority of ingested caffeine via the P450 cytochrome (CYP) 1A2 enzyme.[6] Only ~5% is secreted in the urine by adults. The plasma half-life varies between 3 and 7 hours in adults and increases approximately twofold with elevated estrogen levels in the third trimester of pregnancy or with long term use of OCPs.[7] Cirrhosis, congestive heart failure, and pulmonary edema increase half-life, as does consumption of cimetidine, fluvoxamine, and other CYP1A2 inhibitors. Ciprofloxacin, as a potent inhibitor of 1A2, also increases the half-life of caffeine.[8,9]

Take-Home Points

- Caffeine has a multitude of significant physiological and pharmacologic effects.
- Caffeine is metabolized by CYP1A2.
- Ciprofloxacin and ethinyl estradiol are CYP1A2 inhibitors.
- The ingestion of high doses of caffeine and coadministration of CYP1A2 inhibitors can lead to caffeine toxicity and significant clinical sequelae including seizures and vasospasm.

Summary

Interaction: pharmacokinetic
Substrate: caffeine
Inhibitors: ethinyl estradiol and ciprofloxacin
Enzyme: CYP1A2
Clinical effect: caffeine toxicity

References

1. PDR for herbal medicines. 3rd edn. Montvale: Medical Economics; 2004.
2. Killgore WD, et al. Effects of dextroamphetamine, caffeine and modafinil on psychomotor vigilance test performance after 44 h of continuous wakefulness. J Sleep Res. 2008;17(3):309–21. Epub 2008 Jun 2.
3. Hewlett P. Effects of repeated doses of caffeine on performance and alertness: new data and secondary analyses. Hum Psychopharmacol. 2007;22(6):339–50.
4. Datto C, et al. Augmentation of seizure Induction in electroconvulsive therapy: a clinical reappraisal. J ECT. 2002;18(3):118–25.
5. Marshall JM. Adenosine and muscle vasodilatation in acute systemic hypoxia. Acta Physiol Scand. 2002;168(4):561–73.
6. Miners JO, Birkett DJ. The use of caffeine as a metabolic probe for human drug metabolizing enzymes. Gen Pharmacol. 1996;27(2):245–9.
7. Balogh A, Klinger G, Henschel L, et al. Influence of ethinylestradiol-containing combination oral contraceptives with gestodene or levonorgestrel on caffeine elimination. Eur J Clin Pharmacol. 1995;48(2):161–6.
8. Batty KT, Davis TM, Ilett KF, et al. The effect of ciprofloxacin on theophylline pharmacokinetics in healthy subjects. Br J Clin Pharmacol. 1995;39(3):305–11.
9. Mizuki Y, Fujiwara I, Yamaguchi T. Pharmacokinetic interactions related to the chemical structures of fluoroquinolones. J Antimicrob Chemother. 1996;(37 Suppl A):41–55.

207 Sad Sequelae

Fatal Forty DDI: dong quai, warfarin

Stacy L. Fairbanks MD

Abstract

This case discusses a pharmacodynamic interaction between warfarin and dong quai, resulting in potentiation of the anticoagulant effect of warfarin.

Case

A 31-year-old woman presented to the emergency room with severe abdominal cramping and vaginal bleeding. She described mild nausea and cramping over the past 4 to 6 weeks. She initially attributed this to the timing of her menstrual cycles, but admitted that she did not have a menstrual period last month, and the cramping had continued. On the morning of presentation, the patient awoke with vaginal bleeding and shoulder pain, as well as more severe abdominal pain. She stated that the bleeding was much heavier than her regular cycles.

The patient had undergone replacement of a bicuspid aortic valve with a mechanical prosthesis some years prior. Her warfarin dose and International Normalized Ratio (INR) had been considered stable. She also had a history of pelvic inflammatory disease in the distant past. She was married, with one child, and a nonsmoker.

Vital signs revealed an afebrile, tachycardic patient with an elevated blood pressure. The patient's hematocrit was 29%, and the ß-human chorionic gonadotropin was elevated. Her preoperative INR was 4.5. Abdominal ultrasound disclosed an ectopic pregnancy with severe intra-abdominal bleeding. On further close questioning, the patient admitted that she had begun taking the herbal supplement dong quai at the onset of mild cramping 6 weeks before admission, which was recommended by

S.L. Fairbanks MD
Department of Anesthesiology, University of Colorado, Denver, Denver, CO, USA
e-mail: stacyfairbanks@me.com; STACY.FAIRBANKS@UCDENVER.EDU

C. Marcucci et al. (eds.), *A Case Approach to Perioperative Drug-Drug Interactions*, DOI 10.1007/978-1-4614-7495-1_207

a friend for help with premenstrual syndrome symptoms. The patient was immediately seen by the hematology team, treated with prothrombin-complex concentrates for emergency correction of her coagulopathy and taken to the operating room for an emergency laparotomy.

Discussion

This is an example of a pharmacodynamic interaction.

Dong quai is a Chinese herbal supplement made from the root of *Salvia miltiorrhiza.* It is also known as *Angelica sinensis,* danggui, and tang-kuei. It is used most often for menstrual cramping, irregular menses, premenstrual syndrome and menopausal symptoms.[1,2] It is also used for treatment of infertility, neuralgias, migraines, anemia, hypertension, hepatitis, and is recommended for various cardiovascular diseases. Dong quai is available as tablets, injections, powders, teas, and alcohol extracts.[3]

In Southeast Asia, other *Angelica* species are sometimes substituted for dong quai. Most often these include *Angelica acutiloba*, which is predominantly found in Japan and *Angelica gigas*, which is mainly found in Korea. Though these species are similar, there is significant variation in the chemical composition between them.

Dong quai contains at least six coumarin derivatives and constituents. Coumarins are believed to promote vasodilatation, act as uterine stimulants, and have anti-inflammatory, antipyretic, antispasmodic, immunosuppressant, and estrogen-like effects. In addition, they possess antithrombotic, antiarrhythmic, phototoxic, and carcinogenic effects.[4]

Of the natural coumarin derivatives found in dong quai, ferulic acid and osthole have been show *in vivo* and *in vivo* to possess antithrombotic activity, and while there have been no case reports in the literature, it has been theorized that, in combination with NSAIDS, dong quai may potentiate the risk for bleeding.[2,5,6.]

An animal study revealed that dong quai taken alone did not affect prothrombin (PT) values during a 3-day treatment period in rabbits, but that warfarin and dong quai taken simultaneously caused mean PT values to increase significantly after only 2 days of concurrent dosing. After 4 days of concurrent warfarin and dong quai, PT values tripled. There was no difference in average plasma warfarin steady-state concentrations.[7]

Take-Home Points

- Dong quai can produce clinically significant potentiation of warfarin, with dramatic alterations in INR even in a patient with previously stable INR.
- Herbal supplements are not always pure, and may come in preparations that contain other herbal medications with significant side effects and/or drug interactions.
- If consumed alone, dong quai is not believed to increase INR; however, when combined with other antiplatelet or antithrombotic medications, a significant change in bleeding time may occur.

Summary

Interaction: pharmacodynamic
Substrates: warfarin and dong quai
Sites of action: variable extravascular spaces
Clinical effect: potentiating of the anticoagulant effect of warfarin

References

1. Heck AM, DeWitt BA, Lukes AL. Potential interactions between alternative therapies and warfarin. Am J Health Syst Pharm. 2000;57(13):1221–7.
2. Page RL, Lawrence D. Potentiation of warfarin by dong quai. Pharmacotherapy. 1999;19:870–6.
3. Zhu PDQ. Dong quai. Am J Chin Med. 1987;15:117–25.
4. Hebel SK, editor. The review of natural products. St. Louis: Facts and Comparisons; 1999.
5. Yin ZZ. The effect of dong quai (*Angelica sinsis*) and its ingredient ferulic acid on rat platelet aggregation and release of 5-HT. Acta Pharmaceutica Sinica. 1980;15:321–30.
6. Abebe W. Herbal medication: potential for adverse interactions with analgesic drugs. J Clin Pharm Ther. 2002;27:391–401.
7. Lo ACT, Chan K, Yeung JHK, et al. Danggui (*Angelica sinensis*) affects the pharmacodynamics but not the pharmacokinetics of warfarin in rabbits. Eur J Drug Metab Pharmacokinet. 1995;20:55–60.

The Scary Side of *Ginkgo biloba* Is No Match for an Anesthesia Superstar: Seizures

208

Fatal Forty DDI: *Ginkgo biloba*, phenytoin, CYP2C19

Shreya Patel MD and Kirk Lalwani MD, FRCA, MCR

Abstract

This case discusses the pharmacokinetic interaction between phenytoin and *Ginkgo biloba*, resulting in breakthrough seizures. Phenytoin is a cytochrome P450 2C19 substrate and *Ginkgo biloba* is a 2C19 inducer.

Case

The CA-2 on call one Saturday reported to the Emergency Department (ED) for an airway call. The patient was a 26-year-old female medical student with a history of epilepsy well controlled with phenytoin (Dilantin®, 300 mg/d) who had fallen from a height of 18 feet while bouldering one sunny afternoon in Arizona. The patient had sustained several scrapes and contusions to her right side and head and lost consciousness briefly. She complained of dyspnea, and her exam and conventional radiography revealed a rib fracture. Further questioning of the patient and her friend revealed that the patient did not remember falling, but her friend saw the patient exhibit seizure-like activity. Trying to impress the attending, the patient's friend, also a medical student, suggested hyponatremia and hypoglycemia as differential

S. Patel MD (✉)
Department of Anesthesiology,
University of Arizona College of Medicine, Phoenix, AZ, USA
e-mail: shreyap@email.arizona.edu; shreyap@gmail.com

K. Lalwani MD, FRCA, MCR
Department of Anesthesiology & Perioperative Medicine,
Oregon Health and Science University, Portland, OR, USA

C. Marcucci et al. (eds.), *A Case Approach to Perioperative Drug-Drug Interactions*, DOI 10.1007/978-1-4614-7495-1_208

diagnoses for the patient's seizure. The ED physician seemed convinced, however, the well-read anesthesia resident quietly urged the ED attending to continue to probe the patient about her medication history. It was the anesthesia resident, instead, who looked very impressive when the patient revealed that 2 weeks ago, she had started taking 120 mg/d of *Ginkgo biloba* to improve her memory, while studying for her in-service exams. After treatment and discharge, the patient was instructed to stop the *Ginkgo* supplements, study harder the natural way, and sleep more. She remained seizure-free on her usual dose of phenytoin.

Discussion

This is an example of an inducer added to a substrate.

Many commonly prescribed anticonvulsant drugs including phenytoin and valproate (Depakote®) are either primarily or secondarily metabolized by the cytochrome P450 (CYP) enzymes 2C9 and 2C19 enzyme systems.[1] *Ginkgo biloba* also has a significant inductive effect on CYP2C19.[2,3] The increased metabolism of the patient's anticonvulsant drugs over the course of 2 weeks led to subtherapeutic levels of her medication, with breakthrough seizure and resultant trauma. Furthermore, *Ginkgo* products, including *Ginkgo* nuts and possibly commercially available *Ginkgo biloba* (typically extract from the *Ginkgo biloba* tree leaves), may contain low levels of a potent neurotoxin, 4′-*O*-methoxypyridoxine (4′-MPN). 4′-MPN is capable of inducing convulsions by reducing γ-aminobutyric acid (GABA) levels.[4] Other case reports exist of breakthrough seizures associated with *Ginkgo* use that have proved fatal, and therefore the current recommendation is to not use *Ginkgo* products in conjunction with anticonvulsant medications.

Take-Home Points

- *Ginkgo biloba* is a commonly used herbal supplement to improve memory. It is a 2C19 inducer.
- *Ginkgo biloba* preparations may also contain neurotoxic compounds capable of inducing seizures by a GABA-mediated pathway.
- Phenytoin is a CYP2C19 (and also 2C9 substrate).
- The addition of *Ginkgo biloba* without an increase in phenytoin dose lowered phenytoin levels such that the seizure threshold was broached.

Summary

Interaction: pharmacokinetic
Substrate: phenytoin
Enzyme: CYP2C19
Inducer: *Ginkgo biloba*
Clinical effect: decreased phenytoin levels with resulting breakthrough seizure

References

1. Kupiec T, Raj V. Fatal seizures due to potential herb-drug interactions with Ginkgo Biloba. J Anal Toxicol. 2005;29:755–8.
2. Yin O, Tomlinson B, Waye M, et al. Pharmacogenetics and herb-drug interactions: experience with ginkgo biloba and omeprazole. Pharmacogenetics. 2004;14:841–50.
3. Izzard A, Ernst E. Interactions between herbal medicines and prescribed drugs: an updated systematic review. Drugs. 2009;69:1777–98.
4. Hu Z, Yang X, Ho PCL, et al. Herb-drug Interaction: a literature review. Drugs. 2005;65:1239–82.

209 The Scary Side of *Ginkgo biloba* Is No Match for an Anesthesia Superstar: Sugar

Ginkgo biloba, tolbutamide, CYP2C9

Shreya Patel MD and Kirk Lalwani MD, FRCA, MCR

Abstract
This case discusses the possible pharmacokinetic interaction between tolbutamide and *Ginkgo biloba*. *Ginkgo biloba* should be used with caution in the diabetic population.

Case

The same superstar anesthesia resident was in the Emergency Department (ED) again when a 54-year-old woman with type II diabetes was brought into the ED by her daughter because of increasing confusion and slurred speech. Her daughter reported that her mother took tolbutamide (1 g/d) and that her diabetes was typically managed on that dose. On her last annual checkup 2 weeks earlier, however, her HbA1c was reported as 9.5%; her mother attributed this to a new frozen yogurt shop that opened down the street. The dosage of tolbutamide was increased and the patient promised to watch her diet more carefully. Blood work revealed a blood glucose of 54 mg/dL. The same ED attending tipped his personal computing device at the resident as he asked the patient whether she had been taking *Ginkgo biloba*.

S. Patel MD (✉)
Department of Anesthesiology,
University of Arizona College of Medicine, Phoenix, AZ, USA
e-mail: shreyap@email.arizona.edu; shreyap@gmail.com

K. Lalwani MD, FRCA, MCR
Department of Anesthesiology & Perioperative Medicine,
Oregon Health and Science University, Portland, OR, USA

C. Marcucci et al. (eds.), *A Case Approach to Perioperative Drug-Drug Interactions*, DOI 10.1007/978-1-4614-7495-1_209

The patient revealed that she had been taking *Ginkgo* for 3 months prior to her annual visit and then she discontinued it when her tolbutamide dosage was increased, fearing adverse side effects.

Discussion

This is an example of a possible pharmacokinetic interaction (reversal of induction).

For this interaction we revisit the cytochrome P450 (CYP) system, particularly CYP2C9. The common sulfonylurea, tolbutamide, is partially metabolized by CYP2C9. There are some data suggesting an increase in the hypoglycemic action of tolbutamide *in vitro* and in animal models following exposure to *Ginkgo*.[1–3] These studies showed that *Ginkgo* acted as a 2C9 inhibitor, thus increasing tolbutamide concentrations and hypoglycemic activity. These results, however, have not translated as predictably to human studies. Currently two studies using healthy human volunteers and *Ginkgo* extract present conflicting results; one presenting an attenuation of tolbutamide's effect, which would produce hyperglycemia, and the other presenting a lack of any significant interaction with tolbutamide pharmacokinetics.[1,4]

The story doesn't end there for diabetics and *Ginkgo*. In diet-controlled patients with hyperinsulinemia, *Ginkgo* seems to have little effect. However, in those patients controlled with oral hypoglycemic agents such as glimepiride, glyburide, pioglitazone or rosiglitazone, *Ginkgo* seems to decrease insulin levels and leads to higher blood glucose levels after an oral glucose tolerance test (OGTT).[5] The same researchers also found that in patients with pancreatic exhaustion, *Ginkgo* could actually increase insulin and C-peptide levels, but there was no therapeutic change after an OGTT.[6]

It should be emphasized that the interactions with *Ginkgo* and insulin or other oral hypoglycemic drugs, especially those metabolized by the CYP2C9, are complex and poorly understood. Given the risk for hypoglycemic events similar to those seen in the case above, caution should be exercised when diabetic patients use *Ginkgo*. It should also be emphasized that many patients do not disclose their use of herbal products, and therefore a sudden change in a patient's previous disease course, laboratory results, or symptoms should raise the suspicion of herbal supplementation as a contributory factor.

Take-Home Points

- Tolbutamide is a CYP2C9 substrate.
- *In vivo* human studies show that *Ginkgo* slightly induces the metabolism of tolbutamide.
- *Ginkgo biloba* may act independently to decrease insulin levels
- Patients do not always readily disclose herbal and other supplements.

Summary

Interaction: pharmacokinetic (possible)
Substrate: tolbutamide
Enzyme: CYP2C9
Inducer: *Ginkgo biloba* (possible)
Clinical effect: possible

References

1. Mohutsky MA, Anderson GD, Miller JW, et al. *Ginkgo biloba*: evaluation of CYP2C9 drug interactions *in vitro* and *in vivo*. Am J Ther. 2006;13:24–31.
2. He N, Edeki T. The inhibitory effects of herbal components on CYP2C9 and CYP3A4 catalytic activities in human liver microsomes. Am J Ther. 2004;11:206–12.
3. Sugiyama T, Kubota Y, Shinozuka K, et al. Ginkgo biloba extract modifies hypoglycemic action of tolbutamide via hepatic cytochrome P450 mediated mechanism in aged rats. Life Sci. 2004;75:1113–22.
4. Uchida S, Yamada H, Li XD, et al. Effects of Ginkgo biloba extract on pharmacokinetics and pharmacodynamics of tolbutamide and midazolam in healthy volunteers. J Clin Pharmacol. 2006;46:1290–8.
5. Natural Medicines Comprehensive Database. GINKGO Monograph. http://www.naturaldatabase.com. Last accessed 4 Nov 2009.
6. Kudolo GB. The effect of 3-month ingestion of Ginkgo biloba extract (EGb 761) on pancreatic beta-cell function in response to glucose loading in individuals with non-insulin dependent diabetes mellitus. J Clin Pharmacol. 2001;41:600–11.

The Scary Side of *Ginkgo biloba* Is No Match for an Anesthesia Superstar: Subdural

210

Ginkgo biloba

Shreya Patel MD and Kirk Lalwani MD, FRCA, MCR

Abstract
This case discusses the possible pharmacodynamic interaction between *Ginkgo biloba* and anticoagulant drugs to produce bleeding.

Case

A 42-year-old male Aboriginal person who was an immigrant from Australia came to the Emergency Department (ED) complaining of a worsening headache and blurry vision. The headache started about 10 days earlier and was not associated with sensitivity to light or sound. He reported no recent trauma or stress. His past medical history revealed a mitral valve replacement secondary to rheumatic heart disease 3 years ago. He had since been on stable warfarin therapy with an International Normalized Ratio (INR) of 2.6 the previous month. Fearing an intracranial bleed, the ED physician ordered a head computed tomography (CT) scan and baseline coagulation studies. Surprisingly, the patient's PT, APTT, and platelet counts were all normal but the CT revealed a subdural hematoma. Still perplexed as to the cause of the bleed, the physician ordered detailed coagulation studies, which

S. Patel MD (✉)
Department of Anesthesiology, University of Arizona College of Medicine, Phoenix, AZ, USA
e-mail: shreyap@email.arizona.edu; shreyap@gmail.com

K. Lalwani MD, FRCA, MCR
Department of Anesthesiology & Perioperative Medicine, Oregon Health and Science University, Portland, OR, USA

C. Marcucci et al. (eds.), *A Case Approach to Perioperative Drug-Drug Interactions*, DOI 10.1007/978-1-4614-7495-1_210

revealed decreased platelet aggregation to collagen and prolonged *in vitro* bleeding times (PFA-100). The ED attending, who had been diligently doing his drug–drug interaction (DDI) reading in his off-hours, then thought to further question the patient and determined that he had started taking 85 mg/day of *Ginkgo biloba* 2 months earlier. After letting the surgical resident know he would need to call the posting desk to post the case for the subdural hematoma evacuation, the ED physician decided to write the case up as a case report and also called the anesthesia office to ask where he should have the a cake delivered, with thanks and compliments from the Emergency Department.

Discussion

This is an example of multiple complex pharmacodynamic interactions.

The primary active constituents of *Ginkgo* include flavonoids, terpenoids, and organic acids. Standard preparations of *Ginkgo biloba* extract exist as EGb 761 and contain 24% flavanoids, 6% terpenoids, and no more than 5 parts-million of toxic ginkgolic acids.[1] The terpenoid ginkgolide B is known to potently and directly inhibit platelet-activating factor (PAF) mediated platelet aggregation by binding to PAF receptors on platelet membranes. *Ginkgo* also has been shown to increase concentrations of endothelium-derived thrombolytics, including nitric oxide and prostacyclin.[2] Both of these effects can potentially have dramatic consequences on an already anticoagulated patient.

There are numerous case studies in the literature reporting bleeding with *Gingko* use either alone or in conjunction with anticoagulant drugs. Case reports show patients taking drugs that affect either platelet function or coagulation in addition to *Ginkgo* have experienced substantial bleeding. The most commonly implicated drugs are aspirin, warfarin, and ibuprofen, which have resulted in bilateral subdural hematomas, spontaneous hyphema, fatal intracerebral hemorrhages, perihepatic and vitreous hemorrhages, and postoperative bleeding.[2,3] The causal link between the *Ginkgo* and the bleeding was not definitively suggested in any case, though most cases reported no subsequent bleeding episodes after discontinuing the *Ginkgo*.

Furthermore, there are several reports in the literature of bleeding with *Ginkgo* use in patients who are not on any other anticoagulants. The causal link again cannot be proven, since many patients had other clinical risk factors including increased age, cirrhosis, and hypertension. In addition, the few small, randomized controlled studies that have been carried out did not find any association between *Ginkgo* and an increased risk of bleeding. It should be noted that all of these studies have had small sample sizes and short durations (majority fewer than 100 patients and less than 12 weeks), suggesting insufficient power to detect any association.[2] The current recommendation is to use caution when patients are concurrently using *Ginkgo* and any anticoagulants. *Ginkgo* should definitely be discontinued prior to surgery, but the recommendation varies between 36 hours and 14 days before surgery.[1,4,5]

Take-Home Points

- *Ginkgo biloba* has many pharmacologically active compounds.
- Among these is terpenoid ginkgolide B, which binds to a receptor on platelet membranes.
- Other constituents can increase circulating thrombolytics, including nitric oxide and thrombocyclin.
- Case reports have documented bleeding in anticoagulated patients on *Ginkgo* and in patients on *Ginkgo* alone, however, the causal link cannot be proven.
- Current thought is to discontinue *Ginkgo* before surgery.

Summary

Interactions: pharmacodynamic
Substrates: *Ginkgo biloba* constituents including terpenoid ginkgolide B
Receptor/site of action: platelet activating factor receptor
Clinical effect: possible causal effect of increased anticoagulation

References

1. Sierpina V, Wollschlaeger B, Blumenthal M. *Ginkgo biloba*. Am Fam Physician. 2003;68: 923–6.
2. Bent S, Goldberg H, Padula A, et al. Spontaneous bleeding associated with *Ginkgo biloba*: a case report and systematic review of the literature. J Gen Intern Med. 2005;20:657–61.
3. Bone KM. Potential interaction of *Ginkgo biloba* leaf with antiplatelet or anticoagulant drugs: what is the evidence? Mol Nutr Food Res. 2008;52:764–71.
4. Ang-Lee M, Moss J, Yuan C-S. Herbal medicines and perioperative care. JAMA. 2001;286:208–16.
5. Yagmur E, Piatkowski A, Groger A, et al. Bleeding complication under *Ginkgo biloba* medication. Am J Hematol. 2005;79(4):343–5.

"Khat" Unaware

211

Depletion of central and peripheral endogenous catecholamines

Brian D. Tompkins MD and Kirk Lalwani MD, FRCA, MCR

Abstract
This case discusses several issues pertinent to the perioperative period arising from chronic khat use.

Case

A 29-year-old woman of Somalian descent presented to the labor and delivery unit in active labor. Her nervous husband spoke only a small amount of English, enough for the labor team to learn that the he and his wife had recently immigrated from Somalia and that she was 9 months pregnant.

Following discussions with the patient via a Somalian interpreter, the anesthesia resident was called to place an epidural. The patient was tall and thin and epidural placement was uneventful. However, after the loading dose of bupivacaine, the patient became hypotensive and tachycardic. The resident administered intravenous ephedrine to raise the blood pressure and paged her attending. The hypotension persisted despite another dose of ephedrine, and the patient became diaphoretic, anxious, and pointed to her chest in obvious discomfort. As the tension in the room mounted, the labor nurse noted fetal distress on the monitor and called the obstetric resident who ran into the room, assessed the fetal heart tracing, and called for a stat Ceasarean section. After a rapid-sequence induction and intubation, the anesthesia attending decided to try some phenylephrine to counter the patient's continuing

B.D. Tompkins MD (✉)
Department of Anesthesiology and Critical Care, University of Pennsylvania Health System, Philadelphia, PA, USA
e-mail: brian.tompkins@uphs.upenn.edu; bdtompkins@yahoo.com

K. Lalwani MD, FRCA, MCR
Department of Anesthesiology & Perioperative Medicine, Oregon Health and Science University, Portland, OR, USA

C. Marcucci et al. (eds.), *A Case Approach to Perioperative Drug-Drug Interactions*, DOI 10.1007/978-1-4614-7495-1_211

hypotension. Immediate improvement in the blood pressure was noted, the C-section proceeded uneventfully, and a healthy baby girl was delivered.

Following completion of surgery, the patient had delayed emergence from the anesthetic. As the minutes ticked by, the obstetrician grew increasingly concerned and suggested a CT scan of the brain, but the anesthesia attending calmly picked up the blade of the laryngoscope and displayed it to the operating room team. It was discolored by adherent greenish leafy particles. "She may take a while to wake up. I think I know why all this happened. Let's discuss it later."

Discussion

This is an example of pharmacodynamic interaction at the neurotransmitter level.

More specifically, this case highlights an antagonistic pharmacodynamic interaction and the clinical issues arising from depletion of central and peripheral endogenous catecholamines secondary to chronic khat use resulting in refractory hypotension, resistance to indirect-acting sympathomimetic drugs such as ephedrine, and delayed anesthetic emergence.

Fresh leaves from the khat tree (*Catha edulis*) are chewed habitually by residents of Yemen, Somalia, Ethiopia, and others in East Africa. This habit continues in immigrants in Somali and Ethiopian communities in the United States, United Kingdom, and Europe.

Chewing khat produces a pleasurable, euphoric feeling that is attributed to the amphetamine–like constituents of the plant. Khat contains the pyrrolizidine alkaloids cathinone, cathine, and cathidine. Most of the effects of khat have been attributed to cathinone. Like amphetamines, cathinone causes sympathetic effects through the release of central and peripheral neuronal catecholamines.[1]

Acutely, khat chewing may result in tachycardia, hypertension, arrhythmias, myocardial ischemia, coronary vasospasm, and myocardial infarction.[2,3] These effects are especially pronounced within 4 hours of ingestion. Acute intoxication may also result in an increase in anesthetic requirements, aggressive behavior, and psychosis.[4]

Chronic khat use results in depletion of neuronal catecholamines, refractory hypotension, and resistance to indirect-acting sympathomimetic agents like ephedrine. Chronic use may also lead to the development of tolerance and cross-tolerance to other sympathomimetic agents, as well as hepatitis and nephropathy. Chronic khat users may also have decreased anesthetic requirements and delayed emergence from anesthesia.

Take-Home Points

- Acute ingestion of khat can cause tachycardia, hypertension, arrhythmias, coronary vasospasm, acute myocardial infarction, delayed gastric emptying, and psychosis.
- The pyrrolizidine alkaloids in khat, when used chronically, can cause depletion of central and neuronal catecholamines.
- Khat antagonizes the use of ephedrine and other indirect acting sympathomimetics. In the OR, chronic users of khat are at risk for refractory hypotension that may require treatment with direct-acting sympathomimetic agents.
- Following anesthesia, chronic khat users are at risk for delayed emergence from anesthesia probably as a result of decreased anesthetic requirements.

Summary

Interaction: pharmacodynamic
Substrates: pyrrolizidine alkaloids cathinone, cathine, cathidine
Mechanism/site of action: depletion of central and peripheral catecholamines
Clinical effects: refractory hypotension, tolerance to sympathomimetic agents, decreased anesthetic requirements

References

1. Graziani M, Milella MS, Nencini P. Khat chewing from the pharmacological point of view: an update. Subst Use Misuse. 2008;43(6):762–83.
2. Bamgbade OA. The perioperative implications of khat use. Eur J Anaesthesiol. 2008;25(2): 170–2.
3. Al-Motarreb A, Briancon S, Al-Jaber N, et al. Khat chewing is a risk factor for acute myocardial infarction: a case-control study. Br J Clin Pharmacol. 2005;59(5):574–81.
4. Odenwald M, Neuner F, Schauer M, et al. Khat use as risk factor for psychotic disorders: a cross-sectional and case-control study in Somalia. BMC Med. 2005;12:3–5.

Pain on the Plane

212

Fatal Forty DDI: ginseng, warfarin, CYP2C9

Lei Wu MD and Kirk Lalwani MD, FRCA, MCR

Abstract

This case discusses a pharmacokinetic interaction between warfarin and ginseng resulting in the decreased anticoagulant effect of warfarin. Warfarin is a cytochrome P450 2C9 substrate and ginseng is a 2C9 inducer.

Case

During a 15-hour flight home from a business trip to China, a 60-year-old man felt an intense pain develop in his left calf that reminded him of the deep vein thrombosis (DVT) he suffered 1 year previously. He was very worried, as his father had died of a pulmonary embolism.

In the Emergency Department (ED), he confirmed that because of his family and personal history, he had been on long-term anticoagulant therapy and his International Normalized Ratio (INR) had been well maintained on warfarin at 5 mg/d for the past 11 months. The INR was measured every two to five weeks and had ranged from 2.5 to 3.5 with the last measurement at 3.0 four weeks ago. Unfortunately, venous ultrasonography confirmed the resident's suspicion of DVT and laboratory studies showed a subtherapeutic INR of 1.3 (goal 2–3). The patient insisted he had been taking warfarin as prescribed.

L. Wu MD (✉)
Department of Radiology, USC Medical Center in Los Angeles,
Los Angeles, CA, USA
e-mail: lei.x.wu@gmail.com

K. Lalwani MD, FRCA, MCR
Department of Anesthesiology and Perioperative Medicine,
Oregon Health and Science University,
Portland, OR, USA

C. Marcucci et al. (eds.), *A Case Approach to Perioperative Drug-Drug Interactions*, DOI 10.1007/978-1-4614-7495-1_212

The ED resident was puzzled by the sudden decrease in a previously stable INR. No one answered in the anticoagulation clinic, so the resident called up to the intensive care unit to talk to the pharmacist. The pharmacist asked him to go over all medications, vitamins, and supplements the patient was taking. The patient denied any changes to his diet or medications, but did finally admit that he had started taking American ginseng 3 weeks earlier while in China after a coworker suggested that it would boost his immune system and give him energy. The resident called the ICU pharmacist back and, after a quick literature search, they decided to write up a case report on the herb–drug interaction between ginseng and warfarin.

Discussion

This is an example of an inducer added to a substrate.

The elimination of warfarin is primarily by hepatic metabolism. S-warfarin is metabolized to the inactive 7-hydroxywarfarin by the hepatic cytochrome P450 (CYP) 2C9 enzyme.[1] Its effective half-life ranges from 20 to 60 hours with a mean of 40 hours. Ginsenosides, the principal compounds in American ginseng, have been shown to reduce plasma warfarin levels and INR significantly by inducing hepatic CYP2C9 enzymes; more than 1 week is required to induce hepatic enzymes and to see any significant reduction in plasma warfarin and INR levels.[2]

In this patient's case, he had been taking ginseng for 3 weeks, long enough to induce the 2C9 enzyme and thus increase clearance of warfarin. The fact that he did not start any other new medication eliminates the possibility of other drug–drug interactions. Vitamin K interaction with warfarin also seems unlikely since the patient denied any sudden change in his diet. Discontinuation of ginseng would be expected to raise his INR back to therapeutic range within 2 weeks. In the mean time, the patient was treated acutely for his DVT with low-molecular-weight heparin, and his INR was closely monitored to ensure that discontinuation of ginseng resulted in return to adequate therapeutic levels.

Take-Home Points

- It is important to recognize that almost one in four perioperative patients use herbal supplements, and the majority of these patients will fail to disclose their use of herbs during routine preoperative assessment.[3,4]

- Since ginsenosides are the principal compounds in all ginseng products in various concentrations, other species of ginseng including Asian ginseng (*Panax ginseng*) and Siberian ginseng (*Eleutherococcus senticosus*) can also decrease the efficacy of warfarin and reduce the INR to dangerous levels.[5-7]

Summary

Interaction: pharmacokinetic
Substrate: warfarin
Enzyme: CYP2C9
Inducer: American ginseng
Clinical effect: decreased anticoagulant effect of warfarin

References

1. Kaminsky LS, Zhang ZY. Human P450 metabolism of warfarin. Pharmacol Ther. 1997;73(1):67–74.
2. Yuan CS, Wei G, Dey L, et al. Brief communication: American ginseng reduces warfarin's effect in healthy patients: a randomized, controlled trial. Ann Intern Med. 2004;141(1):23–7.
3. Tsen LC, Segal S, Pothier M, et al. Alternative medicine use in presurgical patients. Anesthesiology. 2000;93(1):148–51.
4. Kaye AD, Clarke RC, Sabar R, et al. Herbal medicines: current trends in anesthesiology practice – a hospital survey. J Clin Anesth. 2000;12(6):468–71.
5. Cui J, Garle M, Eneroth P, et al. What do commercial ginseng preparations contain? Lancet. 1994;344(8915):134.
6. Janetzky K, Morreale AP. Probable interaction between warfarin and ginseng. Am J Health Syst Pharm. 1997;54(6):692–3.
7. Rosado MF. Thrombosis of a prosthetic aortic valve disclosing a hazardous interaction between warfarin and a commercial ginseng product. Cardiology. 2003;99(2):111.

Ca va, c'est Kava

213

Kava, carbidopa-levodopa, dopamine receptors

Solina Tith MD and Kirk Lalwani MD, FRCA, MCR

Abstract

This case discusses a pharmacodynamic interaction between the dopamine agonist levodopa and the dopamine receptor antagonist and supplement kava, resulting in increased Parkinsonian symptoms

Case

A 65-year-old woman originally from the French Polynesian island of Moorea had suffered from Parkinson's disease for the past 15 years. She was a retired seamstress and lived with her daughter, a high school French teacher. The patient's symptoms of tremor, rigidity, shuffling gait, and masked facies had been well controlled with increasing doses of carbidopa-levodopa. At her last annual visit to her primary care physician approximately 7 months ago, the dose of her maintenance carbidopa-levodopa had been increased to 25 to 100 mg 5 times daily.

One night the patient tripped on a rug while setting the table for dinner and broke her arm. Her daughter returned home to find her mother on the floor complaining of arm pain but oddly without painful facial expression, and brought her to the Emergency Department (ED). Apparently the patient had experienced a particularly severe "off" period, which manifested as difficulty walking and rigidity. The daughter reported to the consultant anesthesiologist that her mother had started taking kava a couple of months prior to treat anxiety and leg pain. The patient had not informed her primary care physician of this new remedy, because she did not consider kava to be a drug. However, the patient had noticed "off" periods of

S. Tith MD (✉)
Department of Anesthesiology and Pain Medicine, University of Washington, Seattle, WA, USA
e-mail: solina@uw.edu; solina.tith@gmail.com

K. Lalwani MD, FRCA, MCR
Department of Anesthesiology & Perioperative Medicine, Oregon Health and Science University, Portland, OR, USA

C. Marcucci et al. (eds.), *A Case Approach to Perioperative Drug-Drug Interactions*, DOI 10.1007/978-1-4614-7495-1_213

increasing duration and severity in the past week or so with increasing tremor. The ED physician splinted the patient's arm, and admitted the patient for open reduction and internal fixation of her humeral fracture. The anesthesiologist instructed the patient to discontinue the use of kava indefinitely and to inform her physicians of any new herbal remedies.

Discussion

This is an example of a pharmacodynamic interaction.

Kava is derived from the plant *Piper methysticum*, and has gained popularity as an anxiolytic and sedative. The kavalactones appear to be the source of the pharmacological activity of kava, and have dose-dependent effects on the central nervous system (CNS), including antiepileptic, neuroprotective, and local anesthetic properties.[1–3] Adverse effects generally do not occur at therapeutic dosages of kava. At supra-therapeutic doses, mild gastrointestinal disturbances, visual-accommodation disorders, pupil dilation, and disorders of oculomotor equilibrium have been reported. Toxic dosages can cause progressive ataxia, muscle weakness, and ascending paralysis. "Kava dermopathy," characterized by yellow discoloration of the skin, and fish scale-like lesions on the palms of the hands, soles of the feet, forearms, back, and shins, may also occur following ingestion of toxic doses.[4]

Kava also has central dopamine receptor antagonist activity that reduces the activity of the anti-Parkinsonian drug levodopa.[1,2,5,6] The severe "off" period experienced by the Parkinson's patient was probably caused by its anti-dopaminergic effects. Kava also inhibits cytochrome P450 (CYP) enzymes such as CYP1A2, 2C9, 2C19, 2D6, and 3A4, which are responsible for the metabolism of many pharmaceutical agents.[7]

Studies have suggested that kava has therapeutic potential in the treatment of anxiety.[8,9] A Cochrane meta-analysis found that although kava extract is an effective symptomatic treatment for anxiety when compared to placebo, the size of the effect seems small.[10] Data in several studies suggest that kava is relatively safe for short-term treatment (1 to 24 weeks) of anxiety, and that kava is well tolerated by most users, but long-term trials with larger sample sizes are needed.[10,11] Analysis of several studies found that when taken as recommended, kava was rarely associated with hepatotoxicity; however, overdose, prolonged treatment, and combination with other medications increase the risk.[7] Kava may also be an effective sedative-hypnotic by potentiating γ-aminobutyric acid (GABA) neurotransmission.[3] Thus, kava may have additive effects with benzodiazepines, since both act on the same receptors and on the same areas of the central nervous system. Such an interaction has been reported to cause a semicomatose state.[1,2] Kava may also improve the quality of sleep in humans, and may be used as a centrally acting muscle relaxant.[4]

Take-Home Points

- Kava has antidopaminergic effects that may interact with drugs such as levodopa in patients with Parkinson's disease, resulting in worsening of symptoms or an increase in "off" periods.
- Kava is a popular herbal remedy for anxiety, and is prescribed for its sedative and skeletal muscle relaxant actions.
- Kava may potentiate the effects of alcohol and benzodiazepines, leading to increased levels of sedation and a decreased level of consciousness.
- Kava may play a role in pharmacokinetic drug–drug interactions mediated by a number of P450 subenzymes.[12]

Summary

Interaction: pharmacodynamic
Substrates: levodopa (agonist) and kava (antagonist)
Site of action: central dopamine receptors
Clinical effect: increased Parkinsonian symptoms

References

1. Izzo AA, Ernst E. Interactions between herbal medicines and prescribed drugs: a systematic review. Drugs. 2001;61(15):2163–75.
2. Izzo AA. Herb–drug interactions: an overview of the clinical evidence. Fundam Clin Pharmacol. 2005;19(1):1–16.
3. Ang-Lee MK, Moss J, Yuan CS. Herbal medicines and perioperative care. JAMA. 2001;286(2):208–16.
4. Pepping J. Kava: *Piper methysticum*. Am J Health Syst Pharm. 1999;56(10):957–8, 960.
5. Schelosky L, Raffauf C, Jendroska K, et al. Kava and dopamine antagonism. J Neurol Neurosurg Psychiatry. 1995;58(5):639–40.
6. Meseguer E, Taboada R, Sánchez V, et al. Life-threatening parkinsonism induced by kava-kava. Mov Disord. 2002;17(1):195–6.
7. Teschke R, Schwarzenboeck A, Hennermann KH. Kava hepatotoxicity: a clinical survey and critical analysis of 26 suspected cases. Eur J Gastroenterol Hepatol. 2008;20(12):1182–93.
8. Lindenberg D, Pitule-Schodel H. D. L-kavain in comparison with oxazepam in anxiety disorders. A double-blind study of clinical effectiveness. Fortschr Med. 1990;108(2):49–50,53–4.
9. Woelk H, Kapoula S, Lehrl S, et al. Treatment of patients suffering from anxiety—double-blind study: kava special extract versus benzodiazepines. Z Allgemeinmed. 1993;69:271–7.
10. Pittler MH, Ernst E. Kava extract for treating anxiety. Cochrane Database Syst Rev. 2003;(1):CD003383.
11. Stevinson C, Huntley A, Ernst E. A systematic review of the safety of kava extract in the treatment of anxiety. Drug Saf. 2002;25(4):251–61.
12. Mathews JM, Etheridge AS, Black SR. Inhibition of human cytochrome P450 activities by kava extract and kavalactones. Drug Metab Dispos. 2002;30(11):1153–7.

Summertime and the Herbals are Hot

214

Fatal Forty DDI: goldenseal, amitriptyline, CYP2D6, CYP3A4

Jessica Miller MD, BM and Leelee Thames MD

Abstract
This case discusses the pharmacokinetic interaction between amitriptyline and goldenseal, leading to tricyclic antidepressant toxicity. Amitriptyline is a cytochrome P450 3A4 and cytochrome P450 2D6 substrate and goldenseal is a 3A4 and 2D6 inhibitor.

Case

A 16-year-old girl presented to an ambulatory surgery center for esophago-duodenoscopy and colonoscopy to evaluate functional abdominal pain. The anesthesiologist elicited a history of abdominal pain two to three times a week for the past 6 months. The patient stated that she took amitriptyline and miralax for abdominal pain and had no drug allergies. She also admitted that she visited a naturopathic clinician who prescribes an herbal medication for mouth sores, which the patient thought was caused by the dry mouth associated with amitriptyline.

The patient mentioned a recent episode of lightheadedness and several occasions on which she felt like her heart was racing. She attributed these symptoms to dehydration from the onset of summer weather. On review of her vital signs, the anesthesiologist notice that her heart rate was 115 beats per minute and requested further detail about the herbal medication. The primary ingredient was goldenseal.

J. Miller MD, BM (✉)
Oregon Anesthesiology Group, Providence St. Vincent's Hospital, Portland, OR, USA
e-mail: jmiller@oagpcgroups.com

L. Thames MD
Oregon Anesthesiology Group, Portland, OR, USA

C. Marcucci et al. (eds.), *A Case Approach to Perioperative Drug-Drug Interactions*, DOI 10.1007/978-1-4614-7495-1_214

Discussion

This is an example of an inhibitor added to a substrate.

It can be challenging to elicit a history of herbal medication use and determine active ingredients. Goldenseal (*Hydrastis canadensis*) is an inhibitor of cytochrome P450 (CYP) 2D6 and 3A4 metabolic pathways in the liver. *In vivo* studies demonstrate goldenseal may inhibit these pathways up to 50%.[1,2] CYP2D6 is involved in the metabolism of approximately 30% of all medications, thus this level of inhibition could have significant clinical implications. Amitriptyline relies on both of these enzymes for its metabolic clearance in that it undergoes CYP2D6 hydroxylation and CYP3A4 demethylation.[3]

Goldenseal extract has two principal active components, berberine and hydrastine. These are also termed isoquinoline alkaloids. Berberine has been shown to be more inhibitory than hydrastine *in vitro*, however berberine has low bioavailability.

Goldenseal is packaged as a tea or capsules. It is marketed as a treatment for gastrointestinal problems, mouth sores, and upper respiratory infections. It has also been used to mask illicit substances in urine, specifically marijuana.[4] In this instance, the patient was prescribed a tricyclic antidepressant (TCA), amitriptyline for chronic pain. TCA medications have many side effects including dry mouth, constipation, urinary retention, sexual dysfunction, blurred vision, dizziness, drowsiness, and increased heart rate. In addition, TCAs have a narrow therapeutic window and increased risk of significant and life-threatening toxicity. Cardiovascular collapse and central nervous system toxicity are the most serious consequences of overdose.[5]

The dose of amitriptyline prescribed for chronic pain is usually lower than the dose used for treatment of depression. Goldenseal inhibition of the metabolism of the amitriptyline resulted in larger than expected clinical effect of the medication. In this instance, additional screening with a 12-lead ECG is required to determine if more serious arrhythmias are present. If the patient has any signs of TCA toxicity, she should be admitted for monitoring until symptoms resolve. If there are no signs of toxicity, it would be prudent to delay this elective procedure until the clinical symptoms of palpitations and dizziness have resolved. The patient and her parent should be counseled about drug interactions with the use of herbal medications.

Take-Home Points

- Goldenseal is a CYP2D6 and CYP3A4 inhibitor that can increase plasma levels of medications that utilize these metabolic pathways.
- Patients underestimate the impact of over-the-counter and herbal medications. Careful questioning and a brief review of systems can often uncover subtle symptoms that may reveal drug–drug interactions.
- Drug–drug interactions can commonly effect cardiovascular and central nervous system function. Failure to recognize these interactions prior to delivering anesthesia can have serious consequences.

Summary

Interaction: pharmacokinetic
Substrate: amitriptyline
Enzyme: CYP2D6 and CYP3A4
Inhibitor: goldenseal
Clinical effect: amitriptyline (tricyclic antidepressant) toxicity

References

1. Gurley BJ, Gardner SF, Hubbard MA, et al. In vivo effect of goldenseal, kava kava black cohosh, and valerian on human cytochrome P450 1A2, 2D6, 2E1, and 3A4 phenotypes. Clin Pharmacol Ther. 2005;77(5):415–26.
2. Gurley BJ, Swain A, Hubbard MA, et al. Clinical assessment of CYP2D6-mediated herb-drug interactions in humans: effects of milk thistle, black cohosh, goldenseal, kava kava, St. John's wort, and Echinacea. Mol Nutr Food Res. 2008;52(7):755–63.
3. Venkatakrishnan K, Greenblatt DJ, von Moltke LL, et al. Five distinct human cytochromes mediate amitriptyline N-demethylation in vitro: dominance of CYP 2C19 and 3A4. J Clin Pharmacol. 1998;38(2):112–21.
4. Herbs at a glance: Goldenseal. National Center for Complementary and Alternative Medicine. http://nccam.nih.gov/health/goldenseal. Accessed 21 Sept 2009.
5. Toxicity, Tricyclic Antidepressant. MedScape Reference: Drugs, Diseases & Procedures. http://emedicine.medscape.com/article/1010089-overview. Last accessed 24 Sept 2009.

Garlic I: More Than Just Bad Breath

215

Fatal Forty DDI: garlic, ritonavir, CYP3A4, P-glycoprotein

Vincent Lew MD and Kirk Lalwani MD, FRCA, MCR

Abstract

This case discusses a pharmacokinetic interaction between ritonavir and garlic resulting in abdominal distress. Ritonavir is a cytochrome P450 3A4 and/or P-glycoprotein substrate and garlic is a 3A4 and/or P-glycoprotein inhibitor.

Case

Late one evening, the anesthesia resident and the surgical resident (who had been medical school classmates) were chatting while walking down to the snack machines in the cafeteria when their phones rang at the same time. They were being called about a possible posting for an exploratory laparotomy/appendectomy for a patient complaining of severe abdominal pain. The patient was a 40-year-old man with known human immunodeficiency virus (HIV) infection who believed he had appendicitis. He reported that he was currently on highly active antiretroviral therapy (HAART), but did not know the name of his medications. He also reported taking "some medication" to prevent infections since his "CD4 count is somewhere in the hundreds."

After a complete workup, the surgical resident called the anesthesia resident to tell her that the CT scan was negative for appendicitis, and jokingly asked if she had noticed whether there were any mints in the vending machines as the patient reeked

V. Lew MD (✉)
Department of Anesthesia & Perioperative Care, University of California, San Francisco, San Francisco, CA, USA
e-mail: lewv@anesthesia.ucsf.edu; vincentklew@gmail.com

K. Lalwani MD, FRCA, MCR
Department of Anesthesiology & Perioperative Medicine, Oregon Health and Science University, Portland, OR, USA

C. Marcucci et al. (eds.), *A Case Approach to Perioperative Drug-Drug Interactions*, DOI 10.1007/978-1-4614-7495-1_215

of garlic. The astute anesthesia resident asked the surgical resident to meet her at the patient's bedside to talk to the patient. After questioning, the patient admitted to taking fresh garlic supplement because a friend who was an alternative medicine healer suggested that garlic had antimicrobial properties and he was anxious to avoid HIV-associated opportunistic infections. The residents then inquired as to whether he was taking the protease inhibitor ritonavir, to which the patient responded that that name sounded very familiar. They informed the patient that his stomach pain would likely go away if he stopped taking the garlic supplements. He was discharged from the emergency department in the morning with recommended followup with his outpatient medical care team.

Discussion

This is an example of an inhibitor added to a substrate.

Interactions between large amounts of garlic and antiretroviral medications, specifically ritonavir and saquinavir, have been described. In a case report by Laroche et al. two HIV-positive patients consuming large amounts of garlic supplements developed severe gastrointestinal symptoms after starting HAART containing ritonavir.[1] Curiously, after discontinuing either the garlic supplements or the ritonavir, the gastrointestinal symptoms subsided. Although the mechanism for this toxicity is not clear, a proposed mechanism includes an inhibitory effect of garlic on cytochrome P450 (CYP) 3A4 or P-glycoprotein, resulting in an increased systemic concentration of ritonavir, which is a substrate of both CYP3A4 and P-glycoprotein.[2,3] However, an alternative mechanism for the gastrointestinal toxicity has been proposed, which describes toxic metabolites generated from the direct interaction of garlic with ritonavir.

In a study conducted with healthy volunteers concomitantly taking large amounts of garlic and saquinavir, mean concentrations of saquinavir decreased by more than 50%.[4] Like its interaction with ritonavir, garlic's mechanism for decreased saquinavir concentrations is unclear, though it has been proposed that in addition to its inhibitory effects, garlic also induces several other P450 enzymes.[3]

Take-Home Points

- Physicians will need to keep in mind that herb–drug interactions may mimic other acute medical or surgical symptoms, and a thorough history is essential to avoid misdiagnosis.
- Careful review of antiretroviral regiments for HIV-positive patients also taking garlic supplements is warranted, as garlic may have direct and/or indirect interactions with ritonavir and saquinavir.

Summary

Interaction: pharmacokinetic
Substrate: ritonavir
Enzyme/site of action: CYP3A4 and/or P-glycoprotein pump
Inhibitor: garlic
Clinical effects: abdominal discomfort

References

1. Laroche M, Choudhri S, Gallicano K, et al. Severe gastrointestinal toxicity with concomitant ingestion of ritonavir and garlic. Can J Infect Dis. 1998;9:471P.
2. van den Bout-van den Beukel CJ, Koopmans PP, van der Ven AJ, et al. Possible drug-metabolism interactions of medicinal herbs with antiretroviral agents. Drug Metab Rev. 2006;38:477–514.
3. Hu Z, Yang X, Ho PC, et al. Herb-drug interactions: a literature review. Drugs. 2005;65:1239–82.
4. Piscitelli SC, Burstein AH, Welden N, et al. The effect of garlic supplements on the pharmacokinetics of saquinavir. Clin Infect Dis. 2002;34:234–8.

Garlic II: A Girl Named Allicin

216

Garlic, inhibition of clotting cascade

Vincent Lew MD and Kirk Lalwani MD, FRCA, MCR

Abstract
This case discusses the pharmacodynamic side effect of garlic.

Case

Late one Monday night, the anesthesia resident who was on call for the labor and delivery deck was paged to place an epidural catheter for probable urgent Cesarean section. The patient was a healthy 26-year-old primigravida with mild hyperlipidemia. Her medications included a daily multivitamin and a daily garlic supplement, which a friend suggested would help with her cholesterol levels. Before setting up the epidural tray, the resident checked the patient's laboratory work-up and confirmed that the most recent coagulation panel from 3 hours earlier was normal.

Catheter placement was successful on the first attempt using a loss-of-resistance technique. No paresthesia was elicited during placement, nor was blood or cerebrospinal fluid aspirated. Placement and dosing of the catheter was otherwise uncomplicated and sensory examination confirmed a working catheter. The patient was then whisked to the obstetric operating room where a baby boy was delivered via C-section. Surgery was uneventful, and wound closure was easily performed following achievement of hemostasis.

V. Lew MD (✉)
Department of Anesthesia & Perioperative Care, University of California, San Francisco, San Francisco, CA, USA
e-mail: lewv@anesthesia.ucsf.edu; vincentklew@gmail.com

K. Lalwani MD, FRCA, MCR
Department of Anesthesiology & Perioperative Medicine, Oregon Health and Science University, Portland, OR, USA

C. Marcucci et al. (eds.), *A Case Approach to Perioperative Drug-Drug Interactions*, DOI 10.1007/978-1-4614-7495-1_216

Postoperatively, the patient started to complain of increasing bilateral lower extremity weakness and paresthesia. The astute anesthesia resident quickly surmised that an epidural hematoma could be the culprit, and ordered urgent imaging of the thoracic and lumbar regions. Magnetic resonance imaging confirmed a large epidural hematoma spanning several vertebral levels. The on-call neurosurgery team was alerted for emergency evacuation and spinal decompression. Over the next few days, the patient made a full recovery.

Discussion

This is an example of a pharmacodynamic side effect.

Patients who consume large amounts of garlic that contain the active compound allicin, may be at an increased risk for bleeding even without concomitant anticoagulation or antiplatelet agents. Further, the risk for spontaneous bleeding arising from increased garlic consumption has been documented in several case reports involving postoperative hemostasis.[1,2]

Although the mechanism of increased bleeding has not been fully elucidated, it is generally thought that this increased risk is independent of garlic's interaction with the cytochrome P450 (CYP) system.[3,4] It has been proposed that garlic inhibits platelet aggregation in a dose-dependent fashion, possibly by acting via the ADP pathway (like clopidogrel).[5] There is evidence that one of garlic's constituents, ajoene, may also be irreversible, thereby potentiating the effects of other antiplatelet agents.[5]

In addition to its inherent bleeding risk, diabetic patients who consume large amounts of garlic may be at an increased risk for developing hypoglycemia, especially when taking other oral antihyperglycemic agents. There has been a case report of a diabetic patient on chlorpropamide developing hypoglycemia after consuming large amounts of Indian curry containing garlic.[6] It is currently thought that garlic's hypoglycemic effect stems from its ability to increase insulin levels rather than interacting with other diabetic drugs.

Take-Home Points

- Physicians will need to keep in mind that commonly used herbs such as garlic may interact with other antiplatelet or anticoagulant drugs, or act in an independent fashion to increase the risk for spontaneous and traumatic bleeding.
- Physicians caring for diabetic patients need to advise them about the risk for developing hypoglycemia by consuming large amounts of garlic, especially when antihyperglycemic agents such as chlorpropamide are used.

Summary

Drug effect: pharmacodynamic
Mechanism/site of action: platelets (proposed)
Clinical effects: anticoagulation

References

1. Burnham BE. Garlic as a possible risk for postoperative bleeding. Plast Reconstr Surg. 1995;95:213.
2. German K, Kumar U, Blackford HN. Garlic and the risk of TURP bleeding. Br J Urol. 1995;76:518.
3. Hu Z, Yang X, Ho PC, et al. Herb-drug interactions: a literature review. Drugs. 2005;65:1239–82.
4. Izzo AA, Ernst E. Interactions between herbal medicines and prescribed drugs: a systematic review. Drugs. 2001;61:2163–75.
5. Ang-Lee MK, Moss J, Yuan CS. Herbal medicines and perioperative care. JAMA. 2001;286:208–16.
6. Srinivasan K. Plant foods in the management of diabetes mellitus: spices as beneficial antidiabetic food adjuncts. Int J Food Sci Nutr. 2005;56:399–414.

"Danshen" the Night Away 217

Fatal Forty DDI: Salvia miltiorrhiza, warfarin, CYP2C9, CYP1A2

Tara C. Carey BA, MD and Kirk Lalwani MD, FRCA, MCR

Abstract
This case discusses a mixed pharmacodynamic and pharmacokinetic drug interaction between warfarin and danshen resulting in increased anticoagulation.

Case

Late one Friday night, a 68-year-old woman on chronic anticoagulation with warfarin arrived in the Emergency Department via ambulance, obtunded after a fall. She and her husband had been celebrating their 40th wedding anniversary with an evening of dinner and dancing when she slipped on the dance floor and hit her head. Over the next 2 hours, she became progressively confused, ataxic, with left-sided weakness, and decreased responsiveness. According to her husband, her medical history included atrial fibrillation, hypertension, and stable angina for which she took warfarin and hydrochlorothiazide. Her laboratory studies were significant for an elevated International Normalized Ratio (INR) of 5.9. Computed tomography scan of her head revealed a large right-sided subdural hematoma requiring emergent evacuation following correction of her coagulopathy with human factor VIIa.

Upon interviewing the patient's husband before going back to the operating room, the anesthesia resident learned that the patient had been stable on warfarin for 2 years, with a documented INR of 2.2 a month ago. The husband denied any changes to her

T.C. Carey BA, MD (✉)
Department of Anesthesiology and Perioperative Medicine, Brigham and Women's Hospital, Boston MA, USA
e-mail: tccarey@partners.org

K. Lalwani MD, FRCA, MCR
Department of Anesthesiology & Perioperative Medicine, Oregon Health and Science University, Portland, OR, USA

C. Marcucci et al. (eds.), *A Case Approach to Perioperative Drug-Drug Interactions*, DOI 10.1007/978-1-4614-7495-1_217

Interaction 2: pharmacodynamic
Substrates: warfarin and danshen
Mechanism/site of action: inhibition of platelet adhesion synergizing with increased INR
Clinical effect: increased anticoagulation

References

1. Kam PC, Liew S. Traditional Chinese herbal medicine and anaesthesia. Anaesthesia. 2002;57(11):1083–9.
2. Cheng TO. Warfarin danshen interaction. Ann Thorac Surg. 1999;67(3):894.
3. Chan TY. Interaction between warfarin and danshen (*Salvia miltiorrhiza*). Ann Pharmacother. 2001;35(4):501–4.
4. Izzat MB, Yim AP, El-Zufari MH. A taste of Chinese medicine! Ann Thorac Surg. 1998;66(3):941–2.
5. Tam LS, Chan TY, Leung WK, et al. Warfarin interactions with Chinese traditional medicines: danshen and methyl salicylate medicated oil. Aust N Z J Med. 1995;25(3):258.
6. Yu CM, Chan JC, Sanderson JE. Chinese herbs and warfarin potentiation by 'danshen'. J Intern Med. 1997;241(4):337–9.
7. Chan K, Lo AC, Yeung JH, et al. The effects of Danshen (*Salvia miltiorrhiza*) on warfarin pharmacodynamics and pharmacokinetics of warfarin enantiomers in rats. J Pharm Pharmacol. 1995;47(5):402–6.
8. Hirsh J, Dalen J, Anderson DR, et al. Oral anticoagulants: mechanism of action, clinical effectiveness, and optimal therapeutic range. Chest. 2001;119(1 Suppl):8S–21.
9. Kaminsky LS, Zhang ZY. Human P450 metabolism of warfarin. Pharmacol Ther. 1997;73(1):67–74.
10. Hirsh J, Fuster V, Ansell J, et al. American Heart Association/American College of Cardiology Foundation guide to warfarin therapy. J Am Coll Cardiol. 2003;41(9):1633–52.
11. Wang CM, Cheung WY, Lee PM, et al. Major tanshinones of Danshen (*Salvia miltiorrhiza*) exhibit different modes of inhibition on human CYP1A2, CYP2C9, CYP2E1 and CYP3A4 activities *in vitro*. Phytomedicine. 2010;17:868–75.
12. Qiu F, Zhang R, Sun J, et al. Inhibitory effects of seven components of danshen extract on catalytic activity of cytochrome P450 enzyme in human liver microsomes. Drug Metab Dispos. 2008;36(7):1308–14. Epub 2008 Apr 14.
13. Zhou L, Zuo Z, Chow MS. Danshen: an overview of its chemistry, pharmacology, pharmacokinetics, and clinical use. J Clin Pharmacol. 2005;45(12):1345–59.

Caught Yellow-Handed

218

Fatal Forty DDI: turmeric, warfarin, CYP1A2, CYP2C9

Giorgio Veneziano MD and Michael Mangione MD

Abstract
This case discusses both pharmacokinetic and pharmacodynamics interactions between turmeric and warfarin.

Case

A 67-year-old man arrived in the preoperative area for transurethral resection of the prostate having failed conservative management of an acute episode of acute urinary retention 1 month earlier. He also had a history of atrial fibrillation, hypertension, and coronary artery disease for which he had had a drug-eluting coronary stent placed just over 1 year ago. The anesthesiologist noted the patient was on warfarin and clopidogrel but had stopped both 7 days earlier on instruction from his surgeon. His preoperative International Normalized Ratio (INR) was 1.2. The patient's wife mentioned that 2 months ago his INR had been very high and his warfarin dose had been adjusted. The anesthesiologist began to discuss the risks and benefits of spinal anesthesia when she noticed bright yellow staining on the patient's fingers. The patient mentioned that he had read in a magazine that turmeric could prevent prostate cancer and he had been taking it as a supplement for several months. Unfamiliar with the implications of turmeric therapy, the anesthesiologist checked an online drug and supplement registry. He returned to the patient to inform him that he could not have a spinal anesthetic for his procedure.

G. Veneziano MD (✉)
Department of Anesthesiology & Pain Medicine, University of Pittsburgh Medical Center, Columbus, OH, USA
e-mail: Giorgio.Veneziano@nationwidechildrens.org

M. Mangione MD
Department of Anesthesiology, University of Pittsburgh School of Medicine, VA Pittsburgh Healthcare System, Pittsburgh, PA, USA

C. Marcucci et al. (eds.), *A Case Approach to Perioperative Drug-Drug Interactions*, DOI 10.1007/978-1-4614-7495-1_218

Discussion

This is an example of an inhibitor added to a substrate and also a synergistic pharmacodynamic drug effect.

Turmeric, derived from the rhizome of the *Curcuma longa* plant, is a commonly used spice found in yellow curry dishes. For centuries, turmeric has been used in traditional Asian medicine for a wide variety of ailments, including dyspepsia, wound healing, and rheumatism.

Curcumin, a yellow pigment compound in turmeric, is the major pharmacologically active component of the spice. It has garnered interest because of its anti-inflammatory and antioxidant properties. In the last three decades, curcumin has been extensively investigated *in vitro* and in animal models of specific disease states, though human studies are in most cases lacking. The therapeutic effects of curcumin are being examined in a number of diseases including cancer, Alzheimer's disease, hyperlipidemia, thrombosis, peptic ulcers, psoriasis, rheumatoid arthritis, and HIV/AIDS.[1]

While much has been published of the potential health benefits of curcumin, little has been reported about drug interactions. Based on *in vitro* and animal studies, curcumin may increase the risk for bleeding in patients taking antiplatelet agents. Patients on medications such as aspirin or clopidogrel may develop an exaggerated antiplatelet effect when consuming curcumin. Studies have demonstrated that curcumin inhibits human platelet aggregation by interfering with platelet-activating factor and arachidonic acid-mediated thromboxane formation.[2,3] It appears that curcumin inhibits thromboxane formation induced by these aggregation agonists primarily by interrupting COX activity. This effect on platelets is reversible.[2]

In addition, patients prescribed warfarin may develop excessive anticoagulation after beginning consumption of curcumin. Curcumin has been demonstrated *in vitro* to interact with multiple major human cytochrome P450s (CYP) enzymes including 1A2, 3A4, 2D6, 2C9 and 2B6.[4] Warfarin is primarily metabolized by 2C9 and 1A2, both of which are inhibited by curcumin. The cytochrome P450 inhibition creates the potential for a rising INR in a patient who initiates curcumin while on a stable coumadin regimen.

The National Institute of Health's Internet health service, *Medline Plus*, recommends cessation of turmeric and curcumin prior to scheduled surgery, regardless of concurrent forms of anticoagulation[5] The American Society of Regional Anesthesiology contends that although herbal agents alone do not appear to pose a greater risk of spinal hematoma with neuraxial anesthesia, herbal drugs in combination with other anticoagulants may increase the risk for hemorrhage.[6] Therefore, it is prudent to consider the effects of turmeric in the perioperative patient who is taking or has recently discontinued anticoagulants, especially if a neuraxial anesthetic technique is being considered.

Natural turmeric rhizome is composed of 3% to 5% curcumin. It is estimated the average person in India consumes 2 to 2.5 g turmeric daily.[5] Herbal remedies containing turmeric are widely available commercially and generally contain between 200 and 1000 mg curcumin.

Curcumin has little bioavailability, being poorly absorbed through the gastrointestinal tract and quickly metabolized by liver glucuronidation and sulfation.[1] Detailed pharmacokinetics of curcumin do not exist in humans. However, in a Phase I clinical trial, curcumin blood levels peaked at 1 to 2 hours and gradually declined over the next 12 hours. Toxic effects in humans were not detected in humans in doses up to 8 g daily[7]

Take-Home Points

- Many patients and even some physicians falsely perceive that because they are "natural," food supplements do not have significant adverse effects and drug interactions. Because of this belief, many patients will not inform their providers about regularly consumed supplements.

- It is important not to become complacent in asking the perioperative patient about supplements they may be ingesting, and investigating the potential interactions of those supplements with drugs they are taking or may be exposed to in the perioperative period.

- Turmeric and its active constituent curcumin appear to have intrinsic antiplatelet effects.[2,3] It is important to be mindful of this fact in the perioperative patient where bleeding is a concern. Vigilance in this regard should be heightened when the patient is concurrently taking an antiplatelet medication.

- While curcumin appears to have a short plasma half-life and seems to be a reversible platelet-aggregation inhibitor, detailed pharmacokinetics do not exist for this herb.[2,7] Therefore, it is prudent to advise patients to cease consuming turmeric or curcumin at least 7 days prior to surgery when neuraxial analgesia is contemplated or hemorrhage is a significant risk.

- Curcumin has been demonstrated to be a potent inhibitor of several major human cytochrome P450 enzymes.[4] The full extent of curcumin-drug interactions is far from established, but drug–drug interactions occurring at the cytochrome P450 system are a common mechanism of adverse drug reactions.

Hearing the News

220

Fatal Forty DDI: St. John's wort, oral contraceptives, CYP3A4, P-glycoprotein

Nikki Jaworski MD

Abstract

This case discusses the pharmacokinetic interaction between ethinylestradiol and St. John's wort, leading to decreased contraceptive efficacy. Ethinylestradiol is a cytochrome P450 3A4 and P-glycoprotein substrate and St. John's wort is a 3A4 and P-glycoprotein inducer.

Case

A 24-year-old woman was scheduled for an elective otoplasty and was very excited to finally have her planned plastic surgery. She admitted to no other past medical history and reported that her only medication was oral contraceptives. A routine preoperative urine pregnancy test was positive. The patient was shocked at this result, stating adamantly that she took her birth control pill every morning and never missed a dose. Her case was cancelled and she was referred to an obstetrician.

A repeat pregnancy test was positive and an ultrasound confirmed an early viable intrauterine pregnancy. The patient was quite distressed and adamant that she had been compliant with her oral contraceptives. She inquired if it was safe for her to keep taking her herbal supplement, as she felt that it was helpful in "smoothing things down." Upon questioning, she admitted that she was taking St. John's wort after a friend recommended it when she mentioned that she was feeling depressed but did not like the idea of an antidepressant.

N. Jaworski MD
Department of Anesthesiology & Perioperative Medicine, Oregon Health & Science University, Portland, OR, USA
e-mail: nikkijaworski@gmail.com

C. Marcucci et al. (eds.), *A Case Approach to Perioperative Drug-Drug Interactions*, DOI 10.1007/978-1-4614-7495-1_220

The obstetrician explained to her that although herbal supplements are often thought of as natural, they were in fact chemical compounds that could have interactions with other drugs. In her case, the interaction of St. John's wort with her oral contraceptive may have resulted in her pregnancy.

Discussion

This is an example of an inducer added to a substrate.

St John's wort (SJW) is an herbal supplement most commonly taken for its antidepressant effects. The extracts of St John's wort contain varying amounts of compounds including hypericin, hyperforin, and flavonoids. It is the content of hyperforin contained within the supplement that must be taken into account when contemplating drug–drug interactions (DDIs) with SJW. SJW products may contain a concentration of hyperforin ranging from 0.2% to 5%. Products that contain a concentration of less than one percent are less likely to be implicated in drug interactions than products containing concentrations greater than 4%.[1]

Hyperforin is an inducer of the cytochrome P450 (CYP) enzymes 3A4 and 2C9. In addition, hyperforin increases the expression of the duodenal P-glycoprotein transporter.[1] P-glycoprotein is an ATP-dependent active transporter on the apical surface of enterocytes that pumps absorbed lipophilic compounds back into the intestinal lumen. Oral contraceptives contain ethinylestradiol and a progestin component, which function to inhibit the release follicle-stimulating hormone (FSH) and luteinizing hormone (LH) respectively and ultimately prevent ovulation. Both ethinylestradiol and progestins are primarily metabolized by CYP3A4. Several pharmacologic interaction studies between low dose oral contraceptives and various SJW preparations have been performed to examine the effects of SJW on the blood serum levels of ethinylestradiol, progestins, FSH, and LH as well as the incidence of intracyclic bleeding and possible ovulation.[2–5] The results of these studies varied regarding the effects of hyperforin and the various effects on blood serum levels of these hormones; however, an increased incidence of breakthrough bleeding was a consistent finding. One study demonstrated evidence of follicular maturation and possible ovulation; however, a recent study performed using a SJW preparation with a low hyperforin content (0.2%) found no evidence of interaction with ethinylestradiol or progestin, or increased incidence of intracyclic bleeding.[3,5]

Although intracyclic menstrual bleeding is a well-documented finding among women taking St. John's wort and oral contraceptives, the exact incidence of unwanted pregnancy due to the interaction is unknown. There are case reports in which the drug interaction seemed to be the most likely source of an unplanned pregnancy, but there are no studies clearly demonstrating this result.[6,7]

Take-Home Points

- Hyperforin is the component of St John's wort that induces CYP3A4 resulting in drug–drug interactions.
- The concomitant use of St John's wort with oral contraceptives increases the incidence of irregular menstrual bleeding; however, the number of case reports of unexpected pregnancy remains small.
- The hyperforin content within preparations of St John's wort may vary. Products containing a low concentration of hyperforin are less likely to result in increased metabolism of the hormonal components of oral contraceptives and are less likely to result in intracyclic menstrual bleeding.

Summary

Interaction: pharmacokinetic
Substrate: ethinylestradiol
Enzyme/site of action: CYP3A4 and P-glycoprotein
Inducer: St. John's wort
Clinical effect: decreased blood level of ethinylestradiol leading to decreased contraceptive efficacy

References

1. Madabushi R, Bruno F, Drewelow B, et al. Hyperforin in St. John's wort interactions. Eur J Clin Pharmacol. 2006;62:225–33.
2. Hall SD, Wang Z, Huang SM. The interaction between St John's wort and an oral contraceptive. Clin Pharmacol Ther. 2003;74(6):525–35.
3. Murphy PA, Kern SE, Stanczyk FZ, et al. Interaction of St. John's wort with oral contraceptives: effects on the pharmacokinetics of norethindrone and ethinyl estradiol, ovarian activity and breakthrough bleeding. Contraception. 2005;71(6):402–8.
4. Pfrunder A, Schiesser M, Gerber S, et al. Interaction of St John's wort with low-dose oral contraceptive therapy: a randomized controlled trial. Br J Clin Pharmacol. 2003;56(6):683–90.
5. Will-Shahab L, Bauer S, Kunter U, et al. St John's wort extract (Ze 117) does not alter the pharmacokinetics of a low-dose oral contraceptive. Eur J Clin Pharmacol. 2009;65:287–94.
6. Ernst E. Second thoughts about safety of St John's wort. Lancet. 1999;354(9195):2014–6.
7. Schwarz UI, Buschel B, Kirch W. Unwanted pregnancy on self medication with St John's wort despite hormonal contraception. Br J Clin Pharmacol. 2003;55:112–3.

Index

C. Marcucci et al. (eds.), *A Case Approach to Perioperative Drug-Drug Interactions*, DOI 10.1007/978-1-4614-7495-1

D

F

G

H

N

O

Q

R

U

V

W

Fatal Forty Index

C. Marcucci et al. (eds.), *A Case Approach to Perioperative Drug-Drug Interactions*, DOI 10.1007/978-1-4614-7495-1

Drug Index (Generic)

C. Marcucci et al. (eds.), *A Case Approach to Perioperative Drug-Drug Interactions*, DOI 10.1007/978-1-4614-7495-1

M

N

O

P

Drug Index (Brand)

C. Marcucci et al. (eds.), *A Case Approach to Perioperative Drug-Drug Interactions*, DOI 10.1007/978-1-4614-7495-1

www.ingramcontent.com/pod-product-compliance
Lightning Source LLC
Chambersburg PA
CBHW051149180926
51611CB00001B/1
* 9 7 8 1 4 6 1 4 7 4 9 4 4 *